INFORMATION
ANALYSIS LIBRARY
BLDG. 2001

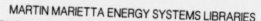

Iron in Immunity, Cancer and Inflammation

Iron in Immunity, Cancer and Inflammation

Edited by

Maria de Sousa
Instituto de Ciencias Biomedicas Abel Salazar,
University of Porto, Portugal

and

Jeremy H. Brock
Department of Bacteriology and Immunology, University of Glasgow, UK

A Wiley–Interscience Publication

JOHN WILEY & SONS
Chichester · New York · Brisbane · Toronto · Singapore

Wiley Editorial Offices

John Wiley & Sons Ltd, Baffins Lane, Chichester,
West Sussex PO19 1UD, England

John Wiley & Sons, Inc., 605 Third Avenue,
New York, NY 10158-0012, USA

Jacaranda Wiley Ltd, G.P.O. Box 859, Brisbane,
Queensland 4001, Australia

John Wiley & Sons (Canada) Ltd, 22 Worcester Road,
Rexdale, Ontario M9W 1L1, Canada

John Wiley & Sons (SEA) Pte Ltd, 37, Jalan Pemimpin #05-04,
Block B, Union Industrial Building, Singapore 2057

Copyright © 1989 by John Wiley & Sons Ltd.

All rights reserved.

No part of this book may be reproduced by any means,
or transmitted, or translated into a machine language
without the written permission of the publisher.

Library of Congress Cataloging-in-Publication Data:

Iron in immunity, cancer, and inflammation/edited by Maria de Sousa
 and Jeremy H. Brock.
   p.   cm.
 'A Wiley–Interscience publication.'
 Includes bibliographies and index.
 ISBN 0 471 92150 5
 1. Iron—Pathophysiology. 2. Iron—Immunology. 3. Cancer—
Pathophysiology. 4. Inflammation—Pathophysiology. I. De Sousa,
Maria. II. Brock, Jeremy H.
   [DNLM: 1. Carrier Proteins. 2. Ferritin—metabolism.
 3. Inflammation—etiology. 4. Iron—immunology. 5. Iron—
metabolism. 6. Neoplasms—etiology. 7. Transferrin—metabolism.
 QV 183 I7145]
 QP535.F4I763 1989
 616.3'9—dc19
 DNLM/DLC
 for Library of Congress   89-5379
                                                           CIP

British Library Cataloguing in Publication Data

Iron in immunity, cancer and inflammation.
 1. Medicine. Drug therapy. Iron
 I. De Sousa, Maria II. Brock, Jeremy H.
 615'.262

 ISBN 0 471 92150 5

Typeset by Acorn Bookwork, Salisbury, Wiltshire
Printed in Great Britain by The Bath Press, Bath, Avon

Dedication

Our collaboration as editors of this book, came about, in a remote way, through the rather unusual decision of a Head of Department of Immunology in a Scottish University to appoint as lecturer in his Department an iron biochemist (JB), remembering somehow that an earlier lecturer in the same Department had developed an interest in iron and the immune system after leaving Scotland (MdS). We wish to dedicate this book to the memory of Professor Robert G. White, a remarkable man whose courage to make unusual decisions contributed to our journey as editors.

Maria de Sousa and Jeremy Brock
Glasgow, 18 July, 1988

Contents

Contributors	xiii
List of Abbreviations	xv
Foreword: A Fast-growing Knowledge	xvii
Part I. Cellular and Molecular Biology of Iron	1
Chapter 1: Iron and the Lymphomyeloid System: a Growing Knowledge	3
M. de Sousa	
Introduction	3
In Search of Ancestors	3
Brief Summary of the Evolution of Iron Recycling	5
Recent Paths and their Guiding Perspectives	7
Where a Frontier Appears Wide Enough to Become a Country	9
This Book and its Two Purposes	10
Conclusion	13
Chapter 2: Recognition and Removal of Senescent Cells	17
M. M. B. Kay	
Role of IgG in Cellular Removal	17
Diminished RBC Lifespan in Old Animals	23
A Senescent Cell Antigen?	24
Characterization of Senescent Cell Antigen as Being Derived from Band 3	25
Evidence for the Role of Oxidation in the Generation of Senescent Red Cell Antigen	26
Concluding Remarks	30
Chapter 3: The Biology of Iron	35
J. H. Brock	
Chemistry of Iron	35
Iron-binding Proteins	36
Iron Metabolism and Recirculation	46
Iron and Bacterial Growth	48

Chapter 4: The Molecular Biology of Iron-binding Proteins 55
P. Arosio, G. Cairo and S. Levi
Introduction 55
Ferritin 56
Transferrin 62
Transferrin Receptor 66
Conclusion 71

Chapter 5: Iron and Cells of the Immune System 81
J. H. Brock
The Interaction of Iron and Iron-binding Proteins with Cells of the Immune System 81
Iron and Immune Function 94
Iron Deficiency and Susceptibility to Infection 98

Part II. Iron and Inflammation 109

Chapter 6: The Anaemia of Inflammation and Chronic Disease 111
A. M. Konijn and C. Hershko
The Anaemia of Malignant Disease 111
RBC Survival and Ineffective Erythropoiesis 112
Erythropoietin 113
The Immune System and the Development of Anaemia of Chronic Disease 116
Iron Metabolism in Inflammation 118
Pathogenesis of the Hypoferraemia of Inflammation 121
Tissue Iron Release and Ferritin Synthesis 124
Serum Ferritin 128
The Role of Interleukin-1 130

Chapter 7: Iron and Joint Inflammation 145
F. J. Andrews, D. R. Blake and C. J. Morris
Iron and Joint Pathology 145
Iron Deficiency and the Joint 150
Biochemistry of Iron Related to Joint Disease 153
Iron, Lymphocytes and the Joint 162
Conclusion 164

Chapter 8: Inflammation and Parasitic Disease 177
I. A. Clark and G. Chaudhri
Introduction 177
The Mediators of Inflammation 178
Interactions Between Mediators 183
Some Roles of Inflammation in Parasitic Disease 186

Part III. Iron and Haematopoiesis — 197

Chapter 9: Iron-binding Proteins and the Regulation of Haematopoietic Cell Proliferation/Differentiation — 199
H. E. Broxmeyer

- Introduction — 199
- Acidic Ferritin — 200
- Lactoferrin — 205
- Transferrin — 210
- Concluding Thoughts — 211

Chapter 10: Iron, the Iron-binding Proteins and Bone Marrow Cell Differentiation — 223
J. Fletcher

- Introduction — 223
- Lactoferrin and Myelopoiesis — 223
- Iron Saturation of Lactoferrin—Active and Inactive Forms of the Molecule — 227
- Lactoferrin Interaction with Cell Surfaces — 230
- Lactoferrin and Chronic Myeloid Leukaemia — 231
- *In Vivo* Evidence for the Importance of Lactoferrin as a Physiological Regulator — 233
- Transferrin — 235
- Ferritin — 237

Part IV. The Immunology of Iron Overload — 245

Chapter 11: The Immunology of Iron Overload — 247
M. de Sousa

- Introduction — 247
- Natural Killer Activity — 248
- Cell Surface Antigens — 248
- Mitogen Responses — 250
- HLA, the Mixed Lymphocyte Reaction and Ferritin Secretion — 251
- The Macrophage in Idiopathic Haemochromatosis — 252
- Phagocytic Cells in Other Situations of Iron Overload — 253
- Concluding Remarks — 255

Part V. Iron and Malignancy — 259

Chapter 12: Iron and Tumor Cell Growth — 261
H. H. Sussman

- Introduction — 261
- Physical Properties of Iron and the Principal Iron Compounds of Cellular Iron Metabolism — 262
- Cellular Metabolism of Iron — 265

Cell Cycle and Cellular Iron	267
Iron-binding Proteins as Modulators of Growth	274

Chapter 13: Ferritin as a Marker of Malignancy — 283
C. Moroz and H. Bessler

The Molecular Structure of Isoferritins Isolated by Monoclonal Antibodies from Human Placenta and Breast Cancer Cells	283
The Immunological Function of Oncofetal Ferritin; its Effect on T Lymphocytes	289
Oncofetal Ferritin as a Marker for Malignancy	291

Chapter 14: Iron-related Markers in Liver Cancer — 301
J. L. Israel, K. A. McGlynn, H.-W. L. Hann and B. S. Blumberg

Introduction	301
Iron, Hepatitis B Virus and Liver Cancer	301
Ferritin as a Marker in Liver Cancer	306
Conclusions	313

Part VI. Implications for Diagnosis and Therapy — 317

Chapter 15: The Iron-binding Proteins in Nuclear Medicine: Uses in Diagnosis and Therapy — 319
M. R. Zalutsky

Introduction	319
Transferrin-mediated ^{67}Ga and ^{111}In Transport	321
Marrow Imaging	322
Cancer-related Applications	322
Inflammation	329
Arthritis	330
Summary	334

Chapter 16: Potential Clinical Uses of Anti-transferrin Receptor Monoclonal Antibodies — 341
I. S. Trowbridge

Introduction	341
Monoclonal Antibodies that Block Transferrin Receptor Function	342
Mechanism by which Monoclonal Antibodies Inhibit Transferrin-mediated Iron Uptake	346
Immunotherapy with Monoclonal Antibodies that Block Transferrin Receptor Function	347
Anti-transferrin Receptor Immunotoxins	353
Concluding Remarks	356

Chapter 17: Clinical Use of Iron Chelation — 361
M. J. Pippard

Introduction	361

Iron Chelation	362
Iron Overload	365
Tissue Damage and Iron Chelation	368
Post-ischaemic Reperfusion Injury	370
Inflammatory and Immune-mediated Diseases	372
Effects on Haem Synthesis	376
Inhibition of Cell Division	378
Toxicity of Iron Chelators	381
Conclusion	382

Chapter 18: Closing Overview 393
A. Jacobs

Appendix: Problems with Iron and Iron-binding Proteins in Tissue Culture 399
J. H. Brock

Introduction	399
Control of Iron Levels in Cell Cultures	400
Control of Levels of Iron-binding Proteins	401
Binding of Iron to Transferrin	402
Removal of Iron from Transferrins	404
Radiolabelling of Transferrins	404
Lactoferrin	405
Ferritin	405

Index 409

Contributors

F. J. Andrews *Department of Surgery, Monash University Medical School, Melbourne 3181, Australia*

P. Arosio *Department of Biomedical Science and Technology, University of Milan, San Raffaele Hospital, Via Olgettina 60, 20132 Milan, Italy*

H. Bessler *Rogoff Medical Research Institute, Beilinson Medical Center and Sackler School of Medicine, Tel-Aviv University, Petah-Tikva, Israel*

D. R. Blake *Bone and Joint Research Unit, London Hospital Medical College, London E1 1AD, UK*

B. S. Blumberg *Division of Population Oncology, Fox Chase Cancer Center, Philadelphia, Pennsylvania 19111, USA*

J. H. Brock *University Department of Bacteriology and Immunology, Western Infirmary, Glasgow G11 6NT, UK*

H. E. Broxmeyer *Departments of Medicine (Hematology/Oncology), Microbiology and Immunology, The Walther Oncology Institute, Indiana University School of Medicine, Indianapolis IN 46223, USA*

G. Cairo *Centro di Studio sulla Patologia Cellulare CNR, Via Mangiagalli 31, 20133 Milan, Italy*

G. Chaudhri
John Curtin School of Medical Research, Australian National University, Canberra ACT 2601, Australia

I. A. Clark *Zoology Department, Australian National University, Canberra ACT 2601, Australia*

M. de Sousa *Instituto de Ciencias Biomedicas Abel Salazar, University of Porto, Portugal*

J. Fletcher *Department of Haematology, City Hospital, Nottingham NG5 1PG, UK*

H.-W. L. Hann *Division of Population Oncology, Fox Chase Cancer Center, Philadelphia, Pennsylvania 19111, USA*

C. Hershko Department of Medicine, Shaare Zedek Medical Centre, Jerusalem Israel

J. L. Israel Division of Population Oncology, Fox Chase Cancer Center, Philadelphia, Pennsylvania 19111, USA

A. Jacobs Department of Haematology, Welsh National School of Medicine, Heath Park, Cardiff CF4 4XN, UK

M. M. B. Kay Department of Medicine, Departments of Medical Biochemistry and Genetics, and Medical Microbiology and Immunology, Texas A&M University, 1901 South First Street, Teague Veterans Center (151), Temple, Texas 76501, USA

A. M. Konijn Department of Nutrition, The Hebrew University Hadassah Medical School, Jerusalem, Israel

S. Levi Department of Biomedical Science and Technology, University of Milan, San Raffaele Hospital, Via Olgettina 60, 20132 Milan, Italy

K. A. McGlynn Division of Population Oncology, Fox Chase Cancer Center, Philadelphia, Pennsylvania 1911, USA

C. Moroz Rogoff Medical Research Institute, Beilinson Medical Center and Sackler School of Medicine, Tel-Aviv University, Petah-Tikva, Israel

C. J. Morris Bone and Joint Research Unit, London Hospital Medical College, London E1 1AD, UK

M. J. Pippard Department of Haematology, Ninewells Hospital and Medical School, Dundee DD1 9SY, UK

H. H. Sussman Stanford University School of Medicine, Stanford, California 94305, USA

I. S. Trowbridge Department of Cancer Biology, The Salk Institute, Post Office Box 85800, San Diego, California 92138, USA

M. R. Zalutsky Department of Radiology, Duke University Medical Center, Box 3808, Durham, North Carolina 27710, USA

List of Abbreviations

AIA	adjuvant induced arthritis
AFP	alpha-fetoprotein
AGEPC	acetyl glycerol ether phosphorylcholine
AICD	anaemia of inflammation and chronic disease
AIF	acidic isoferritin
AIFIA	acidic isoferritin inhibitory activity
ATG	anti-thymocyte globulin
BHA	butylated hydroxyanisole
CFU	colony forming unit
CFU-GEMM	CFU-granulocytic, erythropoietic, monocyte–macrophagic
CFU-GM	CFU-granulocytic–macrophagic
CFU-G	CFU-granulocytic
CIA	colony inhibitory activity
CLD	chronic liver disease
CLL-PRCA	chronic lymphoid leukaemia—pure red cell aplasia
CML	chronic myeloid leukaemia
CSF	colony-stimulating factor
CURL	compartment of uncoupling of receptor–ligand
DF	desferrioxamine
DTPA	diethylene triamine pentaacetic acid
EP	endogenous pyrogen
EPC	erythropoietin responsive cell
Epo	erythropoietin
FAD	flavin adenine dinucleotide
FBL	ferritin bearing lymphocyte
FMN	flavin mononucleotide
FSH	follicle stimulating hormone
G-CSF	granulocyte derived-colony stimulating factor
GM-CSF	granulocyte–macrophage-derived CSF
HBV	hepatitis B virus
HLA	human leucocyte antigens
IH	idiopathic haemochromatosis
IL-1, -2, -3	interleukins -1, -2, -3

IRE	iron-response element
LAF	lymphocyte activating factor
LAI	leukaemia associated inhibitor
LEM	leucocyte endogenous mediator
LIA	leukaemia inhibitory activity
LF	lactoferrin
LT	lymphotoxin, see TNF
M-CSF	macrophage colony-stimulating factor
MLR	mixed lymphocyte reaction
NK	natural killer
nt	nucleotide
PAF	platelet activating factor
PCV	packed cell volume
PGs	prostaglandins
PHA	phytohaemagglutinin
PHC	primary hepatic carcinoma
PIH	pyridoxal isonicotinoyl hydrazone
PLF	placental ferritin
PMN	polymorphonuclear
PVNS	pigmented villonodular synovitis
PWM	pokeweek mitogen
RA	rheumatoid arthritis
RBC	red blood cell
SGPT	serum glutamic-pyruvic transaminase
SOD	superoxide dismutase
TNF	tumour necrosis factor

Foreword: A Fast-growing Knowledge

A number of relevant studies were published in the latter half of 1988 and the early part of 1989, giving some indication of the rapid growth of knowledge in the fields covered by this book. Barbara Bierer's and Gabriel Virella's groups showed that the enhancement of B cell responses provoked by the addition of autologous erythrocytes results from the interaction of CD2 with its LFA-3 ligand expressed by the erythrocytes (Virella et al., Cell. Immunol., **118**, 308–19, 1988), thus clarifying the molecular basis of one form of the regulation of the immune response by erythrocytes, a topic considered in Chapters 1 and 2.

Using chemical and Mössbauer spectroscopy, Yuriv et al. (J. Biol. Chem., **263**, 13508–10, 1988) provided evidence that iron-containing concanavalin A is a ferritin, forcing us to wonder whether one of the most commonly used T cell mitogens will itself fall within the 'hemunology frontier' proposed in Chapter 1.

In a comparative study of the mechanisms by which cachectin/TNFα, IL-1 and endotoxin provoke anaemia in rats, Moldawer et al. (FASEB J., **3**, 1637–43, 1989) found that although TNFα, IL-1 or endotoxin treatment resulted in similar hypoferraemia and shortened plasma iron half-life, only endotoxin or TNF treatment (but not IL-1) reduced significantly the incorporation of ^{59}Fe into newly synthesized red blood cells. Furthermore, Gordeuk et al. (J. Clin. Invest., **82**, 1934–8, 1988) have reported that IL-1 produces hypoferraemia in mice even in animals rendered neutropenic, suggesting that lactoferrin does not play a major role. On the other hand, Taetle and Honeysett (Blood, **71**, 1590–9, 1988) have found that gamma-interferon increases iron release from human macrophages. Thus the complex role played by cytokines in the immune system seems to be extending into the fields of erythropoiesis and iron turnover, and is beginning to answer some of the questions raised in Chapters 5 and 6.

A paper by Stevens et al. has reported the results of the first US National Health and Nutrition Survey of more than 14 000 adults, begun in 1971 with follow-ups between 1981 and 1984, which examined the relationship between iron status and cancer risk. The results of this study (N. Engl. J. Med., **318**, 1047–52, 1988) are consistent with the hypothesis, discussed by

Blumberg and his colleagues in Chapter 14, that high body iron stores increase the risk of cancer.

Chitambar *et al.* (*Blood*, **72**, 1930–6, 1988), examining the inhibitory effect of gallium-transferrin on the growth of leukaemic HL-60 cells *in vitro*, demonstrated by electron spin resonance a decrease in the signal of the tyrosyl radical of the M2 subunit of ribonucleotide reductase, thus clarifying one of the points raised in Chapters 12 and 14. In addition, a drug synergy with hydroxyurea was demonstrated, reinforcing 'the enticing prospect of utilizing our knowledge of iron metabolism for therapeutic intervention in the treatment of leukaemia', as elegantly summed up by Jacobs in the closing chapter of this book (p. 395). The demonstration by Vostrejs *et al.* (*J. Clin. Invest.*, **82**, 331–9, 1988) that transferrin acts as an autocrine growth factor for a lung cancer cell line not only strengthens the link between iron metabolism and cancer, but also adds weight to the idea, discussed in Chapter 5, that in extramedullary tissues and organs iron supply may be regulated by locally synthesized transferrin.

We wish to thank all authors for their prompt response to our invitation to contribute to this book, and to the editorial staff of John Wiley and Sons, particularly Patricia Sharp and Pru Theaker, for their equal promptness in bringing the book to its end.

We gratefully acknowledge Rui Marçal, Raquel Reimão and Anne MacIlveen, whose help proved invaluable in the preparation of this final manuscript.

M.deS.
J.H.B.   April 1989

Part I

Cellular and Molecular Biology of Iron

Iron in Immunity, Cancer and Inflammation
Edited by M. de Sousa and J. H. Brock
© 1989 John Wiley & Sons Ltd

1
Iron and the Lymphomyeloid System: A Growing Knowledge

Maria De Sousa
Abel Salazar Institute for the Biomedical Sciences, Oporto, Portugal

INTRODUCTION

The introductory remarks on the growth of knowledge of a subject usually provide the opportunity to recount a series of enlightening episodes starting from antiquity to the present day. A subject as young as the one to be covered here cannot claim to have a growth of knowledge of that kind. In this chapter, however, I shall retrace briefly the paths that have seduced others and myself into imagining a distant past for the present interest in some aspects of the biology of iron (Brain, 1979; Weinberg, Ell and Weinberg, 1986).

The more recent paths that, in my view, have led to the subject matter of this book, will be considered in greater detail. These paths lie largely on the frontier of immunology with hematology, biochemistry and physiology. 'Walking' them led me to the conclusion that the territory covered by that frontier is now wide enough to become a country in its own right.

In younger years I named that country 'the hemune system' and its study 'hemunology'. Presently, I call it nothing and hope that this book will contribute to presenting the case for its existence.

IN SEARCH OF ANCESTORS

Biologists working on the biochemistry of iron and of the iron-binding proteins start their presentations sometimes with pictures of some of the iron artifacts found in Tutankhamen's treasure. The recognition of iron as a precious metal by the Egyptians seems to have gone beyond the confinement of their rulers' tombs. According to Guido Majno, one ideogram for iron was written 'with the astonishing combination' of a sledge carrying a meteorite indicated by a star; the same ideogram was used to mean 'marvel, astonishment, which tells us that this particular marvel was something to take home' (Majno, 1975).

The subject to be covered by this book, however, cannot truthfully claim to have Egyptian ancestors; although there is some indication that iron rust was used by the Greeks in wound healing (Majno, 1975), it cannot claim ancestors among the Greeks, either. The principal origin of the iron to be considered in this book is not meteorites or warriors' lances but red blood cells and the iron-binding proteins.

The red blood cell appears to have evolved to ensure the iron-dependent function of hemoglobin, and thus of the blood, in the transport and delivery of oxygen to tissues (Lehmann and Huntsman, 1961). One could thus claim William Harvey as an ancestor when he asked whether 'the perpetual motion of the blood' could be for 'the purpose of nutrition'.

The topic 'iron and inflammation' could perhaps find an ancestor in Galen, who adopted venesection as a routine practice in the treatment of acute infection and in the prophylaxis of inflammation based on the realization of 'what great benefits the female sex enjoys' from their 'monthly evacuation of blood' (Brain, 1979): 'a woman who is well cleansed is not seized with gouty or arthritic or pleuritic or peripneumonic disease' (Brain, 1979).

Our search for ancestors in antiquity, however, should not blind us to the fact that, according to Robb-Smith, the association of iron with the blood was not shown until the 18th century, by Menghini, who, in 1747, 'separated it from the ash with the aid of a magnet' (Robb-Smith, 1961). We had to wait 240 years to understand how iron, sitting 'like a jewel' at the center of heme, would answer William Harvey's inspired question (Perutz, 1987). To my knowledge, 231 years were to pass after Menghini's discovery,

TABLE 1.1 Effect of addition of red blood cell lysate, hemoglobin or ferric hydroxide on the mixed lymphocyte reaction (MLR)

Substance added	Concentration	MLR suppression (%)
Red blood cell lysate	12.5 mg/ml	54
	25 mg/ml	59
Hemoglobin	12.5 mg/ml	75
	25 mg/ml	82
Fe	50 μg/ml	39.8
	500 μg/ml	89.2

Translated from Keown and Descamps (1978).

before iron, as a product of red cell breakdown, was shown to have an effect on an immune function *in vitro* (Keown and Descamps, 1978). In experiments motivated by the immunosuppressive effect of blood transfusion, they compared the effect of adding human red blood cells, a red cell lysate, hemoglobin or an iron salt, to the mixed lymphocyte reaction (MLR).The results indicated that a suppressive effect was observed (Table 1.1) with the addition of the red cell lysate or hemoglobin; a similar effect could be provoked by the addition of a ferric salt (Keown and Descamps, 1978).

In vivo, however, the extent of the interaction between red blood cell-derived iron and the immune system far exceeds any experimental models tested *in vitro* so far.

BRIEF SUMMARY OF THE EVOLUTION OF IRON RECYCLING

For reasons that are still unclear to those interested in the principles of molecular evolution (McClendon, 1976), iron has been selected as the most important metal utilized in biological functions. Because an iron atom in a compound can exist in two states of valency, ferrous and ferric, iron became the primordial partner of oxygen in evolution (Cloud, 1978). Like many other long-standing partnerships, this one, to survive, had to use protective devices that would not allow the toxicity of either partner to be expressed in the presence of the other. These devices reach their most refined expression in hemoglobin and the red cell, and their most useful and practical forms in ferritin and transferrin. It is the acknowledged job of those three proteins and of the red blood cell to protect the body from the toxicity of iron in the presence of oxygen, ensuring at the same time that oxygen is transported and delivered to all tissues and that iron is continuously available, not only for the demand of hemoglobin biosynthesis but also for all other enzymatic pathways requiring it (see Chapter 3).

'A most important point that will bear repeating', as stressed by Harris and Kellermeyer (1974), is that 'iron is hardly excreted and tenaciously recycled'. Indeed, with the exception of menstruating women, who lose blood periodically, the amount of iron excreted per day is negligible: 0.5–1 mg. Even in a normal woman with a hemoglobin of 14 mg per 100 ml of blood, with an estimated periodic menstrual loss of 20–23 mg of iron, the daily additional loss is another 0.5–1.4 mg, not exceeding 1.5 mg day^{-1}. During pregnancy, the requirements of the growing fetus impose on the woman an estimated loss of 2.4 mg of iron per day over the three trimesters. These small amounts contrast with the total amount of iron recycled every day, 30–35 mg, of which only 1 mg comes from absorption (Harris and Kellermeyer, 1974). Normally, the amount of iron in the body is kept

TABLE 1.2 Zonal grading of iron absorption and number of IgA-positive cells in the small intestine

Zone	Fe absorption[a]	IgA-positive cells
Duodenum	69.8 ± 6.05	1953 (1588–2429)
Mid-jejunum	28.6 ± 4.08	1235 (1005–1652)
Jejunum–ileum	9.2 ± 3.08	—
Ileum	2.1 ± 0.64	963 (712–1404)

Slightly modified from de Sousa (1981), based on data from Duthie (1964) and Husband and Gowans (1976) in rats.
[a] Expressed as percentage of dose of ^{59}Fe injected directly into the bowel.

constant at absorption which takes place largely through the upper sections of the small intestine (Table 1.2). The total body iron in a 70 kg man has been estimated to be 4.2 g, distributed as follows: hemoglobin (74.3%), ferritin (16.4%), myoglobin (3.3%), haptoglobin–hemoglobin (0.2%), catalase (0.11%), cytochrome c (0.08%), transferrin (0.07%) (Beinert, 1973).

After absorption, iron travels on the serum protein transferrin, which carries it to the bone marrow; in the bone marrow, iron is incorporated in the biosynthetic pathway of hemoglobin. Transferrin, however, has been identified also as a major nutritional requirement for lymphocyte proliferation *in vitro*, in response to stimulation by antigens and mitogens (see Chapter 5) and for the proliferation *in vitro* of malignant T cells (see Chapter 12). Hemoglobin is the almost exclusive constituent of the red cell (95% of its dry weight).

Mammalian hemoglobin free in the plasma would be expected to have a half-life of about 40 minutes and would easily be lost through the kidneys and the reticuloendothelial system (Crosby, 1955). Through having evolved to travel in a cell that acts simultaneously as a protective environment and a carriage, the life-expectancy of hemoglobin increased to the greater life-expectancy of the red blood cell itself; in man this is about 120 days. Human senescent red cells, representing about 0.7% of all erythrocytes, are selectively removed by macrophages; these ensure iron's recycling and re-entry into the circulation pool of transferrin. In the adult, 2–3 million red blood cells are produced and broken down *per second*. The magnitude of recycling of iron that takes place through the macrophage system is not normally mentioned in immunology textbooks. One red blood cell contains 400 million molecules of hemoglobin, which means that 2–3 million times that number of molecules of hemoglobin, containing four times that

Iron and the Lymphomyeloid System

number of iron atoms, are recycled through the immune system *per second*. It is well established that the macrophages of the splenic red pulp play a central role in the removal of effete red cells (Rifkind, 1965; see Chapter 2). What is still under debate is whether the only mechanism in the recognition and removal of the senescent red cell pool is the one described in Chapter 2.

It has been questioned whether high-density red cells are a complete representation of the senescent red cell pool (Mueller *et al.*, 1987); evidence that phagocytosis of high-density red cells can occur independently of antibody should remain under consideration (Clark and Shohet, 1985; Lutz *et al.*, 1987). One might get some further insight into this question from examination of red cell removal in species like fish, in which only IgM has been found in the serum (Jurd, 1985).

Because macrophages are a recognized component of the immune system, their role in the physiological clearance of red blood cells, and their singular ability to discriminate between old and young red cells (see Chapter 2) and to recycle $32-48 \times 10^{12}$ atoms of iron per second, constitute chronologically the first, and perhaps still the most formidable, illustration of the continuous interactions that take place between iron and the immune system in man. For many years, these interactions have been of particular interest to hematologists. As we will see, the interest of immunologists in the interactions between iron, the iron-binding proteins and the cells of the lymphomyeloid system, was not motivated primarily by the physiological clearance of red blood cells.

RECENT PATHS AND THEIR GUIDING PERSPECTIVES

The following description represents my personal view of the development of this field as a comparative latecomer to the decade where most recent paths seem to have begun. Jacobs, in Chapter 18, will have the last word and the opportunity to correct me if I am wrong.

The two perspectives that seem to have influenced the experimental development of the field emerged in the decade 1970–80 from three principal areas of study: hematology, nutrition and immunology. In one perspective, the interaction between iron and cells of the immune system was looked at from the iron side. Those interested primarily in the metal examined its action as a nutrient, as an immunoregulator or as a toxic element. In another perspective, the interaction was looked at from the cell's side. Those interested primarily in the cells examined their ability to synthesize, release and express receptors for the iron-binding proteins.

The hematology and nutrition groups shared an interest in the effects of iron deficiency on immune function (Joynson *et al.*, 1972; Chandra, 1975;

Kulapongs *et al.*, 1974; Jarvis and Jacobs, 1974; Summers and Jacobs, 1976; Dallman, Beutler and Finch, 1978; Brock, 1981) (see Chapter 5). Work from the hematology group of Jacobs reflected an early concern in establishing and quantitating the association of ferritin with monocytes, lymphocytes and neutrophils (Summers, Worwood and Jacobs, 1974, 1975). The immunology groups appeared later within the same decade representing three main interests: in the immunosuppressive effect of blood transfusion (Keown and Descamps, 1978), in the surveillance role of the circulation of lymphocytes (de Sousa, 1978; de Sousa, Smithyman and Tan, 1978; de Sousa and Nishiya, 1978; Nishiya, Chiao and de Sousa, 1980; Dörner *et al.*, 1980) and in the pathogenesis of inflammation (Blake *et al.*, 1981) (see Chapter 7). A significant offshoot of the interest in the iron-binding proteins as molecules of interaction between immune cell sets led to uncovering a possible role for the iron-binding proteins in the regulation of bone marrow cell differentiation (Broxmeyer *et al.*, 1978) (see Chapters 9 and 10).

Other pieces of work published in the same decade demonstrated that macrophages express receptors for lactoferrin (van Snick and Masson, 1976), that activated lymphocytes express receptors for transferrin (Phillips, 1976) and that ferritin could be identified on the surface of a subset of T lymphocytes in breast cancer patients (Moroz *et al.*, 1977) (see Chapter 13). Reviews published in 1978 put together the published evidence for the role of iron on the stimulation of microbial cell growth (Bullen, Rogers and Griffiths, 1978; Payne and Finkelstein, 1978; Weinberg, 1978); in the same year, Fernandez-Pol isolated and characterized a siderophore-like growth factor from mutants of SV-40 transformed cells (Fernandez-Pol, 1978). With the latter finding, the utilization of iron by transformed cells became a process that could be viewed in a manner identical to that previously adopted to view the positive action of iron on microbial cell growth. Since then, the expression of the transferrin receptor by transformed cells has been the focus of much greater attention (see Chapters 12 and 16).

In summary, if one were to locate in time a common root for the paths leading to the topics covered by this book, that root would fall with little doubt within the 1970–80 decade.

Much earlier studies, however, had already illustrated the effect of iron on the development of joint disease (Hiyeda, 1939); Phillips and Thorbecke (1966) had demonstrated that the serum transferrin in rat-into-mouse chimeras had its origin in the repopulating donor bone marrow cells (see Chapter 3); in a study of the migration of neural duct lymphocytes in plaice, Ellis and de Sousa (1974) had shown that labeled lymphocytes migrate to clusters of iron-containing melanomacrophages in fish spleen. Such observations stayed 'unattended' and buried in the literature, as isolated observations often do until a new perspective brings them back to life within the same conjectural territory.

WHERE A FRONTIER APPEARS WIDE ENOUGH TO BECOME A COUNTRY

What new perspective could bring within the boundaries of the same territory the observations made by Hiyeda in the remote rural areas of Manchoukuo that in the spring, people who drank well water with a high iron concentration (more than 0.3 mg l^{-1}) developed arthritic pain (Hiyeda, 1939), the demonstration of rat transferrin production by spleen cells, thymus cells and peritoneal macrophages from mouse radiation chimeras repopulated with rat bone marrow cells (Phillips and Thorbecke, 1966) and the description of the migration of autologous neural duct lymphocytes towards iron-containing melanomacrophages in the plaice spleen (Ellis and de Sousa, 1974)?

Hitherto, the possibilities that iron could contribute to the pathogenesis of inflammation, that cells of the immune system could contribute to the synthesis and secretion of iron-binding proteins, and that lymphocytes migrate to iron-containing sites, have been considered of remote interest and have remained stationed at peripheral outposts of the immunological frontiers. Present dogma at the center of immunology views the immune system as a complex system of interacting cells, prepared, in a military sense, for the attack of external pathogens, whose expansion depends primarily on the recognition of non-self (Klein, 1982). A new dogma is beginning to emerge, which views the development of the immune system depending on the recognition of self antigens; the most powerful lobby of the new dogma sees the idiotype anti-idiotype network as the critical recognition network imparting movement to an otherwise static house of mirrors and self-perpetuating reflected images (Vaz, Martinez and Coutinho, 1984). Neither prevailing nor emerging dogmas see the circulation of the blood or the metabolism of iron as a motivating force for the development of a complex system of surveillance. While searching for evidence for this view, I came to be interested in iron as a target of surveillance by the immune system (de Sousa, 1978; de Sousa *et al.*, 1982). In the course of this search, I was reminded that red blood cells treated with bromelain have been used as tools by those concerned with the regulation of the immune response to self antigens. It is thought that bromelain treatment of mouse red blood cells exposes antigens recognized by IgM autoantibodies produced by spleen cells in unimmunized mice (Cunliffe and Cox, 1979; Cunningham, 1974). Antigens, however, are not usually presented to the immune system at the rate of 10^{12} molecules *per second*. It is hard to imagine this number of molecules of hemoglobin containing four times that number of atoms of iron, with no place to go. The reality nearest to such a picture is perhaps seen in beta-thalassemia major, where the requirement of lifetime blood transfusion leads to the development of an iron load in excess of the phagocytic capacity of the macrophage system and of the binding and storing capacity of transferrin and ferritin, respectively. Such degree of iron overload is incompatible with life and with reproduction; only after the development of an effective iron-chelation therapeutic regimen has the life-expectancy of these patients been extended to the third decade (Orkin, 1987). A more exact illustration of the incompatibility of life with iron overload stems from the studies of rare cases of neonatal hemochromatosis. In a review of 25 published cases, survival ranged from minutes after birth to 9 days, with a mean of 2.7 days (Knisely *et al.*, 1987).

The immune system and the 'red blood cell system' appear thus to have become irrevocably interconnected and interdependent in evolution, rather like a frontier, which with time, could claim a life and a jurisdiction of its own.

THIS BOOK AND ITS TWO PURPOSES

The purpose of this book is two-fold:

(a) To bring together most of the data derived from the work done in the last 10–16 years, illustrating key points of the interaction between iron, the iron-binding proteins and the lymphomyeloid system: cellular and molecular biology (Parts I and III), immunopathology (Parts II and IV), oncology (Part V), and implication for diagnosis and therapy (Part VI).
(b) To bring out, by contrast, the areas about which little seems to be known; not because it could not have been known, but because the questions may not have been asked. I shall conclude these introductory remarks by enumerating some of those questions.

Phylogeny

A view that attributes to the immune system a protective role against the potential toxicity resulting from red cell breakdown and iron accumulation assumes, implicitly, that the appearance of an immune system in evolution would occur in parallel with the development of systems of delivery of oxygen dependent on iron and heme pigments. Likewise, a 'nutritional view', i.e. a view that sees iron acting primarily as an indispensable nutrient for lymphoid cell activation and division, has also to assume an interdependence of the evolution of the two systems. In the latter case, expansion of the immune system would depend, in addition, on the simultaneous exposure to external antigens.

Although the phylogeny of the immune response has been the subject of considerable interest and a great deal is known about the phylogeny of hemoglobin and of oxygen transport (Robb-Smith, 1961), there are practically no studies reflecting an integrated conjectural approach to the examination of the phylogeny of the two systems. Consulting sources on the phylogeny of the immune response, one finds work reflecting largely a persistent preoccupation with the view that the immune system develops in response to exposure to potential external pathogens. One interesting example stems from studies of the development of lymphoid tissues in viviparous and oviparous teleosts (Bly, 1985). Following the hypothesis that 'natural selection will favour individuals in which the development of lymphoid tissues coincides with the first exposure to potential pathogens' (Bly, 1985), it has been anticipated that the immune system in oviparous species would develop at hatching and in viviparous species around parturition. The lymphoid system of viviparous species, however, develops early, 'long before parturition'. The early development of a thymus and a head kidney in the viviparous *Zoarces* coincides with an early development of an efficient oxygen-transport system (Bly, 1985). Moreover, maternal blood components have been described in the gut of *Zoarces* embryos (Kristofferson et al., 1973; Bly, 1985).

Ontogeny and anatomophysiology

Studies of lymphocyte migration during fetal development are, comprehensibly, few. Thanks to the dexterity of Cahill and his coworkers, studies of the fetal lymphocyte circulation have been undertaken in sheep (Cahill et al., 1979; Cahill and Trnka, 1980). Lymphocytes obtained from the intestinal or prescapular lymph in the fetus or in the adult animal were radioisotopically labeled and traced in their respective matched recipients. A comparison of the percentage of the radioactivity recovered in the spleen and the liver in the two groups (Table 1.3) shows that the fetus intestinal lymph and prescapular lymph lymphocytes migrate predominantly to the liver, 32.6% and 23.7% respectively, in contrast to the adult, where recovery in the liver is 4.4% and 2.8% respectively. Recovery of the radioactivity in the fetal spleen is lower than in the liver (12.2% for intestinal lymph, 11.7% for prescapular lymphocytes) and higher in the adult (20% and 25.7%). Studies of the human fetus have demonstrated that the amount of iron in the fetal liver is always significantly higher than that found in the spleen (Singla, Gupta and Agawal, 1985).

In the adult, the critical steps of the metabolism of iron occur at anatomical sites of importance to immune function or cell differentiation, namely, the bone marrow, the duodenum and the red pulp of the spleen. The closest to a direct study of the influence of iron on the development of a section of the immune system *in vivo* is a recent nutritional study of the effect of an iron-fortified formula on secretory IgA of the gastrointestinal

TABLE 1.3 Lymphocyte migration to liver, spleen and the small intestine in adult sheep and the fetal lamb

Source of lymphocytes infused	Liver	Spleen	Small intestine
Fetus			
Intestinal lymph	32.6[a]	12.2	3.0
Prescapular lymph	23.7	11.7	2.5
Adult			
Intestinal lymph	4.4	20.0	12.9
Prescapular lymph	2.8	25.7	1.4

Data from Cahill et al. (1979).
[a]Expressed as mean percentage radioactivity; three animals used in each group.

tract in early infancy (Koutras, Vigorita and Quiroz, 1986). In a study comparing the amount of fecal IgA measured at birth, 2, 4 and 8 weeks in two groups of infants, one receiving a standard formula (Enfamil) and another receiving Enfamil with iron, the authors found significantly higher amounts of IgA at 2, 4 and 8 weeks in the group that had received the iron-fortified formula (Table 1.4); a higher percentage of the infants receiving the iron-fortified formula had demonstrable higher amounts (1 mg dl^{-1}) of fecal IgA from 2 weeks of age onwards.

These results could also indicate that the oral administration of iron stimulated the development of the intestinal microbial flora and can therefore still be viewed within the framework of prevailing immunological thought. However, in a earlier attempt to compare published data on the

TABLE 1.4 Effect of the administration of an iron-fortified formula on amount of fecal secretory IgA in early human life

Group	n[a]	1 (at birth)	Fecal IgA (mg dl^{-1}) 2 (2 weeks)	3 (4 weeks)	4 (8 weeks)
+Fe	15	0	3.8 (0–20)	7.37 (0–30)	23 (6–68)
−Fe	15	0	0	1.62 (0–8.3)	4.4 (0.5–14)

Data from Koutras, Vigorita and Quiroz (1986).
[a]Number of patients followed from birth (stages 1–4) fed iron-fortified (+Fe) or non-iron-fortified (−Fe) formula.

amount of iron absorbed in different sections of the small intestine (Duthie, 1964) with data from separate experiments on numbers of IgA-containing cells seen in the same areas (Husband and Gowans, 1978), it became apparent that there is a similar zonal grading of the two (Table 1.2): the highest amount of iron is absorbed in the duodenum, and the highest average numbers of IgA-positive cells are seen in the same region, followed by the mid-jejunum and the ileum (de Sousa, 1981).

CONCLUSION

Clearly one could continue writing, succumbing to the seduction of listing what one would have liked to know for certain at this stage; readers, quite justifiably, expect to find in books information about what is known. This introduction should not stand in their way.

ACKNOWLEDGEMENTS

I wish to thank Uriel for keeping me chained to thought during the preparation of this chapter, and his master for the large table.

This work was supported by Grants from the American–Portuguese Biomedical Research Fund and the Portuguese National Funding Agency for Science and Technology (JNICT).

REFERENCES

Agius, C. (1985). The melano-macrophage centres of fish: a review. In M. J. Manning and M. F. Tatner (eds) *Fish Immunology*, pp. 85–105. Academic Press, London.
Beinert, H. (1973). Development of the field and nomenclature. In W. Lovenberg (ed.) *Iron-Sulfur Proteins*, Vol. 1, pp. 1–36. Academic Press, New York.
Blake, D. R., Bacon, P. A., Dieppe, P. A., and Gutteridge, J. M. C. (1981). The importance of iron in rheumatoid disease, *Lancet*, **ii**, 1142.
Bly, J. E. (1985). The ontogeny of the immune system in the viviparous teleost. In M. J. Manning and M. F. Tatner (eds) *Fish Immunology*, pp. 327–420. Academic Press, London.
Brain, P. (1979). In defense of ancient blood letting, *S. Afr. Med. J.*, **56**, 149–54.
Brock, J. H. (1981). The effect of iron and transferrin on the response of serum-free cultures of mouse lymphocytes to concanavalin A and lipopolysaccharide, *Immunology*, **43**, 387–92.
Broxmeyer, H. E., Smithyman, A., Eger, R. R., Meyers, P. A., and de Sousa, M. (1978). Identification of lactoferrin as the granulocyte-derived inhibitor of colony-stimulating activity, *J. Exp. Med.*, **148**, 1052–67.

Bullen, J. J., Rogers, H. J., and Griffiths, E. (1978). Role of iron in microbial infection, *Curr. Top. Microbiol. Immunol.*, **80**, 1–35.
Cahill, R. N. P., and Trnka, Z. (1980). Growth and development of recirculating lymphocytes in the sheep fetus, *Monogr. Allergy*, **16**, 38.
Cahill, R. N. P., Poskitt, D. C., Hay, J. B., Heron, I., and Trnka, Z. (1979). The migration of lymphocytes in the fetal lamb, *Eur. J. Immunol.*, **9**, 251–3.
Chandra, R. N. P. (1975). Impaired immunocompetence associated with iron deficiency, *J. Pediatr.*, **86**, 899–902.
Clark, M. R., and Shohet, S. B. (1985). Red cell senescence, *Clin. Haematol.*, **14**, 223–57.
Cloud, P. (1978). *Cosmos, Earth and Man*, Yale University Press.
Cox, K. O., Ramos, T., Cox, J., and Samcewicz, B. (1983). Effects in mice of rat bromelain-treated RBC and lipopolysaccharide on autoantibody production against bromelain-treated isologous RBC, *Int. Arch. Allergy Appl. Immunol.*, **72**, 325–329.
Crosby, W. H. (1955). The metabolism of hemoglobin and bile pigment in hemolytic disease, *Am. J. Med.*, **18**, 112–22.
Cunliffe, D. A., and Cox, K. O. (1979). Effects of bromelain and pronase on erythrocyte membranes, *Mol. Immunol.*, **16**, 427–33.
Cunningham, A. J. (1974). Large numbers of cells in normal mice produce antibody to components of isologous erythrocytes, *Nature*, **252**, 749–51.
Cunningham, A. J. (1976). Self tolerance maintained by active suppressor mechanisms, *Transpl. Rev.*, **31**, 23.
Dallman, P. R., Beutler, E., and Finch, C. A. (1978). Effects of iron deficiency exclusive of anaemia (annotation), *Br. J. Haematol.* **40**, 179–84.
de Sousa, M. (1978). Lymphoid cell positioning: a new proposal for the mechanism of control of lymphoid cell positioning, *Symp. Soc. Exp. Biol.* **32**, 393–409.
de Sousa, M. (1981). *Lymphocyte Circulation: Experimental and Clinical Aspects*, pp. 201–17, John Wiley and Sons, Chichester.
de Sousa, M. (1983). Iron and the lymphomyeloid system: old frontier new perspective, *Microbiology*, **1983**, 322–6.
de Sousa, M., and Nishiya, K. (1978). Inhibition of E-rosette formation by two iron salts, *Cell Immunol.*, **38**, 203–8.
de Sousa, M., Smithyman, A., and Tan, C. T. C. (1978). Suggested models of ecotaxopathy in lymphoreticular malignancy. A role for the iron-binding proteins in the control of lymphoid cell migration, *Am. J. Pathol.*, **90**, 497–520.
de Sousa, M., Martins Da Silva, B., Dörner, M., Munn, C. G., Nishiya, K., Grady, R. W., and Silverstone, A. (1982). Iron and the lymphomyeloid system: rationale for considering iron as a target of immune surveillance. In P. Saltman and J. Hegenauer (eds) *The Biochemistry and Physiology of Iron*, pp. 687, Elsevier, North Holland.
Dörner, M., Silverstone, A., Nishiya, K., de Sostoa, A., Munn, C. G., and de Sousa, M. (1980). Ferritin synthesis by human T lymphocytes, *Science*, **209**, 1019–21.
Duthie, H. L. (1964). The relative importance of the duodenum in the intestinal absorption of iron, *Br. J. Haematol.*, **10**, 59–68.
Ellis, A. E., and de Sousa, M. (1974). Phylogeny of the lymphoid system: study of the fate of circulating lymphocytes in plaice, *Eur. J. Immunol.*, **4**, 338–43.
Fernandez-Pol, J. A. (1978). Siderophore like growth factor synthesized by SV-40 transformed cells adapted to picolinic acid stimulates DNA synthesis in cultured cells, *FEBS Lett.*, **88**, 345–8.

Harris, J. W., and Kellermeyer, R. W. (1974). *The Red Cell*, Harvard University Press.
Hiyeda, K. (1939). The cause of Kaschin-Beck's disease, *Jpn. J. Med. Sci.*, **4**, 91–106.
Husband, A. J., and Gowans, J. L. (1978). The origin and antigen-dependent distribution of IgA containing cells in the intestine, *J. Exp. Med.*, **148**, 1146–60.
Jarvis, J. H., and Jacobs, A. (1974). Morphological abnormalities in lymphocyte mitochondria associated with iron-deficiency anemia, *J. Clin. Pathol.*, **27**, 973–9.
Joynson, D. H. M., Jacobs, A., Walker, D. M., and Dolby, A. E. (1972). Defect of cell-mediated immunity in patients with iron-deficiency anaemia, *Lancet*, **ii**, 1058–9.
Jurd, R. D. (1985). Specialisation in the teleost and anuran immune response: a comparative critique. In M. J. Manning and M. F. Tatner (eds) *Fish Immunology*, pp. 9–28, Academic Press, London.
Keown, P., and Descamps, B. (1978). Suppression de la reaction lymphocytaire mixte par des globules rouges autologues et leurs constituants: une hypothese nouvelle sur l'effet apparemment tolerogene des transfusions sanguines en transplantation. *C. R. Seances Acad. Sci. (D)*, **287**, 749–52.
Klein, J. (1982). *Immunology: The Science of Self/Non-self Discrimination*, John Wiley and Sons, Chichester.
Knisely, A. S., Magid, M. S., Dische, R., and Cutz. E. (1987). Neonatal hemochromatosis, *Birth Defects: Original Article Series*, **23**, 75–102.
Koutras, A. K., Vigorita, V. J., and Quiroz, E. (1986). Effect of iron-fortified formula on SIgA of gastrointestinal tract in early infancy, *J. Pediatr. Gastroenterol. Nutr.*, **5**, 926–30.
Kristopherson, R., Broberg, S., and Pekkarinen, M. (1973). Histology and physiology of embryotrophe formation, embryonic nutrition and growth in the eel-pout *Zoarces viviparus* (L.). *Ann. Zool. Fenn.*, **10**, 467–77.
Kulapongs, P., Vithayasai, V., Suskind, R. (1974). Cell mediated immunity and phagocytosis and killing function in children with severe iron-deficiency anemia, *Lancet*, **ii**, 689–91.
Lehmann, H., and Huntsman, R. G. (1961). Why are red cells the shape they are? The evolution of the human red cell. In A. Macfarlane and A. H. T. Robb-Smith (eds) *The Functions of the Blood*, pp. 73–147, Academic Press, New York.
Lutz, H. U., Bussolino, F., Flepp, R., Fasler, S., Stammler, P., Kazatchine, M. D., and Arese, P. (1987). Naturally occurring anti-band 3 antibodies and complement together mediate phagocytosis of oxidatively stressed human red blood cells, *Proc. Natl Acad. Sci. USA*, **84**, 7368–72.
Majno, G. (1975). *The Healing Hand*, Harvard University Press.
McClendon, J. H. (1976). Elemental abundance as a factor in the origins of mineral nutrient requirements, *J. Mol. Evol.*, **8**, 175–97.
Moroz, C., Giler, S., Kupfer, B., and Urca, I. (1977). Lymphocytes bearing surface ferritin in patients with Hodgkin's disease and breast cancer, *N. Engl. J. Med.*, **297**, 1172–3.
Mueller, T. J., Jackson, C. W., Dockter, M. E., and Morrison, M. (1987). Membrane skeletal alterations during *in vivo* mouse red cell aging. Increase in the band 4.1a:4.1b ratio, *J. Clin. Invest.*, **79**, 492–9.
Nishiya, K., Chiao, J. W., and de Sousa, M. (1980). Iron binding proteins in selected human peripheral blood cell sets: immunofluorescence, *Br. J. Haematol.*, **46**, 235–45.
Orkin, S. H. (1987). Disorders of hemoglobin synthesis: the thalassemias. In G.

Stammatoyannopoulos, A. N. Nienhuis, P. Leder and P. W. Majerus (eds) *The Molecular Basis of Blood Diseases*, p. 122, W. B. Saunders. Philadelphia.

Payne, S. M., and Finkelstein, R. A. (1978). The critical role of iron in host-bacterial interactions, *J. Clin. Invest.*, **61**, 1428–40.

Perutz, M. (1987). Molecular anatomy, physiology and pathology of hemoglobin. In G. Stammatoyannopoulos, A. N. Nienhuis, P. Leder and P. W. Majerus (eds) *The Molecular Basis of Blood Diseases*, pp. 127–78, W. B. Saunders, Philadelphia.

Phillips, J. L. (1976). Specific binding of zinc transferrin to human lymphocytes, *Biochem. Biophys. Res. Commun.*, **72**, 634–9.

Phillips, M. E., and Thorbecke, G. J. (1966). Studies on the serum proteins of chimaeras. Identification and study of the site of origin of donor type serum proteins in adult-rat-into-mouse chimaeras, *Int. Arch. Allergy*, **29**, 553–67.

Rifkind, R. (1966). Destruction of injured red cells *in vivo*, *Am. J. Med.*, **41**, 711–21.

Robb-Smith, A. H. T. (1961). The growth of knowledge of the functions of the blood. In R. G. MacFarlane and A. H. T. Robb-Smith (eds) *Functions of the Blood*, pp. xv–liv. Academic Press, New York.

Singla, P. N., Gupta, V. P., and Agawal, K. N. (1985). Storage iron in human foetal organs, *Acta Pediatr. Scand.*, **74**, 701–6.

Summers, M. R., and Jacobs, A. (1976). Iron uptake and ferritin synthesis by peripheral blood leucocytes from normal subjects and patients with iron deficiency and the anaemia of chronic disease, *Br. J. Haematol.*, **34**, 221–9.

Summers, M., Worwood, M., and Jacobs, A. (1974). Ferritin in normal erythrocytes, lymphocytes, polymorphs and monocytes, *Br. J. Haematol.*, **28**, 19–26.

Summers, M., Worwood, M., and Jacobs, A. (1975). Ferritin synthesis in lymphocytes, polymorphs and monocytes, *Br. J. Haematol.*, **30**, 425–39.

Van Snick, J. L., and Masson, P. L. (1976). The binding of human lactoferrin to mouse peritoneal cells, *J. Exp. Med.*, **144**, 1568–80.

Vaz, N., Martinez, A. C., and Coutinho, A. (1984). The uniqueness and boundaries of the idiotypic self. In H. Kohler, J. Hurbain and P. A. Cazenave (eds), *Idiotypy in Biology and Medicine*, p. 43, Academic Press, New York.

Weinberg, E. D. (1978). Iron and infection, *Microbiol. Rev.*, **42**, 45–66.

Weinberg, R. J., Ell, S. R., and Weinberg, E. D. (1986). Blood-letting, iron homoeostasis and human health, *Med. Hypotheses*, **21**, 441–3.

Iron in Immunity, Cancer and Inflammation
Edited by M. de Sousa and J. H. Brock
© 1989 John Wiley & Sons Ltd.

2
Recognition and Removal of Senescent Cells

Marguerite M. B. Kay

Department of Medicine, Departments of Medical Biochemistry and Genetics, and Medical Microbiology and Immunology, Texas A & M University, 1901 South First Street, Teague Veterans Center (151), Temple, Texas 76501, USA

ROLE OF IgG IN CELLULAR REMOVAL

One of the homeostatic activities vital to the evolution of vertebrates and to the development and survival of individuals is the ability to remove cells programmed for death at the end of their useful lifespan. Daily maintenance of homeostasis in adults requires removal of senescent and damaged cells and tissue repair following trauma. For example, approximately 360 billion senescent red cells are removed daily in humans. An understanding of this basic homeostatic mechanism is essential to both development and ageing, and to the concept of recognition and specificity which permeates disciplines in biomedicine.

Investigation of the mechanism by which senescent cells are removed from the body was approached by postulating that Ig in normal serum attaches to the surface of senescent red cells until a critical level is reached, which results in removal of these cells by macrophages (Kay, 1974, 1975). Stored human red blood cells (RBCs) were incubated in medium, autologous Ig, another individual's allogeneic Ig, or pooled, normal human IgG, IgM and IgA, washed, and incubated with the individual's macrophages. The results of this experiment demonstrated that: (a) the percentage phagocytosis of stored RBCs ('O' RBC) incubated in IgM and IgA is only slightly more than that in medium alone (<10%); (b) the percentage phagocytosis of stored RBCs incubated in autologous IgG was essentially the same as that of stored RBCs incubated in either autologous whole serum or the Ig fraction (42–49%); and (c) allogeneic Ig and IgG (~30% phagocytosis) were not as effective as autologous whole serum, Ig or IgG in promoting phagocytosis, although they had not been tested for blood group compatibility. These results indicate that normal circulating Ig can attach to RBCs and may be required for phagocytosis and suggest that the Ig that attaches is IgG. These experiments support but do not prove the initial working hypothesis which states that immunoglobulins attach to the surface of ageing RBCs until a threshold level is reached at which time macrophages phagocytize the cell.

In an attempt to test this hypothesis directly, and to determine whether the Ig which attached *in situ* was IgG, the following experiments were performed. Freshly drawn human RBCs were separated into young and old populations according to their different densities. Aliquots from each population were incubated with scanning immunoelectron microscopy marker conjugates and prepared for scanning electron microscopy (Kay, 1975, 1977, 1978a, 1978b). At the same time, each population was incubated with macrophages in medium, Ig-depleted serum, or whole serum. Old RBCs were phagocytized regardless of whether the final incubations were performed in medium without serum, in autologous Ig-depleted serum, or whole serum containing Ig (Figure 2.1). This suggested that Ig was attached *in situ* to the RBC and that phagocytic recognition was not inhibited by other serum components. Scanning immunoelectron microscopy of the two populations revealed that young RBCs were essentially unlabeled,

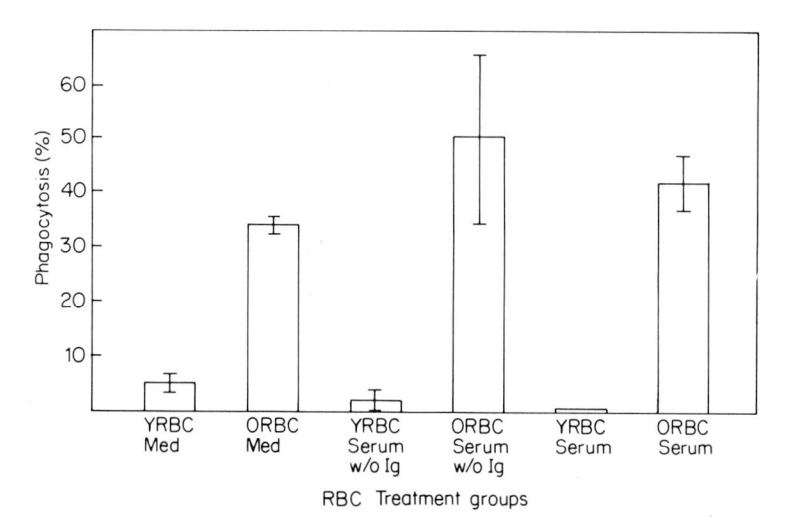

Figure 2.1 Phagocytosis of RBC aged *in situ*. Freshly drawn RBC were separated by density into young and old RBC populations, washed, resuspended in Medium 199 (Med), autologous IgG-depleted serum (Serum w/o Ig), or autologous fresh whole serum (Serum), and incubated with autologous macrophages. Vertical bars indicate 1 SEM

whereas senescent RBCs were labeled with SV-40 anti-human IgG but not with T2 anti-human IgA or with KLH anti-human IgM (Kay, 1975). The number of IgG molecules on senescent RBCs was approximately 100 per cell. On the basis of these findings, it can be concluded that IgG attaches *in situ* to senescent human RBCs.

These results were confirmed *in vivo* using mice which were bred and maintained in a Type I Maximum Security Barrier. RBCs labeled *in situ* with ^{59}Fe were separated on Percoll gradients into young and old populations (Figure 2.2) and injected into separate groups of syngeneic mice (Figure 2.3). Kinetic studies revealed that <90% of the ^{59}Fe-labeled young RBCs were removed from the circulation within 45 days. In contrast, >90% of the ^{59}Fe-labeled old RBCs were removed within 20 days. The difference in the rate of removal of young and old RBCs was statistically significant ($P < 0.001$). Kinetic studies on density-separated spleen cell populations revealed that the radioactivity decreased in the RBC fraction concomitantly with an increase in radioactivity in the splenic macrophage fraction. The radioactivity was found to be inside the macrophages (Bennet and Kay, 1981).

Studies performed *in vitro* with mouse splenic macrophages and autologous young and old RBCs revealed that mouse macrophages phagocytized senescent but not young RBCs ($P < 0.001$). The phagocytosis of middle-aged RBCs (~23%) was intermediate between that of young RBCs (~5%) and old RBCs (~50%). This suggests that the appearance of the antigen to which autologous IgG binds, and, thus, molecular ageing of membranes, may be a cumulative process.

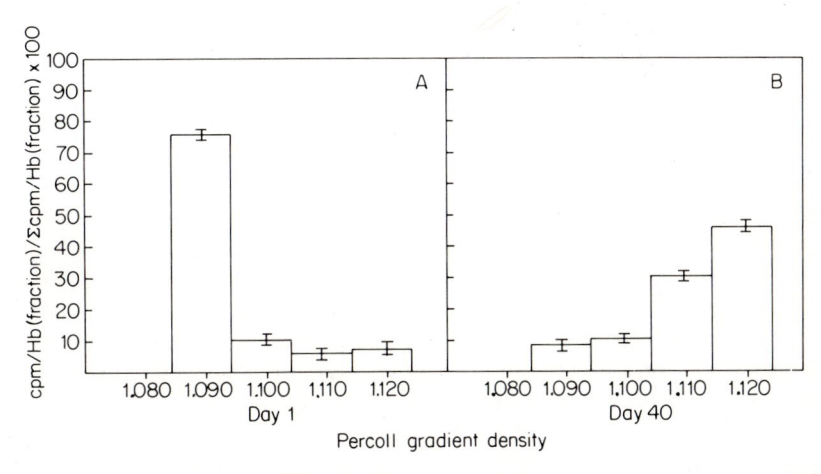

Figure 2.2 Distribution of ^{59}Fe-labeled murine RBC on a Percoll density gradient on Days 1 and 40 after ^{59}Fe pulse-labeling. Seventy-six per cent of the radioactivity is located in the least dense RBC fraction on Day 1 (a). The radioactivity shifts to the most dense fractions by Day 40 (b)

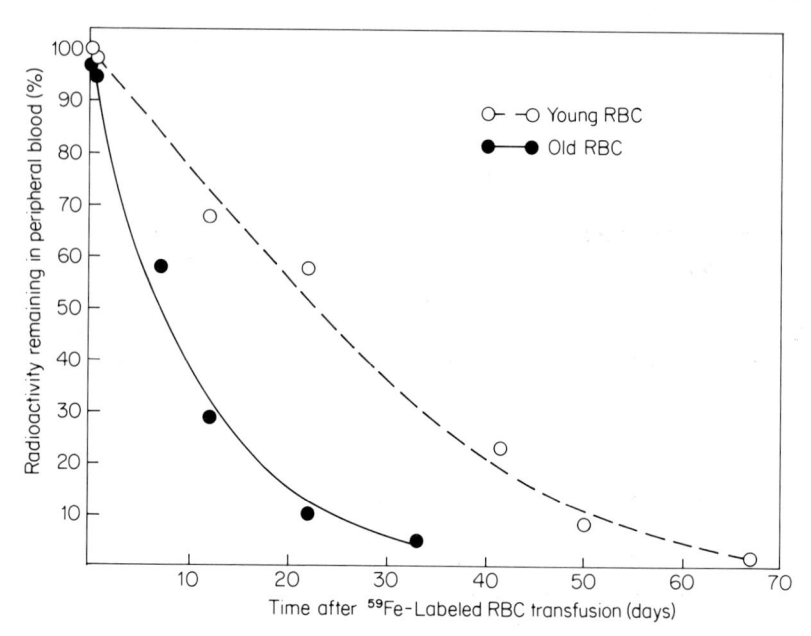

Figure 2.3 Decrease with time of circulating ^{59}Fe-labeled young and senescent RBC after transfusion into mice. Senescent RBC are cleared significantly faster than young RBC ($P \leq 0.001$). Standard deviations for each point are less than unity

The results presented thus far suggest that macrophages distinguish senescent from mature RBCs both *in vitro* and *in vivo* on the basis of selective attachment of autologous IgG to the membrane of senescent RBCs, and suggest that the IgG is an autoantibody. The IgG could be attached by nonspecific absorption or by RBC Fc receptors. Definitive evidence for the role of autoantibodies in the selective removal of senescent cells can be obtained by first dissociating the antibodies from senescent cells and then demonstrating their specific immunologic re-attachment via the Fab portion of the IgG molecule to homologous senescent, but not mature, cells.

IgG was eluted from senescent RBCs and shown to be an IgG free of other immunoglobulins (Kay, 1978b). In order to determine whether the IgG eluted from old RBCs aged *in situ* would re-attach to homologous cells, the eluted IgG was incubated with autologous or allogeneic young, stored RBCs (Kay, 1978b). These RBCs were then washed and incubated with autologous macrophages. The percentage phagocytosis of stored RBCs incubated with autologous IgG and then with autologous macrophages (46 ± 0%) was essentially the same as that of RBCs aged *in situ* (50 ± 4%). Macrophages phagocytized autologous stored RBCs incubated with autologous IgG (27 ± 0% phagocytosis), as well as allogeneic stored RBCs

TABLE 2.1 Phagocytosis of stored RBC (ORBC) incubated with IgG eluted from senescent cells before and after absorption with stored RBC or freshly isolated young RBC (YRBC)

Experiment No.	Quantity*	Phagocytosis (% ± SEM)†		
		Before absorption	After absorption with YRBC	After absorption with ORBC
1	3	49 ± 2	43 ± 9	0
2	3	35 ± 1	34 ± 7	0
3	3	43 ± 11	46 ± 16	0

*Quantity (μg) of IgG added to 1.5×10^8 RBC in 1 ml of Medium 199.
†SEM, standard error of the mean of triplicate or quadruplicate cultures. From Kay (1978).

incubated with autologous IgG (56 ± 4% phagocytosis). However, they did not phagocytize allogeneic cells which had not been incubated with IgG (0% phagocytosis) nor did they phagocytize young allogeneic cells which were incubated with allogeneic IgG (5 ± 3% phagocytosis). IgG was demonstrated on the surface of stored RBCs incubated with IgG eluted from autologous or allogeneic cells with scanning immunoelectron microscopy. Absorption of the eluted IgG with stored RBCs, but not with freshly isolated young RBCs, abolished its phagocytosis-inducing ability (Table 2.1).

These binding and specificity experiments indicate that: (a) IgG is required for phagocytosis of stored autologous and allogeneic RBCs; (b) nonspecific binding of IgG does not play a major role in these experiments because absorption of both pooled normal human IgG and IgG eluted from senescent cells with stored RBCs abolishes its phagocytosis-inducing activity; (c) IgG eluted from senescent RBCs is reactive against stored, but not young, cells; and (d) IgG eluted from senescent RBCs cannot discriminate between autologous and allogeneic cells. The last two findings suggest that the antigen appearing on the surface of cells aged *in situ* and that appearing on stored cells is the same, or closely related, for all individuals.

To determine whether the Fab or Fc portions of IgG attach to RBCs, antigen blockade studies were performed (Kay, 1978b). The results are summarized in Figure 2.4. Stored RBCs were incubated for 30 min with either IgG, its Fab, or its Fc fragment. The RBCs were washed, and all three groups were incubated with IgG for another 30 min. RBCs were washed again and incubated with autologous macrophages (Figure 2.4A). For control cultures, stored RBCs were treated with IgG, Fab, or Fc before they were exposed to mononuclear phagocytes (Figure 2.4B). Control results show that phagocytosis was achieved by exposing the RBCs to IgG.

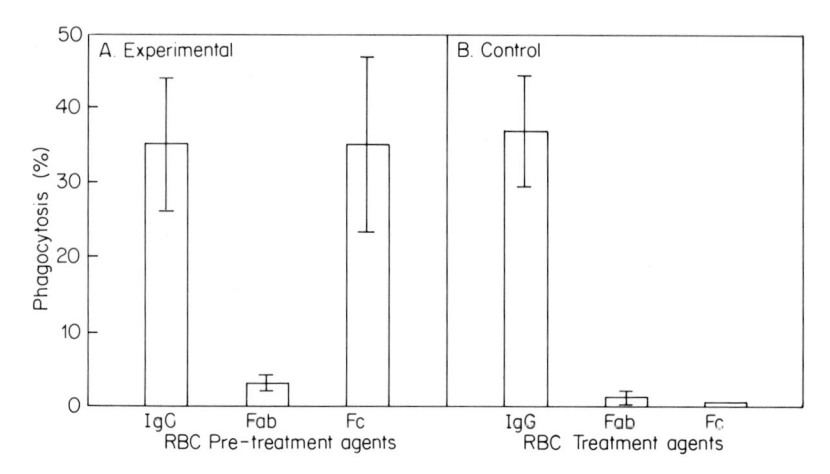

Figure 2.4 (A) Susceptibility to phagocytosis of aged RBC as influenced by their pretreatment with either IgG, Fab, or Fc before exposure to IgG. Stored RBC were incubated with either IgG, Fab, or Fc for 30 min, washed, and incubated with IgG for 30 min. The RBC were washed and incubated with mononuclear phagocytes for 3 hours. (B) Susceptibility to phagocytosis of aged RBC as influenced by their exposure to either IgG, Fab, or Fc. Stored RBC were incubated with either IgG, Fab, or Fc for 30 min, washed, and then incubated with mononuclear phagocytes for 3 hours. Bars indicate standard error of the mean; sample size, 6

Treatment with Fab or Fc did not promote phagocytosis. Experimental results show that treatment of RBCs with Fab prior to incubation with IgG reduced the phagocytosis to essentially zero, whereas pretreatment with Fc did not inhibit phagocytosis (Figure 2.4A). Thus, these blockade studies demonstrate that IgG binds to old RBCs via its Fab region. Binding of Fab but not Fc was also demonstrated with scanning immunoelectron microscopy (Kay, 1978b). Binding of the IgG molecule to aged RBCs via the Fab region is consistent with an immunologic binding of IgG with a surface antigen. The Fc portion of IgG would then be available to the macrophage Fc receptor.

These experiments suggest that the IgG eluted from senescent RBCs is an autoantibody, as it specifically re-attaches to homologous RBCs via its Fab region and initiates their selective destruction by macrophages.

These results indicate that as cells age, new antigens appear on their surface, enabling pre-existing IgG autoantibodies to attach immunologically to them. This provides the necessary signal for macrophages to selectively phagocytize senescent cells. Thus, it would appear that certain autoantibodies are contributing to the maintenance of homeostasis by removing senescent and damaged cells. Autoantibodies of this type have been identified as 'physiologic'.

The IgG autoantibody described here induces phagocytosis of senescent RBCs by macrophages. As a result, senescent cells are removed from the circulation instead of lysing (Jenkin and Karthigasu, 1967; Nelson, 1969; Smith, 1958). Thus, the membranes and hemoglobin of the approximately 1.93×10^{11} senescent cells that are removed daily are enzymatically degraded by macrophages rather than being released into the circulation by lysis, which could be detrimental to an individual's survival. For example, individuals with elevated plasma iron levels, as are seen with overt hemolytic anemia or destruction of ferritin-containing liver cells (e.g. viral hepatitis), are extremely susceptible to even a small inoculum of invading pathogens (Weinberg, 1974). Iron enhances the virulence of bacteria and can neutralize the microbiostatic action of serum (Weinberg, 1974). In addition, iron contributes to oxidative stress of RBCs in three ways (Halliwell and Gutteridge, 1986). It facilitates the decomposition of lipid peroxides and the formation of OH· radicals. Iron is also involved in generation of O_2^- and H_2O_2 by accelerating non-enzymatic oxidation of several molecules. Oxidation is one mechanism of RBC ageing (Kay et al., 1986).

Other investigators have confirmed the presence of IgG on senescent, damaged, and stored RBCs (Glass, Gershon and Gershon, 1983; Bartosz, Sosynski and Kedziona, 1982; Khansari et al., 1983; Khansari and Fudenberg, 1984; Alderman, Fudenberg and Lovins, 1980; Tannert, 1978; Wegner et al., 1980; Smalley and Tucker, 1983; Halhuber et al., 1980; Walker et al., 1984; Singer et al, 1986). IgG has been demonstrated on the surface of senescent and stored RBCs (Wegner et al., 1980; Halhuber et al., 1980) using ^{125}I-labeled anti-IgG. The amount of IgG on the surface of cells increases with storage (Wegner et al., 1980; Kay, Wong and Bolton, 1982). Halhuber et al. (1980) demonstrated IgG on the surface of RBCs stored by the blood bank. Wegner et al. (1980) have calculated that IgG bound to fresh, washed RBCs has an association constant of 1×10^{14} M^{-1}, indicating a high affinity of IgG for the antigen. In addition, they found that there was a seven-fold increase in IgG binding 18 hours after ATP depletion.

DIMINISHED RBC LIFESPAN IN OLD ANIMALS

Glass, Gershon and Gershon (1983) have found a 44% reduction in the mean life span of RBCs in old, specific pathogen-free rats, as compared to the lifespan in young rats, as determined by ^{59}Fe pulse-labeling *in vivo*. There was a 4.5-fold increase in the proportion of young cells circulating in the blood of old animals (9% young cells in young animals and 43% young cells in old animals). In old rats, young as well as old RBCs were heavily labeled with IgG, whereas predominantly old cells carried IgG in young rats (Glass, Gershon and Gershon, 1983). Extending their studies to humans, Glass and Gershon (1985) found a significant increase in reticulocytes in healthy elderly humans even though their hematocrits were the same as those of younger individuals. A significant increase in autologous IgG on fraction III (lower middle-aged) cells was consistently demonstrated in these elderly individuals (Glass and Gershon, 1985). These findings suggest that young cells age prematurely in old individuals. Vomel and Platt (1981) found that transfusion of RBCs of different ages into old rabbits resulted in a decreased lifespan of each RBC age group. Splenectomy of recipient animals prolonged RBC lifespan but resulted in circulating cells with increased fragility. Bartosz, Sosynski and Kedziona (1982) have found increased amounts of cell-membrane-bound IgG on RBCs from patients with Down's syndrome and suggest that accelerated RBC ageing occurs in these individuals. Accelerated ageing of other cells and systems, including the immune system, has been reported in patients with Down's syndrome (Walford, 1980). IgG has been reported on thalassemic RBCs (Galili et al., 1983) and sickle cells (Hebbel and Miller, 1984; Petz et al., 1984).

A SENESCENT CELL ANTIGEN?

The experiments described thus far indicate that macrophages distinguish between mature and senescent cells on the basis of selective IgG binding to the latter. Binding of an IgG autoantibody to senescent RBCs through immunologic mechanisms indicates that antigenic determinants recognized by these IgG autoantibodies appear on the surface of cells as they senesce. However, these experiments do not provide insight into membrane changes during cellular ageing nor do they reveal the mechanism responsible for the appearance of a 'neo-antigen'. In order to obtain this information, it is necessary to isolate and identify the antigen to which IgG binds on senescent RBCs.

Senescent cell antigen was isolated from sialoglycoprotein mixtures with affinity columns prepared with IgG eluted from senescent cells (Kay, 1981a). Material specifically bound by the column was eluted with glycine-HCl buffer. Both glycoprotein and protein stains of gels of the eluted material revealed a band migrating at a molecular weight of ~62 000 in the component 4.5 region. These experiments suggested that the 62 000 M_r glycopeptide carried the antigenic determinants recognized by IgG obtained from freshly isolated senescent cells. The ~62 000 M_r peptide, but not the remaining sialoglycoprotein mixture from which it was isolated, abolished the phagocytosis-inducing ability of IgG eluted from senescent RBCs in the erythrophagocytosis assay (Kay, 1981a, 1981b, 1982). This indicated that the ~62 000 M_r peptide was the antigen which appeared on the membrane of cells as they aged.

Examination of other somatic cells for the antigen which appears on senescent RBCs revealed its presence on lymphocytes, platelets, neutrophils, and cultured human adult liver cells and primary cultures of human embryonic kidney cells as determined by a phagocytosis inhibition assay (Kay, 1981a). Senescent cell antigen was isolated from lymphocytes (Kay, 1981a, 1982) with the senescent RBC IgG affinity column. Gel electrophoresis of the material obtained from the column revealed a band migrating at a M_r of ~62 000 at the same position as the antigen isolated from senescent RBCs. This finding confirmed the results obtained with the phagocytosis inhibition assay, indicating that the antigen which appeared on senescent RBCs also appeared on other somatic cells.

Appearance of the ~62 000 M_r antigen on RBCs initiates binding of IgG autoantibodies *in situ* and phagocytosis of senescent cells by macrophages (Kay, 1974, 1975, 1981a). The antigen is present on stored human lymphocytes, platelets, and neutrophils, and on cultured liver and kidney cells. In addition, IgG autoantibodies in normal serum have been shown to bind to senescent RBCs *in situ* in humans (Kay, 1975), mice (Bennet and Kay, 1981), rats (Glass, Gershon and Gershon, 1983), cows (Bartosz, Sosynski and Wasilewski, 1982), and rabbits (Vomel and Platt, 1981). Thus, the immunologic mechanism for removing senescent and damaged RBCs appears to be a general physiologic process for removing cells programmed for death in mammals and, possibly, other vertebrates (Kay, 1974, 1975; Glass, Gershon and Gershon, 1983).

CHARACTERIZATION OF SENESCENT CELL ANTIGEN AS BEING DERIVED FROM BAND 3

Since mature RBCs cannot synthesize proteins, senescent cell antigen was probably generated by modification of a pre-existing protein of higher molecular weight (Kay, 1981b; Kay, Wong and Bolton, 1982). It was postulated that the senescent cell antigen was a component of the band 4.5 region that was derived from band 3 (Kay, Wong and Bolton, 1982) based on both extraction and isolation conditions, molecular weight, and its characterization as a glycosylated peptide (Kay, 1981a).

Experiments designed to test this hypothesis revealed that senescent cell antigen is immunologically related to band 3 and may represent a physiologically significant proteolytic product of the parent molecule (Kay, Wong and Bolton, 1982; Kay *et al.*, 1983). Both band 3 and senescent cell antigen abolished the phagocytosis-inducing ability of IgG eluted from senescent cells, whereas spectrin, bands 2.1, 4.1, actin, glycophorin A, PAS staining bands 1–4 and desialylated PAS staining bands 1–4 did not (Kay, Wong and Bolton, 1982; Kay *et al.*, 1983; Kay, 1981c). In addition, rabbit antibodies to both purified band 3 and senescent cell antigen reacted with band

3 and its proteolytic products as determined by immunoautoradiography of RBC membranes, indicating that these molecules share common antigenic determinants not possessed by other RBC membrane components (Kay et al., 1983; Kay, 1981c).

Since senescent cell antigen and band 3 share antigenic determinants, the effect of cellular age on the accumulation of band 3 proteolytic products was investigated using the immunoblotting technique (Kay, 1984a, 1984b). Antibodies to band 3 and senescent cell antigen were used to determine the relative amount of band 3 breakdown products in the membranes of young, middle-aged, and old cells, by immunoautoradiography using gel overlay and immunoblotting procedures (Kay, 1984a, 1984b). Results revealed that antibodies both to band 3 and IgG eluted from senescent cells bind to a polypeptide migrating at $M_r \sim 62\,000$ in membranes of old but not young cells. IgG eluted from senescent cells did not bind to band 3 polypeptide $M_r \sim 40\,000$ to which antibodies to band 3 bound. These results indicated that band 3 breakdown products increase with cell age and that antigenic determinants recognized by IgG eluted from senescent cells reside on a $M_r \sim 62\,000$ fragment of band 3. The finding that senescent cell IgG does not bind to band 3 fragment $M_r \sim 40\,000$ suggests that this fragment may be a cytoplasmic segment that does not extend through the membrane and/or that it is a degradation product of the $M_r \sim 62\,000$ fragment representing the cytoplasmic portion.

EVIDENCE FOR THE ROLE OF OXIDATION IN THE GENERATION OF SENESCENT RED CELL ANTIGEN

We have postulated that generation of senescent cell antigen may result from oxidation-induced cross-linking followed by proteolysis (Kay, Wong and Bolton, 1982; Kay et al., 1983). As an approach to evaluating oxidation as a possible mechanism responsible for generation of senescent cell antigen, we studied RBCs from vitamin E-deficient rats (Kay et al., 1986). The importance of vitamin E as an antioxidant, providing protection against free radical-induced membrane damage, has been well documented (McCay and King, 1980; Menzel, 1980; Walton and Packer, 1980; Farrell et al., 1977). Vitamin E is primarily localized in cellular membranes, and a major role of vitamin E is the termination of free radical chain reactions propagated by the polyunsaturated fatty acids of membrane phospholipids. Vitamin E-deficient RBCs are defective in their ability to scavenge free radicals (Farrel et al., 1977; Dodge et al., 1967).

The RBC has many potential sources for generating free radicals. Hemoglobin is known to catalyze lipid peroxidation as well as enhance the decomposition of lipid hydroperoxides to the corresponding free radicals

(Chiu, Lubin and Shohet, 1982). Auto-oxidation of oxyhemoglobin results in the generation of a superoxide radical (Tapple, 1953; Koppenol and Butler, 1977). The reaction of a superoxide radical with peroxides in the RBCs produces highly reactive intermediates, such as the hydroxyl radical (OH·). These radicals in turn react with the lipid and protein components of the membrane, damaging its integrity and leading to eventual hemolysis of the cell (Chiu, Lubin and Shohet, 1982). Lipid peroxidation in the RBC membrane can result in accumulation of an aldehyde, which can cause a reduction in deformability (Pfafferott, Meiselman and Hochstein, 1982; Jain et al., 1983) and formation of irreversibly sickled cells (Jain and Shohet, 1984).

In humans, vitamin E deficiency shortens RBC lifespan, causing a compensated hemolytic anemia in patients with cystic fibrosis (Jain and Shohet, 1984). In newborns, vitamin E deficiency causes a hemolytic anemia that develops by 4–6 weeks of age (Oski, 1983).

Specific biochemical alterations in the membrane of RBCs from vitamin E-deficient rhesus monkeys have been described (Shapiro, Mott and Machlin, 1982a, 1982b). Furthermore, vitamin E deficiency represents a 'physiologic' method for rendering cells susceptible to free radical damage and may simulate conditions encountered *in situ*. In contrast, methods that have been used to induce oxidative damage *in vitro*, such as exposing cells to malondialdehyde, peroxide, etc., result in numerous pronounced membrane changes that are not observed in cells aged *in situ* (unpublished observations). We used vitamin E deficiency as a method for inducing oxidation of RBCs *in situ* so that we could determine the contribution of oxidation to RBC ageing.

The role of free radical damage in ageing has received a great deal of attention. It is interesting that there is a correlation between lifespan and natural antioxidant levels in a variety of species and that the level of such antioxidants appears to correlate with metabolic activity of individual species (Cutler, 1976). Evidence for free radical damage associated with ageing is the presence of lipofuscin and ceroid, so-called ageing pigments, which represent accumulated breakdown products of polyunsaturated fatty acids and proteins. It has been suggested that free radicals may be mediators of ageing and specific pathologies, such as inflammation, arthritis, adult respiratory distress syndrome, and other conditions (Autor, 1982; Packer, 1984). Free radicals have also been implicated as causative agents in mutagenesis and carcinogenesis as well as causing cross-linking of macromolecules and the formation of age pigments (Packer, 1984).

Clinical studies of vitamin E-deficient rats indicated accelerated destruction of RBCs and were consistent with the vitamin E-deficient rats having a compensated hemolytic anemia as is observed in vitamin E-deficient humans.

TABLE 2.2 Phagocytosis of unfractionated and age-separated RBCs from vitamin E-deficient and normal rats

Vitamin E diet	RBC fraction	Percentage phagocytosis
Normal (50 mg/kg)	Young	2 ± 3
	Middle-aged	1 ± 1
	Old	72 ± 3
	Unfractionated	13 ± 3
Deficient (0 mg/kg)	Young	89 ± 1
	Middle-aged	88 ± 1
	Old	99 ± 0
	Unfractionated	87 ± 1

The phagocytosis assay was performed with U937 cells. RBCs were incubated with macrophages overnight at 37°C in a humidified atmosphere containing 5% CO_2. Data are presented as the mean ± 1 SD, $n = 3$. Diet is expressed as mg of vitamin E per kg of diet. From Kay et al. (1986).

The phagocytosis assay was performed on both age-separated and unseparated RBCs from rats fed a diet containing normal amounts of vitamin E or a diet deficient in vitamin E (Table 2.2). Old RBCs obtained from rats fed a diet containing normal amounts of vitamin E were phagocytized, whereas young and middle-aged RBCs were not. In contrast, young and middle-aged as well as old RBCs were phagocytized when obtained from vitamin E-deficient rats. There was a significant difference in phagocytosis between RBCs obtained from normal rats and vitamin E-deficient rats, even when unfractionated RBCs were used for the assay (Table 2.2).

We suspected that anion transport might be altered with cellular ageing because our previous studies had indicated that senescent cell antigen is derived from band 3 by cleavage in the transmembrane anion-transport region (Kay, Wong and Bolton, 1982; Kay et al., 1983; Kay, 1982, 1984a, 1984b). If this suspicion proved to be correct, then we would have a functional assay for ageing of band 3, the major anion transport protein of the RBC membrane.

Transport studies on age-separated rat RBCs indicated that anion transport decreased with age (Table 2.3). The kinetic Michaelis constant (K_m) increased and the maximal velocity (V_{max}) decreased in old RBCs as compared to middle-aged RBCs.

These data provided us with an assay of cellular function to use to determine whether RBCs from vitamin E-deficient rats exhibited characteristics of old RBCs prematurely. Results of the anion-transport studies on RBCs from vitamin E-deficient rats revealed that their anion transport was impaired, as was transport in old RBCs (Table 2.3).

TABLE 2.3 Effect of cellular aging and vitamin E deficiency on anion transport system of rat RBCs

	K_m (mM)	V_{max} (mol $\times$ 10^{-8} per 10^8 cells per min)
Cell age		
Middle-aged	0.5 ± 0.2	41.8 ± 1.9
Old	1.6 ± 0.4*	17.3 ± 3.8*
Vitamin E diet		
Normal	0.7 ± 0.1	41.2 ± 3.7
Deficient	2.0 ± 0.3*	16.2 ± 2.0*
Deficient + vitamin E	2.0 ± 0.3*	12.1 ± 1.7*

Results are presented as the mean ± 1 SD. There is no statistical difference between deficient, deficient + vitamin E, and old cells. K_m, concentration at half-maximal exchange, corresponding to an apparent Michaelis–Menten constant (in mM); V_{max}, maximal flux, determined at 37°C and pH 7.2.
*$P \leq 0.01$. From Kay et al. (1986).

Differences were not detected in protein or glycoprotein composition of RBC membranes from control and vitamin E-deficient rats. Although high molecular weight polypeptides or polymers were detected with Coomassie blue staining of 2–16% polyacrylamide gels, there were no differences in the number or amount of these polypeptides between control and experimental samples. Immunoblotting studies revealed increased breakdown products of band 3 in cells from vitamin E-deficient rats. Thus, vitamin E deficiency leads to accelerated RBC ageing, presumably through oxidation. As a mechanism for cellular ageing and generation of senescent cell antigen, free radical reactions and oxidation are considered probable candidates (Kay, Wong and Bolton, 1982). Most free radical reactions involve the reduction of molecular oxygen, leading to the formation of highly reactive oxygen species such as superoxide anion (O_2^-), hydroxyl radical (OH·), hydrogen peroxide (H_2O_2), and singlet oxygen (O_2^*). The production of these highly reactive oxygen species as metabolic intermediates appears to be an evolutionary consequence of aerobic existence because the spin state of oxygen favors univalent pathways of reduction (Fridovich, 1975).

We used vitamin E deficiency as a model for studying oxidation because studies show that, in mammals, vitamin E functions as an antioxidant, and because vitamin E deficiency simulates conditions encountered *in situ* more closely than does chemical treatment of cells *in vitro*.

The results presented here indicate that vitamin E deficiency causes premature ageing of RBCs and IgG binding. RBCs from vitamin E-deficient rats behave like old RBCs in the phagocytosis assay, and in anion transport and glyceraldehyde 3-phosphate dehydrogenase activity. In addition, increased breakdown products of band 3 were observed in RBC membranes from vitamin E-deficient rats. We have not observed high molecular weight complexes containing band 3 in membranes from vitamin E-deficient rats or old cells aged *in situ*, except under conditions that precipitate IgG (unpublished observations). Similar results were obtained with RBCs from copper-deficient chickens (Bosman, Harris and Kay, unpublished). This suggests that any oxidative system may cause premature RBC ageing.

CONCLUDING REMARKS

Investigations into the mechanisms(s) responsible for the removal of RBCs indicate that a physiologic IgG autoantibody attaches to senescent cells, initiating their removal by macrophages. Since this mechanism is responsible for the removal of senescent cells in a number of species, including mice, rats, rabbits, cows and chickens, it appears that the immunologic mechanism for removing senescent and damaged cells may be a general physiologic process for removing cells programmed for death in vertebrates.

Senescent cell IgG autoantibody recognizes a 'neo-antigen' called 'senescent cell antigen', that appears on old cells. This antigen appears to be derived from band 3, the major anion-transport protein of RBCs. Band 3 appears to undergo degradation as RBCs age, leading to generation of senescent cell antigen. Oxidation appears to be a mechanism leading to degradation of band 3 and appearance of senescent cell antigen. Future studies are expected to focus on clinical conditions caused by either premature or delayed appearance of senescent cell antigen.

REFERENCES

Alderman, E. M., Fudenberg, H. H., and Lovins, R. E. (1980). Binding of immunoglobulin classes to subpopulations of human red blood cells separated by density-gradient centrifugation, *Blood*, **55**, 817–22.

Autor, A. P. (1982). *Pathology of Oxygen*, Academic Press, New York.

Bartosz, G., Sosynski, M., and Kedziona, J. (1982). Aging of the erythrocyte, VI. Accelerated red cell membrane aging in Down's syndrome? *Cell. Biol. Int. Rep.*, **6**, 73–7.

Bartosz, G., Sosynski, M., and Wasilewski, A. (1982). Aging of the erythrocyte, XVII. Binding of autologous immunoglobulin, *Mech. Ageing Dev.*, **20**, 223–32.

Bennet, G., and Kay, M. M. B. (1981). Homeostatic removal of senescent murine erythrocytes by splenic macrophages, *Exp. Hematol.*, **9**, 295.

Chiu, D., Lubin, B., and Shohet, S. B. (1982). Peroxidative reactions in red cell biology. In W. A. Pryor (ed.) *Free Radicals in Biology*, Vol. 5, pp. 115–60, Academic Press, New York.

Cutler, R. G. (1976). Nature of aging and life maintenance processes, *Interdiscip. Top. Gerontol.*, **9**, 83–133.
Dodge, J. T., Cohen, G., Kayden, H. J., and Phillips, G. B. (1967). Peroxidative hemolysis of red blood cells from patients with abetalipoproteinemia, *J. Clin. Invest.*, **46**, 357–68.
Farrell, P., Bieri, J. G., Fratantoni, J. F., Wood, R. E., and Disant'Agree, P. A. (1977). The occurrence and effects of human vitamin E deficiency, *J. Clin. Invest.*, **60**, 233–41.
Fridovich, I. (1975). Superoxide dismutase, *Nutr. Rev. Biochem.*, **44**, 147–59.
Galili, U., Korkesh, A., Kahane, I., and Rachmilewitz, E. A. (1983). Demonstration of a natural antigalactosyl IgG antibody on thalassemic red blood cells, *Blood*, **61**, 1258–64.
Glass, G. A., and Gershon, H. (1985). Some characteristics of the human erythrocyte as a function of donor and cell age, *Exp. Hematol.*, **13**, 1122–6.
Glass, G. A., Gershon, H., and Gershon, D. (1983). The effect of donor and cell age on several characteristics of rat erythrocytes, *Exp. Hematol.*, **11**, 987–95.
Halhuber, K. T., Stibenz, D., Feuerstein, H. et al. (1980). *9th International Symposium on the Structure and Function of Erythroid Cells*, Berlin, GDF. Abstracts, 66.
Halliwell, B., and Gutteridge, J. M. C. (1986). Iron and free radical reactions: two aspects of antioxidant protection, *Trends Biochem. Sci.*, **11**, 372–5.
Hebbel, R. P., and Miller, W. J. (1984). Phagocytosis of sickle erythrocytes: immunologic and oxidative determinants of hemolytic anemia, *Blood*, **64**, 733–41.
Jain, S. K., and Shohet, S. B. (1984). A novel phospholipid in irreversibly sickled cells: Evidence for *in vivo* peroxidative membrane damage in sickle cell disease, *Blood*, **63**, 326–67.
Jain, S. K., Mohandas, N., Clark, M. R., and Shohet, S. B. (1983). The effect of malonyldialdehyde, a product of lipid peroxidation, on the deformability, dehydration and ^{51}Cr survival of erythrocytes, *Br. J. Haematol.*, **53**, 247–55.
Jenkin, C. R., and Karthigasu, K. (1967). Elimination hepatique des erythrocytes agés et alterés chez le rat, *C. R. Soc. Biol.*, **161**, 1006–7.
Kay, M. M. B. (1974). Mechanisms of macrophage recognition of senescent red cells, *Gerontologist*, **14**, 33.
Kay, M. M. B. (1975). Mechanism of removal of senescent cells by human macrophages *in situ*, *Proc. Natl Acad. Sci. USA*, **72**, 3521–5.
Kay, M. M. B. (1977). High resolution scanning electron microscopy and its application to research on immunity and aging. In Makinodan, T. (ed.) *Immunity and Aging*, pp. 135–50, Plenum Press, New York.
Kay, M. M. B. (1978a). Multiple labeling technique for scanning electron microscopy. In M. A. Hayat (ed.) *Principles and Techniques of Scanning Electron Microscopy*, pp. 338–57, Van Nostrand-Reinhold, New York.
Kay, M. M. B. (1978b). Role of physiological autoantibody in the removal of senescent human red cells, *J. Supramol. Struct.*, **9**, 555.
Kay, M. M. B. (1981a) Isolation of the phagocytosis inducing IgG-binding antigen on senescent somatic cells, *Nature*, **289**, 491–4.
Kay, M. M. B. (1981b). The IgG autoantibody binding determinant appearing on senescent cells resides on a 62,000 MW peptide, *Acta Biol. Medica Germ.*, **40**, 385–91.
Kay, M. M. B. (1981c). The senescent cell antigen is not a desialylated glycoprotein, *Blood*, **58**, 90a.
Kay, M. M. B. (1982). Accumulation of band 3 breakdown products is a function of cell age, *Blood*, **60**, 21 (abstract).

Kay, M. M. B. (1984a). Band 3, the predominant transmembrane polypeptide, undergoes proteolytic degradation as cells age, *Monogr. Dev. Biol.*, **17**, 245-53.

Kay, M. M. B. (1984b). Localization of senescent cell antigen on band 3, *Proc. Natl Acad. Sci. USA*, **81**, 5753-7.

Kay, M. M. B., Wong, P., and Bolton, P. (1982). Antigenicity, storage and aging: Physiologic autoantibodies to cell membrane and serum proteins, *Mol. Cell. Biochem.*, **49**, 65-85.

Kay, M. M. B., Goodman, S., Sorensen, K., Whitfield, C., Wong, P., Zaki, L., and Rudoloff, V. (1983). The senescent cell antigen is immunologically related to band 3, *Proc. Natl Acad. Sci. USA*, **80**, 1631-5.

Kay, M. M. B., Bosman, G. J. C. G. M., Shapiro, S. S., Bendich, A., and Bassel, P. S. (1986). Oxidation as a possible mechanism of cellular aging: Vitamin E deficiency causes premature aging and IgG binding to erythrocytes, *Proc. Natl Acad. Sci. USA*, **83**, 2463-7.

Khansari, N., and Fudenberg, H. H. (1984). Phagocytosis of senescent erythrocytes by autologous monocytes: Requirement of membrane-specific autologous IgG for immune elimination of aging red blood cells, *Cell. Immunol.*, **78**, 114-21.

Khansari, N., Springer, G. F., Merler, E., and Fudenberg, H. H.(1983). Mechanisms for the removal of senescent human erythrocytes from circulation: Specificity of the membrane-bound immunoglobulin G, *Mech. Ageing Dev.*, **21**, 49-58.

Koppenol, W. H., and Butler, J. (1977). Mechanism of reactions involving singlet oxygen and the superoxide anion, *FEBS Lett.*, **83**, 1-6.

McCay, P. B., and King, M. M. (1980). In L. J. Machlin (ed.) *Vitamin E: a Comprehensive Treatise*, pp. 289-317, Dekker, New York.

Menzel, D. B. (1980). In L. J. Machlin (ed) *Vitamin E: a Comprehensive Treatise*, pp. 473-494, Dekker, New York.

Nelson, D. S. (1969). Macrophages in auto-immunity, the disposal of effete cells and chronic inflammation. In D. S. Nelson (ed.) *Macrophages and Immunity*, pp. 247-268. North-Holland, Amsterdam.

Oski, F. A. (1983). Anemia related to nutritional deficiencies other than vitamin B_{12} and folic acid. In Williams (ed.) *Hematology*, pp. 532-7, McGraw-Hill, New York.

Packer, L. (1984). Vitamin E, physical exercise and tissue damage in animals, *Med. Biol.*, **62**, 105-9.

Petz, L. D., Yam, P., Wilkinson, L., Garratty, G., Lubin, B., and Mentzer, W. (1984). Increased IgG molecules bound to the surface of red blood cells of patients with sickle cell anemia, *Blood*, **64**, 301-4.

Pfafferott, C., Meiselman, H. J., and Hochstein, P. (1982). The effect of malonyldialdehyde on erythrocyte deformability, *Blood*, **59**, 12-15.

Shapiro, S. S., Mott, D. J., and Machlin, L. J. (1982a). Alterations of enzymes in red blood cell membranes in vitamin E deficiency, *Ann. N. Y. Acad. Sci.*, **393**, 263-76.

Shapiro, S. S., Mott, D. J., and Machlin, L. J. (1982b). Altered binding of glyceraldehyde-3-phosphate dehydrogenase to its binding site in vitamin E-deficient red blood cells, *Nutr. Rep. Int.*, **25**, 507-17.

Singer, J. A., Jennings, L. K., Jackson, C. W., Dockter, M. E., Morrison, M., and Walker, W. S. (1986). Erythrocyte homeostasis: Antibody-mediated recognition of the senescent state by macrophages, *Proc. Natl Acad. Sci. USA*, **83**, 5498-501.

Smalley, C. E., and Tucker, E. M. (1983). Blood group A antigen site distribution and immunoglobulin binding in relation to red cell age, *Br. J. Heamatol.*, **54**, 209-19.

Smith, F. (1958). Erythrophagocytosis in human lymph-glands, *J. Path. Bact.*, **78**, 383-92.

Tannert, C. H. (1978). Untersuchungen zum altern roter blutzellen. Ph.D. Dissertation, Humbolt University, Berlin, GDR.
Tapple, A. L. (1953). The mechanism of oxidation of unsaturated fatty acids catalyzed by hematin compounds, *Arch. Biochem. Biophys.*, **44**, 378–95.
Vomel, T. H., and Platt, D. (1981). Phagocytic activity of reticulohistiocyte system in rabbits after splenectomy and activation with ink, *Mech. Ageing Dev.*, **17**, 267–73.
Walford, R. L. (1980). Immunology and aging. *Am. J. Clin. Pathol.*, **74**, 147–53.
Walker, W. S., Singer, J. A., Morrison, M., and Jackson, C. W. (1984). Preferential phagocytosis of *in vivo* aged murine red blood cells by a macrophage-like cell line, *Br. J. Haematol.*, **58**, 259–66.
Walton, J. R., and Packer, L. (1980). In L. J. Machlin (ed.) *Vitamin E: A Comprehensive Treatise*, pp. 495–518, Dekker, New York.
Wegner, G., Tannert, C. H., Maretzki, D., Schossler, W., and Strauss, D. (1980). IXth International Symposium on the Structure and Function of Erythroid Cells, Berlin, GDR. Abstracts, 57.
Weinberg, E. D. (1974). Iron and susceptibility to infectious disease, *Science*, **148**, 952–6.

Iron in Immunity, Cancer and Inflammation
Edited by M. de Sousa and J. H. Brock
© 1989 John Wiley & Sons Ltd.

3
The Biology of Iron

J. H. Brock
University Department of Bacteriology and Immunology, Western Infirmary, Glasgow G11 6NT, Scotland

Iron is the most abundant transition metal in living organisms. The characteristic chemistry of this element has endowed it with a series of properties which make it uniquely able to fulfil certain biological reactions, particularly those involving redox mechanisms. As a result iron is essential to almost all forms of life. However, these properties may, if uncontrolled, give rise to harmful oxidation or free radical reactions. Consequently, evolution has ensured that iron normally remains bound to carrier molecules such as haem or proteins, which prevent these undesirable reactions while allowing the biologically useful features of the chemistry of iron to be exploited.

The aim of this chapter is to provide a background to the more specialized topics dealt with in subsequent chapters. It is not intended to provide exhaustive treatment of the chemistry and biology of iron, which would itself require a whole book. Nor is it intended to give equal emphasis to all aspects, but to concentrate on those areas of iron metabolism which are of most relevance to the lymphomyeloid system, immunological function, and cancer. For a more general coverage of iron metabolism the reader is referred to Jacobs and Worwood (1980).

CHEMISTRY OF IRON

This section will briefly mention those aspects of the chemistry of iron which are important for its function in biological systems. Iron is in group VII of the periodic table and two main valence states occur, the divalent ferrous form and the trivalent ferric form. Both form salts with common anions, but ferrous salts, although quite stable in the solid state, are oxidized to the ferric form in solution in the presence of oxygen. Likewise, ferric salts are stable as solids, and in strongly acidic solutions, but at pH values approaching neutral they are rapidly hydrolysed to insoluble polymeric hydroxides, so that at neutral pH the equilibrium concentration of free Fe^{3+} is only about 10^{-18} M (Spiro, 1977). It is thus evident that under physiological conditions, neither Fe^{2+} nor Fe^{3+} are likely to exist as free ions in solution in significant amounts. Indeed, it would be harmful if the situation were otherwise, because ionic iron, or iron atoms whose co-ordination sites are not all occupied by an appropriate electron donor, are capable of mediating a univalent reduction of oxygen, giving rise to unstable intermediates with unpaired electrons. Such intermediates, if capable of independent existence, are known as free radicals and are extremely reactive. Under controlled conditions their existence may be beneficial, e.g. in the intralysosomal killing of bacteria in phagocytic cells, but in other situations they can cause host damage. This is particularly likely to occur when abnormal levels of iron build up, either locally during inflammation (see Chapters 6 and 7), or as a generalized condition in iron overload (see Chapter 11). The mechanisms and significance of free radical formation are dealt with in more detail in those chapters, and are reviewed in detail by Halliwell and Gutteridge (1985, 1986).

The ability of iron to form co-ordination compounds is responsible for its binding to many organic molecules. In most of these the iron atom forms an octahedral complex. The groups to which iron can co-ordinate include amino acid side-chains, as in transferrins, and pyrrole groups in haem compounds. One or more of the co-ordination sites may be linked to water molecules, or to molecular oxygen, the latter being of critical importance for the oxygen-transporting property of haemoglobin.

Co-ordination may also occur to small molecules, giving rise to iron chelates. These chelates, which normally involve Fe^{3+}, may be of moderate affinity, such as those with citrate or nitrilotriacetate, or of high affinity, such as those with desferrioxamine or enterochelin. The former group probably do not occur *in vivo*, though they provide useful sources of soluble unpolymerized Fe^{3+} for experimental work. The latter group are synthesized by micro-organisms for the purpose of scavenging iron (see p. 48). These compounds, and synthetic analogues, have found clinical use in iron overload and may be of use in inflammation (Chapter 17).

IRON-BINDING PROTEINS

Iron transport proteins: the transferrins

The transferrins are a group of closely related proteins found in all vertebrates, and related proteins are also found in insects and their allies.

The structure and molecular biology of these proteins is dealt with in Chapter 4, so this discussion will centre on their iron-binding properties and their physiological function. Several comprehensive reviews of the transferrins have been published (Morgan, 1981; Brock, 1985; Huebers and Finch, 1987). Transferrin itself (sometimes called serotransferrin, and formerly known as siderophilin) is a serum protein, and is the most widely studied member of the group. A variant differing only in the composition of the glycan chains occurs in avian egg white (ovotransferrin or conalbumin) and in the milk (and perhaps other secretions) of some mammals. In many mammals, however, milk contains little or no transferrin, but instead a distinct, albeit closely related, protein called lactoferrin (or sometimes lactotransferrin) is present. This protein also occurs in other external secretions, and in the secondary granules of neutrophils. Finally there are three more recently discovered members of this group of proteins known as melanotransferrin, the *Blym*-1 proteins and uteroferrin.

Transferrin

The existence of a non-haem iron-binding protein in plasma was first described at the end of the last century (Häuserman, 1899), and transferrin was first isolated and characterized by Laurell and Ingleman (1947). All mammalian transferrins so far characterized are single-chain glycoproteins of molecular weight 75 000–80 000, and the polypeptide chain is folded to give two globular domains, each of which contains a specific binding site for a single Fe^{3+} (Williams, 1982; Bailey et al., 1988). It is possible to proteolytically cleave some transferrins into single-domain half-molecules, suggesting that a bridging region analogous to the hinge region of immunoglobulins is present (Williams, 1982; Brock, 1985). The transferrins are glycosylated, but the number and composition of the glycan chain(s) varies among different species. Furthermore, heterogeneity in the degree of branching and number of sialic acid residues is found among transferrin molecules within each species (Hatton et al., 1979). There is some evidence that in man the degree of sialylation is related to certain disease states; in particular, a variant with abnormally low numbers of sialic acid residues is found in the serum of chronic alcoholics and may be a useful diagnostic marker (Stibler, Borg and Allgulander, 1979).

Binding of iron by transferrin requires the concomitant binding of a synergistic anion. Under *in vivo* conditions this is normally carbonate or bicarbonate, but a large number of other anions, mostly α-hydroxy carboxylic acids, can substitute for bicarbonate *in vitro* (Schlabach and Bates, 1975). The nature of the residues involved in the iron-binding site has been the subject of much research over the past two decades using chemical modification and related methods, and this has led to the conclusion that the iron atom was co-ordinated to two histidines, two tyrosines, a water molecule and the (bi)carbonate anion, which also binds to an arginine or tyrosine residue in the polypeptide chain (Chasteen, 1983). However, more recently a crystallographic study of lactoferrin at 3.2 Å resolution by Anderson *et al.* (1987) and a similar study on rabbit transferrin by Bailey *et al.* (1988), shows that only one histidine is involved, the other co-ordination site being an aspartic acid residue. Interestingly, in a rare variant of human transferrin which binds iron only poorly at the site in the C-terminal domain, a glycine residue at position 392 is replaced by an arginine which is thought to interact with the critical aspartic acid residue at position 394 (Evans *et al.*, 1988).

The binding of iron by transferrin results in the formation of a red-brown complex. Under physiological conditions the iron is bound with high affinity but this decreases rapidly as the pH is lowered, so that at pH 5 iron will be removed by relatively low-affinity chelating agents such as citrate. This feature plays an important role in the mechanism of cellular uptake of transferrin-bound iron (see p. 42). Since the two domains of the transferrin molecule are not identical, differences in the iron-binding properties of the two sites might be expected, and slight spectral differences (Brock and Arzabe, 1976), as well as differences in affinity and the effect of pH, are known to exist (Lestas, 1976). Over 20 years ago Fletcher and Huehns (1968) proposed that the two sites might have different functional properties, but despite intense investigation over the next 15 years no clear evidence for such a functional difference was unequivocally shown. Nevertheless, the undoubted chemical differences between the sites suggest that some as yet undiscovered functional difference might exist.

The main function of transferrin is the transport of iron from sites of absorption, and erythrocyte catabolism and storage, to iron-requiring cells and tissues, principally erythroid precursors in the bone marrow. Cellular acquisition of transferrin-bound iron occurs by a process of receptor-mediated endocytosis, described in detail on p. 42. Some transferrin-bound iron is delivered to hepatocytes, the main iron-storage cells, which incorporate the metal into ferritin (Young and Aisen, 1981). This iron may later be released for metabolic activity, though the factors controlling release are not well understood. A third category of cells acquiring iron from transferrin consists of actively proliferating cells such as fibroblasts, endothelial cells and activated lymphocytes. Delivery of iron is essential for proliferation, probably because of the involvement of the iron-containing enzyme ribonucleotide reductase in DNA synthesis (see Chapter 12). There have been suggestions that transferrin may play additional roles in cell proliferation independent of iron delivery, and this is dealt with in Chapter 12.

The delivery of iron to transferrin has been much less studied than the uptake of transferrin-bound iron. In general, it is thought that transferrin acts as a passive recipient of iron released by cells and tissues, the control of which is regulated intracellularly. A report that macrophages possess receptors which preferentially bind apotransferrin has not been confirmed (see Chapter 5), and transferrin saturation does not appear to directly influence the rate of return of iron to the circulation (Fillet, Cook and Finch, 1974).

Lactoferrin

Lactoferrin closely resembles transferrin in its molecular weight, three-dimensional structure and iron-binding properties, and its structure has recently been elucidated in crystallographic studies (Anderson *et al.*, 1987) (see Chapter 4). Human lactoferrin exhibits a 59% sequence homology with human transferrin (Metz-Boutigue *et al.*, 1984). Its physicochemical properties differ from those of transferrin in three important respects. Firstly, the distribution and composition of the two glycan chains differ, those of lactoferrin being distributed one on each domain (Spik *et al.*, 1982), whereas both the transferrin glycan chains are bound to the C-terminal domain (this applies to the human proteins: the situation in other species may be different). The lactoferrin glycans also contain terminal fucose residues, absent from transferrin. Secondly, lactoferrin has an unusually high isoelectric point, the p*I* being 8.0 or more (see Brock, 1985), compared with about 5.9 for transferrin. Perhaps because of its high p*I*, lactoferrin shows a marked tendency to bind non-covalently to a wide range of molecules, and the possible significance of this is discussed in Chapter 5.

The third difference between lactoferrin and transferrin lies in the iron-binding properties. The affinity of lactoferrin for Fe^{3+} is somewhat higher than that of transferrin, and results in lactoferrin being able to retain its iron in the presence of chelators such as citrate down to pH 4 or lower (Masson and Heremans, 1968). This may be important in assessing the function of lactoferrin.

The function of lactoferrin is less well defined than that of transferrin. In particular, there is no clear evidence of an iron-transport role. Originally its major function was thought to be as a bacteriostatic agent in the gut and other secretory surfaces (see p. 48). It has also been proposed that lactoferrin mediates transfer of iron into mucosal cells (Lönnerdal, 1985), but evidence that lactoferrin enhances iron absorption is not convincing, and some reports suggest an inhibitory effect (Brock, 1980). Lactoferrin may enhance cell proliferation (Amouric *et al.*, 1984), but this does not appear to be due to iron donation (Oria *et al.*, 1988). A further proposal postulates a role for lactoferrin in the hypoferraemia of inflammation. As discussed in Chapter 6, this is not proven, and controversy also surrounds its proposed role in myelopoiesis (discussed in Chapters 9 and 10).

Uteroferrin, the Blym-1 proteins and melanotransferrin

Uteroferrin is an iron-containing protein found in the amniotic fluid of ungulates, which appears to function both as an alkaline phosphatase and as an iron-transport protein for the transfer of iron from mother to fetus (Buhi *et al.*, 1982). Its structural relationship to other transferrins is unclear, and no human analogue has yet been characterised.

The *Blym*-1 proteins have not been identified as such but are the predicted products of genes isolated from chicken (Goubin *et al.*, 1983) and human (Diamond, Devine and Cooper, 1984) lymphomas. They show homology with the N-terminal sequences of other transferrins, but are only about one-tenth of the size.

Melanotransferrin is the name recently given to the melanoma-associated p97 cell-surface antigen which shows sequence homology with transferrin and probably binds iron (Brown *et al.*, 1982). Its function is unknown.

Iron storage: ferritin and haemosiderin

Whereas transferrin is primarily an extracellular protein whose main function is iron transport, ferritin is essentially an intracellular protein, and is concerned with iron storage and detoxification. For reviews of ferritin see Theil (1987) and Drysdale (1988).

The structure of ferritin, which is described in detail in Chapter 4, is that of a hollow sphere composed of 24 subunits, each of approximately 20 000 molecular weight. Within the hollow protein shell, iron can accumulate in the form of a polymeric iron hydroxide, to which some phosphate groups may also be attached. The interior is about 70–80 Å in diameter, which allows for up to about 4500 iron atoms to be accommodated, though about half this number are normally present. Thus ferritin has a very high iron-binding capacity, and the protein serves to limit the degree of iron hydroxide polymerization to a size at which the polymer remains soluble. Considerable study has been made of the way in which iron enters and leaves the interior of the molecule (Rice *et al.*, 1983). For iron to enter the ferritin molecule it must initially be in the ferrous form. The arrangement of the subunits leaves a number of channels 3–4 Å wide through which ferrous ions may be able to pass, aided by amino acid side-chains at the surface of these channels. Once in the interior the iron is oxidized to the ferric form by the catalytic action of amino acid side-chains, and polymerizes. However, once the iron core has begun to be formed, the core itself plays the major role in oxidizing incoming ferrous ions. Release of iron *in vitro* requires the presence of reducing and/or chelating agents, and is enhanced at low pH. The last iron atoms to enter the molecule are those most readily liberated, suggesting that the atoms at the surface of the polymeric core are the most labile (Treffry and Harrison, 1984). Thus the apoferritin core not only serves to limit the size of the polynuclear iron hydroxide core, but also plays an active role in transporting and allowing oxidation of the metal.

The degree of iron loading can affect the electrophoretic properties of ferritin and give rise to heterogeneity. However, of far more significance has been the heterogeneity resulting from the existence of two distinct subunits (Arosio, Adelman and Drysdale, 1978). The heavy (H) and light (L) subunits differ not only in their molecular weights (21 099 versus 19 766 respectively for the human proteins; see also Chapter 4), but also in their tissue distribution; the H subunit is particularly prevalent in Heart and the L in Liver. However, the H subunit tends to also predominate in cells of the lymphomyeloid system, other than macrophages involved in iron storage. Furthermore, recent work on ferritin gene structure suggests that the two-subunit model may be an oversimplification (Theil, 1987).

Ferritin is present in all types of mammalian cells so far studied, though the amount varies considerably, being greatest in cells such as macrophages and hepatocytes that are involved in iron storage. It may be present both in the cytoplasm and in lysosomes. In the latter case degradation may occur, and this gives rise to haemosiderin, particularly if ferritin is iron-loaded (Richter, 1984). Haemosiderin is a heterogeneous compound consisting essentially of insoluble polymerized ferric hydroxide containing variable amounts of phosphate and protein. The latter is thought to consist of ferritin degradation products (Weir, Gibson and Peters, 1984). Removal of iron from haemosiderin occurs more slowly than from ferritin, and the compound is generally considered to be a relatively inactive form of storage iron (O'Connell *et al.*, 1986a, 1986b). It is haemosiderin that is responsible for the strong staining with Perl's reagent seen when iron-overloaded tissues are examined.

It has generally been considered that the main function of ferritin is to store iron not immediately required for metabolic activity and release it to metabolic iron pools when required. It is well known that cells and tissues, when loaded with iron, incorporate the metal into ferritin, the synthesis of which is itself stimulated by iron (see Chapter 4). Theil (1987) has suggested that three functionally distinct types of ferritin exist: 'housekeeping' ferritin for subsequent use by the cell itself, specialized iron-storage ferritin in those cells such as macrophages and Kupffer cells which release iron for use elsewhere, and stress ferritin, for detoxifying abnormal amounts of iron entering the cell. However, it is not yet possible to relate this proposal to the actual types of ferritin observed in different cells. Furthermore, although release of iron from ferritin can be achieved *in vitro* by the use of suitable chelators and/or reducing agents, there is little evidence for any controlled release of iron from ferritin within cells or tissues (Crichton, 1984). This tends to argue against the idea that release of iron from ferritin is directly regulated by the metabolic needs of the particular cell or tissue concerned. Increasing attention is therefore being paid to the importance of ferritin in detoxification of excess intracellular iron (Joshi and Zimmerman, 1988).

It should also be noted that, while iron is the traditional stimulus for ferritin synthesis (see Chapter 4), increased synthesis also occurs during inflammation (see Chapter 6) and during cell differentiation (Fibach, Konijn and Rachmilewitz, 1985). The underlying control mechanisms in these situations are unknown.

While ferritin is essentially an intracellular protein, small amounts also occur in serum. This has received much attention over the past decade because serum ferritin levels can often be used as a clinical indicator of iron status (Worwood, 1986). Some of the serum ferritin molecules in man are glycosylated, suggesting that a specific secreted form of ferritin exists. The origin of serum ferritin is discussed in Chapter 5. As far as is known, serum ferritin plays no major role in iron recirculation, though the more acidic serum ferritin molecules may regulate myelopoiesis (see Chapter 9). Ferritin is also found in small amounts in milk (Arosio, Adelman and Drysdale, 1984), though again its function here is unknown.

Cellular iron uptake—the transferrin receptor cycle

The fact that transferrin binds iron with extremely high affinity, yet is able to release the metal upon interaction with iron-requiring cells, has excited the interests of a growing number of research workers over the past 15 years. The problem was first seriously addressed by Speyer and Fielding (1974), who demonstrated that transferrin was bound to reticulocyte membranes and that the iron/transferrin ratio increased with incubation time. However, studies by a number of groups over the next few years, almost all of whom worked with reticulocytes, failed to conclusively identify a transferrin receptor, and led to conflicting opinions as to whether iron release from transferrin occurred at the cell membrane or required internalization. The subsequent demonstration of receptor-mediated binding of transferrin on non-erythroid cell lines opened the way for studies using more homogeneous cell populations, and led to the molecular characterization of the transferrin receptor (Sutherland *et al.*, 1981). This consists of a transmembrane molecule of approximately 180 000 molecular weight, composed of two identical subunits. The structure of the transferrin receptor and the way in which its expression is controlled are described in Chapter

4, and this discussion will therefore be concerned with the way in which it enables transferrin-bound iron to be delivered to cells. Detailed reviews of the function and structure of the transferrin receptor have been published (May and Cuatrecasas, 1985; Dautry-Varsat, 1986; Hunt, 1986; Huebers and Finch, 1987).

It is now known that the uptake of iron from transferrin occurs by a rather special type of receptor-mediated endocytosis. The initial event is the binding of transferrin to the extracellular portion of the receptor. One transferrin molecule can bind to each subunit of the receptor. At physiological pH the affinity of the receptor for transferrin depends upon the degree of iron binding; the affinity constants are approximately 1.1×10^8 M^{-1} for diferric transferrin, 2.6×10^7 M^{-1} for monoferric, and 4.6×10^{-6} M^{-1} for apotransferrin (Young, Bomford and Williams, 1984). Thus under normal circumstances only iron-containing transferrin molecules will be bound, though this may not be true in iron deficiency when transferrin saturation is reduced.

The receptor–transferrin complexes are then clustered together and eventually localize in clathrin-coated pits, which eventually bud off to form coated vesicles. It is probable that this process occurs independently of whether transferrin is bound to the receptor (Watts, 1985), though contrary findings have been reported (Klausner, Harford and van Renswoude, 1984). There is also controversy over whether phosphorylation is required for internalization, the evidence against (Zerial et al., 1987; Davis and Meisner, 1987) being somewhat more convincing than the evidence in favour (May and Tyler, 1987), although the situation may vary among different cells. The vesicles lose their clathrin coat and fuse to form an endosome or 'compartment of uncoupling of receptor from ligand' (CURL), in which the intravesicular pH is lowered to about 4.8 by means of a proton pump. As a result, iron is released from transferrin. Unusually, however, the interaction between transferrin and its receptor is strengthened rather than lost as a result of the pH change. The receptor–transferrin complexes are segregated into a small dumb-bell shaped vesicle which buds off from the main portion of the endosome, which contains the iron. The vesicle containing the receptor–transferrin complex passes through the Golgi, at which point its pathway intersects with that of newly synthesized receptors, and is then returned to the cell membrane, with which it fuses. However, as the receptor–transferrin complexes are now exposed to physiological pH, the recycled transferrin molecules, which have lost their iron, are displaced by new iron-containing transferrin molecules from the extracellular fluid, and the process is repeated. The transferrin cycle is shown in Figure 3.1.

Although the main features of the transferrin cycle are now well established, a number of important areas await clarification. It is still not known

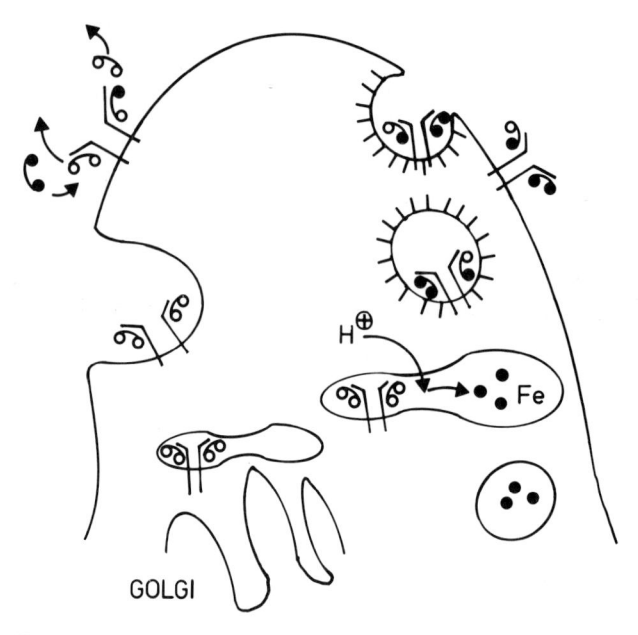

Figure 3.1 Receptor-mediated endocytosis of transferrin. Transferrin, containing one or two atoms of iron (right), enters clathrin-coated pits and these then form coated vesicles. These vesicles are converted to an endosome, where a proton pump causes acidification and loss of iron from transferrin. The receptor–apotransferrin complex segregates into a dumb-bell-shaped vesicle which passes through the Golgi and is finally exocytosed. The apotransferrin is then displaced by fresh iron-containing transferrin molecules

which structural features of the transferrin molecule are involved in the interaction with the receptor, although the failure of individual transferrin half-molecules to act as iron donors (Esparza and Brock, 1980; Brown-Mason and Woodworth, 1984) suggests that an inter-domain region may be involved. It is also far from clear how iron moves from the endosome to its final destination, such as the mitochondria or ferritin. Finally, there continues to be some evidence that internalization of transferrin may not always be essential for iron delivery to cells (Nuñez and Glass, 1983).

Other iron-containing proteins

Haemoglobin and myoglobin

The biology and chemistry of haemoglobin and myoglobin have been extensively studied, and the fundamental role of haemoglobin in oxygen transport is one of the cornerstones of mammalian biochemistry. Extensive reviews of haemoglobin structure and function are available (Antonini, Rossi-Bernardi and Chiancone, 1981; Dickerson and Geis, 1983) and because these proteins are somewhat peripheral to the theme of this book, only a brief mention of their properties will be given. Myoglobin is present in tissue, serves to store oxygen, and consists of a single polypeptide chain plus a haem group, with a molecular weight of 18 000. Haemoglobin consists of four polypeptide chains, two α-chains of molecular weight 15 126 and two β-chains of molecular weight 15 867. Each polypeptide chain is associated with a haem group. The iron atoms in haemoglobin are co-ordinated to the four nitrogens of the porphyrin ring and the imidazole group of a histidine residue in the polypeptide chain. A sixth co-ordination site links to the oxygen molecule.

Other haem-containing proteins

Although haemoglobin and myoglobin are by far the most important haem proteins in quantitative terms, a number of other haem-containing proteins, mainly enzymes, play important roles in electron transport and oxygen metabolism. Peroxidases, which inactivate some of the reactive intermediates formed from hydrogen peroxide, are important because they constitute part of a microbicidal system of phagocytic cells. In this system peroxidase catalyses a reaction between hydrogen peroxide and halide or pseudohalide which results in the formation of a toxic oxyhalide (Klebanoff, 1975). Defects in this activity may occur in iron deficiency (see Chapter 5). Other haem-containing enzymes include catalase, which decomposes hydrogen peroxide to oxygen, cytochrome *c* oxygenase, which is involved in the utilization of oxygen, and various other oxygenases which convert oxygen to hydroxyl groups in organic compounds. Haem is also present in various non-phosphorylating electron transport enzymes, and in cytochromes. The latter are involved in electron transport, in which the iron atom is reversibly oxidized and reduced between the Fe^{2+} and the Fe^{3+} states.

Iron–sulphur proteins

A number of redox enzymes belong to a class of compounds known as iron–sulphur proteins. These proteins, reviewed by Thomson (1985), generally mediate one-electron transport reactions. They usually contain either two or four iron atoms closely linked to a similar number of sulphide ions, and to the sulphydryl side-chains of cysteine residues. The simplest and best-characterized iron–sulphur proteins are the ferredoxins and rubredoxins, found predominantly in bacteria and plants. The more complex iron–sulphur proteins also contain molybdenum, flavin compounds or haem groups. In mammals, ferredoxins exist in the adrenal cortex and other steroidogenic tissues (adrenodoxins) and in the kidney and liver. These are involved in the conversion of cholesterol to steroid hormones. The complex type of iron–sulphur proteins include mitochondrial NADH dehydrogenase, which contains multiple iron–sulphur units and a mole of FMN, and succinate dehydrogenase, which contains one mole of FAD. These, together with a high-potential (HIPIP) type of ferredoxin, are typically found in the heart and are involved in oxidative phosphorylation. Xanthine oxidase, found in liver and milk, and aldehyde oxygenase, from liver, are also complex-type iron–sulphur proteins involved in electron transport. Finally, there are two mammalian iron–sulphur proteins which mediate non–redox types of reaction; these are aconitase, a Krebs cycle enzyme, and amidophosphoribosyl transferase, which is involved in the early stages of purine biosynthesis.

Other non-haem iron-containing proteins

There are a number of other miscellaneous iron-containing proteins. One of these is the enzyme ribonucleotide reductase, which reduces ribonucleotides to deoxyribonucleotides, an essential step in DNA synthesis. This enzyme is unusual in that it contains two subunits held together by a relatively loosely bound non-haem ferric ion (Atkin *et al.*, 1973). The enzyme appears to turn over rapidly and needs a continuous supply of iron to maintain activity. It is therefore not surprising that the role played by iron in cell proliferation (see Chapters 5 and 12) has been linked to the need for ribonucleotide reductase activity. The activity of monoamine oxidase appears to be iron-dependent (Symes, Missala and Sourkes, 1971), though the exact role of the metal is unclear. Finally, several groups of workers have identified low levels of iron-containing peptides in human serum, which promote growth of both bacteria and mammalian cells (Fernandez-Pol, 1978; Jones *et al.*, 1986; Pickhart and Thaler, 1980). Their significance is unclear, though it is possible that they may be intracellular iron-transport intermediates which are liberated extracellularly under certain conditions.

The activity of a number of these iron-containing enzymes is impaired in iron deficiency, and this aspect has been reviewed by Galan, Hercberg and Touitou (1984).

IRON METABOLISM AND RECIRCULATION

A fundamental aspect of iron metabolism in man is that it is highly conservative, most iron being recycled within the body. There is no controlled excretory mechanism, and iron status is maintained by control of the absorption of dietary iron.

Iron absorption

Over 50 years have elapsed since McCance and Widdowson (1937) demonstrated that iron balance was regulated at the absorption stage. Yet despite intensive research, reviewed more extensively by Charlton and Bothwell (1983) and by Huebers and Finch (1985), the mechanisms involved in iron absorption remain unclear, as do the ways in which uptake is related to body needs. Of the total body iron content of 4–5 g, only about 1 mg in men or 2 mg in women is taken up per day into plasma from dietary sources. Only a small percentage of dietary iron is absorbed under normal conditions, the proportion depending not only upon body iron needs, but also upon the nature of the iron carrier and the other dietary substances present. Iron is most readily absorbed when it can be easily released from carrier molecules at the acidic pH found in the upper gastrointestinal tract, which is the region in which iron absorption occurs. Iron in the form of haem is absorbed more efficiently, and is only released from the porphyrin ring when it has entered the mucosal cell. Consequently absorption of haem iron is less affected by intraluminal factors. It has been suggested that entry of iron to mucosal cells is mediated by lactoferrin (Lönnerdal, 1985) or by transferrin (Huebers and Finch, 1985). Neither of these views is universally accepted, as the presence of transferrin receptors on mucosal cells may relate more to the highly proliferative nature of these cells than to a role in iron absorption, and there is evidence that lactoferrin diminishes rather than enhances iron absorption (Brock, 1980). Alternatively, iron may enter mucosal cells without any carrier molecule (Charlton and Bothwell, 1983).

Once within mucosal cells, iron may either be stored in mucosal ferritin, or transported across the mucosal cell, perhaps by a transferrin-like protein (Pollack and Lasky, 1976), and released to the plasma. Not all iron entering the mucosal cell reaches the plasma, and the amount retained may depend upon the levels of mucosal ferritin. It has also been proposed that mucosal macrophages may control the fate of iron entering mucosal cells (Refsum and Schreiner, 1984). This latter theory is compatible with the fact that iron release from the mucosa and iron release from reticuloendothelial cells appear to share common control mechanisms, both being reduced during inflammation (see Chapter 6).

Iron absorption is normally increased during iron deficiency, and decreased in individuals with replete iron stores. An exception occurs in the case of idiopathic haemochromatosis (dealt with in more detail in Chapter 11), in which a failure to regulate iron absorption appears to be responsible for the development of iron overload. The mechanisms linking iron absorption to iron status are not understood, but may involve the degree of erythropoiesis and levels of mucosal ferritin (Huebers and Finch, 1985). It does not appear to be mediated by the degree of saturation of serum transferrin.

Iron recirculation

Iron released from the intestinal mucosa is bound by circulating transferrin, where it joins a much larger pool of iron in transit from sites of storage and erythrocyte catabolism to the bone marrow. The major portion of this iron is destined for incorporation into haemoglobin, while smaller amounts are taken up by non-erythroid cells. This latter portion is of particular relevance to the topics dealt with in this book. As described in more detail in Chapter 2, erythrocytes are eventually taken up and degraded by macrophages in the liver and spleen, which either store the iron obtained from degraded haemoglobin as ferritin, or release it to the circulation where it is bound by transferrin. Under normal circumstances the rate of erythropoiesis is controlled by the hormone erythropoietin, though iron supply may become a limiting factor in iron deficiency and perhaps also in inflammation. There is normally a large reservoir of storage iron present in the hepatocytes, most of which is in the form of ferritin, though these stores largely disappear during iron deficiency. Uptake of iron by hepatocytes may occur from transferrin, or from haemoglobin–haptoglobin or haem–haemopexin complexes which may form as a result of haemolysis and liberation of haemoglobin.

Cellular uptake of iron is normally regulated by the expression of transferrin receptors. The mechanism by which iron is released from hepatocytes, macrophages and intestinal mucosal cells is not well understood, but is in some way regulated by erythropoietic needs, though this may not be the case in inflammation (see Chapter 6).

As mentioned above, the body possesses no controlled mechanism for iron excretion, such losses as do occur being the result of cellular desquamation, particularly of intestinal mucosal cells, and through sweat. It is for this reason that an abnormally large iron uptake, due either to a lack of control of absorption, as occurs in idiopathic haemochromatosis, or to repeated blood transfusions, results in severe iron overload.

IRON AND BACTERIAL GROWTH

One of the earliest properties attributed to the transferrin class of proteins was their ability to inhibit microbial growth. This property is due to their high affinity for iron, which renders the metal unavailable for microbial metabolism. To counter the effects of iron limitation thus imposed on bacteria within mammalian tissues, these organisms produce low molecular weight high-affinity iron chelators known as siderophores, which are able to successfully compete with host iron-binding proteins. The majority of these siderophores are derivatives of catechol or hydroxamic acid, and a large number of different types have now been identified. It is thus considered that transferrin and lactoferrin serve as nonspecific antimicrobial agents which protect against systemic and secretory surface infections respectively. Lactoferrin is also thought to contribute to the antibacterial activity of neutrophils by a similar mechanism (see Chapters 5 and 10). The whole area of the role of iron-binding proteins as antimicrobial agents has been extensively studied over the past 40 years, and detailed reviews are available, including a recent book on the subject by Bullen and Griffiths (1987). This topic will therefore not be dealt with further in this volume.

REFERENCES

Amouric, M., Marvaldi, J., Pichon, J., Bellot, F., and Figarella, C. (1984). Effect of lactoferrin on the growth of a human adenocarcinoma cell line—comparison with transferrin, *In Vitro*, **20**, 543–8.

Anderson, B. F., Baker, H. M., Dodson, E. J., Norris, G. E., Rumball, S. V., Waters, J. M., and Baker, E. N. (1987). Structure of human lactoferrin at 3.2Å resolution, *Proc. Natl Acad. Sci. USA*, **84**, 1768–74.

Antonini, E., Rossi-Bernardi, L., and Chiancone, E. (eds) (1981). Hemoglobins, *Methods Enzymol.*, **76**.

Arosio, P., Adelman, T. G., and Drysdale, J. W. (1978). On ferritin heterogeneity. Further evidence for heteropolymers, *J. Biol. Chem.*, **253**, 4451–8.

Atkin, C. L., Thelander, L., Reichard, P., and Lang, G. (1973). Iron and free radical in ribonucleotide reductase, *J. Biol. Chem.*, **248**, 7464–72.

Bailey, S., Evans, R. W., Garratt, R. C., Gorinsky, B., Hasnain, S., Horsburgh, C., Jhoti, H., Lindley, P. F., Mydin, A., Sarra, R., and Watson, J. L. (1988). Molecular structure of serum transferrin at 3.3Å resolution, *Biochemistry*, **27**, 5804–12.

Brock, J. H. (1980). Lactoferrin in human milk: its role in iron absorption and protection against enteric infection in the newborn infant, *Arch. Dis. Child.* **55**, 417–21.

Brock, J. H. (1985). The transferrins. In P. M. Harrison (ed.) *Metalloproteins*, Part 2, pp. 183–262, Macmillan. London.

Brock, J. H., and Arzabe, F. R. (1976). Cleavage of diferric bovine transferrin into two monoferric fragments, *FEBS Lett.*, **69**, 63–6.

Brown, J. P., Hewick, R. M., Hellström, I., Hellström, K. E, Doolittle, R. F., and Dreyer, W. J. (1982). Human melanoma-associated antigen p97 is structurally and functionally related to transferrin, *Nature*, **296**, 171–3.

Brown-Mason, A., and Woodworth, R. C. (1984). Physiological levels of binding

and iron donation by complementary halves of ovotransferrin to transferrin receptors on chick reticulocytes, *J. Biol. Chem.*, **259**, 1866–73.
Buhi, W. C., Ducsay, C. A., Bazer, F. W., and Roberts, R. M. (1982). Iron transfer between the purple phosphatase uteroferrin and transferrin and its possible role in iron metabolism in the fetal pig, *J. Biol. Chem.*, **257**, 1712–23.
Bullen, J. J., and Griffiths, E. (1987). *Iron and Infection. Molecular, Physiological and Clinical Aspects*, Wiley, Chichester.
Charlton, R. W., and Bothwell, T. H. (1983). Iron absorption, *Annu. Rev. Med.*, **34**, 55–68.
Chasteen, N. D. (1983). The identification of the probable locus of iron and anion binding in the transferrins, *Trends Biochem. Sci.*, **8**, 272–5.
Crichton, R. R. (1984). Iron uptake and utilization by mammalian cells. II. Intracellular iron utilization, *Trends Biochem. Sci.*, **9**, 283–6.
Dautry-Varsat, A. (1986). Receptor-mediated endocytosis: the intracellular journey of transferrin and its receptor, *Biochimie*, **68**, 375–81.
Davis, R. J., and Meisner, H. (1987). Regulation of transferrin receptor recycling by protein kinase C is independent of receptor phosphorylation at serine 24 in Swiss 3T3 fibroblasts, *J. Biol. Chem.*, **262**, 10641–7.
Diamond, A., Devine, J. M., and Cooper, G. M. (1984). Nucleotide sequence of a human *Blym* transforming gene activated in a Burkitt's lymphoma, *Science*, **225**, 516–9.
Dickerson, R. E., and Geis, I. (1983). *Hemoglobin Structure, Function. Evolution and Pathology*, Benjamin, Menlo Park, California.
Drysdale, J. W. (1988). Human ferritin gene expression, *Prog. Nucleic Acids Res.*, **35**, 127–55.
Esparza, I., and Brock, J. H. (1980). The interaction of bovine transferrin and monoferric transferrin fragments with rabbit reticulocytes, *Biochim. Biophys. Acta*, **624**, 479–89.
Evans, R. W., Meilak, A., Patel, K. J., Wong, C., Garratt, R. C., and Chitnavis, B. (1988). Characterisation of the amino acid change in a variant transferrin. *Biochem. Soc. Trans.*, **16**, 834–5.
Fernandez-Pol, J. A. (1978). Isolation and characterization of a siderophore-like growth factor from mutants of SV40-transformed cells adapted to picolinic acid, *Cell*, **14**, 489–99.
Fibach, E., Konijn, A. M., and Rachmilewitz, E. A. (1985). Changes in cellular ferritin content during myeloid differentiation of human leukemic cell lines, *Am. J. Hematol.*, **18**, 143–51.
Fillet, G., Cook, J. D., and Finch, C. A. (1974). Storage iron kinetics. VII. A biological model for reticuloendothelial iron transport, *J. Clin. Invest.*, **53**, 1527–33.
Fletcher, J., and Huehns, E. R. (1968). Function of transferrin, *Nature*, **218**, 1211–14.
Galan, P., Hercberg, S., and Touitou, Y. (1984). The activity of tissue enzymes in iron-deficient rat and man: an overview, *Comp. Biochem. Physiol.*, **77B**, 647–53.
Goubin, G., Goldman, D. S., Luce, J., Neiman, P. E., and Cooper, G. M. (1983). Molecular cloning and nucleotide sequence of a transforming gene detected by transfection of chicken B-cell lymphoma DNA, *Nature*, **302**, 114–19.
Halliwell, B., and Gutteridge, J. M. C. (1985). The importance of free radicals and catalytic metal ions in human disease, *Mol. Aspects Med.*, **8**, 89–193.
Halliwell, B., and Gutteridge, J. M. C. (1986). Oxygen free radicals and iron in relation to biology and medicine: some problems and concepts, *Arch. Biochem. Biophys.*, **246**, 501–14.

Hatton, M. W. C., März, L., Berry, L. R., Debanne, M. T., and Regoeczi, E. (1979). Bi- and tri-antennary human transferrin glycopeptides and their affinities for the hepatic lectin specific for asialo-glycoproteins, *Biochem. J.*, **181**, 633–8.
Häuserman, H. (1899). Uber den Eisengehalt des Blutplasmas und der Leukocyten, *Hoppe Seylers Z. Physiol. Chem.*, **26**, 436–7.
Huebers, H. A., and Finch, C. A. (1985). Molecular aspects of iron absorption and its control. In G. Spik, J. Montreuil, R. R. Crichton and J. Mazurier (eds) *Proteins of Iron Metabolism*, pp. 263–74. Elsevier, Amsterdam.
Huebers, H. A., and Finch, C. A. (1987). The physiology of transferrin and transferrin receptors, *Physiol. Rev.*, **67**, 520–82.
Hunt, R. C. (1986). Endocytosis and control of expression of transferrin receptor, *Dev. Comp. Immunol.*, **10**, 273–7.
Jacobs, A., and Worwood, M. (eds) (1980). *Iron in Biochemistry and Medicine 2*, Academic Press, London.
Jones, R. L., Grady, R. W., Sorette, M. P., and Cerami, A. (1986). Host associated iron transfer factor in normal humans and patients with transfusion siderosis, *J. Lab. Clin. Med.*, **107**, 431–8.
Joshi, J. G., and Zimmerman, A. (1988). Ferritin: an expanded role in metabolic regulation, *Toxicology*, **48**, 21–9.
Klausner, R. D., Harford, J., and van Renswoude, J. (1984). Rapid internalization of the transferrin receptor in K562 cells is triggered by ligand binding or treatment with a phorbol ester, *Proc. Natl Acad. Sci. USA*, **81**, 3005–9.
Klebanoff, S. (1975). Antimicrobial mechanism in neutrophil polymorphonuclear leukocytes, *Semin. Hematol.*, **12**, 117–42.
Laurell, C. B., and Ingleman, D. (1947). Fe-binding protein of swine serum, *Acta Chem. Scand.*, **1**, 770–6.
Lestas, A. N. (1976). The effect of pH upon human transferrin: selective labelling of the two iron-binding sites, *Br. J. Haematol.*, **32**, 341–50.
Lönnerdal. B. (1985). Biochemistry and physiological function of human milk proteins, *Am. J. Clin. Nutr.*, **42**, 1299–317.
Masson, P. L., and Heremans, J. F. (1968). Metal-combining properties of human lactoferrin (red milk protein). I. The involvement of bicarbonate in the reaction, *Eur. J. Biochem.*, **6**, 579–84.
May, W. S., and Cuatrecasas, P. (1985). Transferrin receptor: its biological significance, *J. Membr. Biol.*, **88**, 205–15.
May, W. S., and Tyler, G. (1987). Phosphorylation of the surface transferrin receptor stimulates receptor internalization in HL60 leukemia cells. *J. Biol. Chem.*, **262**, 16710–8.
McCance, R. A., and Widdowson, E. M. (1937). Absorption and excretion of iron, *Lancet*, **ii**, 680–4.
Metz-Boutigue, M-H., Jollès, J., Mazurier, J., Schoentgen, F., Legrand, D., Spik, G., Montreuil, J., and Jollès, P. (1984). Human lactotransferrin: amino acid sequence and structural comparisons with other transferrins, *Eur. J. Biochem.*, **145**, 659–76.
Morgan, E. H. (1981). Transferrin: biochemistry, physiology and clinical significance, *Mol. Aspects Med.*, **4**, 1–123.
Nuñez, M. T., and Glass, J. (1983). The transferrin cycle and iron uptake in rabbit reticulocytes. Pulse studies using ^{59}Fe, ^{125}I-labelled transferrin, *J. Biol. Chem.*, **258**, 9676–80.
O'Connell, M. J., Ward, R. J., Baum, H., and Peters, T. J. (1986a). In vitro and in vivo studies on the availability of iron from storage proteins to stimulate

membrane lipid peroxidation. In C. Rice-Evans (ed.) *Free Radicals. Cell Damage and Disease*, pp. 29–37, Richelieu Press, London.

O'Connell, M. J., Halliwell, B., Moorhouse, C. P., Aruoma, O. I., Baum, H., and Peters, T. J. (1986b). Formation of hydroxyl radicals in the presence of ferritin and haemosiderin. Is haemosiderin formation a biological protection mechanism? *Biochem. J.*, **234**, 727–31.

Oria, R., Alvarez-Hernández, X., Licéaga, J., and Brock, J. H. (1988). Uptake and handling of iron from transferrin, lactoferrin and immune complexes by a macrophage cell line, *Biochem. J.*, **251**, 221–5.

Pickhart, L., and Thaler, M. M. (1980). Growth-modulating tripeptide (glycyl-histidyllysine): association with copper and iron in plasma, and stimulation of adhesiveness and growth of hepatoma cells in culture by tripeptide–metal ion conjugates, *J. Cell. Physiol.*, **102**, 129–39.

Pollack, S., and Lasky, F. D. (1976). A new iron-binding protein isolated from intestinal mucosa, *J. Lab. Clin. Med.*, **87**, 670–9.

Refsum, S. B., and Schreiner, B.-I. (1984). Regulation of iron balance by absorption and excretion. A critical view and a new hypothesis, *Scand. J. Gastroenterol*, **19**, 867–74.

Rice, D. W., Ford, G. C., White, J. L., Smith, J. M. A., and Harrison, P. M. (1983). The spatial structure of horse spleen ferritin, *Adv. Inorg. Biochem.*, **5**, 39–50.

Richter, G. W. (1984). Studies on iron overload. Rat liver siderosome ferritin, *Lab. Invest.*, **50**, 26–35.

Schlabach, M. R., and Bates, G. W. (1975). The synergistic binding of anions and Fe^{3+} by transferrin, *J. Biol. Chem.*, **250**, 2182–8.

Speyer, B. E., and Fielding, J. (1974). Chromatographic fractionation of human reticulocytes after uptake of doubly-labelled [^{59}Fe, ^{125}I] transferrin, *Biochim. Biophys. Acta*, **332**, 192–200.

Spik, G., Strecker, G., Fournet, B., Bouquelet, S., Montreuil, J., Dorland, L., Van Halbeek, H., and Vliegenthart, J. F. G. (1982). Primary structure of the glycans from human lactotransferrin, *Eur. J. Biochem.*, **121**, 413–19.

Spiro, T. G. (1977). Chemistry and biochemistry of iron. In E. B. Brown, P. Aisen, J. Fielding and R. R. Crichton (eds) *Proteins of Iron Metabolism*, pp. xxiii–xxxii, Grune and Stratton, New York.

Stibler, H., Borg, S., and Allgulander, C. (1979). Clinical significance of abnormal heterogeneity of transferrin in relation to alcohol consumption, *Acta Med. Scand.*, **206**, 275–81.

Sutherland, R., Delia, D., Schneider, C., Newman, R., Kemshead, J., and Greaves, M. (1981). Ubiquitous cell-surface glycoprotein on tumor cells is proliferation-associated receptor for transferrin, *Proc. Natl Acad. Sci. USA*, **78**, 4515–19.

Symes, A. L., Missala, K., and Sourkes, T. L. (1971). Iron and riboflavin-dependent metabolism of a monoamine in the rat *in vivo*, *Science*, **174**, 153–5.

Theil, E. C. (1987). Ferritin: structure, gene regulation, and cellular function in animals, plants and microorganisms, *Annu. Rev. Biochem.*, **56**, 289–315.

Thomson, A. J. (1985). Iron–sulphur proteins. In P. M. Harrison (ed.) *Metalloproteins*, Part 1, pp. 79–120. Macmillan, London.

Treffry, A., and Harrison, P. M. (1984). Non-random distribution of iron entering rat liver ferritin *in vivo*, *Biochem. J.*, **220**, 857–9.

Watts, C. A. (1985). Rapid endocytosis of the transferrin receptor in the absence of bound transferrin, *J. Cell Biol.*, **100**, 633–7.

Weir, M. P., Gibson, J. F., and Peters, T. J. (1984). Biochemical studies on the isolation and characterisation of human spleen haemosiderin, *Biochem. J.*, **223**, 31–8.

Williams, J. (1982). The evolution of transferrin, *Trends Biochem. Sci.*, **7**, 394–7.
Worwood, M. (1986). Serum ferritin, *Clin. Sci.*, **70**, 215–20.
Young, S. P., and Aisen, P. (1981). Transferrin receptors and the uptake and release of iron by isolated hepatocytes, *Hepatology*, **1**, 114–19.
Young, S. P., Bomford, A., and Williams, R. (1984). The effect of iron saturation of transferrin on its binding and uptake by rabbit reticulocytes, *Biochem. J.*, **219**, 505–10.
Zerial, M., Suomalainen, M., Zanetti-Schneider, M., Schneider, C., and Garoff, H. (1987). Phosphorylation of the human transferrin receptor by protein kinase C is not required for endocytosis and recycling in mouse 3T3 cells, *EMBO J.*, **6**, 2661–7.

Iron in Immunity, Cancer and Inflammation
Edited by M. de Sousa and J. H. Brock
© 1989 John Wiley & Sons Ltd.

4
The Molecular Biology of Iron-binding Proteins

Paolo Arosio*, Gaetano Cairo† and Sonia Levi*
*Department of Biomedical Science and Technology, University of Milano, c/o San Raffaele Hospital, Via Olgettina 60, 20132 Milan, Italy
†Centro di Studio sulla Patologia Cellulare CNR, Via Mangiagalli 31, 20133 Milan, Italy

INTRODUCTION

Ferritin, transferrin and the transferrin receptor are the major proteins of iron metabolism. They have been studied for a considerable time, and their characteristics and functions have been reviewed extensively (Munro and Linder, 1978; Harrison, Clegg and May, 1980; Aisen and Listowsky, 1980; Seligman, 1983; Ford et al., 1984; Trowbridge et al., 1984; Williams, 1985; Bomford and Munro, 1985; Schneider and Williams, 1985; May and Cuatrecasas, 1985; Testa, 1985).

Interest in these proteins has recently increased, as there are indications that they have other functions besides recycling iron for haemoglobin synthesis. In particular they appear to directly or indirectly affect cell proliferation and differentiation.

Recently, the application of molecular biology techniques has greatly increased our knowledge of these proteins, as the corresponding cDNAs and genes have been isolated, permitting the determination of their primary structures and providing probes to study their expression at the molecular level. Moreover, these techniques have permitted the identification of proteins which are structurally related to the well-characterized iron-binding proteins, but whose functions are obscure.

In this chapter we will briefly review the fast-growing data on the molecular biology of ferritins, transferrins and transferrin receptors, with particular attention to molecular aspects of protein structure, gene organization and gene expression.

FERRITIN

Ferritin protein structure

Iron is stored in tissues in the core of soluble ferritin and in insoluble haemosiderin, which is probably a degradation product of the former (Munro and Linder, 1978). Ferritin is found in all living organisms from bacteria to mammals, with a remarkably consistent structure, this being an almost spherical protein shell that surrounds an iron core of variable size (Harrison, Clegg and May, 1980). Thanks to the long and extensive crystallographic work of Harrison's group in Sheffield, the three-dimensional structure of mammalian ferritin has been resolved and recently reviewed (Ford *et al.*, 1984). The protein is composed of 24 subunits and is roughly spherical, with an outer diameter of about 125 Å and a central cavity about 80 Å across (Ford *et al.*, 1984). The inner space can readily communicate with the outside, as shown by exchange analysis (Collawn and Fish, 1985), through two types of channels 3–4 Å wide. There are six channels on the four-fold symmetry axes that are aligned with hydrophobic residues, and eight pores on the three-fold symmetry axes, aligned with hydrophilic residues (Ford *et al.*, 1984). Unless the protein breathes (which is unlikely, given its rigid structure), only small molecules can penetrate the inner cavity and have access to the iron core, which is formed by crystalline aggregates of ferric hydroxyphosphate (Ford *et al.*, 1984). The iron is segregated in the central cavity and does not appear to affect the conformation of the molecule; consequently, the immunological and surface properties of the protein are not influenced by iron loading (Harrison, Clegg and May, 1980). The oxidation and uptake of ferrous iron is catalysed by ferritin, and iron is readily released upon reduction (Harrison, Clegg and May, 1980; see also Chapter 3).

The subunits are folded in a bundle of four tightly packed α-helices of similar length (named A, B, C and D), plus a fifth short helix (named E) at an acute angle to the bundle. Peptide folding is ensured by hydrophobic and ionic interactions, and protein assembly is stabilized mainly by hydrophobic interactions that make ferritin exceptionally stable to thermal and chemical denaturation (Stefanini, Vecchini and Chiancone, 1987). Ferritin can be dissociated only at extreme pH values (below 3 or above 11) or in hot sodium dodecyl sulphate.

Ferritins show a large degree of surface charge heterogeneity; horse spleen ferritin, for instance, can be separated into some five components on conventional isoelectric focusing (Arosio, Adelman and Drysdale, 1978) and into more than ten components in narrow pH range Immobiline isoelectric focusing (Righetti *et al.*, 1987). This heterogeneity is partially explained by the existence of multiple subunit types that assemble in different proportions in the protein shell (Arosio, Adelman and Drysdale, 1978). Three subunit types have been identified so far: the L (light or liver subunit) of 19 900 M_r; the H (heavy or heart subunit) of 21 000 M_r; and the G (glycosylated subunit) of 23 000 M_r. The L chain is predominant in iron (and ferritin) rich tissues such as liver and spleen, and was the first to be recognized and crystallized (Granick, 1942). The ferritin subunit structure described above refers to the L chain. The H chain is widespread in all tissues, and the G chain is mainly found in serum. The sequences of the subunits have been determined from protein sequencing (Wustfeld and Crichton, 1982; Addison *et al.*, 1983) or from the nucleotide sequences of the corresponding cDNAs (Costanzo *et al.*, 1984; Costanzo, Santoro and Cortese, 1984; Leibold *et al.*, 1984; Boyd *et al.*, 1985; Dörner *et al.*, 1985; Jain *et al.*, 1985a; Chou *et al.*, 1986). The H chain is made up of 182 and the L of 174 amino acids. L chains from horse, rat and human share about 85% of sequence homology, while human H and L chains differ by about 45% (Costanzo, Santoro and Cortese, 1984; Leibold *et al.*, 1984; Boyd *et al.*, 1985). In the absence of crystallographic data the H chain structure has been studied by computer simulation, which indicated that it has a similar folding to the L chain (Leibold *et al.*, 1984; Boyd *et al.*, 1985), in agreement with preliminary crystallographic data that showed that the H-rich isoferritins crystallize with identical symmetry and space group as the L-rich (Bolognesi *et al.*, 1984).

The glycosylated G subunit has been isolated only from human serum (Cragg, Wagstaff and Worwood, 1981; Santambrogio *et al.*, 1987), even though small amounts may also be present in tissues. It has immunochemical properties similar, but not identical, to the L chain (Santambrogio *et al.*, 1987) and probably carries a single glycosidic residue of the complex type (Campanini *et al.*, in preparation). It is presently unclear whether it originates from post-translational modification of the L chain or from a specific transcript.

The functional significance of the H and L subunit types has not been completely clarified, but it appears to be important, as they are both present in all vertebrate species studied and also in some invertebrates (Arosio *et al.*, 1984). A library of monoclonal antibodies for the two subunits has been obtained (Luzzago *et al.*, 1986), and more recently the cDNA for the human H chain has been cloned into a vector of overexpression in *E. coli* (Levi *et al.*, 1987). The study of recombinant ferritins and of mutants, obtained by site-directed mutagenesis, will probably clarify the functional and structural properties of the two chains. Preliminary data indicate that the H subunit takes up and releases iron faster than the L, probably as a consequence of its higher ferro-oxidase activity (Levi *et al.*, 1988) and work is in progress to clarify whether iron enters the molecule through its hydrophilic channels, as suggested by Wardeska,

Viglione and Chasteen (1986). We postulate that in the intracellular environment the H chain is involved mainly in iron detoxification and short-term storage, while the L chain is involved in long-term iron storage (see also Chapter 3).

Ferritin transcripts

Various laboratories have cloned (sometimes serendipitously) cDNAs for human (Costanzo *et al.*, 1984; Costanzo, Santoro and Cortese, 1984; Boyd *et al.*, 1985; Dörner *et al.*, 1985; Jain *et al.*, 1985a; Chou *et al.*, 1986; Santoro *et al.*, 1986), rat (Leibold *et al.*, 1984), tadpole (Didsbury *et al.*, 1986) and chicken (Stevens, Dodgson and Engel, 1987) ferritins. All the cDNAs share common characteristics. The coding regions as well as the 3' and 5' non-coding regions are of similar size, and they hybridize to mRNAs of similar dimensions, of 870–1100 nucleotides (nt). Near the end of the 3' flanking region they all show a single polyadenylation signal. At medium and high stringency, H and L cDNAs hybridize only with the corresponding mRNAs (Jain *et al.*, 1985b), even of different species, allowing the quantitation of H and L transcripts.

The sequences of human H chain cDNAs determined in various laboratories are essentially identical. The cDNA has an open reading frame of 552 nt that codes for 183 amino acids, including the N-terminal methionine that is not present in the mature protein, flanked by 208 and 160 nt at the 5' and 3' non-coding regions respectively. H chain mRNA is about 1050 nt long, with some minor heterogeneity in size, possibly caused by variability in polyadenylation (Costanzo *et al.*, 1984; Boyd *et al.*, 1985; Chou *et al.*, 1986).

The sequences of human L chain cDNA obtained in three different laboratories (Costanzo, Santoro and Cortese, 1984; Boyd *et al.*, 1985; Chou *et al.*, 1986) are identical, while the one determined in a fourth laboratory (Dörner *et al.*, 1985) has a major difference in the 5' flanking region and a nucleotide substitution in the coding region that determines a switch Thr→Ala at codon 101. This finding suggests genetic polymorphisms of the L chain, if it does not originate from cloning artifacts. The mRNA is composed of an open reading frame of 528 nt that encodes 175 residues, including the initial methionine, flanked by 198 and 146 nt at the 5' and 3' ends respectively (Boyd *et al.*, 1985; Dörner *et al.*, 1985; Chou *et al.*, 1986).

Rat and human L chain cDNA sequences of the coding region have 85% homology, while human H and L share 64% homology (Leibold *et al.*, 1984; Dörner *et al.*, 1985). Tadpole sequence seems intermediate between the two subunits, as it shares 59–66% homology with the two human cDNAs (Didsbury *et al.*, 1986). Based on these data, it was suggested that H and L genes diverged more than 2.5 million years ago (Dörner *et al.*, 1985). There is also a highly conserved sequence of 28 nt at the 5' untranslated region of all the ferritin mRNAs which, as discussed below, is essential for the iron-mediated translational regulation of ferritin expression (Leibold and Munro, 1988).

It is a common finding that in Northern blotting human H cDNA also hybridizes with a high molecular weight RNA that does not appear to be related to ferritin expression. In a detailed analysis it was found that this cDNA contains a GC-rich sequence of 67 nt in the 5' flanking region that is complementary to a sequence on the 28 S ribosomal RNA (Jain *et al.*, 1985b). This complementarity is not found in the L chain cDNA, and may play a role in stabilizing the transcript.

Structure of the ferritin genes

With the cloning of cDNAs, it became evident that human and rat genomes carry a large number of sequences complementary to ferritin cDNAs, indicating that the two subunits are encoded by complex families of genes or pseudogenes (Costanzo *et al.*, 1984; Costanzo, Santoro and Cortese, 1984; Leibold *et al.*, 1984; Boyd *et al.*, 1985; Dörner *et al.*, 1985; Jain *et al.*, 1985a; Chou *et al.*, 1986; McGill *et al.*, 1987). Increasing the stringency in Southern blot experiments does not select the various fragments since they have a high degree of homology (Jain *et al.*, 1985a). Various techniques were used to localize the fragments on human chromosomes, using chromosome sorting (Lebo *et al.*, 1985), *in situ* hybridization (McGill *et al.*, 1984) and Southern blotting of human–rodent hybridoma cell lines (Cragg, Drysdale and Worwood, 1985). They showed that the DNA fragments hybridizing with ferritin cDNAs are spread all over the human genome; in particular, L chain genes or pseudogenes are located on chromosomes 19–22 and X, and H chain on chromosomes 1–3, 6, 11, 14, 20 and X. The expression of ferritin is associated with the presence of chromosome 11 for the H chain and 19 for the L chain (Cragg, Drysdale and Worwood, 1985).

It is now well established that essentially only one gene is active for each subunit. The lines of evidence for this conclusion can be summarized as follows: (a) nucleotide sequences and primer extension analyses of ferritin transcripts from various human tissues and cell lines indicate the presence of only one messenger type for H and one for L chains (Costanzo, Santoro and Cortese, 1984; Costanzo *et al.*, 1984; Dörner *et al.*, 1985; Jain *et al.*, 1985a; Chou *et al.*, 1986; Santoro *et al.*, 1986); (b) Southern blots of chicken DNA with H chain probes revealed a single gene in the haploid genome (Stevens, Dodgson and Engel, 1987); (c) the active genes for H and L have been cloned and sequenced (Costanzo *et al.*, 1986; Santoro *et al.*, 1986; Hentze *et al.*, 1986) and some subclones hybridize to a single DNA fragment (Santoro *et al.*, 1986); (d) the cloned gene for the H subunit was shown to be active in the transcription of ferritin mRNA, and located on chromosome 11 (Hentze *et al.*, 1986); (e) some of the fragments hybridizing with ferritin cDNAs have been cloned and sequenced, and they have characteristics typical of pseudogenes that arose from retrotranscription of mRNA—they are intronless or have misplaced introns and have a poly-A stretch at the 3' region (Santoro *et al.*, 1986). Therefore there is no doubt that H and L chains are encoded by two distinct genes located on chromosomes 11 and 19 respectively, and that the heterogeneity of ferritin subunits may arise from post-translational modifications.

However, some questions are still open regarding ferritin genes. On chromosome 3 the genes for transferrin and its receptor are mapped, and the presence of a ferritin gene may be not casual. Moreover, idiopathic haemochromatosis, a genetic disease with altered iron absorption, is associated with the expression of some HLA phenotypes, whose genes are located on chromosome 6. It is therefore possible that this disease is linked to alterations of the ferritin gene (or pseudogene) located there. However, the studies so far performed have failed to find any relationships between idiopathic haemochromatosis and ferritin genetic polymorphism (Sampietro *et al.*, 1987). The study of ferritin genes has been further stimulated by the finding that two pseudogenes have an uninterrupted coding sequence that may direct the synthesis of a functional protein (Santoro *et al.*, 1986). The significance of this finding is not clear, but raises the hypothesis that, if in abnormal circumstances the gene can be activated, a different ferritin could be synthesized.

Ferritin H and L chain genes contain three introns which split the coding sequences in equivalent places in the two subunits. The resulting four exons roughly correspond to four structural domains of the protein: the α-helices A, B, C and D plus E (Costanzo *et al.*, 1986; Santoro *et al.*, 1986). The introns of H and L genes show no similarity in size and sequence. The two genes have the canonic TATA box 29–31 nt upstream of the start of transcription, and do not share obvious homologies in the 5' non-transcripted regions that are rich in GC content as is commonly found in 'housekeeping' proteins (Santoro *et al.*, 1986).

Ferritin gene expression

Ferritin synthesis in tissues and cell lines is readily stimulated by iron, in keeping with the protein's function of sequestering and storing surplus iron. Iron induction is not inhibited by actinomycin D (Drysdale and Munro, 1966) or other agents that block RNA synthesis (Menozzi, Hanotte and Miller, 1985), indicating that it acts at a post-transcriptional level.

Based on this and other evidence, a model was proposed in which the translation of the ferritin mRNA is prevented by adhering ferritin free subunits in the post-ribosomal fraction, and iron administration removes the inhibition by prompting the assembly of ferritin subunits (Zahringer, Baliga and Munro, 1976). Ferritin would therefore prevent iron entering the nucleus and damaging DNA. This model was essentially confirmed by recent findings showing that when iron is administered to rats, a large proportion of H and L ferritin mRNAs (detected by cDNA probes) moves from the post-ribosomal to the polyribosomal fraction in various tissues (Aziz and Munro, 1986). These results indicate that both H and L subunits are under the control of iron, and are in keeping with data showing that iron induces a similar increase of H and L ferritin chains in HeLa cells (Cairo et al., 1985). Recent studies have identified a potential stem-loop structure in the 5' untranslated region of rat and human ferritin mRNA (Aziz and Munro, 1987; Hentze et al., 1987) which confers translational responsiveness to iron. The mechanism may involve iron-mediated suppression of synthesis of a cytoplasmic protein which blocks translation by binding to the iron-response element (Leibold and Munro, 1988; Rouault et al., 1988). Structurally similar potential stem-loop sequences are also present in the 3' untranslated region of the transferrin receptor mRNA (see below), and can confer ferritin-like translational regulation of an indicator gene transcript when cloned into the 5' untranslated region of the mRNA (Casey et al., 1988).

Other effectors, besides iron, regulate ferritin synthesis, and the regulation occurs at various levels. In HeLa cells iron administration causes an increase in synthesis and of the total amounts of H and L transcripts (Cairo et al., 1985). The degree of this transcriptional stimulus is not sufficient to explain the large induction of ferritin protein synthesis, but indicates that iron acts on various levels. During chemically induced cellular differentiation, the levels of H and L mRNAs are modulated (Chou et al., 1986), in keeping with the findings that different tissues contain different amounts and proportions of H and L chains (Arosio, Adelman and Drysdale, 1978). Lymphoid cells contain different levels of H and L ferritins, according to their lineage, proliferation status and anatomical site (Dörner et al., 1983; Vezzoni et al., 1986) and their ferritin mRNA levels correlate with the corresponding protein content (Cairo et al., 1986). Therefore, some factors related to cell differentiation/proliferation regulate the transcription of ferritins. Furthermore, hormones may affect ferritin expression, as suggested by recent findings that during the first weeks of lactation the ferritin content of milk changes dramatically (Arosio et al., 1986). Finally, inflammation may affect ferritin synthesis, and the possible mechanisms involved are discussed in Chapter 6.

TRANSFERRIN

Transferrin protein structure

The transferrin family comprises a class of single-chain proteins of about 80 kDa, with two iron-binding sites. They are widely distributed in the biological fluids of vertebrates (Aisen and Listowsky, 1980). Transferrins developed later than ferritins during evolution and are found only in the phylum Chordata. The most studied transferrins have been isolated from mammalian sera (serum transferrin or simply transferrin), or milk (lactotransferrin or lactoferrin), and from egg white (ovotransferrin or conalbumin). Recently the family was enlarged to a superfamily (Williams, 1985), as new proteins with structural similarities to transferrins were identified. These are: p97, a membrane-bound glycoprotein of 97 kDa (recently renamed melanotransferrin) found in human melanomas, which shows a large degree of sequence homology with transferrins (Rose et al., 1986); the oncogene Blym-1 found in chicken B cells (Goubin et al., 1983) and in human Burkitt's lymphomas (Diamond et al., 1983), which shares sequence homology with the N-terminal of transferrin; and an iron-binding protein of 40 kDa found in prochordates (Martin et al., 1984), which is thought to be a half-sized ancestor of vertebrate transferrin.

A low resolution (6 Å) three-dimensional structure was obtained for rabbit serum transferrin (Gorinsky et al., 1979), and crystallization of an N-terminal fragment of this molecule is in progress (Sarra and Lindley, 1986). More recently the human lactoferrin structure has been resolved at 3.2 Å resolution (Anderson et al., 1987). Transferrin has dimensions of 100 × 50 × 50 Å, and consists of two ellipsoid lobes at an angle of about 30° to each other. The two iron-binding sites are located in the two lobes. Upon iron binding, the molecule undergoes a conformational transition, becoming more compact (Kilar and Simon, 1985). The conformational change is accompanied by higher resistance to denaturation (Azari and Feeney, 1961), and may explain the different affinities of the two forms for the receptor.

The amino acid sequences of some transferrins have been obtained from sequencing of either the proteins or their cDNAs (Jeltsch and Chambon, 1982; Williams et al., 1982; MacGillivray et al., 1983; Metz-Boutique et al., 1984; Yang et al., 1984; Uzan et al., 1984). The most important feature is that the N-terminal and C-terminal halves of the sequence are imperfect copies, and share sequence homology of 35–40% (Williams, 1985). This strongly suggests that the present transferrins originated from gene duplication of an ancestral half-sized protein. The same feature is present also in p97, which displays an even greater homology between the two halves (46%) (Rose et al., 1986). The sequences of transferrins of different origin share some 40–50% homology (Williams, 1985).

In ovotransferrin the N-terminal half of the molecule has six disulphide bridges, five of which are local, i.e. join residues less than 50 amino acids apart. The C-terminal half has nine disulphide bridges, four of which are long-range (Montreuil *et al.*, 1985). This basic 6 + 9 pattern of disulphide bridges of ovotransferrin is modified to 6 + 10 in human lactoferrin, 6 + 13 in serum transferrin (Montreuil *et al.*, 1985), and to a putative 7 + 7 in p97 (Rose *et al.*, 1986). The variability of disulphide bridges is rather unusual, and is possibly a device acquired during evolution to preserve and stabilize the conformation of the molecule (Williams, 1985).

The recent definition of lactoferrin structure (Anderson *et al.*, 1987) confirmed the two-fold internal homology. The two lobes, which are connected by a short α-helix, show essentially the same folding, which is stabilized by six pairs of disulphide bridges. The lobes are subdivided into two domains of similar size and supersecondary structures. The two iron atoms occupy equivalent locations in the two lobes, at the interface between the two domains and in a highly hydrophilic environment. Each iron is co-ordinated to four protein ligands: Tyr-93 and Tyr-191 in the N lobe (Tyr-447 and Tyr-540 in C), His-252 (His-609) and Asp-62 (Asp-407). All these residues are conserved in all the transferrins so far sequenced, as are two other residues, Tyr-83 (427) and His-117 (472), which are close to the iron site. Thus four of the six iron co-ordination sites are occupied by protein ligands. The remaining two may be occupied by carbonate, which probably interacts also with Arg-121 (477). A similar arrangement of iron-binding ligands has very recently been reported for rabbit transferrin (Bailey *et al.*, 1988).

The sequence of p97 has been recently determined by sequencing its cDNA (Rose *et al.*, 1986). It shares a striking homology with the human transferrins, and in addition it contains an extra 25-amino acid peptide at the C-terminus that has highly hydrophobic characteristics and is the putative site of anchorage of the protein to the cell membrane (Rose *et al.*, 1986). The structural similarity to transferrin, and its capacity to bind iron, indicate that p97 has some function in cellular iron transport.

The Blym-1 oncogenes found in chicken and in Burkitt lymphomas encode a short peptide of 56 residues, 20 of which are homologous with the N-terminal sequence of human transferrin (Goubin *et al.*, 1983; Diamond *et al.*, 1983). Their structures do not appear to contain iron-binding sites, so they are probably not directly involved in iron metabolism.

Transferrin transcripts

Full-length cDNAs have been cloned for human and rat serum transferrins (Yang *et al.*, 1984; Uzan *et al.*, 1984; Levin *et al.*, 1984), chicken ovotransferrin (Jeltsch and Chambon, 1982) and p97 (Rose *et al.*, 1986). All the sequences of human serum transferrin so far obtained are virtually identical (MacGillivray *et al.*, 1983; Yang *et al.*, 1984; Uzan *et al.*, 1984). Human transferrin cDNA has an open reading frame that encodes a protein of 679 amino acids, plus a leading sequence of 19 amino acids that is not found in the mature protein and probably constitutes a signal for protein secretion. The nucleotide leader sequences of human transferrins, p97 and ovotransferrin are 56% homologous but have little homology with that of Blym-1.

Human transferrin cDNA hybridizes with a mRNA of about 2400 nt (Uzan *et al.*, 1984). Rat (Uzan *et al.*, 1984) and chicken (Jeltsch and Chambon, 1982) messengers are of similar size. The messenger contains a 5' untranslated sequence of 150–200 nt, and a 3' untranslated sequence of 166 nt with one polyadenylation signal (Uzan *et al.*, 1984). The protein p97 appears to have a larger transcript of about 4000 nt, as its 3' untranslated region is 1617 nt long (Brown, Rose and Plowman, 1985). No apparent analogies in the untranslated sequences of the various transferrin cDNAs have been noted so far. The homology of nucleotide sequences of the various transferrins is higher than that of the amino acid sequences, indicating that the functional activity of the molecule does not impose strong structural constraints.

Transferrin gene structures

In 1979 the chicken transferrin gene was cloned by Cochet *et al.*, (1979) and found to be composed of 17 exons of about 60–200 base pairs. Exon 1 encodes the 5' end of mRNA, and exon 17 the 3' end of mRNA. The entire messenger is encoded by a genomic region of 10.3 kb (Cochet *et al.*, 1979). The leader sequence is synthesized on the first two exons, unlike other genes. An AT-rich region was found 25 bases upstream from the ovotransferrin cap site, as a possible promoter. More recently, genomic clones for about 70% of the human serum transferrin mRNA sequence were isolated from a liver DNA library (Park *et al.*, 1985). The part of the gene examined so far contains 12 exons of 33–181 base pairs, separated by introns of 700–4900 base pairs. The complete gene seems to have a similar organization to that of chicken, as the exons have identical size and distribution. In the human gene the dimension of the introns is larger than in chicken, making the full gene 24 kb long, about double the size of the avian gene.

Most exons encoding the N-terminal domain of the protein are of similar size to the corresponding exons coding for the C-terminal domain, and the sequences at the border of the corresponding introns are extremely well conserved. These findings allowed the construction of a model showing how the present-day transferrin gene originated by gene duplication (Park et al., 1985).

The p97 gene has been cloned and sequenced (Brown, Rose and Plowman, 1985). It contains at least 16 introns, and spans 26 000 nt. The gene of p97 does not have a consensus TATA box at the 5' flanking region, but has direct repeats that resemble known enhancer elements (Brown, Rose and Plowman, 1985).

The transferrin genes are represented only once in the haploid genome. Previous linkage of serum transferrin variants with chromosomal markers assigned the transferrin gene to chromosome 3. More recently, using an *in situ* hybridization technique applied on man–rodent hybridoma cell lines, it was found that the gene maps on the long arm of chromosome 3 at 21–25 (Yang et al., 1984). The melanotransferrin p97 gene is localized in a nearby site, as detected by *in situ* hybridization studies (Le Beau et al., 1986). Mouse transferrin gene maps on chromosome 9, a homologue of human chromosome 3 (Naylor et al., 1982). Some polymorphisms of the human transferrin gene have been found to be associated with electrophoretic variants of serum transferrin (Schaeffer et al., 1985).

Transferrin gene expression

In humans distinct genes are present for the three transferrin types, i.e. serum, lacto- and melanoma transferrins. In contrast, in chicken the same gene expresses serum and ovotransferrins which have the same amino acid sequence and are encoded by identical mRNAs (Thibodeau, Lee and Palmiter, 1978), and differ only in their carbohydrate moiety. The chicken is an interesting model of how the same gene can express proteins with different functions in different tissues which are under different metabolic controls. Steroid hormones and nutritional iron deficiency are known to modulate the expression of circulating transferrin. In the oviduct, oestrogen and progesterone readily stimulate transferrin synthesis by increasing mRNA transcription (McKnight, Lee and Palmiter, 1980). Oestrogen also affects transferrin synthesis in the liver, but the response is delayed, and is less pronounced than in the oviduct, despite the fact that the liver carries receptors for oestradiol (McKnight et al., 1980). Iron deprivation causes an increase in serum transferrin levels by stimulating synthesis in liver but not in the oviduct (Morgan, 1969). Moreover, in liver, iron and oestrogen have additive effects on transferrin expression, suggesting that they act on different mechanisms of induction (McKnight et al., 1980).

In human and rat the major source of transferrin is liver, where its synthesis is stimulated by nutritional iron deficiency and steroid hormones (Morgan, 1969). In addition, transferrin is expressed in lower amounts by many other tissues (Idzerda *et al.*, 1986). Iron status affects transferrin gene expression in liver, but not in brain, kidney or testis (Idzerda *et al.*, 1986), while in Sertoli cells transferrin synthesis is regulated by various hormones, such as follicle-stimulating hormone (FSH), testosterone and insulin (Skinner and Griswold, 1982). In addition, during development the expression of transferrin mRNA follows strikingly different time courses in various tissues: in liver it steadily increases in fetal life, reaching a plateau shortly after birth, in brain it is low at birth and gradually increases during postnatal development, and in muscle it is maximal just before birth (Levin *et al.*, 1984). A further step in the understanding of transferrin gene expression came from the recent work of Adrian *et al.* (1986), who found in the 5′ flanking region sequences homologous with regulatory elements responding to heavy metals, glucocorticoid receptor and putative acute-phase reaction signal.

Recent studies have shown that the expression of p97 (melanotransferrin) is increased by addition of melanocyte-stimulating hormone to human melanoma cell lines, and that its expression is not co-ordinated with the expression of transferrin receptor (Seligman *et al.*, 1986).

Transferrin enters cells by receptor-mediated endocytosis. It is therefore difficult to distinguish exogenous from endogeneous transferrin. This problem is overcome by the use of cDNA probes, which clearly show that transferrin is synthesized by a large number of different cell types, such as T lymphocytes (Lum, Yang and Bowman, 1985), brain oligodendrocytes (Bloch *et al.*, 1985), muscle (Levin *et al.*, 1984) and testis (Skinner and Griswold, 1982). Moreover, it was reported that transferrin acts as a fetal growth factor in embryonic induction (Ekblom *et al.*, 1983) and as a neurotrophic factor (Beach, Popiela and Festoff, 1983). These findings suggest that transferrin has other functions besides recycling iron for erythropoiesis.

TRANSFERRIN RECEPTOR

Structure of the transferrin receptor

Receptors for transferrin were originally identified in tissues with high iron uptake such as haemoglobin-forming cells and the placenta (Jandl and Katz, 1963; Morgan, 1964; Aisen and Brown, 1979; Seligman, Schleicher and Allen, 1979). The availability of large quantities of placenta permitted the isolation and purification of the receptor (Seligman, Schleicher and Allen, 1979). It is a membrane protein of approximately 180 000 molecular weight (Enns and Sussman, 1981a), and consists of two equal subunits of about 90 000 molecular weight linked by disulphide bond(s) (Wada, Hass and Sussman, 1979; Enns and Sussman, 1981a). The disulphide bridges must lie in proximity to the cell membrane, as treatment of the cells with trypsin releases a peptide of 70 000 molecular weight that binds transferrin. The receptors purified from placenta and reticulocytes (Enns and Sussman, 1981b), and from malignant and non-malignant cells (Stein and Sussman, 1983), have similar proteolytic digest maps. Thus the transferrin receptor is probably identical in all tissues. The transferrin receptor undergoes various post-translational modifications, as it is glycosylated (Enns and Sussman, 1981a; Schneider *et al.*, 1982), phosphorylated (Davis *et al.*, 1986) and has covalently bound fatty acids (Omary and Trowbridge, 1981a). The carbohydrate moiety accounts for about 5% by weight of the receptor (Enns and Sussman, 1981a), and consists of three N-asparagine-linked oligosaccharides, two of the high-mannose type and one of the complex type (Schneider *et al.*, 1982). Phosphorylation, catalysed by protein kinase C, occurs on serine residue(s) on the cytoplasmic part of the molecule, and appears important for regulation of transferrin receptor activity (Davis *et al.*, 1986). Melanoma cells synthesize within minutes an 88 000 molecular weight species with carbohydrate chains of the high-mannose type; later (within hours) this species matures to the final product with high-mannose- and complex-type oligosaccharides and fatty acids (Omary and Trowbridge, 1981b). The half-life of the transferrin receptor (about 60 hours) is longer than that of the linked fatty acids (Omary and Trowbridge, 1981b). The fatty acids may play some role in anchoring the receptor to the membrane, or in recycling the receptor during transferrin-mediated iron uptake.

The receptor binds diferric transferrin with an affinity constant of about 10^9 M^{-1} (Wada, Hass and Sussman, 1979). Its affinity for apotransferrin and monoferric transferrin is lower, but does not appear to differ for the two monoferric types, i.e. with iron on either the N- or the C-terminal binding site (Huebers *et al.*, 1981). Each receptor subunit binds one transferrin molecule (Schneider *et al.*, 1982).

Cloning of transferrin receptor cDNAs (Schneider, Kurkinen and Greaves, 1983; Kuhn, McClelland and Ruddle, 1984; Stearne, Pietersz and Goding, 1985) permitted the elucidation of the amino acid sequence and clarification of the structure (Schneider *et al.*, 1984; McClelland, Kuhn and Ruddle, 1984). The mRNAs encode a peptide of 760 residues, the calculated molecular weight being in good agreement with analytical results (Schneider *et al.*, 1984; McClelland, Kuhn and Ruddle, 1984). The receptor lacks the N-terminal hydrophobic signal sequence present in most membrane and secreted proteins. However, at a short distance from the N-terminus there is a cluster of basic hydrophilic residues followed by a highly hydrophobic region, which probably represent the stop-transfer sequence and transmembrane fragment. Thus the molecule is divided into three domains: the cytoplasmic domain consists of the first 62 amino acids of the N-terminal sequence, and this is followed by the transmembrane domain of 26 amino acids, and finally by the extracellular domain that covers the last 656 amino acids on the C-terminus (Schneider et al., 1984; McClelland, Kuhn and Ruddle, 1984). This is a rather unusual structure for a transmembrane protein, as most are orientated in the opposite way, i.e. with the C-terminus on the cytoplasmic side. The long extracellular domain contains three possible sites for N-linked glycosylation, all of which appear to carry glycan chains. The full sequence has eight cysteines, four around the transmembrane sequence and the remainder in the extracellular domain. The transmembrane Cys-62 is involved in the formation of thioester bonds with fatty acids, and Cys-89 and Cys-98 are involved in interchain bonds (Jing and Trowbridge, 1987). A cluster of three basic residues located close to the transmembrane domain is the likely site of trypsin cleavage.

The cytoplasmic sequence is relatively short in comparison with other transmembrane proteins. It contains four serines as candidates for protein kinase C-mediated phosphorylation, but the enzyme appears to act only on serine 24, which is a long way from the membrane (Davis et al., 1986). A detailed study showed that the transmembrane sequence also functions as a signal for protein insertion into the membrane, and its deletion confines the full receptor to the cytoplasm (Zerial et al., 1986).

A partial amino acid sequence of the murine transferrin receptor has been deduced from cDNA cloning (Stearne, Pietersz and Goding, 1985). It shows a high degree of homology with the human protein, particularly in the transmembrane domain. It differs in having two instead of three glycosylation sites and a lower number of cysteines. In addition, the previously identified trypsin cleavage site is modified, and consequently the extracellular part of the murine receptor is not released by trypsin treatment. The estimated total size of the murine receptor is similar to that of the human receptor, but with a possibly longer cytoplasmic sequence (Stearne, Pietersz and Goding, 1985).

Transcript and gene of the transferrin receptor

Human transferrin receptor cDNAs have been cloned in two laboratories from libraries of placenta and fibroblast cDNAs (Schneider et al., 1984; McClelland, Kuhn and Ruddle, 1984). The sequences obtained are essentially the same, giving further proof that the transferrin receptor is the same in all human cells. The cDNAs cloned by Schneider et al. (1984) reach a length of about 5 kb, and appear to cover essentially the full length of the mRNA. It is composed of a 5' non-coding region of about 280 nucleotides, an open reading frame encoding a peptide of 760 amino acids, and an unusually long 3' non-coding region of about 2500 nucleotides. In the 3' non-coding region an initiation codon is present that is apparently not used, as also occurs in the 5' region, where there are several unused polyadenylation signals. It is interesting that the genomic clone obtained by McClelland, Kuhn and Ruddle (1984) is actively expressed, even though it lacks most of the 3' non-coding sequences. The cloned murine transferrin receptor cDNA encodes about half of the coding region (Stearne, Pietersz and Goding, 1985).

Transferrin receptor cDNAs hybridize with a messenger of 4.6–5.5 kb, which is approximately the size of the sequenced cDNAs (Schneider *et al.*, 1984). In addition it was found that murine cDNA hybridizes with a 2.7 kb messenger in some murine myelomas but not in other cell lines (Stearne, Pietersz and Goding, 1985). The significance of this shorter transcript is unknown. Human and murine cDNAs appear to cross-hybridize, but give weak signals (Stearne, Pietersz and Goding, 1985).

The gene for the human transferrin receptor has been identified and almost entirely cloned (McClelland, Kuhn and Ruddle, 1984). It covers a length of more than 31 kb, and is constituted by at least 19 exons of about 70–650 bases. The 5' non-coding region of the receptor cDNA is encoded by the first exon, and most of all the 3' non-coding region is encoded by a single exon (McClelland, Kuhn and Ruddle, 1984). The organization of the gene was studied by heteroduplex analysis, and the precise localization of exon–intron splicing sites is not yet available.

Previous immunological analyses on hybrid cell lines showed that the transferrin receptor is mapped on chromosome 3 (Enns *et al.*, 1983). A more recent study using *in situ* hybridization showed that the gene is mapped on the long arm of chromosome 3, at q26.2–ter, and therefore in close proximity to transferrin and p97 genes (Rabin *et al.*, 1985). Apparently, a single gene exists for haploid genoma.

Transferrin receptor gene expression

The transferrin receptor is expressed at a high level (up to 250 000 molecules per cell) in immature reticulocytes, but not in mature red cells (Seligman, 1983). In placenta there is a direct correlation between transferrin binding sites and fetal iron requirements (McArdle and Morgan, 1982). These findings indicate that transferrin receptor expression is related to cellular iron requirements. However, a high density of transferrin receptors is found in most actively proliferating cells, malignant or not, that appear to require low amounts of iron (Sutherland *et al.*, 1981). It is therefore not clear whether either transferrin or iron is required for cellular proliferation and differentiation (see Chapter 12). The hypothesis that the transferrin receptor acts mainly on iron transport is substantiated by the findings that iron-chelating agents inhibit cellular proliferation (Gurley and Jett, 1981) in a similar way to blocking by anti-transferrin receptor antibodies (Fitzgerald et al., 1983). However, not all cell types are equally sensitive to the growth-inhibitory effect of anti-transferrin receptor antibodies (Trowbridge et al., 1984; see Chapter 16).

There is clear evidence that most cell types express transferrin receptors, and that this expression can be regulated. In general, a highly proliferative status of cells is associated with a high density of transferrin receptors (Sutherland et al., 1981). In addition, the level of intracellular iron regulates the expression of the receptor, as iron-chelating agents induce, and iron and haemin depress, its synthesis (Testa, 1985). This pattern of regulation appears to be analogous to that of low-density lipoprotein receptors, whose expression is regulated by cytoplasmic levels of cholesterol metabolites.

The molecular mechanisms of regulation of transferrin receptor expression are now under analysis in various laboratories. Louache et al. (1985) showed that the effects of iron on transferrin receptor synthesis are abrogated by actinomycin D, and Mattia et al. (1984) found that the amounts of translatable transferrin receptor mRNA are directly related to intracellular iron levels. Moreover, Rao et al. (1986) showed that desferrioxamine treatment of K562 cells causes an early increase in transferrin receptor mRNA, as detected by hybridization with a cDNA probe, while haemin treatment has the opposite effect. Transcriptional assays on isolated nuclei indicate that iron acts at a transcriptional level (Rao et al., 1986). Ho, King and Sartorelli (1986) studied transferrin gene expression during chemically induced differentiation of HL-60 leukaemic cells, and found that mRNA levels decreased earlier than those of the protein; moreover, they indicated that the decrease in transferrin receptor expression which occurs when cells reach the confluent status (Pelosi-Testa et al., 1986) is associated with a lowered level of mRNA (Ho, King and Sartorelli, 1986). In addition, Hirata et al. (1986) found detectable levels of the receptor protein and transcript in active alveolar macrophages, but not in circulating monocytes. The 3' untranslated region of the transferrin receptor mRNA contains potential stem-loop sequences similar to the iron-response element (IRE) of ferritin mRNA (Casey et al., 1988; Müllner and Kühn, 1988; see also p. 61). These IREs probably protect the mRNA from degradation during iron limitation, perhaps, as with iron regulation of ferritin translation, by the binding of a cytoplasmic protein to the IRE.

The present data, therefore, indicate that both iron and proliferative status regulate transferrin receptor expression and they appear to act on different mechanisms, as deletion of sequences on the 3' non-coding region of the cDNA abolishes the iron-dependent, but not the proliferation dependent, regulation (Owen and Kuhn, 1987).

To accomplish their function, the receptors, after binding transferrin, cluster in plasma membrane coated pits, enter the cell via coated vesicles, and move to endosomes, where the acidic pH induces iron release. The receptor–transferrin complex returns to the cell surface, where transferrin is released and the receptor used for another cycle (Klausner, Harford and Van Renswoude, 1984a; see also Chapter 3). The functional activity of the receptor is therefore also modulated by the rate of cycling. For instance, addition of tumour-promoting phorbol esters to K562 cells causes a rapid internalization of receptors, resulting in a decreased cell surface expression (Klausner, Harford and Van Renswoude, 1984b). Fibroblasts exposed to mitogens rapidly increase the level of surface expression of transferrin receptors, probably by redistribution from internal compartments to the plasma membrane (Davis and Czech, 1986).

The understanding of transferrin receptor regulation appears to be a complex matter, as many agents affect the cellular redistribution and cycling in vesicles, and, moreover, this receptor appears to recycle in at least two different pathways (Stein and Sussman, 1986).

CONCLUSION

Present data on molecular characteristics of human ferritins, transferrins and the transferrin receptor are summarized in Table 4.1. These three families of proteins have different primary structures and gene organizations; thus they are structurally and genetically unrelated. However, the genes for transferrin, transferrin receptor and a (pseudo) gene for ferritin are clustered near the end of the long arm of chromosome 3, and the expression of all of these proteins appears to be regulated by intracellular

TABLE 4.1 Molecular characteristics of human iron-binding proteins

	Protein[a] (kDa)	Subunit (amino acids)	Transcript (kb)	Gene (kb)	Exons (number)	Gene localization (chromosome)	Iron effect on protein synthesis
Ferritins							
H	550	182	1.0	3	4	11	Positive
L	480	174	1.0	3	4	19	Positive
Transferrins							
Serum	88	679	2.4	24	17	3q21–25	Negative
Melano-	97	719	3.8	26	16	3q28–29	ND
Lacto-	80	703	ND	ND	ND	3q21–23	ND
Transferrin receptor	180	760	4.9	31	19	3q26.2–qter	Negative

ND = not determined.
[a]Excluding leader sequences of transferrins.

iron levels. It is possible that the regulation of their synthesis is somehow related, and they may share some common mechanisms. Moreover, the expression of transferrin receptor, ferritins, and p97 is affected by malignant transformation and cellular proliferation, suggesting again that they respond to common regulatory factors. However, detailed and integrated analyses of the expression of these proteins in the same cell systems and in the same circumstances are only now starting to be performed and will probably help to clarify the mechanisms underlying the expression of these genes.

The use of molecular biology techniques has clearly established that human transferrins and ferritins form classes of genetically distinct proteins with closely related structures. The possibility of manipulating the genes encoding for these proteins, and performing site-directed mutagenesis on them, will probably permit clarification of the functional significance of the presence of two gene products for ferritin (H and L chain) and of three gene products for transferrin (serum, lacto- and melanotransferrin).

REFERENCES

Addison, J. M., Fitton, J. E., Lewis, W. G., May, K., and Harrison, P. M. (1983). The amino acid sequence of human liver apoferritin, *FEBS Lett.*, **164**, 139–44.

Adrian, G. S., Korinek, B. W., Bowman, B. H., and Yang, F. (1986). The human transferrin gene: 5' region contains conserved sequences which match the control elements regulated by heavy metals, glucocorticoids and acute phase reaction, *Gene*, **49**, 167–75.

Aisen, P., and Brown, E. B. (1979). Structure and function of transferrin, *Prog. Hematol.*, **9**, 25–6.

Aisen, P., and Listowsky, I. (1980). Iron transport and storage proteins, *Annu. Rev. Biochem.*, **49**, 357–93.

Anderson, B. F., Baker, H. M., Dodson, E. J., Norris, G. E., Rumball, S. V., Waters, J. M., and Baker, E. N. (1987). Structure of human lactoferrin at 3.2 Å resolution, *Proc. Natl Acad. Sci. USA*, **84**, 1769–73.

Arosio, P., Adelman, T. G., and Drysdale, J. W. (1978). On ferritin heterogeneity—further evidence for heteropolymers, *J. Biol. Chem.*, **253**, 4451–8.

Arosio, P., Levi, S., Gabri, E., Stefanini, S., Finazzi-Agro, A., and Chiancone, E. (1984). Properties of ferritin from the earth worm *Ochtolasion complanatum*, *Biochim. Biophys. Acta*, **787**, 264–9.

Arosio, P., Ponzone, A., Ferrero, R., Renoldi, I., and Levi, S. (1986). Characteristics of ferritins in human milk secretions: similarities to serum and tissue isoferritins, *Clin. Chim. Acta*, **161**, 201–8.

Azari, P. R., and Feeney, R. E. (1961). The resistances of conalbumin and its iron complex to physical and chemical treatments, *Arch. Biochem. Biophys.*, **92**, 44–52.

Aziz, N., and Munro, H. N. (1986). Both subunits of rat liver ferritin are regulated at translational level by iron induction, *Nucl. Acids Res.*, **14**, 915–27.

Aziz, N., and Munro, H. N. (1987). Iron regulates ferritin mRNA translation

through a segment of its 5' untranslated region, *Proc. Natl. Acad. Sci. USA*, **84**, 8478–82.
Bailey, S., Evans, R. W., Garratt, R. C., *et al.* (1988). Molecular structure of serum transferrin at 3.3 Å resolution. *Biochemistry*, **27**, 5804–12.
Beach, R. L., Popiela, H., and Festoff, B. W. (1983). The identification of neurotrophic factor as transferrin, *FEBS Lett.*, **156**, 151–6.
Bloch, B., Popovici, T., Levin, M. J., Tuil, D., and Kahn, A. (1985). Transferrin gene expression visualized in oligodendrocytes of the rat brain by using *in situ* hybridization and immunohistochemistry, *Proc. Natl Acad. Sci. USA*, **82**, 6706–10
Bolognesi, M., Gatti, G., Levi, S., Gabri, E., and Arosio, P. (1984). Crystallographic data for horse heart ferritin, *FEBS Lett.*, **165**, 63–6.
Bomford, A. B., and Munro, H. N. (1985). Transferrin and its receptor: their roles in cell function, *Hepatology*, **5**, 870–5.
Boyd, D., Vecoli, C., Belcher, D. M., Jain, S. K., and Drysdale, J. W. (1985). Structural and functional relationships of human ferritin H and L chains deduced from cDNA clones, *J. Biol. Chem.*, **260**, 11755–61.
Brown, J. P., Rose, I. M., and Plowman, G. D. (1985). Human melanoma antigen p97, a membrane-associated transferrin homologue. In G. Spik, J. Montreuil, R. R. Crichton, and J. Mazurier (eds) *Proteins of Iron Storage and Transport*, pp. 39–46, Elsevier, Amsterdam.
Cairo, G., Bardella, L., Schiaffonati, L., Arosio, P., Levi, S., and Bernelli-Zazzera, A. (1985). Multiple mechanisms of iron-induced ferritin synthesis of HeLa cells, *Biochem. Biophys. Res. Commun.*, **133**, 314–21.
Cairo, G., Vezzoni, P., Bardella, L., Schiaffonati, L., Rappocciolo, E., Levi, S., Arosio, P., and Bernelli-Zazzera, A. (1986). Regulation of ferritin synthesis in malignant and non-malignant lymphoid cells, *Biochem. Biophys. Res. Commun.*, **139**, 652–7.
Casey, J. L., Hentze, M. W., Koeller, D. M., Caughman, S. W., Rouault, T. A., Klausner, R. D., and Harford, J. B. (1988). Iron-responsive elements: regulatory RNA sequences that control mRNA levels and translation, *Science*, **240**, 924–8.
Chou, C. C., Gatti, R. A., Fuller, M. L., Concannon, P., Wong, A., Chada, S., Davis, R. C., and Salser, W. A. (1986). Structure and expression of ferritin genes in a human promyelocytic cell line that differentiates in vitro, *Mol. Cell. Biol.*, **6**, 566–73.
Cochet, M., Gannon, F., Hen, R., Maroteaux, L., Perrin, F., and Chambon, P. (1979). Organization and sequence studies of the 17-piece chicken conalbumin gene, *Nature*, **282**, 567–74.
Collawn, J. F., and Fish, W. W. (1985). Hydrogen–tritium exchange by apoferritin and ferritin, *Arch. Biochem. Biophys.*, **240**, 242–5.
Costanzo, F., Santoro, C., and Cortese, R. (1984). The structure of human apoferritin genes. In A. Albertini, P. Arosio, E. Chiancone and J. W. Drysdale (eds) *Ferritins and Isoferritins as Biochemical Markers*, pp. 79–85, Elsevier, Amsterdam.
Costanzo, F., Santoro, C., Colantuoni, V., Bensi, G., Raugei, G., Romano, V., and Cortese, R. (1984). Cloning and sequencing of a full length cDNA coding for a human apoferritin H chain: evidence for a multigene family, *EMBO J.*, **3**, 23–7.
Costanzo, F., Colombo, M., Staempflis, S., Santoro, C., Marone, M., Frank, R., Delius, H., and Cortese, R. (1986). Structure of gene and pseudogenes of human apoferritin H, *Nucl. Acids Res.*, **14**, 721–36.
Cragg, S. J., Drysdale, J., and Worwood, M. (1985). Genes for the 'H' subunit of human ferritin are present on a number of human chromosomes, *Hum. Genet.*, **71**, 108–12.

Cragg, S. J., Wagstaff, M., and Worwood, M. (1981). Detection of a glycosylated subunit in human serum ferritin, *Biochem. J.*, **199**, 565-71.
Davis, R. J., and Czech, M. P. (1986). Regulation of transferrin receptor expression at the cell surface by insulin-like growth factors, epidermal growth factor and platelet-derived growth factor, *EMBO J.*, **5**, 653-8.
Davis, R. J., Johnson, G. L., Kelleher, D. J., Anderson, J. K., Mole, J. E., and Czech, M. P. (1986). Identification of serine 24 as the unique site on the transferrin receptor phosphorylated by protein kinase C., *J. Biol. Chem.*, **261**, 9034-41.
Diamond, A., Cooper, G. M., Ritz, J., and Lane, M. A. (1983). Identification and molecular cloning of the Human Blym transforming gene activated in Burkitt's lymphomas, *Nature*, **305**, 112-15.
Didsbury, J. R., Theil, E. C., Kaufman, R. E., and Dickey, L. F. (1986). Multiple red cell ferritin mRNAs, which code for an abundant protein in the embryonic cell type, analyzed by cDNA sequence and by primer extension of the 5' untranslated regions, *J. Biol. Chem.*, **261**, 949-55.
Dörner, M. H., Silverstone, A. E., De Sostoa, A., Munn, G., and de Sousa, M. (1983). Relative subunit composition of the ferritin synthesised by selected human lymphomyleloid cell populations, *Exp. Hematol.*, **11**, 866-72.
Dörner, M. H., Salfeld, J., Will, H., Leibold, E. A., Vass, J. K., and Munro, H. N. (1985). Structure of human ferritin light subunit messenger RNA. Comparison with heavy subunit message and functional implications, *Proc. Natl Acad. Sci. USA*, **82**, 3139-43.
Drysdale, J. W., and Munro, H. N. (1966). Regulation of synthesis and turnover in rat liver, *J. Biol. Chem.*, **241**, 3630-4.
Ekblom, P., Thesleff, I., Saxen, L., Miettinen, A., and Timpl, R. (1983). Transferrin as a fetal growth factor: acquisition of responsiveness related to embryonic induction, *Proc. Natl Acad. Sci. USA*, **80**, 2651-5.
Enns, C. A., and Sussman, H. H. (1981a). Physical characterization of the transferrin receptor in human placentae, *J. Biol. Chem.*, **256**, 9820-3.
Enns, C. A., and Sussman, H. H. (1981b). Similarities between the transferrin receptor proteins on human reticulocytes and human placentae, *J. Biol. Chem.*, **256**, 12620-3.
Enns, C. A., Suomalainen, H., Gebhardt, J., Schroder, J., and Sussman, H. H. (1982). Human transferrin receptor: expression of the receptor is assigned to chromosome 3, *Proc. Natl Acad. Sci. USA*, **79**, 3241-5.
Fitzgerald, D. P. P., Trowbridge, I. S., Pastan, I., and Willingham, M. C. (1983). Enhancement of toxicity of antitransferrin receptor antibody–*Pseudomonas* exotoxin conjugated by adenovirus, *Proc. Natl Acad. Sci. USA*, **80**, 4134-8.
Ford, G. C., Harrison, P. M., Rice, D. W., Smith, J. M. A., Treffry, A., White, J. L., and Yariv, J. (1984). Ferritin: design and formation of an iron-storage molecule, *Philos. Trans. R. Soc. Lond. (Biol.)*, **304**, 551-65.
Gorinsky, B., Horsburgh, C., Lindley, P. F., Moss, D. S., Parkar, M., and Watson, J. L. (1979). Evidence for the bilobal nature of diferric rabbit plasma transferrin, *Nature*, **281**, 157-8.
Goubin, G., Goldman, D. S., Luce, J., Neiman, P. E., and Cooper, G. M. (1983). Molecular cloning and nucleotide sequence of a transforming gene detected by transfection of a chicken B-cell lymphoma DNA, *Nature*, **302**, 114-19.
Granick, S. (1942). Ferritin: 1. Physical and chemical properties of horse spleen ferritin, *J. Biol. Chem.*, **146**, 451-61.
Gurley, L. R., and Jett, J. H. (1981). Cell cycle kinetics of Chinese hamster (cho) cells treated with the iron chelating agent picolinic acid, *Cell Tissue Kinet.*, **14**, 269-83.

Harrison, P. M., Clegg, G. A., and May, K. (1980). Ferritin structure and function. In A. Jacobs and M. Worwood (eds) *Iron in Biochemistry and Medicine*, pp. 131–62, Academic Press.
Hentze, M. W., Keim, S., Papadopoulos, P., O'Brien, S., Modi, W., Drysdale, J., Leonard, W. J., Harford, J. B., and Klausner, R. D. (1986). Cloning characterization, expression, and chromosomal localization of a human ferritin heavy-chain gene, *Proc. Natl Acad. Sci. USA*, **83**, 7226–30.
Hentze, M. W., Rouault, T. A., Caughman, S. W., Dancis, A., Harford, J. B., and Klausner, R. D. (1987). A *cis*-acting element is necessary and sufficient for translational regulation of human ferritin expression in response to iron, *Proc. Natl. Acad. Sci. USA*, **84**, 6730–4.
Hirata, T., Bitterman, P. B., Mornex, J. F., and Crystal, R. G. (1986). Expression of the transferrin receptor gene during the progress of mononuclear phagocyte maturation, *J. Immunol.*, **136**, 1339–45.
Ho, P. T. C., King, I., and Sartorelli, A. C. (1986). Transcriptional regulation of the transferrin receptor in differentiating HL-60 leukemic cells, *Biochem. Biophys. Res. Commun.*, **138**, 995–1000.
Huebers, H. A., Csiba, E., Josephson, B., Huebers, E., and Finch, C. A. (1981). Interaction of diferric human transferrin with reticulocytes, *Proc. Natl Acad. Sci. USA*, **78**, 621–5.
Idzerda, K. L., Huebers, H., Finch, C. A., and McKnight, G. S. (1986). Rat transferrin gene expression: tissue-specificity regulation by iron deficiency, *Proc. Natl Acad. Sci. USA*, **83**, 3723–7.
Jain, S. K., Barrett, K. J., Boyd, D., Favreau, M. F., Crampton, J., and Drysdale, J. W. (1985a). Ferritin H and L chains are derived from different multigene families, *J. Biol. Chem.*, **260**, 11762–8.
Jain, S. K., Crampton, J., Gonzalez, I. L., Schmickel, R. D., and Drysdale, J. W. (1985b). Complementarity between ferritin H mRNA and 28 S ribosomal RNA, *Biochem. Biophys. Res. Commun.*, **131**, 863–7.
Jandl, J. H., and Katz, J. H. (1963). The plasma-to-cell cycle of transferrin, *J. Clin. Invest.*, **42**, 314–26.
Jeltsch, J. M., and Chambon, P. (1982). The complete nucleotide sequence of the chicken ovotransferrin mRNA, *Eur. J. Biochem.*, **122**, 291–5.
Jing, S., and Trowbridge, I. S. (1987). Identification of the intermolecular disulfide bonds of the human transferrin receptor and its lipid attachment site, *EMBO J.*, **6**, 327–31.
Kilar, F., and Simon, I. (1985). The effect of iron binding on the conformation of transferrin. A small angle X-ray scattering study, *Biophys. J.*, **48**, 799–802.
Klausner, R. D., Harford, J. B., and Van Renswoude, J. (1984a). Binding of apotransferrin to K562: explanation of the transferrin cycle, *Proc. Natl Acad. Sci. USA*, **80**, 2263–6.
Klausner, R. D., Harford, J. B., and Van Renswoude, J. (1984b). Rapid internalization of the transferrin receptor in K562 cells is triggered by ligand binding or treatment with a phorbol ester, *Proc. Natl Acad. Sci. USA*, **81**, 3005–9.
Kuhn, L. C., McClelland, A., and Ruddle, F. H. (1984). Gene transfer, expression and molecular cloning of the human transferrin receptor gene, *Cell*, **37**, 95–103.
Le Beau, M. M., Diaz, M. O., Plowman, G. D., Brown, J. P., and Rowley, J. D. (1986). Chromosomal sublocalization of human p97 melanoma antigen, *Hum. Genet.*, **72**, 294–6.
Lebo, R. V., Kan, Y. W., Cheung, M. C., Jain, S. K., and Drysdale, J. (1985). Human ferritin light chain gene sequences mapped to several sorted chromosomes, *Human Genet.*, **71**, 325–8.

Leibold, E. A., and Munro, H. N. (1988) Cytoplasmic protein binds *in vitro* to a highly conserved sequence in the 5' untranslated region of ferritin heavy- and light-subunit mRNAs, *Proc. Natl. Acad. Sci.*, **85**, 2171–5.

Leibold, E. A., Aziz, N. N., Brown, A. J., and Munro, H. N. (1984). Conservation in rat liver of light and heavy subunit sequences of mammalian ferritins. Presence of unique octapeptide, *J. Biol. Chem.*, **259**, 4327–34.

Levi, S., Cesareni, G., Arosio, P., Lorenzetti, R., Soria, M., Sollazzo, M., Albertini, A., and Cortese, R. (1987). Characterization of human ferritin H chain synthetized in Escherichia coli, *Gene*, **51**, 267–72.

Levi, S., Luzzago, A., Cesareni, G., Lozzi, A., Franceschinelli, F., Albertini, A., and Arosio, P. (1988). Mechanism of ferritin iron uptake: activity of the H-chain and deletion mapping of the ferro-oxidase site. *J. Biol. Chem.*, **263**, 18086–92.

Levin, M. J., Tuil, D., Uzan, G., Dreyfus, J. C., and Kahn, A. (1984). Expression of the transferrin gene during development of non-hepatic tissues: High levels of transferrin mRNA in fetal muscle and adult brain, *Biochem. Biophys. Res. Commun.*, **122**, 212–17.

Louache, F., Pelosi, E., Titeux, M., Peschle, C., and Testa, U. (1985). Molecular mechanisms regulating the synthesis of transferrin receptors and ferritin in human erythroleukaemic cell lines, *FEBS Lett.*, **183**, 223–7.

Lum, J. B., Yang, F., and Bowman, B. H. (1985). Molecular biology of the human transferrin gene. In G. Spik, J. Montreuil, R. R. Crichton, and J. Mazurier (eds) *Proteins of Iron Storage and Transport*, pp. 357–60, Elsevier, Amsterdam.

Luzzago, A., Arosio, P., Iacobello, C., Ruggeri, G., Capucci, L., Brocchi, E., De Simone, F., Gamba, D., Gabri, E., Levi, S., and Albertini, A. (1986). Immunochemical characterization of human liver and heart ferritins with monoclonal antibodies, *Biochim. Biophys. Acta*, **872**, 61–71.

MacGillivray, R. T., Mendez, E., Shewale, J. G., Sinha, S. K., Lineback-Zins, J., and Brew, K. (1983). The primary structure of human serum transferrin. The structures of seven cyanogen bromide fragments and the assembly of the complete structure, *J. Biol. Chem.*, **258**, 3543–53.

Martin, A. W., Huebers, E., Huebers, H., Webb, J., and Finch, C. A. (1984). A mono-sited transferrin from a representative deuterostome: the ascidian *Pyura stolonifera* (subphylum urochordata), *Blood*, **64**, 1047–52.

Mattia, E., Rao, K., Shapiro, D. S., Sussman, H. H., and Klausner, R. D. (1984). Biosynthetic regulation of the human transferrin receptor by desferrioxamine in K562 cells, *J. Biol. Chem.*, **259**, 2689–92.

May, W. S., and Cuatrecasas, P. (1985). Transferrin receptor: its biological significance, *J. Membr. Biol.*, **88**, 205–15.

McArdle, M. J., and Morgan, E. H. (1982). Transferrin and iron movements in rat conceptus during gestation, *J. Reprod. Fertil.*, **66**, 529–36.

McClelland, A., Kuhn, L. C., and Ruddle, F. H. (1984). The human transferrin receptor gene: genomic organisation and the complete primary structure of the receptor deduced from a cDNA sequence, *Cell*, **39**, 267–74.

McGill, J. E., Boyd, D., Barrett, K. J., Drysdale, J. W., and Moore, C. M. (1984). Localization of ferritin H (heavy) and L (light) subunits by *in situ* hybridization, *Am. J. Hum. Genet.*, **36**, 146S.

McGill, J. R., Naylor, S. L., Sakaguchi, A. Y., Moore, C. M., Boyd, D., Barrett, K. J., Shows, T. B., and Drysdale, J. W. (1987). Human ferritin H and L sequences lie on ten different chromosomes, *Hum. Genet.*, **76**, 66–70.

McKnight, G. S., Lee, D. C., and Palmiter, R. D. (1980). Transferrin gene expression. Regulation of mRNA in chick liver by steroid hormones and iron deficiency, *J. Biol. Chem.*, **255**, 148–53.

McKnight, G. S., Lee, D. C., Hemmaplardh, D., Finch, C. A., and Palmiter, R. D.

(1980). Transferrin gene expression. Effects of nutritional iron deficiency, *J. Biol. Chem.*, **255**, 144–7.

Menozzi, F. D., Hanotte, O., and Miller, A. O. A. (1985). Stimulation of protein accumulation in HeLa cells by inhibitors of DNA replication, *FEBS Lett.*, **193**, 49–53.

Metz-Boutigue, M. H., Jolles, J., Mazurier, J., Schoentgen, F., Legrand, D., Spik, G., Montreuil, J., and Jolles, P. (1984). Human lactotransferrin: amino acid sequence and structural comparisons with other transferrins, *Eur. J. Biochem.*, **145**, 659–76.

Montreuil, J., Mazurier, J., Legrand, D., and Spik, G. (1985). Human lactotransferrin: structure and function. In G. Spik, J. Montreuil, R. R. Crichton, and J. Mazurier (eds) *Proteins of Iron Storage and Transport*, pp. 25–38, Elsevier, Amsterdam.

Morgan, E. H. (1964). Interaction between rabbit, human and rat transferrin and reticulocytes, *Br. J. Haematol.*, **10**, 442–52.

Morgan, E. H. (1969). Factors affecting the synthesis of transferrin by rat liver slices, *J. Biol. Chem.*, **244**, 4193–9.

Müllner, E. W., and Kühn, L. C. (1988). A stem-loop in the 3' untranslated region mediates iron-dependent regulation of transferrin receptor mRNA stability in the cytoplasm, *Cell*, **53**, 815–25.

Munro, H. N., and Linder, M. C. (1978). Ferritin: Structure, biosynthesis and role in iron metabolism, *Physiol. Rev.*, **58**, 314–96.

Naylor, S. L., Elliott, R. W., Brown, J. A., and Shows, T. B. (1982). Mapping of aminoacylase-1 and β-galactosidase-A to homologous regions of human chromosome 3 and mouse chromosome 9 suggests location of additional genes, *Am. J. Hum. Genet.*, **34**, 235–44.

Omary, M. B., and Trowbridge, I. S. (1981a) Covalent binding of fatty acid to the transferrin receptor in cultured human cells, *J. Biol. Chem.*, **256**, 4715–18.

Omary, M. B., and Trowbridge, I. S. (1981b). Biosynthesis of the human transferrin receptor in cultured cells, *J. Biol. Chem.*, **256**, 12888–92.

Owen, D., and Kuhn, L. C. (1987). Noncoding 3' sequences of the transferrin receptor gene are required for mRNA regulation by iron, *EMBO J.*, **6**, 1287–95.

Park, I., Schaeffer, E., Sidoli, A., Baralle, F. E., Cohen, G. N., and Zakin, M. M. (1985). Organization of the human transferrin gene: direct evidence that it originated by gene duplication, *Proc. Natl Acad. Sci. USA*, **82**, 3149–53.

Pelosi-Testa, E., Testa, U., Samoggia, P., Salvo, G., Camagna, A., and Peschle, C. (1986). Expression of transferrin receptor in human erythroleukemic lines: regulation in the plateau and exponential phase of growth, *Cancer Res.*, **46**, 5330–4.

Rabin, M., McClelland, A., Kuhn, L., and Ruddle, F. H. (1985). Regional localization of human transferrin receptor gene to 3q26.2 → ter, *Am. J. Hum. Genet.*, **37**, 1112–16.

Rao, K., Harford, J. B., Rouault, T., McClelland, A., Ruddle, F. H., and Klausner, R. D. (1986). Transcriptional regulation by iron of the gene for the transferrin receptor, *Mol. Cell. Biol.*, **6**, 236–40.

Righetti, P. G., Gelfi, C., Bossi, M. L., and Boschetti, E. (1987). Isoelectric focusing and non-isoelectric precipitation of ferritin in immobilized pH gradients: an improved protocol overcoming protein–matrix interactions, *Electrophoresis*, **8**, 62–70.

Rose, I. M., Plowman, G. D., Teplow, D. B., Dreyer, W. J., Hellstrom, K. E., and Brown, J. P. (1986). Primary structure of the human melanoma-associated antigen p97 (melanotransferrin) deduced from the mRNA sequence, *Proc. Natl Acad. Sci. USA*, **83**, 1261–5.

Rouault, T. A., Hentze, M. W., Caughman, S. W., Harford, J. B., and Klausner, R. D.

(1988). Binding of a cytosolic protein to the iron-responsive element of human ferritin messenger RNA, *Science*, **241**, 1207–10.
Sampietro, M., Cairo, G., Piperno, A., Fargion, S., Bardella, L., Schåaffonati, L., and Fiorelli, G. (1987). Analysis of the genes for transferrin, transferrin receptor as well as H and L subunits of ferritin in idiopathic hemochromatosis, *Ric. Clin. Lab.*, **17**, 209–214.
Santambrogio, P., Cozzi. A., Levi, S., and Arosio, P. (1987). Human serum ferritin G peptide is recognized by anti-L ferritin subunit antibodies and concanavalin A, *Br. J. Haematol.*, **64**, 235–7.
Santoro, C., Marone, M., Ferrone, M., Costanzo, F., Colombo, M., Minganti, C., Cortese, R., and Silengo, L. (1986). Cloning of the gene coding for human L apoferritin, *Nucl. Acids Res.*, **14**, 2863–76.
Sarra, R., and Lindley, P. F. (1986). Preliminary X-ray data for an N-terminal fragment of rabbit serum transferrin, *J. Mol. Biol.*, **188**, 727–8.
Schaeffer, E., Park, I., Cohen, G. N., and Zakin, M. M. (1985). Organization of the human serum transferrin gene. In G. Spik, J. Montreuil, R. R. Crichton, and J. Mazurier (eds) *Proteins of Iron Storage and Transport*, pp. 361–4, Elsevier, Amsterdam.
Schneider, C., Kurkinen, M., and Greaves, M. (1983). Isolation of cDNA clones for the human transferrin receptor, *EMBO J.*, **2**, 2259–63.
Schneider, C., and Williams, J. C. (1985). Molecular dissection of the human transferrin receptor, *J. Cell Sci.*, **3**, 139–49.
Schneider, C., Sutherland, R., Newman, R., and Greaves, M. (1982). Structural features of cell surface receptor for transferrin that is recognised by the monoclonal antibody OKT9, *J. Biol. Chem.*, **257**, 8516–22.
Schneider, C., Owen, M. J., Banville, D., and Williams, J. G. (1984). Primary structure of human transferrin receptor deduced from the mRNA sequence, *Nature*, **311**, 675–80.
Seligman, P. A. (1983). Structure and function of the transferrin receptor, *Prog. Hematol.*, **13**, 131–47.
Seligman, P. A., Schleicher, R. B., and Allen, R. H. (1979). Isolation and characterization of transferrin receptor from human placenta, *J. Biol. Chem.*, **254**, 9943–7.
Seligman, P. A., Butler, C. D., Massey, E. J., Kaur, J. A., Brown, J. P., Plowman, G. D., Miller, Y., and Jones, C. (1986). The p97 antigen is mapped to the q24-ter region of chromosome 3; the same region as the transferrin receptor, *Am. J. Hum. Genet.*, **38**, 540–8.
Skinner, M. K., and Griswold, M. D. (1982). Secretion of testicular transferrin by cultured Sertoli cells is regulated by hormones and retinoids, *Biol. Reprod.*, **27**, 211–21.
Stearne, P. A., Pietersz, G. A., and Goding, J. W. (1985). cDNA cloning of the murine transferrin receptors: sequence of trans-membrane and adjacent regions, *J. Immunol.*, **134**, 3474–9.
Stefanini, S., Vecchini, P., and Chiancone, E. (1987). On the mechanism of horse spleen apoferritin assembly: a sedimentation velocity and circular dichroism study, *Biochemistry*, **26**, 1831–8.
Stein, B. S., and Sussman, H. H. (1983). Peptide mapping of human transferrin receptor in normal and transformed cells, *J. Biol. Chem.*, **258**, 2668–73.
Stein, B. S., and Sussman, H. H. (1986). Demonstration of two distinct transferrin receptor recycling pathways and transferrin-independent receptor internalization in K562 cells, *J. Biol. Chem.*, **261**, 10319–31.

Stevens, P. W., Dodgson, J. B., and Engel, J. D. (1987). Structure and expression of the chicken ferritin H-subunit gene, *Mol. Cell Biol.*, **7**, 1751–8.
Sutherland, R., Delia, D., Schneider, C., Newman, R., Kemshead, J., and Greaves, M. (1981). Ubiquitous cell surface glycoprotein on tumor cells is proliferation associated receptor for transferrin, *Proc. Natl Acad. Sci. USA*, **78**, 4515–19.
Testa, U. (1985). Transferrin receptor: structure and function, *Curr. Top. Hematol.*, **5**, 127–59.
Thibodeau, S. N., Lee, D. C., and Palmiter, R. D. (1978). Identical precursors for serum transferrin and egg white conalbumin, *J. Biol. Chem.*, **253**, 3771–4.
Trowbridge, I. S., Newman, R. A., Domingo, D. L., and Sauvage, C. (1984). Transferrin receptors: Structure and function, *Biochem. Pharmacol.*, **6**, 925–32.
Uzan, G., Frain, M., Park, I., Besmond, C., Maessen, G., Trepat, J. S., Zakin, M. M., and Kahn, A. (1984). Molecular cloning and sequence analysis of cDNA for human transferrin, *Biochem. Biophys. Res. Commun.*, **119**, 273–81.
Vezzoni, P., Levi, S., Gabri, E., Pozzi, M. R., Spinazze, S., and Arosio, P. (1986). Ferritins in malignant and non-malignant lymphoid cells, *Br. J. Haematol.*, **62**, 105–10.
Wada, H. D., Hass, P. E., and Sussman, H. H. (1979). Transferrin in human placental brush border membranes, *J. Biol. Chem.*, **254**, 12629–35.
Wardeska, J. G., Viglione, B., and Chasteen, N. D. (1986). Metal ion complexes of apoferritin, evidence for initial binding in the hydrophilic channels, *J. Biol. Chem.*, **261**, 6677–83.
Williams, J. (1985). The structure of transferrins. In G. Spik, J. Montreuil, R. R. Crichton, and J. Mazurier (eds) *Proteins of Iron Storage and Transport*, p. 13, Elsevier, Amsterdam.
Williams, J., Elleman, T. C., Kingston, I. B., Wilkins, A. G., and Kuhn, K. A. (1982). The primary structure of hen ovotransferrin, *Eur. J. Biochem.*, **122**, 297–303.
Wustfeld, C., and Crichton, R. R. (1982). The amino acid sequence of human spleen apoferritin, *FEBS Lett.*, **150**, 43–8.
Yang, F., Lum, J. B., McGill, J. R., Moore, C. M., Naylor S. L., van Bragt, P. H., Baldwin, W. D., and Bowman, B. H. (1984). Human transferrin: cDNA characterization and chromosomal localization, *Proc. Natl Acad. Sci. USA*, **81**, 2752–6.
Zahringer, J., Baliga, B. S., and Munro, H. N. (1976). Novel mechanism for translational control in regulation of ferritin synthesis by iron, *Proc. Natl Acad. Sci. USA*, **73**, 857–61.
Zerial, M., Melancon, P., Schneider, C., and Garoff, H. (1986). The transmembrane segment of the human transferrin receptor functions as a signal peptide, *EMBO J.*, **5**, 1543–50.

Iron in Immunity, Cancer and Inflammation
Edited by M. de Sousa and J. H. Brock
© 1989 John Wiley & Sons Ltd.

5
Iron and Cells of the Immune System

J. H. Brock
University Department of Bacteriology and Immunology, Western Infirmary, Glasgow G11 6NT, Scotland

A decade ago a review of the interaction of iron and iron-binding proteins with cells of the immune system would have run to little more than a page or two. However, the past ten years have seen an enormous increase in the interaction between biochemists with an interest in iron metabolism and immunologists who wished to understand in more detail how immunological phenomena might be explained at the cellular and molecular level. This has led not only to a realization that iron and iron-binding proteins play a role in immune function but, perhaps more importantly, also to an understanding of how and why this is so. This chapter will cover two aspects of these developments. Firstly, it will describe how iron and iron-binding proteins interact with cells involved in the immune system (mainly lymphocytes, macrophages and neutrophils). Secondly, it will discuss how iron affects immune function.

THE INTERACTION OF IRON AND IRON-BINDING PROTEINS WITH CELLS OF THE IMMUNE SYSTEM

Lymphocytes

Lymphocytes play a number of diverse roles in the immune system, many of them mediated by distinct cell subsets. A common feature of almost all lymphocyte activities is, however, their need to undergo a process of activation and proliferation in order to give rise to the daughter effector cells. It has become evident in recent years that iron-binding proteins can affect these events.

Transferrin and lymphocyte proliferation

A major area of interest in the interaction of iron metabolism and lymphocyte function has been the role of transferrin in lymphocyte proliferation. Although some early studies had suggested that transferrin might be required for lymphocyte proliferation (Vogt, Mishell and Dutton, 1969; Tormey, Imrie and Mueller, 1972), their interpretation was complicated by the uncertain role of the transferrin present in fetal calf serum used in the culture medium. More convincing evidence was provided by Phillips and Azari (1975), who showed that lymphocytes cultured in serum-free medium proliferated in response to phytohaemagglutinin (PHA) when iron-containing transferrin was added to the medium, but not if iron-free (apo) transferrin were used, nor if the iron was added as ferric citrate. The presence of transferrin receptors on PHA-stimulated lymphocytes was first demonstrated by Larrick and Cresswell (1979), and it was subsequently shown that proliferating lymphocytes acquired iron from transferrin by a mechanism similar to that described for other cells (Brock and Rankin, 1981; Hamilton, 1983). Iron uptake was shown to precede DNA synthesis (Brock and Rankin, 1981), probably because production of the iron-containing enzyme ribonucleotide reductase is a rate-limiting step in lymphocyte proliferation (Hoffbrand *et al.*, 1976; Leberman *et al.*, 1984; Kay and Benzie, 1986), and it is now generally agreed that acquisition of iron is essential to allow activated lymphocytes to proceed from G1 to S phase. In common with studies using transformed cell lines, it has been found that the degree of expression of transferrin receptors on lymphocytes is related to proliferative activity. Little binding of transferrin occurs in resting lymphocytes (Brock and Rankin, 1981; Galbraith *et al.*, 1980; Khalfoun *et al.*, 1986), although transferrin receptors may exist intracellularly (Weiel and Hamilton, 1984). Similarly, treatment of mitogen-stimulated lymphocytes with substances that inhibit proliferation such as interferon-α (Besancon, Bourgeade and Testa, 1985), cyclosporine (Prince and John, 1986) or calcium channel-blocking agents (Neckers *et al.*, 1986), also reduces expression of transferrin receptors. The availability of transferrin-bound iron in the extracellular medium also influences expression of transferrin receptors, their number decreasing if the culture medium is supplemented with additional iron (Ward *et al.*, 1984) and increasing if iron availability is reduced by addition of a high-affinity iron-chelating agent such as picolinic acid (Pelosi *et al.*, 1986).

Blockade of transferrin-mediated iron uptake inhibits lymphocyte proliferation. Anti-transferrin receptor monoclonal antibodies that block transferrin binding and iron uptake in activated lymphocytes inhibit proliferation, whereas antibodies that bind to the transferrin receptor but do not block transferrin binding are without effect (Mendelsohn, Trowbridge and Castagnola, 1983; Brock, Mainou-Fowler and Webster, 1986; Taetle, Castagnola and Mendelsohn, 1986; Kemp *et al.*, 1987). These effects are discussed in more detail in Chapter 16. Similarly, proliferation of murine lymphocytes in medium containing fetal calf serum can be blocked by addition of mouse apotransferrin, which presumably binds to the murine transferrin receptors and prevents iron uptake from the more weakly bound bovine transferrin in the medium (Brock, Mainou-Fowler and Webster, 1986).

Is transferrin the obligatory iron donor to proliferating lymphocytes? While many studies have reported that other iron donors such as chelates either cannot support proliferation or are much less effective (Phillips and Azari, 1975; Brock, 1981; Mendelsohn, Trowbridge and Castagnola, 1983), others have reported good proliferation in the absence of transferrin (Tanno and Takashima, 1982; Titeux *et al.*, 1984). The reasons for these differences are not clear, but may be explained in some cases by the fact that lymphocytes can themselves synthesize transferrin (see below), which may then mediate proliferation. Although chelates such as nitrilotriacetate and citrate donate large amounts of iron to lymphocytes (Brock and Rankin, 1981), it is possible that they may be toxic to the cells, particularly if polymers are present (Soyano, Fernandez and Romano, 1985), as much of this iron is subsequently found in an insoluble intracellular (or perhaps membrane-bound) form (A. Djeha and J. H. Brock, unpublished observations). Excess ferric citrate also reduces the cloning efficiency of human memory CD4+ and cytotoxic CD8+ T cells, but not of CD8− helper cells (Good *et al.*, 1986; Good, Powell and Halliday, 1987). However, the lipophilic iron chelator pyridoxal isonicotinoyl hydrazone (PIH) can support lymphocyte proliferation (Brock and Stevenson, 1987) and is known to donate iron to cells by a transferrin-independent mechanism (Ponka, Schulman and Wilczynska, 1982). Furthermore, a low-affinity iron-uptake system not involving transferrin has recently been described in leukaemic cells (Basset, Quesneau and Zwiller, 1986) and might also operate in lymphocytes if large quantities of non-transferrin-bound iron are present, e.g. in idiopathic haemochromatosis.

The induction of transferrin receptor expression is generally thought to be dependent upon depletion of intracellular iron pools (see Chapter 3). In PHA-stimulated T lymphocytes, expression of transferrin receptors is dependent upon prior expression of interleukin-2 (IL-2) receptors (Tac) and the subsequent binding of IL-2 itself (Hamilton, 1982; Neckers and Cossman, 1983). How this then triggers transferrin receptor expression is not known, although Pelosi *et al.* (1986) have proposed that proliferation acts as a stimulus for synthesis of transferrin receptors, and their actual expression is then determined by iron availability rather than by proliferation *per se*. Recent studies on the molecular biology of the transferrin receptor, discussed in Chapter 4, tend to support this proposal. However, a study by Kumagai *et al.* (1988) has shown that while IL-2 is required for production of transferrin receptor mRNA in PHA-stimulated lymphocytes, in phorbol ester-stimulated cells, transferrin receptor mRNA expression occurs by an IL-2 independent mechanism.

One feature of transferrin receptor expression on activated lymphocytes that has aroused comment is the fact that the number of receptors expressed is very large in relation to the amount of iron taken up, particularly if comparison is made with erythroid precursors (Brock and Mainou-Fowler, 1983; Young and Bomford, 1984), and indeed the amount of iron taken up by lymphocytes is not necessarily related to the number of transferrin receptors expressed (Bomford et al., 1983). It has been suggested that this hyperexpression of transferrin receptors may permit normal immune function to be maintained when transferrin saturation is reduced, e.g. in inflammation or iron deficiency. However, it must be remembered that lymphocyte activation *in vivo* probably occurs mainly in the spleen or lymph nodes, and that transferrin saturation in these environments may not be the same as in plasma. The fact that activated CD4+ (helper) T lymphocytes synthesize transferrin (Lum et al., 1986) suggests that some local control of the supply of transferrin-bound iron might occur. Clearly the large amount of *in vitro* work carried out on the role of iron and transferrin in lymphocyte proliferation needs to be complemented with *in vivo* studies.

The foregoing discussion has dealt with the role of iron in lymphocyte proliferation in general, nearly all the data relating to human or murine cells stimulated with the T cell mitogens PHA or concanavalin A. A similar requirement for transferrin has been reported for mixed lymphocyte reactions (Rammensee et al., 1985; Kemp et al., 1987) and B lymphocyte proliferation (Brock, 1981; Neckers, Yenokida and James, 1984). However, some immunoglobulin synthesis by B cells appears to occur in advance of expression of transferrin receptors (Neckers, Yenokida and James, 1984). With regard to T cell subsets it is known that cloning efficiency is differentially affected by non-transferrin-bound iron (see above), but there is otherwise little information on whether the degree of iron saturation of transferrin can regulate the ratio of lymphocyte subsets. Preliminary experiments have, however, shown that when murine lymphocytes respond to concanavalin A the CD4/CD8 ratio increases in the presence of transferrin 80% saturated with iron, but remains unchanged at 50% or lower iron saturation (C. Harrigan and J. H. Brock, unpublished). Further work in this area would be of interest.

Other effects of transferrin on lymphocyte activation

While it is generally agreed that DNA synthesis is the main event dependent upon transferrin and/or iron in lymphocyte function, there is evidence that some other events may also be affected. In some cases, it may be that other cellular metabolic events are also iron-dependent, and this is discussed in Chapter 12. However, it has also been proposed that binding of transferrin to its receptor is in itself a proliferation-promoting signal (Brock and Mainou-Fowler, 1983). This now seems unlikely given that, as mentioned above, the chelator PIH can promote proliferation by donating iron via a transferrin-independent route (Brock and Stevenson, 1987). However, Navas *et al.* (1986) have identified a diferric transferrin reductase in cell membranes which can act upon receptor-bound transferrin and stimulate cell growth, and it is possible that other forms of iron, including Fe–PIH, might have a similar effect. A possibly related mechanism involving the production of reactive oxygen intermediates has been demonstrated by Novogrodsky *et al.* (1982). There is also evidence that iron and/or transferrin may control events prior to Tac expression: Carotenuto *et al.* (1986) have reported that stimulated lymphocytes incubated with desferrioxamine expressed less Tac than controls, although Pelosi *et al.* (1986) found no such effect when picolinic acid was used as chelator. Both these studies reported normal production of IL-2 in the presence of chelators. The actual role of iron and transferrin in these events remains to be elucidated.

It has been reported that the inhibitory effect of low-density lipoproteins (LDLs) on lymphocyte proliferation can be reversed by transferrin (Cuthbert and Lipsky, 1984; Scupham, McCarthy and Harmony, 1987), perhaps by effects on the intracellular routing of the relevant receptors. However, part of the inhibitory effect of LDLs appears to be an artifact arising from the presence of EDTA (Cuthbert and Lipsky, 1986).

The role of transferrin and the transferrin receptor in natural killer (NK) activity

A further possible role for the transferrin receptor in lymphocyte function is as a target structure recognized by natural killer (NK) cells. This was originally proposed by Vodinelich *et al.* (1983), who showed that affinity-purified proteolysis fragments of the human transferrin receptor inhibited the killing of K562 cells by NK cells. Subsequent studies have produced conflicting results. Some workers have shown that there is a correlation between the degree of expression of transferrin receptors on target cells and their susceptibility to NK cells (Newman, Warner and Dennert, 1984; Brieva and Stevens, 1984; Lazarus and Baines, 1985), while others have reported contrary findings (Dokhélar *et al.*, 1984; Bridges and Smith, 1985). It has also been suggested that while there may indeed be a correlation between transferrin receptor expression and susceptibility to NK lysis, other target structures such as the low-affinity Fc receptor may also be involved (Perl *et al.*, 1986; Borysiewicz, Graham and Sissons, 1986). The ability of anti-transferrin antibodies to block NK-mediated lysis has led to a proposal that transferrin itself may act as a bridge between target and effector cell (Baines, Lafleur and Holbein, 1983; Alarcon and Fresno, 1985), which would suggest that receptors may also be present, perhaps at low levels, on the NK cells themselves. The reduced activity of NK cells from thalassaemic patients (Akbar et al., 1986, 1987) would support this suggestion. However, Shau, Shen and Golub (1986) have reported that the role of transferrin is to enhance development of NK activity *per se* rather than an involvement in target recognition. Thus the latest evidence tends to suggest that the transferrin receptor may not be a target for NK recognition, or is certainly not the only such structure.

Interaction of ferritin with lymphocytes

Although ferritin is generally considered to be an intracellular iron-storage protein, small amounts are normally present in serum, and levels of serum ferritin increase during iron overload or inflammatory disease. It is therefore of interest that membrane-bound ferritin may be found on lymphocytes (Cragg, Hoy and Jacobs, 1984). These workers found that mainly B cells were involved, and that there was no difference between CD4+ and CD8+ T cells. However, surface ferritin increased following stimulation with PHA (Pattanapanyasat, Hoy and Jacobs, 1987), though whether this is acquired exogenously or is synthesized by the cells themselves is not clear. Although evidence has been presented for the existence of specific ferritin receptors on hepatocytes (Mack, Powell and Halliday, 1983) and on some cell lines (Fargion et al., 1988), there is as yet no good evidence for their existence on lymphocytes. Nevertheless, exposure of lymphocytes to ferritin reduces the proliferative response to T-cell mitogens (Matzner et al., 1979, 1985; Bryan and Leech, 1983), with acidic isoferritins being more active than basic isoferritins (Matzner et al., 1985). Indeed, acidic isoferritin-bearing lymphocytes are reported to act as suppressor cells (Moroz and Kupfer, 1981) and this is discussed in detail in Chapter 13.

Synthesis of iron-transport and iron-storage proteins by lymphocytes

As well as synthesizing transferrin receptors, whose function is discussed above, lymphocytes can synthesize ferritin and transferrin. They do not synthesize lactoferrin although, as discussed in the section on macrophages and in Chapter 10, they may bind this protein.

Synthesis of transferrin was first reported by Soltys and Brody (1970), and has been confirmed by Lum et al. (1986), who detected transferrin mRNA in activated CD4+ lymphocytes. However, transferrin may also be produced by CD8+ cells (Broxmeyer, Lu and Bognacki, 1983; see also Chapters 9 and 10), though this study did not demonstrate the synthesis of transferrin directly. It is possible that transferrin synthesis by lymphocytes represents a regulatory autocrine loop (Lum *et al.*, 1986), and information on the iron saturation of the newly synthesized transferrin would be of interest in this respect.

While it is well established that lymphocytes synthesize ferritin (Dörner *et al.*, 1980), there is some controversy over how synthesis is controlled. Much evidence suggests that in contrast to most other types of cells so far studied, addition of iron to lymphocyte cultures does not increase synthesis (Summers, White and Jacobs, 1975; Summers and Jacobs, 1976; Lema and Sarcione, 1981; Dörner *et al.*, 1983), although iron may decrease the rate of catabolism, thereby increasing intracellular ferritin levels in response to iron (Pattanapanyasat, Hoy and Jacobs, 1988). In studies of this type it is important to check the degree of contamination with monocytes, as these cells synthesize much more ferritin than lymphocytes and show a large increase in response to iron (Summers, White and Jacobs, 1975; Dörner *et al.*, 1983). Synthesis of ferritin by lymphocytes is increased by *in vitro* culture, irrespective of whether or not mitogens are present (Pattanapanyasat, Hoy and Jacobs, 1987, 1988). The stimulus for ferritin synthesis in lymphocytes is intriguing; if exogenous iron is ineffective, this raises the possibility that synthesis is promoted either by a redistribution of intracellular iron pools, or by a totally iron-independent event. It is also noteworthy that lymphocytes, and particularly lymphoblasts, preferentially synthesize the acidic H subunit (Dörner *et al.*, 1980; Cairo *et al.*, 1985; Vezzoni *et al.*, 1986), and the possible significance of this is discussed in Chapter 9.

Pattanapanyasat, Hoy and Jacobs (1987, 1988) have reported that cultured lymphocytes may secrete ferritin. However, there was a concomitant loss of cell viability, which raises the possibility of leakage from moribund cells; and, as discussed below, it may be that any active secretion was due to the presence of small numbers of monocytes.

Macrophages

Whereas interactions between lymphocytes and proteins of iron metabolism have only been recognized in recent years, macrophages have a well-established role in iron metabolism due to their involvement in the catabolism of effete erythrocytes, as well as playing an important part in immune function. However, it is not certain that those macrophages most actively involved in iron recirculation, principally Kupffer cells and macrophages in the red pulp of the spleen, also carry out immunological functions such as antigen processing and presentation. Nevertheless, the phagocytic nature of macrophages means that these cells may acquire iron by a number of different routes, and this will be discussed below.

Expression of transferrin receptors by macrophages

There has been some controversy over whether or not macrophages express transferrin receptors. In non-erythroid cells, expression of transferrin receptors is generally associated with proliferation, and as it is generally agreed that macrophages and monocytes undergo little if any proliferation once they leave the bone marrow, one would not expect these cells to express transferrin receptors to any extent. While expression of transferrin receptors on normal blood monocytes is indeed low or non-existent (Andreesen *et al.*, 1984, 1986; Björn-Rasmussen *et al.*, 1985), Hamilton, Weiel and Adams (1984), using ligand-binding assays, reported low numbers (<1000 per cell) on mouse peritoneal macrophages, and somewhat higher numbers (3400 per cell) on inflammatory macrophages. Nevertheless, these numbers are much lower than those normally expressed on proliferating cells. Expression of transferrin receptors on inflammatory macrophages was decreased by exposure to γ-interferon (Hamilton, Gray and Adams, 1984; Weiel, Adams and Hamilton, 1985), suggesting that the expression may be related to the relative immaturity of inflammatory cells, which may have only recently finished undergoing proliferative activity. In contrast, when normal transferrin receptor-negative human monocytes were cultured *in vitro*, transferrin receptors became detectable by immunofluorescence after 5–6 days (Andreesen *et al.*, 1984; Hirata *et al.*, 1986). These studies did not investigate whether the transferrin receptor-positive populations were undergoing proliferation. However, human peritoneal macrophages from patients undergoing continuous ambulatory peritoneal dialysis for renal failure were found to express transferrin receptors but did not show any proliferative activity (S. J. McGregor and J. H. Brock, unpublished), suggesting that in macrophages, expression of transferrin receptors may not be linked to proliferation. Increased expression of transferrin receptors may be found on monocytes of patients with hereditary haemochromatosis (Björn-Rasmussen *et al.*, 1985), though this does not seem to result in increased iron uptake (Sizemore and Bassett, 1984). Nevertheless, normal alveolar macrophages do express a relatively high level of transferrin receptors (Andreesen *et al.*, 1984; McGowan, Murray and Parrish, 1986; Hirata *et al.*, 1986), and take up transferrin-bound iron (Wyllie, 1977; Sato *et al.*, 1986; McGowan, Murray and Parrish, 1986), which is consistent with the idea that these macrophages are to some extent a self-replicating population which will therefore be undergoing proliferation.

The above-mentioned studies all refer to transferrin receptors reactive with monoclonal antibodies such as OKT9 produced against the well-characterized transferrin receptor of erythroid and proliferating cells. This receptor is known to bind preferentially to iron-containing transferrin (see Chapter 3). However, Nishisato and Aisen (1982) reported that macrophages possessed receptors which preferentially bound apotransferrin, and suggested that these might be involved in iron release. Subsequent studies by this group (Saito et al., 1986) as well as work by other groups (Esparza and Brock, 1981; Baynes et al., 1987) have, however, failed to provide any evidence for such a function. Since this apotransferrin receptor was never characterized, it seems more likely that interaction was due to the well-known ability of macrophages to bind a variety of macromolecules by relatively non-selective mechanisms.

In conclusion, therefore, it appears that normal monocytes and macrophages (other than alveolar) express, at most, only low levels of transferrin receptors, but these increase during *in vitro* culture or in certain pathological conditions. It has been pointed out that since macrophages, particularly those involved in erythrocyte catabolism, acquire iron by phagocytic activity, the expression of transferrin receptors might seem superfluous (Baynes et al., 1987). A possible explanation comes from the work of Oria et al. (1988), who showed that in a macrophage-like cell line, iron acquired by a phagocytic route was handled differently from iron acquired via transferrin. Iron acquired by phagocytosis might therefore not be readily available for the cell's own metabolic needs.

Interaction of lactoferrin with macrophages

The ability of macrophages to interact with lactoferrin was first reported by Van Snick and Masson (1976), who showed that lactoferrin bound to mouse peritoneal macrophages (and to a lesser extent to peritoneal lymphocytes). They subsequently reported that the protein was internalized and degraded by the cells, with the iron being incorporated into ferritin (Van Snick, Markowetz and Masson, 1977). The ability of lactoferrin to bind to cells of the monocyte series has been confirmed by others (Bennett and Davis, 1981; Steinmann et al., 1982; Bennett et al., 1983; Birgens et al., 1983, 1984; Goavec et al., 1985; Bartal, Padeh and Passwell, 1987; Oria et al., 1988) and is now well established. What is less clear is the nature of this interaction, and its biological significance. As regards the nature of lactoferrin–macrophage interactions, some workers have claimed that a specific receptor exists on monocytes (Birgens et al., 1983; Bartal, Padeh and Passwell, 1987), but no receptor molecule has so far been isolated, nor have factors regulating expression of the putative receptor been investigated. On the other hand, the interaction is reported to involve membrane-bound DNA (Bennett et al., 1983; Moguilevsky, Courtoy and Masson, 1985), to be competitively inhibited by elastase (Moguilevsky, Courtoy and Masson, 1985) and to be mediated via the glycan moiety of lactoferrin (Goavec et al., 1985), none of which are consistent with a specific receptor–protein interaction. In view of this, and of the known ability of the highly cationic lactoferrin to bind nonspecifically to a variety of molecules (Hekman, 1971), it seems most likely that a specific lactoferrin receptor is not involved.

However, this does not mean to say that lactoferrin–macrophage interactions may not be of biological significance. In particular, it has been proposed that such an interaction is involved in the control of myelopoiesis, and this is discussed in Chapters 9 and 10. A further possible role arose from the work of Van Snick, Masson and Heremans (1974), who proposed that lactoferrin might short-circuit transferrin-bound iron to macrophages in the liver and spleen and thus contribute to the hypoferraemia of inflammation (see Chapter 6). However, the rate of uptake of lactoferrin-bound iron is at best extremely slow (Van Snick, Markowetz and Masson, 1977; Oria et al., 1988), and in no way compares with the rate of acquisition of iron from transferrin via transferrin receptors. A role in iron redistribution therefore seems unlikely. Binding may, however, trigger intracellular events, as lactoferrin increases the rate of proliferation of a murine macrophage cell line (Oria et al., 1988), though this is clearly not related to iron uptake. Lima and Kierszenbaum (1985, 1987) have shown that exposure of mouse peritoneal macrophages to either apo- or iron-containing lactoferrin enhanced their phagocytic activity, but that intracellular killing was only enhanced when iron was present. Other effects on monocyte or macrophage functions include inhibition of accessory cell function in antibody production (Duncan and McArthur, 1981), stimulation of production of migration-inhibition factor (Kijlstra and Broersma, 1984), modulation of cytotoxic activity (Nishiya and Horwitz, 1982) and inhibition of prostaglandin E_2 production (Bartal, Padeh and Passwell, 1987). In none of these studies was the mode of action of lactoferrin investigated. The biological significance of lactoferrin–macrophage interactions, which are discussed further in Chapter 10, and indeed of lactoferrin itself (see Chapter 3), must therefore await further work.

Synthesis and release of ferritin by macrophages

As mentioned above, monocytes and macrophages, unlike lymphocytes, show a well-defined increase in ferritin synthesis in response to iron (Summers, White and Jacobs, 1975; Doolittle and Richter, 1981; Dörner et al., 1983; Alvarez-Hernández, Felstein and Brock, 1986). However, there is some evidence that ferritin synthesis by monocytes and macrophages may be triggered by events occurring during maturation and differentiation.

The ferritin content of inflammatory mouse peritoneal macrophages is only about 2% of that of the more mature resident or activated cells (Alvarez-Hernández, Felstein and Brock, 1986), and human alveolar macrophages contain over 100 times more ferritin than blood monocytes (Andreesen *et al.*, 1984). Furthermore, the ferritin content of the latter increases markedly during *in vitro* culture, the kinetics being similar to those of the development of transferrin receptors discussed above (Andreesen *et al.*, 1984, 1986). The reason for this increase in ferritin content is not clear, but it is tempting to speculate that it may be related to the scavenging functions of macrophages, which would clearly require them to be able to deal with any iron acquired during this activity. There is also evidence that inflammation causes an increase in ferritin synthesis which is not necessarily triggered by iron, and this is discussed in Chapter 6.

Interest in ferritin release by macrophages has been stimulated by investigations into the source of ferritin in serum (see Chapter 6). High serum ferritin levels occur in those conditions in which storage iron is increased, and it has been suggested that the iron-rich macrophages release increased amounts of ferritin to the circulation (Birgegård, 1980). Cultured macrophages and monocytes release ferritin to the culture medium (Kleber *et al.*, 1978; Esparza and Brock, 1981; Worwood, Hourahane and Jones, 1984), and release from monocytes can also be detected by the haemolytic plaque assay (Pollack *et al.*, 1983; Ohnishi, Shimizu and Yamada, 1984). However, in none of the cell culture studies can leakage from moribund cells be excluded as a source of extracellular ferritin, though a relatively greater amount of glycosylated ferritin in the extracellular medium points to a secretory mechanism. On the other hand, macrophages cultured in the presence of the glycosylation inhibitor tunicamycin released the same amount of ferritin as controls (Alvarez-Hernández, 1986). The best evidence for secretion comes from the study of Ohnishi, Shimizu and Yamada (1984), who showed that inhibitors of protein synthesis reduced ferritin-specific haemolytic plaque formation. It is noteworthy that when unseparated mononuclear cells were used in the haemolytic plaque technique, plaques were associated with monocytes rather than lymphocytes (Pollack *et al.*, 1983). However, only about 2% of monocytes yielded plaques, suggesting that a subpopulation of cells may be involved. Thus although there is strong circumstantial evidence for serum ferritin originating from a secretory activity of macrophages, further data are still required.

Synthesis of transferrin by macrophages

Although it has been known for some time that macrophages can synthesize transferrin (Phillips and Thorbecke, 1966; Haurani, Meyer and

O'Brien, 1973), little is known about its significance or control. It has been suggested that endogenous transferrin might act as a vehicle for the release of iron from macrophages (Haurani and Ballas, 1984), which is discussed below.

Release of iron by macrophages

Because macrophages are involved in the processing of senescent erythrocytes and the subsequent return of iron to the circulation, there has been some interest in the mechanism of iron release by these cells. The release of ferritin has already been discussed above, and several studies have shown that this ferritin contains iron (Kleber *et al.*, 1978; Esparza and Brock, 1981; Custer, Balcerzak and Rinehart, 1982; Saito *et al.*, 1986). However, it is well known that most iron released from liver and spleen is bound by serum transferrin. While it is possible that endogenously synthesized transferrin might account for some of this release, it is clear that the majority must be bound by the extracellular transferrin pool, as macrophages are at best only a minor source of transferrin. *In vitro* systems for studying macrophage iron release following ingestion of erythrocytes have shown that some of the released iron binds to extracellular transferrin (Haurani and O'Brien, 1972; Kleber *et al.*, 1978; Custer, Balcerzak and Rinehart, 1982; Saito *et al.*, 1986). However, peritoneal macrophages do not readily liberate iron from haemoglobin due to low levels of haem oxygenase (Kleber *et al.*, 1978), and significant amounts of haemoglobin are therefore released, presumably through exocytosis or leakage. To avoid this problem, labelled transferrin–anti-transferrin immune complexes have been used to load macrophages with iron (Esparza and Brock, 1981). In this system the majority of iron released is bound to extracellular transferrin, though the availability of extracellular apotransferrin does not affect the rate of release (Esparza and Brock, 1981; Saito *et al.*, 1986). If no apotransferrin is available, the released iron polymerizes or binds nonspecifically to other extracellular proteins (Brock, Esparza and Logie, 1984), and it has been proposed that iron may cross the cell membrane as Fe^{2+}. Less iron is released by inflammatory macrophages than by resident cells (Esparza and Brock, 1981; Saito *et al.*, 1986; Alvarez-Hernández, Felstein and Brock, 1986; McGowan, Murray and Parrish, 1986), which may help to explain the development of hypoferraemia during inflammation (see Chapter 6), and release can also be reduced by preincubating the macrophages with the inflammatory cytokine tumour necrosis factor (Brock and Alvarez-Hernández, 1989). It is thus evident that macrophages may possess more than one mechanism for releasing iron, though again the problem of distinguishing active release from leakage needs to be addressed.

Neutrophils

Unlike macrophages and lymphocytes, neutrophils synthesize only small amounts of ferritin (Summers, White and Jacobs, 1975) and do not apparently express transferrin receptors. The major area of interest in these cells as far as iron-binding proteins is concerned with their synthesis of lactoferrin.

Lactoferrin synthesis and function

The discovery by Baggiolini *et al.* (1970) of lactoferrin in the secondary granules of neutrophils was important, because until that time lactoferrin had been recognized only as a protein of external secretions such as milk, saliva and tears, whose function was primarily concerned with antimicrobial activity. It thus became evident that possible functions of lactoferrin needed to be considered in a wider context than just the protection of secretory surfaces from infection.

Lactoferrin biosynthesis occurs at the myelocyte stage of maturation and is largely complete by the time the band stage is reached (Rado *et al.*, 1984; Rado, Wei and Benz, 1987). There is no synthesis by mature neutrophils, which thus contain their full complement of lactoferrin in their secondary granules. No replenishment is therefore possible after degranulation, which leads to the extracellular release of about 80% of cellular lactoferrin (Leffell and Spitznagel, 1975).

Evidence for the antimicrobial role of neutrophil lactoferrin comes from the work showing that phagocytosis of ferritin, but not of apoferritin, caused neutrophil lactoferrin to become iron-saturated and impaired subsequent antimicrobial activity (Bullen and Armstrong, 1979; Bullen and Wallis, 1977). In addition, patients with congenital lactoferrin deficiency are prone to bacterial infections (Breton-Gorius *et al.*, 1980; Boxer *et al.*, 1982a). The extracellular release of lactoferrin during degranulation suggests that the protein may also serve to prevent extracellular bacterial growth, particularly in an inflammatory lesion where the lower pH would tend to make transferrin less effective. The antimicrobial role of lactoferrin in neutrophils is discussed in detail by Bullen (1987).

It is now evident that lactoferrin released by neutrophils may have functions beyond that of antimicrobial activity, and in particular may control the production of neutrophils themselves. This is discussed in detail in Chapters 9 and 10. The interaction of lactoferrin with macrophages is discussed above. There is also some evidence that lactoferrin binds to neutrophils themselves (Bennett and Davis, 1981; Maneva, Sirakov and Manev, 1983), and that this may affect their migratory and adhesive properties (Oseas *et al.*, 1981; Boxer *et al.*, 1982b).

Transferrin binding

A curious and as yet unexplained property of transferrin is its ability to promote the adherence of pollen grains to neutrophils (Sass-Kuhn *et al.*, 1984; Mackay *et al.*, 1986). The mechanism of this interaction is specific insofar as other types of cells do not react, nor do inert particles such as latex, but the interaction does not involve the classical transferrin receptor. Varying the degree of iron saturation of transferrin also had no effect, and lactoferrin, despite its ability to adhere to neutrophils, was ineffective. The interaction did not cause release of lysosomal enzymes by neutrophils, and it has been proposed (Mackay *et al.*, 1986) that transferrin might help to promote removal of pollen grains from the respiratory tract.

Mast cells

Transferrin may be involved in the inhibition of IgE-mediated release of inflammatory mediators from mast cells by serum from mice treated with a pollen protein (Mécheri *et al.*, 1987). The activity required transferrin of high iron saturation, and could also be demonstrated using iron salts. Transferrin is clearly not the only factor involved, as normal mouse serum was much less inhibitory. The mechanisms involved, other than an evident requirement for iron, remain to be investigated.

IRON AND IMMUNE FUNCTION

The first part of this chapter has discussed how iron and iron-binding proteins interact with and affect the function of cells involved in the immune system. It therefore follows that abnormalities in iron status or metabolism may alter immune responsiveness. Some of these effects, such as iron overload and inflammatory disease, are discussed in detail elsewhere in this volume and will not therefore be dealt with here. The main function of this section will therefore be to discuss the effects of iron deficiency on the immune system. This topic has been regularly reviewed over the past few years, for example by Brock and Mainou-Fowler (1986), Dallman (1987) and Kuvibidila (1987), so this section will concentrate on relating clinical and experimental observations to the specific cellular functions of iron discussed above.

Cell-mediated immunity

The assessment of cell-mediated immunity in iron-deficient patients has usually been carried out either by skin tests or by examining the proliferative response of lymphocytes. A number of studies have shown that skin test responses to a variety of antigens were reduced in iron-deficient patients (Joynson *et al.*, 1972; MacDougall *et al.*, 1975; Chandra, 1975; Krantman *et al.*, 1982), and in some cases normal responses were restored after iron therapy (Jacobs and Joynson, 1974; MacDougall *et al.*, 1975). However, tuberculin testing seems to be unaffected by iron deficiency (Joynson *et al.*, 1972; Chandra, 1975).

A major difficulty in clinical studies is excluding effects of other nutritional deficiencies and of concomitant infections. In consequence, experimental animal models have been used, as these two variables can then be much more closely controlled. Kuvibidila, Baliga and Suskind (1981) examined the skin test responses of iron-deficient mice to dinitrofluorobenzene and found them to be reduced, which supports the majority of the clinical evidence.

Given the known role of iron in lymphocyte proliferation, one might expect to find this function decreased in iron deficiency, but in fact conflicting results have been reported, some studies reporting normal responses (Kulapongs *et al.*, 1974; Gupta, Dhatt and Singh, 1982; Krantman *et al.*, 1982; Grosch-Wörner *et al.*, 1984) and others reduced proliferation (Joynson *et al.*, 1972; Fletcher *et al.*, 1975; MacDougall *et al.*, 1975; Sawitsky, Kanter and Sawitsky, 1976). Again, recourse to animal models has yielded more consistent results, depressed responses being observed (Soyano, Candellet and Layrisse, 1982; Kuvibidila *et al.*, 1983a, 1983b; Mainou-Fowler and Brock, 1985). In particular, it has been demonstrated that the availability of transferrin-bound iron has a critical effect (see above) and that in iron-deficient mice, serum iron levels are inadequate for promoting optimal proliferation (Mainou-Fowler and Brock, 1985). In contrast, protein synthesis was unaffected. Use of iron-replete culture media to test the responses of lymphocytes from iron-deficient patients could therefore lead to erroneous results and might explain some of the conflicting results of clinical studies.

Antibody responses

The effect of iron deficiency on antibody levels and responses is uncertain. Clinical studies have generally shown normal (or elevated) immunoglobulin levels in iron-deficient subjects, even in patients where cell-mediated immunity was found to be depressed (MacDougall *et al.*, 1975; Chandra, 1975; Bagchi, Mohanram and Reddy, 1980; Prema *et al.*, 1982), although in one study (MacDougall and Jacobs, 1978) a small sample of iron-deficient children failed to respond normally to diphtheria immunization. In contrast, data from experimental animal studies suggest that iron deficiency may depress antibody responses. Nalder *et al.*, (1972) reported decreased responses to tetanus toxoid in iron-deficient rats, and reduced levels of immunoglobulins (Kochanowski and Sherman, 1985) or of antibody-secreting cells have been found in rats and mice (Kuvibidila, 1982; Kochanowski and Sherman, 1985). An effect on mucosal immunity is also suggested by a report that numbers of sIgA- and IgM-secreting cells were reduced in the intestinal mucosa of iron-deficient rats (Perkkiö et al., 1987).

As discussed above, antibody production by B cells may occur without prior acquisition of iron from transferrin, and one might therefore expect antibody production to be less affected by iron deficiency than cell-mediated immunity. While this seems to be the case in man, animal studies are tending to favour the opposite conclusion. Possibly iron is more critical for antibody production by rodent B cells than for human cells.

Lymphocyte abnormalities

While the foregoing indicates that lymphocyte effector functions may be depressed in iron deficiency, most of these observations do not distinguish between a lack of available iron to support metabolic activity during an immune response and a more fundamental impairment of lymphocyte function. Studies that have attempted to distinguish between priming and effector activities have tended to show that only the latter are affected (Cummins et al., 1978; Kuvibidila, Baliga and Suskind, 1981). Nevertheless, there is evidence for more fundamental defects. Some studies have reported actual reductions in the number of lymphocytes, or alterations in the ratio of subpopulations in humans (Srikantia et al., 1976; Bagchi, Mohanram and Reddy, 1980) and rats (Rothenbacher and Sherman, 1980; Soyano, Candellet and Layrisse, 1982). Mitochondrial abnormalities have been detected by electron microscopy of lymphocytes from iron-deficient human subjects (Jarvis and Jacobs, 1974; Jiménez et al., 1982), suggesting long-term damage to these cells, and this could explain the findings of Kochanowski and Sherman (1985), who reported that the impaired antibody production found in rat pups born to iron-deficient mothers was not improved by subsequent iron repletion.

Natural killer cell activity

Iron-deficient rat pups were found to have impaired splenic NK cell activity (Sherman and Lockwood, 1987). Since no characterization of the spleen cell populations was carried out, it is impossible to say whether reduced recruitment of NK cells to the spleen or intrinsic defects in NK cytotoxic activity is involved.

Macrophage function

Few studies have attempted to demonstrate impaired macrophage function in iron deficiency. However, Kuvibidila and Wade (1987) found that clearance of polyvinylpyrrolidone (PVP) was impaired in iron-deficient mice, the defect being partially restored by prior iron repletion. The data suggested that defective macrophage function rather than reduced numbers of macrophages in the liver and spleen was responsible. How iron deficiency could affect phagocytosis of an inert molecule such as PVP is unclear, and is unlikely to be due, as suggested by the authors, to a deficiency in myeloperoxidase, as this enzyme is involved in intracellular post-phagocytic events rather than ingestion *per se*. Kuvibidila, Baliga and Suskind (1983) have also reported reduced tumoricidal activity of splenic macrophages from iron-deficient mice. Again, the reason for the defect is not clear, but in this case it might relate to inadequate intracellular iron levels in macrophages, as depletion of intracellular iron *in vitro* leads to impaired production of reactive oxygen intermediates (Thompson and Brock, 1986). Impaired IL-1 production has also been found (Helyar and Sherman, 1987), and this might play a part in reduced cell-mediated and humoral responses. The cause of decreased IL-1 production is unknown.

Neutrophil function

There have been a number of investigations into the effect of iron deficiency on neutrophil function. The commonest findings have suggested that defects exist in the production or activity of reactive oxygen species. These include impaired reduction of nitroblue tetrazolium by neutrophils from iron-deficient patients (Chandra, 1973, 1975; Celada *et al.*, 1979) and experimental animals (Moore and Humbert, 1984), and defective myeloperoxidase levels and/or activity in both patients (Prasad, 1979; Yetgin *et al.*, 1979; Turgeon-O'Brien *et al.*, 1985) and experimental animals (Mackler *et al.*, 1984). Interestingly, Turgeon-O'Brien *et al.* (1985) reported that defective myeloperoxidase activity was confined to patients with nutritional iron deficiency and did not occur in patients with anaemia of chronic disease. However, some clinical studies failed to find any abnormalities in these functions (Kulapongs *et al.*, 1974; Van Heerden *et al.*, 1981). The reported defects probably relate to the fact that iron-containing enzymes are involved in oxygen metabolism, and suggest that inadequate iron levels were available during neutrophil maturation. Since reactive oxygen species and myeloperoxidase play an important role in neutrophil bactericidal activity, it is not surprising that defective bacterial killing has also been reported in iron deficiency (Chandra, 1973, 1975; Macdougall *et al.*,

1975; Srikantia et al., 1976; Yetgin et al., 1979; Moore and Humbert, 1984; Walter et al., 1986), although actual uptake of bacteria was unimpaired (Walter et al., 1986).

Other activities of neutrophils have been less often investigated, and generally seem to be normal. Thus chemotaxis (Van Heerden et al., 1981) and lysozyme production (Celada et al., 1979) were unaffected.

IRON DEFICIENCY AND SUSCEPTIBILITY TO INFECTION

Whether the above-mentioned defects in immune cell function associated with iron deficiency lead to an increased susceptibility to infection remains a contentious issue. Clinical studies almost always involve subjects from low socio-economic groups, and raise problems of the existence of other predisposing factors. These difficulties of interpretation have been reviewed by Dallman (1987). Furthermore, it has been argued that iron deficiency may actually be protective because of reduced iron availability to invading micro-organisms (Weinberg, 1984). At present it seems best to conclude that the weight of evidence showing an involvement of iron in immune cell function is considerable, and that *a priori* one would expect iron deficiency to impair immunological mechanisms involved in defence against infection. Iron deficiency is therefore likely to be a contributory factor in predisposing to susceptibility to infection.

REFERENCES

Akbar, A. N., Fitzgerald-Bocarsly, P. A., De Sousa, M., Giardina, P. J., Hilgartner, M. W., and Grady, R. W. (1986). Decreased natural killer activity in thalassemia major: a possible consequence of iron overload, *J. Immunol.*, **136**, 1635–40.

Akbar, A. N., Fitzgerald-Bocarsly, P. A., Giardina, P. J., Hilgartner, M. W., and Grady, R. W. (1987). Modulation of the defective natural killer activity seen in thalassaemia major with desferrioxamine and gamma-interferon, *Clin. Exp. Immunol.*, **70**, 345–53.

Alarcón, B., and Fresno, M. (1985). Specific effect of anti-transferrin antibodies on natural killer cells directed against tumor cells. Evidence for the transferrin receptor being one of the target structures recognized by NK cells, *J. Immunol.*, **134**, 1286–91.

Alvarez-Hernández, J. (1986). Iron metabolism in macrophages. Ph.D. thesis, University of Glasgow.

Alvarez-Hernández, X., Felstein, M. V., and Brock, J. H. (1986). The relationship between iron release, ferritin synthesis and intracellular iron distribution in mouse peritoneal macrophages. Evidence for a reduced level of metabolically-available iron in elicited macrophages, *Biochim. Biophys. Acta*, **886**, 214–22.

Andreesen, R., Osterholz, J., Bodemann, H., Bross, K. J., Costabel, U., and Löhr,

G. W. (1984). Expression of transferrin receptors and intracellular ferritin during terminal differentiation of human monocytes, *Blut*, **49**, 195–202.

Andreesen, R., Bross, K. J., Osterholz, J., and Emmrich, F. (1986). Human macrophage maturation and heterogeneity: analysis with a newly generated set of monoclonal antibodies to differentiation antigens, *Blood*, **67**, 1257–64.

Bagchi, K., Mohanram, M., and Reddy, V. (1980). Humoral immune response in children with iron-deficiency anaemia, *Br. Med. J.*, **208**, 1249–51.

Baggiolini, M., de Duve, C., Masson, P. L., and Heremans, J. F. (1970). Association of lactoferrin with specific granules in rabbit heterophil leucocytes, *J. Exp. Med.*, **131**, 559–70.

Baines, M. G., Lafleur, F. L., and Holbein, B. E. (1983). Involvement of transferrin and transferrin receptors in human natural killer effectors target interaction, *Immunol. Lett.*, **7**, 51–5.

Bartal, L., Padeh, S., and Passwell, J. H. (1987). Lactoferrin inhibits prostaglandin E_2 secretion by breast milk macrophages, *Pediatr. Res.*, **21**, 54–7.

Basset, P., Quesneau, Y., and Zwiller, J. (1986). Iron-induced L1210 cell growth: evidence of a transferrin-independent iron transport, *Cancer Res.*, **46**, 1644–7.

Baynes, R. D., Bukofzer, G., Bothwell, T. H., and Bezwoda, W. R. (1987). Apo-transferrin receptors and the delivery of iron from cultured human blood monocytes, *Am. J. Hematol.*, **25**, 417–25.

Bennett, R. M., and Davis, J. (1981). Lactoferrin binding to human peripheral blood cells: an interaction with a B-enriched population of lymphocytes and a subpopulation of adherent mononuclear cells, *J. Immunol.*, **127**, 1211–16.

Bennett, R. M., Davis, J., Campbell, S., and Portnoff, S. (1983). Lactoferrin binds to cell membrane DNA. Association of surface DNA with an enriched population of B cells and monocytes, *J. Clin. Invest.*, **71**, 611–18.

Besancon, F., Bourgeade, M-F., and Testa, U. (1985). Inhibition of transferrin receptor expression by interferon-α in human lymphoblastoid cells and mitogen-induced lymphocytes, *J. Biol. Chem.*, **260**, 13074–80.

Birgegård, G. (1980). The source of serum ferritin during infection. Studies with concanavalin A–Sepharose absorption, *Clin. Sci.*, **59**, 385–7.

Birgens, H. S., Hansen, N. E., Karle, M., and Kristensen, L. Ø. (1983). Receptor binding of lactoferrin by human monocytes, *Br. J. Haematol.*, **54**, 383–91.

Birgens, H. S., Karle, H., Hansen, N. E., and Kristensen, L. Ø. (1984). Lactoferrin receptors in normal and leukaemic blood cells, *Scand. J. Haematol.*, **33**, 275–80.

Björn-Rasmussen, E., Hageman, J., Van Den Dungen, P., Prowit-Ksiazek, A., and Biberfeld, P. (1985). Transferrin receptors on circulating monocytes in hereditary haemochromatosis, *Scand. J. Haematol.*, **34**, 308–11.

Bomford, A., Young, S. R., Nouri-Aria, K., and Williams, R. (1983). Uptake and release of transferrin and iron by mitogen-stimulated human lymphocytes, *Br. J. Haematol.*, **55**, 93–101.

Borysiewicz, L. K., Graham, S., and Sissons, J. G. P. (1986). Human natural killer cell lysis of virus-infected cells. Relationship to expression of the transferrin receptor, *Eur. J. Immunol.*, **16**, 405–11.

Boxer, L. A., Coates, T. D., Haak, R. A., Wolach, J. B., Hoffstein, S., and Baehner, R. L. (1982a). Lactoferrin deficiency associated with altered granulocyte function, *N. Engl. J. Med.*, **303**, 404–10.

Boxer, L. A., Haak, R. A., Yang, H. H., Wolach, J. B., Whitcomb, J. A., Butterick, C. J., and Baehner, R. L. (1982b). Membrane-bound lactoferrin alters the surface properties of polymorphonuclear leukocytes, *J. Clin. Invest.*, **70**, 1049–57.

Breton-Gorius, J., Mason, D. Y., Buriot, D., Vilde, J-L., and Griscelli, C. (1980).

Lactoferrin deficiency as a consequence of a lack of specific granules in neutrophils from a patient with recurrent infections, *Am. J. Pathol.*, **99**, 413–28.

Bridges, K. R., and Smith, B. R. (1985). Discordance between transferrin receptor expression and susceptibility to lysis by natural killer cells, *J. Clin. Invest.*, **76**, 913–18.

Brieva, J. A., and Stevens, R. M. (1984). Involvement of the transferrin receptor in the production and NK-induced suppression of human antibody synthesis, *J. Immunol.*, **133**, 1288–92.

Brock, J. H. (1981). The effect of iron and transferrin on the response of serum-free cultures of mouse lymphocytes to concanavalin A and lipopolysaccharide, *Immunology*, **43**, 387–92.

Brock, J. H., and Alvarez-Hernández, X. (1989). Modulation of macrophage iron metabolism by tumour necrosis factor and interleukin 1, *FEMS Microbiol. Immunol.*, **47**, 309.

Brock, J. H., Esparza, I., and Logie, A. C. (1984). The nature of iron released by resident and stimulated mouse peritoneal macrophages, *Biochim. Biophys. Acta*, **797**, 105–11.

Brock, J. H., and Mainou-Fowler, T. (1983). The role of iron and transferrin in lymphocyte transformation, *Immunol. Today*, **4**, 347–51.

Brock, J. H., and Mainou-Fowler, T. (1986). Iron and immunity, *Proc. Nutr. Soc.*, **45**, 305–15.

Brock, J. H., Mainou-Fowler, T., and Webster, L. M. (1986). Evidence that transferrin functions only as an iron donor in promoting lymphocyte proliferation, *Immunology*, **57**, 105–10.

Brock, J. H., and Rankin, M. C. (1981). Transferrin binding and iron uptake by mouse lymph-node cells during transformation in response to concanavalin A, *Immunology*, **43**, 393–8.

Brock, J. H., and Stevenson, J. (1987). Replacement of transferrin in serum-free cultures of mitogen-stimulated mouse lymphocytes by a lipophilic iron chelator, *Immunol. Lett.*, **15**, 23–5.

Broxmeyer, H. E., Lu, L., and Bognacki, J. (1983). Transferrin, derived from an OKT8-positive subpopulation of T-lymphocytes, suppresses the production of granulocyte-macrophage colony-stimulating factors from mitogen-activated T lymphocytes, *Blood*, **62**, 37–50.

Bryan, C. F., and Leech, S. H. (1983). The immunoregulatory nature of iron. 1. Lymphocyte proliferation, *Cell. Immunol.*, **75**, 71–9.

Bullen, J. J. (1987). Iron and the antibacterial function of polymorphonuclear leucocytes. In J. J. Bullen and E. Griffiths (eds) *Iron and Infection*, p. 211–41. Wiley, Chichester.

Bullen, J. J., and Armstrong, J. A. (1979). The role of lactoferrin in the bactericidal function of polymorphonuclear leucocytes, *Immunology*, **36**, 781–91.

Bullen, J. J., and Wallis, S. N. (1977). Reversal of the bactericidal effects of polymorphs by a ferritin-antibody complex. *FEMS Microbiol, Lett.* **1**, 117–20.

Cairo, G., Bardella, L., Schiaffonati, L., Arosio, P., Levi, S., and Bernelli-Zazzera, A. (1985). Multiple mechanisms of iron-induced ferritin synthesis in HeLa cells, *Biochem. Biophys. Res. Commun.* **133**, 314–21.

Carotenuto, P., Pontesilli, O., Cambier, J. C., and Hayward, A. R. (1986). Desferoxamine blocks IL2 receptor expression on human T lymphocytes, *J. Immunol.*, **136**, 2342–7.

Celada, A., Herreros, V., Pugin, P., and Rudolf, M. (1979). Reduced leucocyte alkaline phosphatase activity and decreased NBT reduction test in induced iron deficiency, *Br. J. Haematol.* **43**, 457–63.

Chandra, R. K. (1973). Reduced bactericidal capacity of polymorphs in iron deficiency, *Arch. Dis. Child.*, **48**, 864–6.
Chandra, R. K. (1975). Impaired immunocompetence associated with iron deficiency, *J. Pediatr.*, **86**, 899–902.
Cragg, S. J., Hoy, T. G., and Jacobs, A. (1984). The expression of cell surface ferritin by peripheral blood lymphocytes and monocytes, *Br. J. Haematol.*, **57**, 679–84.
Cummins, A. G., Duncombe, V. M., Bolin, T. D., Davis, A. E., and Kelly, J. D. (1978). Suppression of rejection of *Nippostrongylus brasiliensis* in iron and protein deficient rats: effect of syngeneic lymphocyte transfer, *Gut*, **19**, 823–6.
Custer, G., Balcerzak, S., and Rinehart, J. (1982). Human macrophage hemoglobin-iron metabolism in vitro, *Am. J. Hematol.*, **13**, 23–36.
Cuthbert, J. A., and Lipsky, P. E. (1984). Immunoregulation by low density lipoproteins in man. Inhibition of mitogen-induced T-lymphocyte proliferation by interference with transferrin metabolism, *J. Clin. Invest.*, **73**, 992–1003.
Cuthbert, J. A., and Lipsky, P. E. (1986). Low-density lipoprotein (LDL) and lymphocyte responses: direct suppression by native LDL and indirect inhibition from zinc chelation by contaminating EDTA, *Biochim. Biophys. Acta*, **876**, 210–19.
Dallman, P. R. (1987). Iron deficiency and the immune response, *Am. J. Clin. Nutr.*, **46**, 329–34.
Dokhélar, M-C., Garzon, D., Testa, U., and Tursz, T. (1984). Target structure for natural killer cells: evidence against a unique role for transferrin receptor, *Eur. J. Immunol.* **14**, 340–4.
Doolittle, R. L., and Richter, G. W. (1981). Isoferritins in rat Kupffer cells, hepatocytes and extrahepatic macrophages. Biosynthesis in cell suspensions and cultures in response to iron, *Lab. Invest.*, **45**, 567–74.
Dörner, M. H., Silverstone, A., Nishiya, K., De Sostoa, A., Munn, G., and De Sousa, M. (1980). Ferritin synthesis by human T lymphocytes, *Science*, **209**, 1019–21.
Dörner, M. H., Silverstone, A. E., De Sostoa, A., Munn, G., and De Sousa, M. (1983). Relative subunit composition of the ferritin synthesized by selected human lymphomyeloid cell populations, *Exp. Hematol.*, **11**, 866–72.
Duncan, R. L., and McArthur, W. P. (1981). Lactoferrin-mediated modulation of mononuclear cell activities. 1. Suppression of the murine *in vitro* primary antibody response, *Cell. Immunol.*, **63**, 308–20.
Esparza, I., and Brock, J. H. (1981). Release of iron by resident and stimulated mouse peritoneal macrophages following ingestion and digestion of transferrin-antitransferrin immune complexes, *Br. J. Haematol.*, **49**, 603–14.
Fargion, S., Arosio, P., Fracanzani, A. L., Cislaghi, V., Levi, S., Cozzi, A., Piperno, A., and Fiorelli, G. (1988). Characteristics and expression of binding sites specific for ferritin H-chain on human cell lines, *Blood*, **71**, 753–7.
Fletcher, J., Mather, J., Lewis, M. J., and Whiting, G. (1975). Mouth lesions in iron-deficient anemia: relationship to *Candida albicans* in saliva and to impairment of lymphocyte transformation, *J. Infect. Dis.*, **131**, 44–50.
Galbraith, G. M. P., Goust, J. M., Mercurio, S. M., and Galbraith, R. M. (1980). Transferrin binding by mitogen-activated human peripheral blood lymphocytes, *Clin. Immunol. Immunopathol.*, **16**, 387–95.
Goavec, M., Mazurier, J., Montreuil, J., and Spik, G. (1985). Rôle des glycannes dans la fixation de la serotransferrine et de la lactotransferrine humaines sur les macrophages alvéolaires humains, *C. R. Seances Acad. Sci. (III)*, **301**, 689–94.
Good, M. F., Powell, L. W., and Halliday, J. W. (1987). The effect of non-transferrin-bound iron on murine T lymphocyte subsets: analysis by clonal techniques, *Clin. Exp. Immunol.*, **70**, 164–47.

Good, M. F., Chapman, D. E., Powell, L. W., and Halliday, J. W. (1986). The effect of iron (Fe^{3+}) on the cloning efficiency of human memory T4+ lymphocytes, *Clin. Exp. Immunol.*, **66**, 340–72.

Grosch-Wörner, I., Grosse-Wilde, H., Bender-Götze, C., and Schäfer, K. H. (1984). Lymphozytenfunktionen bei Kindern mit Eisenmangel, *Klin. Wochenschr.*, **62**, 1091–3.

Gupta, K. K., Dhatt, P. S., and Singh, H. (1982). Cell-mediated immunity in children with iron-deficiency anaemia, *Indian. J. Pediatr.*, **49**, 507–10.

Hamilton, T. A. (1982). Regulation of transferrin receptor expression in concanavalin A stimulated and Gross virus transformed rat lymphoblasts, *J. Cell. Physiol.*, **113**, 40–6.

Hamilton, T. A. (1983). Receptor-mediated endocytosis and exocytosis of transferrin in concanavalin-A stimulated rat lymphoblasts, *J. Cell. Physiol.*, **114**, 222–8.

Hamilton, T. A., Gray, P. W., and Adams, D. O. (1984). Expression of the transferrin receptor on murine peritoneal macrophages is modulated by *in vitro* treatment with interferon gamma, *Cell. Immunol.*, **89**, 478–88.

Hamilton, T. A., Weiel, J. E., and Adams, D. O. (1984). Expression of the transferrin receptor in murine peritoneal macrophages is modulated in the different stages of activation, *J. Immunol.*, **132**, 2285–90.

Haurani, F. I., and Ballas, S. K. (1984). Iron metabolism. In S. M. Reicherd and J. P. Filkins (eds) *The Reticuloendothelial System*, Vol. 7A, pp. 353–77, Plenum, New York.

Haurani, F. I., Meyer, A., and O'Brien, R. (1973). Production of transferrin by the macrophage, *J. Reticuloendothelial Soc.*, **14**, 309–16.

Haurani, F. I., and O'Brien, R. (1972). A model system for release of iron from the reticuloendothelial system. *J. Reticuloendothelial Soc.*, **12**, 29–34.

Hekman, A. (1971). Association of lactoferrin with other proteins, as demonstrated by changes in electrophoretic mobility, *Biochim. Biophys. Acta*, **251**, 380–7.

Helyar, L., and Sherman, A. R. (1987). Iron deficiency and interleukin 1 production by rat leukocytes, *Am. J. Clin. Nutr.*, **46**, 346–52.

Hirata, T., Bitterman, P. B., Mornex, J-F., and Crystal, R. G. (1986). Expression of the transferrin receptor gene during the process of mononuclear phagocyte maturation, *J. Immunol.*, **136**, 1339–45.

Hoffbrand, A. V., Ganeshaguru, K., Hooton, J. W. L., and Tattersall, M. H. N. (1976). Effect of iron deficiency and desferrioxamine on DNA synthesis in human cells, *Br. J. Haematol.*, **33**, 517–26.

Jacobs, A., and Joynson, D. H. M. (1974). Lymphocyte function and iron-deficiency anaemia, *Lancet*, **ii**, 844.

Jarvis, J. H., and Jacobs, A. (1974). Morphological abnormalities in lymphocyte mitochondria associated with iron-deficiency anaemia, *J. Clin. Pathol.*, **27**, 973–9.

Jiménez, A., Sánchez, A., Vázquez, R., and Olmos, J. M. (1982). Alteraciones mitocondriales en los linfocitos de pacientes con anemia ferropénica, *Morfol. Norm. Patol.*, **6B**, 279–87.

Joynson, D. H. M., Jacobs, A., Walker, D. M., and Dolby, A. F. (1972). Defect in cell mediated immunity in patients with iron-deficiency anaemia, *Lancet*, **ii**, 1058–9.

Kay, J. E., and Benzie, C. R. (1986). The role of the transferrin receptor in lymphocyte activation, *Immunol. Lett.*, **12**, 55–8.

Kemp, J. D., Thorson, J. A., McAlmont, T., Horowitz, M., Cowdery, J. S., and Ballas, Z. K. (1987). Role of the transferrin receptor in lymphocyte growth: a rat IgG monoclonal antibody against the murine transferrin receptor produces highly selective inhibition of T and B cell activation protocols, *J. Immunol.*, **138**, 2422–6.

Khalfoun, B., Degenne, B., Crouzat-Reynes, G., and Bardos, P. (1986). Effect of human syncytiotrophoblast plasma membrane-soluble extracts on in vitro mitogen-induced lymphocyte proliferation. A possible inhibition mechanism involving the transferrin receptor, *J. Immunol*, **137**, 1187–93.

Kijlstra, A., and Broersma, L. (1984). Lactoferrin stimulates the production of leucocyte migration inhibitory factor by human peripheral mononuclear leucocytes, *Clin. Exp. Immunol.*, **55**, 459–64.

Kleber, E. E., Lynch, S. R., Skikne, B., Torrance, J. D., Bothwell, T. H., and Charlton, R. W. (1978). Erythrocyte catabolism in the inflammatory peritoneal monocyte, *Br. J. Haematol.*, **39**, 41–54.

Kochanowski, B. A., and Sherman, A. R. (1985). Decreased antibody formation in iron-deficient rat pups—effect of iron repletion, *Am. J. Clin. Nutr.*, **41**, 278–84.

Krantman, H. J., Young, S. R., Ank, B. J., O'Donnell, C. M., Rachelefsky, G. S., and Stiehm, E. R. (1982). Immune function in pure iron deficiency, *Am. J. Dis. Child.*, **136**, 840–4.

Kulapongs, P., Vithayasai, V., Suskind, R., and Olson, R. E. (1974). Cell mediated immunity and phagocytosis and killing function in children with severe iron-deficiency anaemia, *Lancet*, **ii**, 689–91.

Kumagai, N., Benedict, S. H., Mills, G. B., and Gelfland, E. W. (1988). Comparison of phorbol ester/calcium ionophore and phytohemagglutinin-induced signaling in human T lymphocytes. Demonstration of interleukin 2-independent transferrin receptor gene expression, *J. Immunol.*, **40**, 37–43.

Kuvibidila, S. (1987). Iron deficiency, cell-mediated immunity and resistance against infection: present knowledge and controversies, *Nutr. Res.*, **7**, 989–1003.

Kuvibidila, S. R., Baliga, B. S., and Suskind, R. M. (1981). Effects of iron deficiency anemia on delayed cutaneous hypersensitivity in mice, *Am. J. Clin. Nutr.*, **34**, 2635–40.

Kuvibidila, S. R., Baliga, R. S., and Suskind, R. M. (1982). Generation of plaque forming cells in iron deficient anemic mice, *Nutr. Rep. Internat.*, **26**, 861–71.

Kuvibidila, S. R., Baliga, B. S., and Suskind, R. M. (1983). The effect of iron-deficiency anemia on cytolytic activity of mice spleen and peritoneal cells against allogenic tumor cells, *Am. J. Clin. Nutr.*, **38**, 238–44.

Kuvibidila, S., and Wade, S. (1987). Macrophage function as studied by the clearance of ^{125}I-labelled polyvinylpyrollidone in iron-deficient and iron replete mice, *J. Nutr.*, **117**, 170–6.

Kuvibidila, S., Nauss, K. M., Baliga, B. S., and Suskind, R. M. (1983a). Impairment of blastogenic response of splenic lymphocytes from iron-deficient mice: in vivo repletion, *Am. J. Clin. Nutr.*, **37**, 15–25.

Kuvibidila, S. R., Nauss, K. M., Baliga, B. S., and Suskind, R. M. (1983b). Impairment of blastogenic response of splenic lymphocytes from iron-deficient mice. In vitro repletion by hemin, transferrin and ferric chloride, *Am. J. Clin. Nutr.*, **37**, 557–65.

Larrick, J. W., and Cresswell, P. (1979). Modulation of cell surface iron transferrin receptors by cellular density and state of activation, *J. Supramol. Struct.*, **11**, 579–86.

Lazarus, A. H., and Baines, M. G. (1985). Studies on the mechanism of specificity of human natural killer cells for tumour cells: correlation between target cell transferrin receptor expression and competitive activity, *Cell. Immunol.*, **96**, 255–66.

Leberman, H. M., Cohen, A., Lee, J. W. W., Freedman, M. H., and Gelfand, E. W. (1984). Deferoxamine: a reversible S-phase inhibitor of human lymphocyte proliferation, *Blood*, **64**, 748–53.

Leffel, M. S., and Spitznagel, J. K. (1975). Fate of human lactoferrin and myeloperoxidase in phagocytizing human neutrophils: effects of immunoglobulin G subclasses and immune complexes coated on latex beads, *Infect. Immun.*, **12**, 813–20.

Lema, M. J., and Sarcione, E. J. (1981). A comparison of iron induction of rat lymphocyte ferritin synthesis *in vivo* and *in vitro*, *Comp. Biochem. Physiol.*, **69B**, 287–90.

Lima, M. F., and Kierszenbaum, F. (1985). Lactoferrin effects on phagocytic cell function. I. Increased uptake and killing of an intracellular parasite by murine macrophages and human monocytes, *J. Immunol.*, **134**, 4176–83.

Lima, M. F., and Kierszenbaum, F. (1987). Lactoferrin effects on phagocytic cell function. II. The presence of iron is required for the lactoferrin molecule to stimulate intracellular killing by macrophages but not to enhance the uptake of particles and microorganisms, *J. Immunol.*, **139**, 1647–51.

Lum, J. B., Infante, A. J., Makker, D. M., Yang, F., and Bowman, B. H. (1986). Transferrin synthesis by inducer T lymphocytes, *J. Clin. Invest.*, **77**, 841–9.

MacDougall, L. G., and Jacobs, M. R. (1978). The immune response in iron-deficient children. Isohaemagglutinin titres and antibody response to immunisation, *South Afr. Med. J.*, **53**, 405–7.

Macdougall, L. G., Anderson, R., McNab, G. M., and Katz, J. (1975). The immune response in iron-deficient children: Impaired cellular defense mechanisms with altered humoral components, *J. Pediatr.*, **86**, 833–43.

Mack, U., Powell, L. W., and Halliday, J. W. (1983). Detection and isolation of a hepatic membrane receptor for ferritin, *J. Biol. Chem.*, **258**, 4672–5.

Mackay, J. A., Sass-Kuhn, S., Moqbel, R., Walsh, G. M., and Kay, A. B. (1986). The requirements for transferrin-dependent adherence of human granulocytes to pollen grains, *Allergy*, **41**, 169–78.

Mackler, B., Person, R., Ochs, H., and Finch, C. A. (1984). Iron deficiency in the rat: effects on neutrophil activation and metabolism, *Pediatr. Res.*, **18**, 549–51.

Mainou-Fowler, T., and Brock, J. H. (1985). Effect of iron deficiency on the response of mouse lymphocytes to concanavalin A: The importance of transferrin-bound iron, *Immunology*, **54**, 325–32.

Maneva, A. I., Sirakov, L. M., and Manev, V. V. (1983). Lactoferrin binding to neutrophilic polymorphonuclear leucocytes, *Int. J. Biochem.*, **15**, 981–4.

Matzner, Y., Hershko, C., Polliack, A., Konijn, A., and Izak, G. (1979). Suppressive effect of ferritin on *in vitro* lymphocyte function, *Br. J. Haematol.*, **42**, 345–53.

Matzner, Y., Konijn, A. M., Shlomai, Z., and Ben-Basset, H. (1985). Differential effect of isolated placental isoferritins on *in vitro* T-lymphocyte function, *Br. J. Haematol.*, **59**, 443–8.

McGowan, S. E., Murray, J. J., and Parrish, M. G. (1986). Iron binding, internalization and fate in human alveolar macrophages, *J. Lab. Clin. Med.*, **108**, 587–95.

Mécheri, S., Peltre, G., Lapeyre, J., and David, B. (1987). Biological effect of transferrin on mast cell mediator release during the passive cutaneous anaphylaxis reaction: a possible inhibition mechanism involving iron, *Ann. Inst. Pasteur Immunol. (Paris)*, **138**, 213–21.

Mendelsohn, J., Trowbridge, I., and Castagnola, J. (1983). Inhibition of human lymphocyte proliferation by monoclonal antibody to transferrin receptor, *Blood*, **62**, 821–6.

Moguilevsky, N., Courtoy, P. J., and Masson, P. L. (1985). Study of lactoferrin-binding sites at the surface of blood monocytes. In G. Spik J. Montreuil, R. R. Chrichton, and J. Mazurier (eds) *Proteins of Iron Storage and Transport*, pp. 199–202, Elsevier, Amsterdam.

Moore, L. L., and Humbert, J. R. (1984). Neutrophil bactericidal dysfunction towards oxidant radical-sensitive microorganisms during experimental iron deficiency, *Pediatr. Res.*, **18**, 684–9.

Moroz, C., and Kupfer, B. (1981). Suppressor cell activity of ferritin-bearing lymphocytes in patients with breast cancer, *Isr. J. Med. Sci.*, **17**, 879–81.

Nalder, B. N., Mahoney, A. W., Ramakrishnan, R., and Hendricks, D. G. (1972). Sensitivity of the immunological response to the nutritional status of rats, *J. Nutr.*, **102**, 535–42.

Navas, P., Sun, I. L., Morré, D. J., and Crane, F. L. (1986). Decrease of NADH in HeLa cells in the presence of transferrin or ferricyanide, *Biochem. Biophys. Res. Commun*, **135**, 110–15.

Neckers, L. M., and Cossman, J. (1983). Transferrin receptor induction in mitogen-stimulated human T lymphocytes is required for DNA synthesis and cell division and is regulated by interleukin 2, *Proc. Natl Acad. Sci, USA*, **89**, 3494–8.

Neckers, L. M., Yenokida, G., and James, S. P. (1984). The role of the transferrin receptor in human B-lymphocyte activation, *J. Immunol.*, **133**, 2437–41.

Neckers, L. M., Bauer, S., McGlennen, R. C., Trepel, J. B., Rao, K., and Greene, W. C. (1986). Diltiazem inhibits transferrin receptor expression and causes GI arrest in normal and neoplastic T cells, *Mol. Cell Biol.*, **6**, 4244–50.

Newman, R. A., Warner, J. F., and Dennert, G. (1984). NK recognition of target structures. Is the transferrin receptor the NK target structure? *J. Immunol.*, **133**, 1841–5.

Nishisato, T., and Aisen, P. (1982). Uptake of transferrin by rat peritoneal macrophages, *Br. J. Haematol.*, **52**, 631–40.

Nishiya, K., and Horwitz, D. A. (1982). Contrasting effect of lactoferrin on human lymphocyte and monocyte natural killer cell activity and antibody-dependent cell-mediated cytotoxicity, *J. Immunol.*, **129**, 2519–23.

Novogrodsky, A., Ravid, A., Glaser, T., Rubin, A. L., and Stenzel, K. H. (1982). Role of iron in transferrin-dependent lymphocyte mitogenesis in serum free medium, *Exp. Cell Res.*, **139**, 419–22.

Ohnishi, K., Shimizu, K., and Yamada, M. (1984). Enumeration of circulating ferritin-secreting cells by a reverse hemolytic plaque assay, *Acta Haematol.*, **71**, 39–44.

Oria, R., Alvarez-Hernández, X., Licéaga, J., and Brock, J. H. (1988). Uptake and handling of iron from transferrin, lactoferrin and immune complexes by a macrophage cell line, *Biochem. J.*, **251**, 221–5.

Oseas, R., Yang, H-H., Baehner, R. L., and Boxer, L. A. (1981). Lactoferrin: A promoter of polymorphonuclear leukocyte adhesiveness, *Blood*, **57**, 939–45.

Pattanapanyasat, K., Hoy, T. G., and Jacobs, A. (1987). The response of intracellular and surface ferritin after T-cell stimulation *in vitro*, *Clin. Sci.*, **73**, 605–11.

Pattanapanyasat, K., Hoy, T. G., and Jacobs, A. (1988). Effect of phytohaemagglutinin on the synthesis and secretion of ferritin in peripheral blood lymphocytes, *Br. J. Haematol*, **69**, 565–70.

Pelosi, E., Testa, U., Louache, F., Thomopoulos, P., Salvo, G., Samoggia, P., and

Peschle, C. (1986). Expression of transferrin receptors in phytohemagglutinin-stimulated human T-lymphocytes, *J. Biol. Chem.*, **261**, 3036–42.

Perkkiö, M. V., Jansson, L. T., Dallman, P. R., Siimes, M. A., and Savilahti, E. (1987). sIgA and IgM-containing cells in the intestinal mucosa of iron-deficient rats, *Am. J. Clin. Nutr.*, **46**, 341–5.

Perl, A., Looney, R. J., Ryan, D. H., and Abraham, G. N. (1986). The low affinity 40,000 Fc-gamma receptor and the transferrin receptor can be alternative or simultaneous target structures on cells sensitive for natural killing, *J. Immunol.*, **136**, 4714–20.

Phillips, J. L., and Azari, P. (1975). Effect of iron transferrin on nucleic acid synthesis in phytohemagglutinin-stimulated human lymphocytes, *Cell. Immunol,.* **15**, 94–9.

Phillips, M. E., and Thorbecke, G. J. (1966). Studies on the serum proteins of chimeras. I. Identification and study of the site of origin of donor type serum proteins in rat-into-mouse chimeras, *Int. Arch. Allergy Appl. Immunol.*, **29**, 553–67.

Pollack, M. S., Martins da Silva, B., Moshief, R. D., Groshen, S., Bognacki, J., Dupont, B., and de Sousa, M. (1983). Ferritin secretion by human mononuclear cells: association with HLA phenotype, *Clin. Immunol. Immunopathol.*, **27**, 124–34.

Ponka, P., Schulman, H. M., and Wilczynska, A. (1982). Ferric pyridoxal isonicotinoyl hydrazone can provide iron for heme synthesis in reticulocytes, *Biochim. Biophys. Acta*, **718**, 151–6.

Prasad, J. S. (1979). Leucocyte function in iron-deficiency anemia, *Am. J. Clin. Nutr.*, **32**, 550–2.

Prema, K., Ramalakshmi, B. A., Madhava Peddi, R., and Babu, S. (1982). Immune status of anaemic pregnant women, *Br. J. Obstet. Gynaecol.*, **89**, 222–5.

Prince, H. E., and John, J. K. (1986). Cyclosporine inhibits the expression of receptors for interleukin 2 and transferrin on mitogen-activated human T lymphocytes, *Immunol. Invest.*, **15**, 463–72.

Rado, T. A., Wei, X., and Benz, E. J. (1987). Isolation of lactoferrin cDNA from a human myeloid library and expression of mRNA during normal and leukemic myelopoiesis, *Blood*, **70**, 989–93.

Rado, T. A., Bollekens, J., St Laurent, G., Parker, L., and Benz, E. J. (1984). Lactoferrin biosynthesis during granulocytopoiesis, *Blood*, **64**, 1103–9.

Rammensee, H-G., Lesley, J., Trowbridge, I. S., and Evan, M. J. B. (1985). Antibodies against the transferrin receptor block the induction of cytotoxic T lymphocytes. A new method for antigen-specific negative selection *in vitro*, *Eur. J. Immunol.*, **15**, 687–92.

Rothenbacher, H., and Sherman, A. R. (1980). Target organ pathology in iron deficient suckling rats, *J. Nutr.*, **110**, 1648–54.

Saito, K., Nishisato, T., Grasso, J. A., and Aisen, P. (1986). Interaction of transferrin with iron-loaded rat peritoneal macrophages, *Br. J. Haematol.*, **62**, 275–86.

Sass-Kuhn, S. P., Moqbel, R., Mackay, J. A., Cromwell, O., and Kay, A. B. (1984). Human granulocyte/pollen binding protein. Recognition and identification as transferrin, *J. Clin. Invest.*, **73**, 202–10.

Sato, H., Kubota, Y., Takahashi, S., and Matsuoka, O. (1986). ^{59}Fe release from alveolar macrophages ingested ^{59}Fe-iron dextran—enhancement by combination of Ca-DTPA and macrophage activating substances, *J. Radiat. Res.*, **27**, 105–11.

Sawitsky, B., Kanter, R., and Sawitsky, A. (1976). Lymphocyte response to phytomitogens in iron deficiency, *Am. J. Med. Sci.*, **272**, 153–60.

Scupham, D. W., McCarthy, B. M., and Harmony, J. A. K. (1987). The regulation

by low-density lipoprotein of activation of oxidative enzyme primed lymphocytes is governed by transferrin, *Cell. Immunol.*, **108**, 378–95.
Shau, H., Shen, D., and Golub, S. H. (1986). The role of transferrin in natural killer cell and IL-2 induced cytotoxic cell function, *Cell. Immunol.*, **97**, 121–30.
Sherman, A. R., and Lockwood, J. F. (1987). Impaired natural killer cell activity in iron-deficient rat pups, *J. Nutr.*, **117**, 567–71.
Sizemore, D. J., and Bassett, M. L. (1984). Monocyte transferrin-iron uptake in hereditary hemochromatosis, *Am. J. Hematol*, **16**, 347–54.
Soltys, H. D., and Brody, J. I. (1970). Synthesis of transferrin by human peripheral blood lymphocytes, *J. Lab. Clin. Med.*, **75**, 250–7.
Soyano, A., Candellet, D., and Layrisse, M. (1982). Effect of iron deficiency on the mitogen-induced proliferative response of rat lymphocytes, *Int. Arch. Allergy Appl. Immunol.*, **69**, 353–7.
Soyano, A., Fernandez, E., and Romano, E. (1985). Suppressive effect of iron on in vitro lymphocyte function: formation of iron polymers as a possible explanation, *Int. Arch. Allergy Appl. Immunol.*, **76**, 376–8.
Srikantia, S. G., Prasad, J. S., Bhaskaram, C., and Krishnamachari, K. A. V. R. (1976). Anaemia and immune response, *Lancet*, **i**, 1307–9.
Steinmann, G., Broxmeyer, H. E., De Harven, E., and Moore, M. A. S. (1982). Immuno-electron microscopic tracing of lactoferrin, a regulator of myelopoiesis, into a subpopulation of human peripheral blood monocytes, *Br. J. Haematol.*, **50**, 75–84.
Summers, M., White, G., and Jacobs, A. (1975). Ferritin synthesis in lymphocytes, polymorphs and monocytes, *Br. J. Haematol.*, **30**, 425–34.
Summers, M. R., and Jacobs, A. (1976). Iron uptake and ferritin synthesis by peripheral blood leucocytes from normal subjects and patients with iron deficiency and the anaemia of chronic disease, *Br. J. Haematol.*, **34**, 221–9.
Taetle, R., Castagnola, J., and Mendelsohn, J. (1986). Mechanisms of growth inhibition by anti-transferrin receptor monoclonal antibodies, *Cancer Res.*, **46**, 1759–63.
Tanno, Y., and Takashima, T. (1982). Enhancing effect of saccharated ferric oxide on human lymphocyte transformation in serum-free medium, *Tohoku J. Exp. Med.*, **136**, 463–4.
Thompson, H. L., and Brock, J. H. (1986). The effect of iron and agar on production of hydrogen peroxide by stimulated and activated mouse peritoneal macrophages, *FEBS Lett.*, **200**, 283–6.
Titeux, M., Testa, U., Louache, F., Thomopoulos, P., Rochant, H., and Breton-Gorius, J. (1984). The role of iron in the growth of human leukemic cell lines, *J. Cell. Physiol.*, **121**, 251–6.
Tormey, D. C., Imrie, R. C., and Mueller, G. C. (1972). Identification of transferrin as a lymphocyte growth promoter in human serum, *Exp. Cell Res.*, **74**, 163–9.
Turgeon-O'Brien, H., Amiot, J., Lemieux, L., and Dillon, J.-C. (1985). Myeloperoxidase activity of polymorphonuclear leukocytes in iron deficiency anaemia and anaemia of chronic disorders, *Acta Haematol.*, **74**, 151–4.
Van Heerden, C., Oosthuizen, R., Van Wyk, H., Prinsloo, P., and Anderson, R. (1981). Evaluation of neutrophil and lymphocyte function in subjects with iron deficiency, *S. Afr. Med. J.*, **24**, 111–13.
Van Snick, J. L., Markowetz, B., and Masson, P. L. (1977). The ingestion and digestion of human lactoferrin by mouse peritoneal macrophages and the transfer of its iron to ferritin, *J. Exp. Med.*, **146**, 817–27.

Van Snick, J. L., and Masson, P. L. (1976). The binding of human lactoferrin to mouse peritoneal cells, *J. Exp. Med.*, **144**, 1568–80.

Van Snick, J. L., Masson, P. L., and Heremans, J. F. (1974). The involvement of lactoferrin in the hyposideremia of acute inflammation, *J. Exp. Med.*, **141**, 1068–84.

Vezzoni, P., Levi, S., Gabri, E., Pozzi, M. R., Spinazze, S., and Arosio, P. (1986). Ferritins in malignant and non-malignant lymphoid cells, *Br. J. Haematol.*, **62**, 105–10.

Vodinelich, L., Sutherland, R., Schneider, C., Newman, R., and Greaves, M. (1983). Receptor for transferrin may be a 'target' structure for natural killer cells, *Proc. Natl Acad. Sci. USA*, **86**, 835–9.

Vogt, A., Mishell, R. I., and Dutton, R. W. (1969). Stimulation of DNA synthesis of mouse spleen cell suspensions by bovine transferrin, *Exp. Cell Res.*, **54**, 195–200.

Walter, T., Arredondo, S., Arévalo, M., and Stekel, A. (1986). Effect of iron therapy on phagocytosis and bactericidal activity in neutrophils of iron deficient infants, *Am. J. Clin. Nutr.*, **44**, 877–82.

Ward, J. H., Jordan, I., Kushner, J. P., and Kaplan, J. (1984). Heme regulation of HeLa cell transferrin receptor, *J. Biol. Chem.*, **259**, 13231–40.

Weiel, J. E., Adams, D. O., and Hamilton, T. A. (1985). Biochemical models of gamma-interferon action: altered expression of transferrin receptors on murine peritoneal macrophages after treatment *in vitro* with PMA or A23187, *J. Immunol.*, **134**, 293–8.

Weiel, J. E., and Hamilton, T. A. (1984). Quiescent lymphocytes express intracellular transferrin receptors, *Biochem. Biophys. Res. Commun.*, **119**, 598–602.

Weinberg, E. D. (1984). Iron withholding; a defense against infection and neoplasia, *Physiol. Rev.*, **64**, 65–102.

Worwood, M., Hourahane, D., and Jones, B. M. (1984). Accumulation and release of isoferritins during incubation *in vitro* of human peripheral blood mononuclear cells, *Br. J. Haematol.*, **56**, 31–43.

Wyllie, J. C. (1977). Transferrin uptake by rabbit alveolar macrophages in vitro, *Br. J. Haematol.*, **37**, 17–24.

Yetgin, S., Altay, C., Ciliv, G., and Laleli, Y. (1979). Myeloperoxidase activity and bactericidal function of PMN in iron deficiency, *Acta Haematol.*, **61**, 10–14.

Young, S., and Bomford, A. (1984). Transferrin and cellular iron exchange, *Clin. Sci.*, **67**, 273–8.

Part II

Iron and Inflammation

Iron in Immunity, Cancer and Inflammation
Edited by M. de Sousa and J. H. Brock
© 1989 John Wiley & Sons Ltd.

6
The Anaemia of Inflammation and Chronic Disease

Abraham M. Konijn* and Chaim Hershko†
*Department of Nutrition, The Hebrew University Hadassah Medical School, Jerusalem, Israel
†Department of Medicine, Shaare Zedek Medical Center, Jerusalem, Israel

The anaemia of inflammation and chronic disease (AICD) is probably the most common type of anaemia encountered in hospitalized patients. It received renewed attention following the annotation of Cartwright and Lee (1971) and has recently been reviewed extensively in several publications (Lee, 1983; Roeser, 1980). AICD is usually manifested in a normocytic and normochromic anaemia or, occasionally, hypochromic anaemia in patients with long-standing disease. This variant of anaemia may be associated with inflammation caused by infection, connective tissue disorders such as rheumatoid arthritis, or malignancies. Many of the features of AICD resemble iron deficiency anaemia; serum iron is low and red cell protoporphyrins are elevated (Cartwright and Lee, 1971). However, total iron-binding capacity tends to be high in iron deficiency anaemia and low in AICD.

THE ANAEMIA OF MALIGNANT DISEASE

Anaemia secondary to malignant disease may be directly associated with the malignant process, such as pure red cell aplasia, microangiopathic haemolytic anaemia, autoimmune haemolytic anaemia of the cold or warm antibody type, anaemia caused by trapping circulating red blood cells (RBCs) in an enlarged spleen or even phagocytosis of RBCs by malignant cells. The various types of anaemia associated with specific neoplastic disorders have been described in detail in recent reviews by Doll and Weiss (1985) and Zucker (1985) and will not be dealt with further.

The most common type of anaemia associated with cancer is similar to that observed in infectious and inflammatory diseases and has likewise been attributed to multiple pathogenic mechanisms. Such mechanisms involve decreased iron availability for erythropoiesis, decreased RBC survival, suppressed RBC formation due to decreased erythropoietin levels and/or a reduced response of the bone marrow to erythropoietin, or the presence of humoral factors inhibiting erythropoiesis.

RBC SURVIVAL AND INEFFECTIVE ERYTHROPOIESIS

A moderately reduced RBC survival time has been observed in some studies in patients and animals with inflammatory conditions or following injection of endotoxin. Patients with rheumatoid arthritis, whether iron-deficient or iron-replete, have reduced RBC survival (Cavill and Bentley, 1982; Dinant and de Maat, 1978).

Reduced RBC survival was also reported in patients with other chronic inflammatory diseases (Cavill, Ricketts and Napier, 1977). Cats, in which a sterile abscess was induced by a subcutaneus turpentine injection, had reduced ^{51}Cr-labelled RBC survival time and a reduced packed cell volume (Weiss, Krehbiel and Lund, 1983). There seems to be an inverse correlation between the duration of the inflammatory condition and RBC survival; RBC survival was normal in dogs given two turpentine injections but was shortened in dogs who received six injections over 28 days (Rigby et al., 1962). Similarly, in rats one turpentine injection did not cause a significant reduction in RBC survival (Konijn and Hershko, 1977), but in rats with chronic experimental adjuvant-induced disease, RBC lifespan was reduced (Mikolajew et al., 1969). Normal syngeneic ^{51}Cr-labelled RBCs injected into mice infected with Bacillus Calmette Guerin (BCG) had a normal lifespan during the first 14 days of infection but a shorter lifespan thereafter (Marchal and Milon, 1981a). However, the development of anaemia preceded the phase of reduced RBC lifespan.

There is no simple explanation for the reduced RBC lifespan encountered in inflammation. Cartwright and Lee (1971) attributed the decrease in RBC survival, at least in part, to the existence of an extracorpuscular haemolytic factor; normal RBCs transfused into patients had a moderately shortened lifespan, but RBCs from patients transfused into healthy people had a normal survival time. This may be caused by the removal of RBCs from the circulation by a hyperactive reticuloendothelial (RE) system (Lee, 1983).

Inflammation is usually associated with fever. Experimentally induced fever in rabbits (Karle, 1968, 1974), produced by the injection of endotoxin, heated milk, or external body heating, caused an increased destruction of

RBCs, resulting in a 15% reduction of peripheral RBC cell mass within a few days. The loss of RBCs was preferentially due to the destruction of old cells. *In vitro* exposure of RBCs to slightly elevated temperatures for a few hours caused an increase in their osmotic fragility, accelerated spontaneous haemolysis, and a reduced survival following reinfusion. The increase in temperature induced changes in the RBC membrane and altered the rheologic properties of the RBCs due to a decrease in cell plasticity (Karle and Hansen, 1970). Thus, heat-damaged RBCs are prone to phagocytosis and to destruction in the spleen (Karle, 1968). However, in mice infected with BCG, increased phagocytosis of RBCs was excluded as a cause of the anaemia (Marchal and Milon, 1981a).

The anaemia of inflammation and chronic disease is mainly the result of a negative balance between the destruction and production of RBCs. Erythropoiesis is not able to compensate for the shortened RBC survival. A number of investigators attributed the anaemia of inflammation and chronic disease to unavailability of iron for erythropoiesis due to increased sequestration in the RE and parenchymal system (Freireich *et al.*, 1957; Hershko, Cook and Finch, 1974; Lee, 1983; Mikolajew *et al.*, 1969; Noyes, Bothwell and Finch, 1960; Roeser, 1980). This aspect of the anaemia will be discussed later in some detail. However, other mechanisms have also been explored: decreased erythropoietin (Epo) production and secretion resulting in inappropriately low Epo levels; decreased bone marrow response to Epo; a reduction in the number of erythroid bone marrow cells; and modulation of haematopoiesis by sensitized T lymphocytes (Marchal and Milon, 1986).

ERYTHROPOIETIN

An inverse relationship between serum Epo levels or its urinary secretion, and haemoglobin levels, has been found in patients with iron deficiency anaemia (Erslev *et al.*, 1980; Hammond, Shore and Movassaghi, 1968; Movassaghi, Shore and Hammond, 1967; Ward, Kurnick and Pysarczyk, 1971), thalassaemia major and congenital hypoplastic anaemia (Hammond, Shore and Movassaghi, 1968; Movassaghi, Shore and Hammond, 1967). Epo synthesis is influenced by blood haemoglobin levels and by tissue anoxia (Berglund, Hemmingsson and Birgegård, 1987; Jelkman, 1982; Zucker, Freidman and Lysik, 1974). The role of Epo in the anaemia of inflammation has been examined in a number of studies.

Exogenous Epo administered in rats abolished the mild anaemia induced by turpentine abscess (Gutinsky and Van Dyke, 1963; Zarrabi, Lysik and Zucker, 1977). Epo given to hypertransfused rats with adjuvant-induced arthritis restored ^{59}Fe incorporation into RBCs to control levels (Lukens, 1973). Cobalt injection and iron infusion corrected the anaemia of inflammation in cats with sterile turpentine abscesses (Weiss, Krehbiel and Lund, 1983). These experiments point to a defect in Epo secretion in inflammation and not to a decreased response of the bone marrow to Epo. On the other hand, endotoxin suppressed in a log dose-dependent manner the incorporation of ^{59}Fe into mouse RBCs following Epo administration (Schade and Fried, 1976). Studies of serum or urinary Epo levels in patients with inflammatory and malignant diseases yielded conflicting results. Some investigators found inappropriately low Epo secretion or plasma levels in relation to the haemoglobin concentration in patients suffering from inflammatory diseases (Alexanian, 1972; Douglas and Adamson, 1975; Erslev *et al.*, 1980; Mahmood, Robinson and Vautrin, 1977; Ward, Gordon and Picket, 1969; Ward, Kurnick and Pysarczyk, 1971), lung cancer (Cox, Musial and Gyde, 1986) and malignant lymphoma (Ward, Kurnick and Pysarczyk, 1971). These results conflict with the findings of more recent studies in which Epo responses in chronic disease or inflammation were normal. Kaaba *et al.* (1984) and Alexanian (1972) reported normal responses of Epo to anaemia in patients with lung cancer and other malignancies. Similarly, in patients with other, non-haematological inflammatory diseases, Epo responses to anaemia were normal (Cotes *et al.*, 1980; Wallner *et al.*, 1977). A detailed study of serum Epo levels in various chronic inflammatory conditions by Birgegård, Hällgren and Caro (1987) showed a close dependence of serum Epo levels on haemoglobin levels. This in turn was influenced by the degree of inflammatory activity. Thus, higher inflammatory activity yielded lower haemoglobin levels and, accordingly, higher serum Epo. A positive correlation was found between serum Epo levels and RBC sedimentation rate. In contrast to the studies cited above, these authors found an appropriate Epo response relative to haemoglobin levels. Corticosteroid treatment suppressed inflammatory activity but did not increase serum Epo. Thus, Epo levels were regulated only by haemoglobin levels. The main difference between the earlier studies showing a normal response was the assay method employed for measuring serum Epo. In studies using *in vivo* assays or *in vitro* bioassays, decreased serum Epo levels were found in disease. In later studies, where a normal Epo response was found, radioimmunoassays were employed. This apparent contradiction may be resolved by the following explanations:

(1) *Epo secreted in inflammatory disease has normal immunoreactivity but its bioactivity is reduced*. Experiments to confirm or reject this assumption have not been performed yet.

(2) *An impaired marrow response to Epo in chronic diseases*. Experiments performed to test this hypothesis have shown a normal marrow response *in vivo* to exogenous Epo in inflamed patients (Lukens, 1973; Walner *et al.*,

1977; Zarrabi, Lysik and Zucker, 1977) and a normal *in vitro* response of bone marrow from patients with malignant disease without anaemia (Zucker, Freidman and Lysik, 1974) but a decreased response in cancer patients with anaemia. Zucker, Freidman and Lysik (1974) have shown that the induction of [^{59}Fe]haem synthesis by Epo in human bone marrow cell cultures, taken from anaemic patients with malignancy but without bone marrow involvement, was significantly less than in normals or in patients with malignancy without anaemia, or in patients with anaemia of inflammation. Dainiak *et al.* (1983) tested the *in vitro* response of erythroid progenitors BFU-e and CFU-e from cancer patients to Epo. They found that colony formation was normal at all Epo concentrations tested in 91% of the patients. These studies conflict with those of Zucker, Freidman and Lysik (1977), who found, in rats with transplantable tumours, a decreased erythropoiesis *in vivo* and a decreased marrow response to Epo *in vitro*. Comparable results were reported by Chandler and Fletcher (1973) in chicken. However, different parameters were investigated; Zucker, Freidman and Lysik (1974) studied haem synthesis and Dainiak *et al.* (1983) erythroid colony formation. Zucker (1985) concluded that cancer alters only the more mature, differentiated, haemoglobinized erythroid cells. There seems to be some resemblance between the anaemia of malignancy and BCG infection. Anaemic BCG-infected mice had increased Epo levels but a decreased incorporation of ^{59}Fe into bone marrow haem (Marchal and Milon, 1981b). This was apparently due to a decreased population of Epo-responsive cells in their bone marrow. A lower than normal number of CFU-e was also observed in the bone marrow of mice bearing turpentine abscesses (Reissman and Udupa, 1978), but the number of bone marrow BFU-e and CFU-e in anaemic, rheumatoid arthritic patients did not differ significantly from those in normal controls (Reid *et al.*, 1984).

(3) *An inhibitor of erythropoiesis in the serum of patients with malignancy or chronic inflammatory disease*. This inhibitor may mask the *in vivo* or *in vitro* Epo bioassay. Reid *et al.* (1984) added serum from anaemic and non-anaemic rheumatoid arthritis patients to cultures of bone marrow cells or peripheral blood cells depleted of T cells, B cells and monocytes, and found that serum from anaemic patients, but not from non-anaemic patients, inhibited or failed to stimulate BFU-e growth. Kaaba *et al.* (1984) examined the effect of sera from thirteen patients with disseminated bronchial cancer on the *in vitro* growth of erythroid progenitors isolated from normal human bone marrow. More than half of the cultures containing cancer serum showed no growth of either CFU-e or BFU-e, in contrast to the growth observed with normal sera. Zucker (1985) analysed the results of studies undertaken by his group (Zucker and Lysik, 1977; Zucker, Lysik and Di Stefano, 1977) and of those by Roodman, Horadam and Wright (1983) and

proposed that macrophages in cancer may become activated and release soluble substances capable of inhibiting erythropoiesis. Thus, acidic isoferritins have been shown to be secreted from T cells and/or macrophages in leukaemia and to inhibit erythropoiesis (Broxmeyer et al., 1981) (see also Chapter 9). Broxmeyer et al. (1986) have demonstrated the inhibitory effect of acidic isoferritin on colony formation of erythroid (BFU-e) progenitor cells. Serum ferritin is elevated in inflammatory conditions (Baynes et al., 1986; Birgegård et al., 1978; Elin, Wolff and Finch, 1977; Pelkonen, Swanljung and Siimes, 1986; Roeser, 1980) and malignancies (Marcus and Zinberg, 1975; Matzner, Konijn and Hershko, 1980; Niitsu et al., 1984; Pagé, Thériault and Caron, 1979; Worwood, 1979; Wurz, Von Moers and Zippel, 1985). In certain malignant diseases acidic isoferritins were found to be elevated in the serum (Cazzola et al., 1983; Niitsu et al., 1980, 1984). Whether acidic isoferritins may also be elevated in the sera of patients with inflammatory diseases has yet to be determined.

Recently, Schooley, Kullgren and Allison (1987) found that interleukin-1 (IL-1), a protein factor secreted mainly by stimulated monocytes and macrophages (Dinarello, 1984), inhibited the action of Epo on Epo-responsive cells (EPCs) recovered from spleens and bone marrow of mice made anaemic by intraperitoneal injections of phenylhydrazine hydrochloride. The proliferative response of EPCs was inhibited by purified and cloned human IL-1 as well as by cloned murine IL-1. IL-1 does not inhibit the binding of Epo to receptors since the proliferative response was inhibited even when the IL-1 was added 17 hours after the administration of the Epo.

THE IMMUNE SYSTEM AND THE DEVELOPMENT OF ANAEMIA OF CHRONIC DISEASE

The multifactorial pathogenesis of the anaemia associated with malignancy and chronic inflammatory disease is underlined by the observations indicating a possible role for the immune system in the regulation of erythropoiesis in disease. In a case of T cell chronic lymphocytic leukaemia, anaemia was attributed to T cell suppression of erythropoiesis (Hoffman et al., 1978). Resumption of normal in vitro erythroid proliferation in marrow cells in this patient with T cell chronic lymphatic leukaemia (CLL) was only possible after treatment with anti-thymocyte-globulin (ATG) and complement. ATG inactivated or destroyed a cell population interfering with the normal proliferative or differentiative response of erythroid stem cells to Epo.

T cells obtained from patients with B cell CLL who developed pure red cell aplasia (CLL-PRCA) inhibited in vitro marrow CFU-e growth (Mangan,

Chikkappa and Farley, 1982); removal of T cells by E-rosette techniques augmented CFU-e growth ten-fold. Only T cells or B cells (bearing Fc receptors for IgG) obtained during the active phase of CLL-PRCA suppressed *in vitro* CFU-e growth in autologous or allogeneic marrows. Recently, NK cells were shown to be able to inhibit *in vitro* CFU-e proliferation (Mangan *et al.*, 1984). Interferon boosting of NK cells augmented their suppressive effect on both marrow CFU-e and blood BFU-e proliferation (Mangan, Chikkappa and Farley, 1982). By analogy with CLL, in inflammatory diseases it is also possible that the immune system may participate in the pathogenesis of anaemia. Janossy *et al.* (1980) have shown that the immunoregulatory system is hyperactive in rheumatoid arthritis and there is a possibility that hyperactive T cells are involved in the suppression of erythropoiesis in rheumatoid arthritis (Reid *et al.*, 1984).

In a series of articles, Marchal and Milon (Marchal and Milon, 1981a, 1981b, 1986; Milon and Marchal, 1981; Milon, Lebastard and Marchal, 1985) analysed the mechanism of BCG-induced anaemia in mice. BCG-induced anaemia in mice is associated with peripheral granulomonocytosis occurring only in euthymic mice. Anaemia and a decreased number of erythroid bone marrow cells were observed in the first week following intravenous injection of viable BCG into normal mice but not in athymic nu/nu mice. Anaemia developed in BCG-infected athymic mice only following prior grafting with thymus cells from newborn normal mice or i.v. injection of spleen cells from BCG-infected normal mice (Marchal and Milon, 1981b; Milon and Marchal, 1981). That T cells were involved in the generation of the anaemia was demonstrated by loss of the effect of the graft in athymic mice, following lysis of T cells with anti-Thy-1 serum and complement. Thus, the condition necessary for the development of anaemia during BCG infection correlated with the conditions allowing an immune response against infection (Milon and Marchal, 1981). The role of T cells in the development of BCG anaemia was proven again by using two genetically different strains of mice; C3H/He mice resistant to haematopoietic modification by BCG infection, and C57BL/6 mice responding to BCG with anaemia. Marchal and Milon (1986) have shown that in the bone marrow of C57BL/6 mice the number of BCG-specific T cells was 50–100 times higher than in C3H/He mice. Using monoclonal antibodies, they found that haematopoiesis in the BCG-infected mice was under the control of L3T4+Lyt2− BCG-specific T lymphocytes. Because an increased production of short-lived phagocytes and monocytes was found concomitant with decreased packed cell volume (PCV), Marchal and Milon (1986) attributed the decreased erythropoiesis and T lymphocyte-induced enhancement of phagocyte production to a more effective competition of late phagocyte progenitors for IL-3, which is secreted by L3T4+ lymphocytes.

However, other explanations are possible. Lectin-activated T lymphocytes secrete haematopoietic suppressor activity (Bacigalupo et al., 1981; Podesta et al., 1982), which may be related to interferon-γ secreted by T lymphocytes (Zoumbos, Djue and Young, 1984; Linch, 1985). Interferon-γ is also produced by NK cells, but most relevant to marrow function are activated T cells of the CD8+ type, because this subset preferentially populates the marrow (Nakao et al., 1984).

T cells are also able to produce and secrete ferritin rich in the H-type acidic subunit (Dörner et al., 1980). H-type subunits have recently been shown to inhibit colony formation by normal human erythroid (BFU-e) progenitor cells (Broxmeyer et al., 1986). Thus, T cells may have a potential role in the regulation of erythropoiesis in disease by secreting factors suppressing erythropoiesis.

IRON METABOLISM IN INFLAMMATION

In spite of the mechanisms described above, reduced RBC survival, inadequate Epo effect, or abnormal immune function cannot be fully responsible for the anaemia of inflammation and chronic disease, and it is most likely that in the majority of cases the erythroid proliferation is limited primarily by the availability of iron (Douglas and Adamson, 1975).

The profound changes in iron metabolism in response to inflammation or neoplasia are characterized by a blockade of iron release from tissues, resulting in a reduction in circulating iron levels (Lee, 1983; Roeser, 1980). Invading organisms, neoplasia, and experimental conditions causing inflammation, such as the injection of bacterial endotoxins or the administration of turpentine or carrageenan, all have similar effects on iron metabolism and other non-immune responses to inflammation. These changes will ultimately result in decreased haemoglobin levels, a drop in the PCV, and an increase in free and zinc RBC protoporphyrin concentrations (Gorodetski et al., 1985, 1986). The haematological events associated with iron metabolism in inflammation and chronic disease are summarized in Table 6.1. The most important parameter is a decrease in tissue iron release leading to hypoferraemia and iron-deficient erythropoiesis. It has been suggested that such hypoferraemia may represent a defensive mechanism against invading organisms or malignant cells by depriving them of vital iron (Kochan, 1973; Weinberg, 1975, 1978, 1986). Thus, the term 'nutritional immunity' was introduced by Kochan (1973) and adopted by others (Weinberg, 1975).

Release of radioiron labels from parenchymal or RE cells is characterized by a rapid early phase and a slower late phase of cellular transport (Hershko, Cook and Finch, 1974; Fillet, Cook and Finch, 1974). The early phase represents release of iron from a labile intracellular pool, whereas

TABLE 6.1 The effect of inflammation on parameters of iron metabolism

Tissue iron release	Decreased
Tissue storage iron	Increased
Iron absorption	Decreased
Serum iron	Decreased
Total iron-binding capacity	Decreased
Plasma iron turnover	Decreased
Haemoglobin	Decreased
Packed cell volume	Decreased
RBC protoporphyrins	Increased
Plasma lactoferrin	Increased
Serum ferritin	Increased

the late release is derived from iron stored in ferritin. These two distinct phases of release account for the exchange of iron between tissues and plasma. In experimental animals, inflammation induced by turpentine or endotoxin is characterized by a marked reduction in the fraction of iron released in the early phase, probably reflecting a reduction in the 'labile iron pool' (Figure 6.1) and an increase in the fraction of iron stored in ferritin. A part of the intracellular ferritin is denatured to form haemosiderin (Hoy and Jacobs, 1981; Jacobs, 1980). This process is accelerated by inflammation, probably due to intracellular events activated by inflammatory mediators. Thus, lysosomal enzymes may be discharged due to the destabilizing effect of intracellular mediators of inflammation on the lysosomal membrane, and may cause enhanced haemosiderin formation from ferritin, with the net effect of making iron less available to the labile pool and thus to the plasma iron pool and for erythropoiesis. Thus, in chronic disease an increased portion of the intracellular iron may be found in haemosiderin (Hershko, Cook and Finch, 1974; Hershko, 1977; Roeser, 1980) (Figure 6.1).

Using ^{59}Fe-labelled heat-damaged nonviable RBCs, Konijn and Hershko (1977) found increased radioiron retention in the RE cells of inflamed rats, leading to a decrease in plasma iron turnover, thus confirming earlier studies (Freireich *et al.*, 1957; Karle, 1974; Noyes, Bothwell and Finch, 1960; Quastel and Ross, 1966). Likewise, in parenchymal cells, Hershko, Cook and Finch (1974) found increased retention of radioiron in turpentine-inflamed rats following injection of ^{59}Fe-labelled haemoglobin–haptoglobin complexes. More recently, Esparza and Brock (1981) and Alvarez-Hernandez, Felstein and Brock (1986) studied the *in vitro* uptake of iron from ^{59}Fe–transferrin–anti-transferrin immune complexes and the subsequent release of iron from mouse peritoneal macrophages. They have shown that following labelling of thioglycolate-elicited macrophages, the

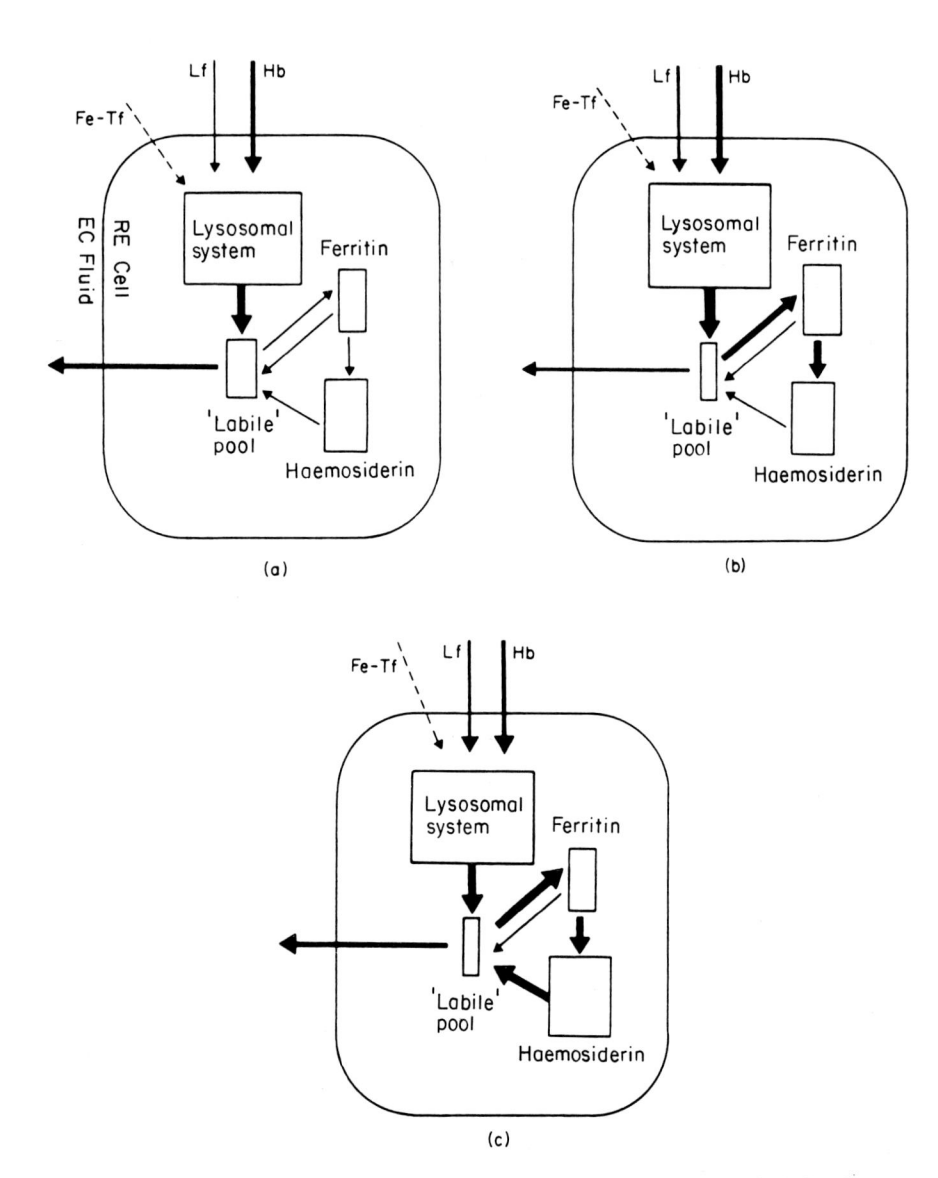

Figure 6.1 Suggested scheme for iron turnover in reticuloendothelial cells: (a) under normal conditions; (b) during unsteady state in acute inflammation; (c) during steady state in chronic inflammation. Hb: haemoglobin in red blood cells; Lf: lactoferrin; Fe-Tf: transferrin-bound iron; RE cell: reticuloendothelial cell; EC fluid: extracellular fluid. From Roeser (1980) with permission of the author and Academic Press

iron label was preferentially incorporated into haemosiderin-like compounds and soluble compounds other than ferritin. Thioglycolate-elicited macrophages released less iron *in vitro* than resident macrophages or macrophages activated by an immunological agent (*Corynebacterium parvum*). Others (Nishisato and Aisen, 1983) have shown that after stimulation with methaemalbumin or peptone broth, rat peritoneal macrophages failed to release detectable amounts of iron to transferrin. Iron uptake by inflammatory macrophages is increased. In thioglycolate-stimulated mouse peritoneal macrophages or in macrophages obtained from turpentine-inflamed mice, transferrin radioiron uptake is four times greater than in macrophages from normal mice (Birgegård and Caro, 1984). Likewise, uptake of transferrin iron by pulmonary macrophages obtained from rabbits with acute turpentine inflammation (Macdonald, MacSween and Pechet, 1969) was increased in comparison to pulmonary macrophages from normal rabbits. Thus, increased tissue uptake and retention of iron in inflammation, quantitatively most important in the RE system, and reduced intestinal iron absorption (Hershko, Cook and Finch, 1974), will ultimately result in hypoferraemia and anaemia.

PATHOGENESIS OF THE HYPOFERRAEMIA OF INFLAMMATION

At the site of the inflammation, the noxious agents responsible, such as invading organisms, tumour tissue, trauma, endotoxin and turpentine, will cause the release of chemotactic factors and accumulation of polymorphonuclear cells (PMNs) and monocytes. Neutrophils will be provoked to discharge their specific granules by the same chemotactic factors which, at lower concentrations, have been responsible for their initial local accumulation. The specific granules contain a protease which cleaves complement component C5 into C5a, a 74-residue glycopolypeptide. C5a is a powerful chemotactic factor (Fernandez *et al.*, 1978). Chemotactic factors will therefore be released by the first few neutrophils which, in turn, will release more chemotactic factors, attracting yet more neutrophils and monocytes, thus causing the inflammatory response to have an explosive character if uninterrupted. Matzner, Partridge and Babior (1983) described the existence of a protein inhibitor of neutrophil chemotaxis in synovial fluid. The primary effect of its activity appears to be directed against C5a chemotaxis. This inhibitor also exists in the abdominal fluid and is probably secreted from fibroblasts (Matzner and Brzezinski, 1984). The complement component C5a is a potent mediator of the acute inflammatory response. In addition to stimulating neutrophil chemotaxis, C5a has also been shown to induce, *in vitro*, exocytosis of lysosomal granular enzymes, to enhance the formation of oxygen radical species, and to promote neutrophil adherence and autoaggregation (Chenoweth and Hugli, 1980; Craddock et al., 1977; Fernandez et al., 1978; O'Flaherty, Kreutzer and Ward, 1977; Webster et al., 1980). Specific receptors for C5a have been demonstrated on macrophages (Chenoweth, Goodman and Weigle, 1982). C5a promotes the secretion of IL-1 from these cells (Chenoweth, Goodman and Weigle, 1982; Goodman, Chenoweth and Weigle, 1982). The putative role of IL-1 in the hypoferraemia of inflammation will be discussed later. Apolactoferrin is among the materials released by the PMNs at the site of inflammation. It is an iron-binding protein similar to but distinct from transferrin (see Chapters 3 and 10). Within the PMN this protein exists in an iron-free state and binds iron avidly at acid pH, in contrast to apotransferrin, which is unable to bind iron at low pH. Release of apolactoferrin by the PMN was proposed by Van Snick, Masson and Heremans (1974) to be responsible for the hypoferraemia of inflammation. Apolactoferrin secreted at the inflammatory site by the PMN (Figure 6.2) in response to stimulation by C5a and/or IL-1 (Webster et al., 1980) is capable of exchanging iron with transferrin at acid pH, a condition often existing at the site of inflammation. The iron–lactoferrin complex is rapidly taken up by macrophages. Lactoferrin iron is transported to the liver but not to erythropoietic cells in the bone marrow. However, even minute amounts of endotoxin will cause a fall in serum iron without a corresponding reduction in tissue or plasma pH and, at physiological pH, iron in serum remains bound to transferrin. Administration of IL-1 (leukocytic pyrogen, leukocyte endogenous mediator, lymphocyte-activating factor) also causes a remarkable reduction in serum iron without changing the pH (Bailey et al., 1976; Kampschmidt and Upchurch, 1962, 1969; Pekarek and Beisel, 1971; Pekarek, Wannemacher and Beisel, 1972; Van Miert et al., 1984). Indeed, a low pH may only be found at the site of inflammation in tissues due to release of lactic acid and other metabolic products by accumulating PMNs. Thus, only at the site of inflammation may iron exchange between lactoferrin and transferrin take place, and this could therefore explain only a small fraction of the hypoferraemia associated with inflammation. Letendre and Holbein (1983) studied the hypoferraemia of experimental *Neisseria meningitidis* infection in mice and did not find an increased rate of plasma iron clearance during the hypoferraemic phase.

The Van Snick hypothesis is based on the observation that intravenous injection of 15 mg of human apolactoferrin into rats caused a 46% decrease in the plasma iron level within 4 hours. However, this study was criticized because of the unphysiological amounts of lactoferrin used (Roeser, 1980). Sawatzki, Hoffman and Kubanek (1983) repeated these experiments using intravenous doses of 3 mg of mouse apolactoferrin in mice. This treatment caused hypoferraemia in association with increased plasma lactoferrin levels. The effect was maintained by multiple injections. Taking into

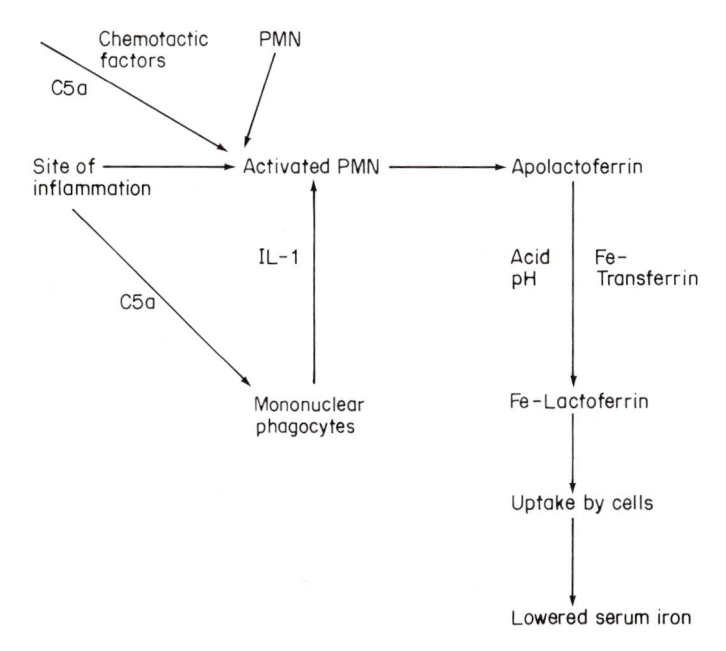

```
              Chemotactic    PMN
              factors
        C5a              \   /
                          \ /
    Site of ─────────→ Activated PMN ─────────→ Apolactoferrin
    inflammation              ↑                       │
                              │                       │
                             IL-1              Acid  │  Fe-
                              │                pH    │  Transferrin
          C5a                 │                      │
             \                │                      ↓
              ↓               │                 Fe-Lactoferrin
         Mononuclear                                 │
         phagocytes                                  ↓
                                                Uptake by cells
                                                     │
                                                     ↓
                                              Lowered serum iron
```

Figure 6.2 Proposed scheme for the mechanism of action of lactoferrin in the altered iron metabolism in inflammation and the production of hypoferraemia

account the size of mice, this amount of lactoferrin will bring plasma lactoferrin concentrations well above physiologically obtainable levels. During the acute phase of infection, endogenous plasma lactoferrin is only slightly increased to about three times normal values (Hansen et al., 1976), and this response is proportional to the amount of injected bacteria (Sawatzki, Hoffman and Kubanek, 1983). Because of its short half-life, the actual low level of serum lactoferrin is misleading, as the iron-loaded lactoferrin is rapidly removed from the circulation by the monocyte–macrophage system and from there to the liver. Thus, in theory the actual amounts of iron that can be removed from the serum by lactoferrin may be significant. The lactoferrin hypothesis cannot explain the decreased iron absorption associated with inflammation (Hershko, Cook and Finch, 1974; Lee, 1983). Baynes et al. (1986) reached the conclusion that lactoferrin plays no role in the hypoferraemic response to inflammation: lactoferrin concentrations in plasma parallel blood neutrophil counts (Hansen et al., 1976), and in patients with neutropenic sepsis, lactoferrin concentrations are low in the presence of reduced plasma iron concentrations. Similarly, in patients with rheumatoid arthritis, variations in plasma lactoferrin and serum ferritin concentrations were independent.

In contrast to the lack of convincing evidence for the role of lactoferrin in the pathogenesis of hypoferraemia, lactoferrin has an obvious role in host defence against bacterial infections. Sawatzki, Hoffman and Kubanek (1984) demonstrated that lactoferrin administration to mice prior to *Salmonella typhimurium* infection resulted in a reduced splenic bacterial count of 24 hours compared with mice without lactoferrin. The mechanism of this protective action is most probably by competition of lactoferrin with bacterial siderophores for iron, or a bactericidal effect of lactoferrin. Iron bound to lactoferrin has been shown to augment superoxide anion production by human monocytes in response to zymosan induction. Apolactoferrin, iron-saturated transferrin and free trivalent iron ions were inactive (Ito *et al.*, 1983). Thus iron-saturated lactoferrin enhances the microbicidal and tumoricidal activity of monocytes.

TISSUE IRON RELEASE AND FERRITIN SYNTHESIS

The reduction in release of iron from the labile iron pool in inflammation, and its increased diversion into ferritin stores, can be explained by one or more of the following mechanisms: (a) increased cellular uptake of iron, with subsequent expansion of the labile iron pool stimulating ferritin synthesis and diverting incoming iron into ferritin stores (Lynch *et al.*, 1974); (b) a primary membrane effect, blocking the entrance of cellular iron into the plasma, increasing the labile iron pool and stimulating ferritin synthesis; and (c) a primary enhancement of ferritin synthesis, resulting in the diversion of labile iron into ferritin stores and reducing the pool of iron available for immediate release.

Measurements of plasma iron turnover and the relative hepatic uptake of transferrin iron in inflammation did not indicate increased iron uptake by parenchymal cells (Konijn and Hershko, 1977).

Apoferritin is an inducible protein whose synthesis is stimulated by intracellular labile iron (Drysdale and Munro, 1966; Konijn, Baliga and Munro, 1973; Zähringer, Baliga and Munro, 1976; see also Chapter 4). *In vivo* iron administration to rats results in increased hepatic ferritin synthesis occurring at about 5 hours after iron injection (Drysdale and Munro, 1966). Consequently, in the case of a primary membrane block of iron release, a delay of several hours would be expected between the reduction in serum iron and plasma iron turnover and an increase in ferritin synthesis caused by an increased labile iron pool. Konijn and Hershko (1977) studied the sequential changes in serum iron and hepatic ferritin synthesis (Figure 6.3A) in rats following the induction of inflammation with turpentine. Alterations in the rate of apoferritin synthesis preceded the changes in serum iron throughout the study. [^{3}H]Leucine incorporation into ferritin at 4 hours of inflammation was twice normal, whereas serum iron and

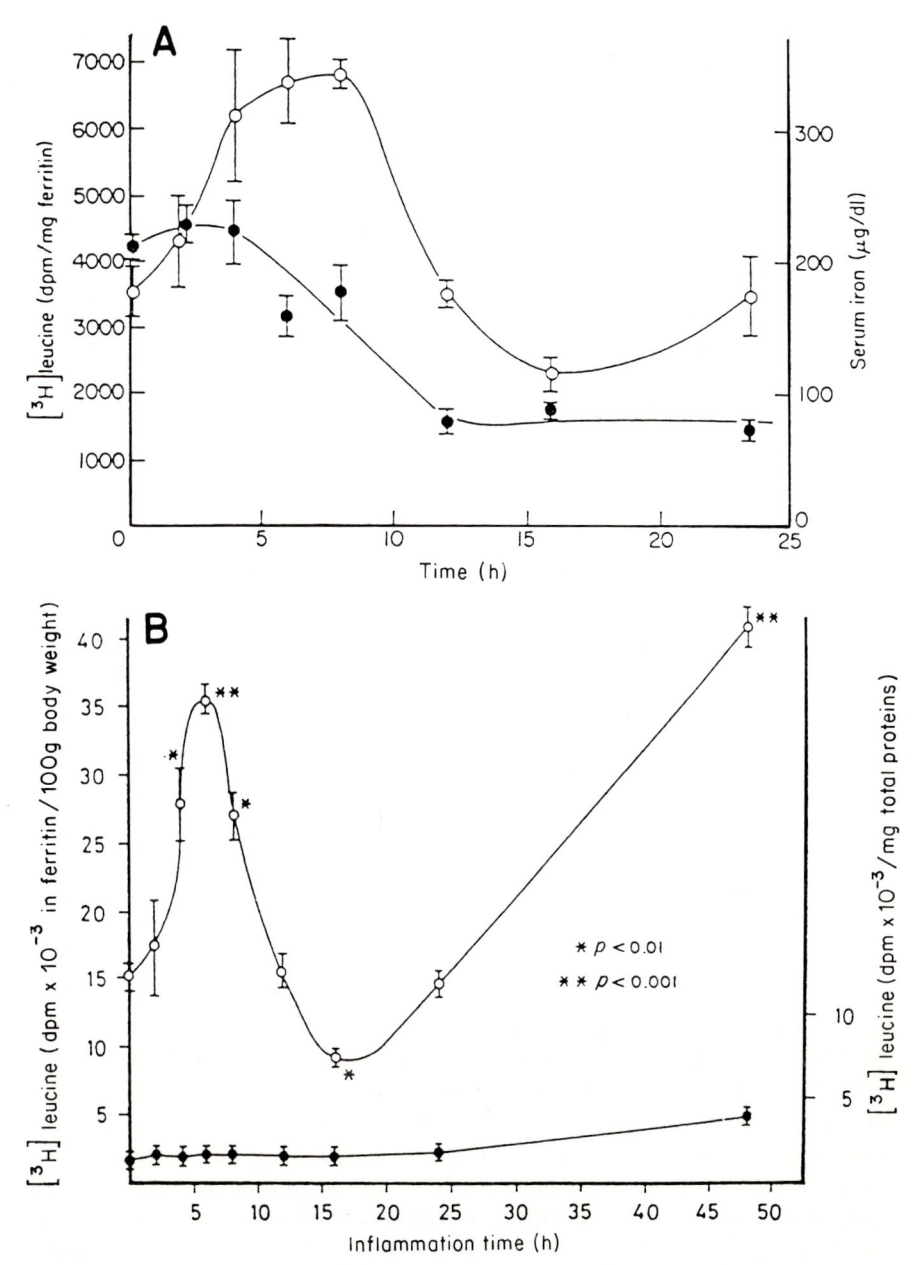

Figure 6.3 (A) Sequential changes in serum iron (●) and hepatic apoferritin synthesis (○) during the first 24 hours of turpentine-induced inflammation in rats. (B) Sequential changes in hepatic apoferritin synthesis (○) and total hepatic protein synthesis (●) 0–48 hours following turpentine-induced inflammation in rats. From Konijn and Hershko (1977) (A) and Konijn et al. (1981) (B) with permission of the British Journal of Haematology

plasma iron turnover were still unchanged. Ferritin synthesis remained elevated up to 8 hours after induction of inflammation. Conversely, maximal reduction in serum iron levels occurred at 12 hours of inflammation, at a time when apoferritin synthesis has already declined to the initial rate. These findings indicate that the increase in apoferritin synthesis in inflammation is not the result of a preceding block in iron release, and thus not the result of iron induction.

Apoferritin synthesis is regulated not only by iron supply but also by other, presumably humoral, factors. Thus, in developing erythroid cells the phase of maximal apoferritin synthesis precedes the phase of maximal iron uptake (Konijn, Hershko and Izak, 1979), indicating that ferritin may play a role not only in the storage of iron, but also in regulating cellular iron uptake and release. In another study, induction of human myeloid cell line differentiation has been shown to cause an increase in intracellular apoferritin synthesis and intracellular apoferritin concentrations (Fibach, Konijn and Rachmilewitz, 1985), irrespective of rates of iron uptake. It is possible that the increased apoferritin synthesis rates observed in inflammation are the result of direct stimulation by the inflammatory response, probably through IL-1, by analogy with other acute-phase-reacting proteins. Such increase in apoferritin synthesis probably directly causes the iron block in inflammation by diverting iron from the labile pool to ferritin stores. According to this hypothesis, the fall in serum iron is caused by an enlarged apoferritin pool which is able to trap iron from the labile iron pool, making it unavailable for release to transferrin. This hypothesis is compatible with ferrokinetic data indicating a reduced flow into the plasma (Konijn and Hershko, 1977; Hershko, Cook and Finch, 1974).

In rats with turpentine abscess, two waves of increased ferritin synthesis have been observed (Konijn et al., 1981) (Figure 6.3B), the second wave starting about 24 hours after the induction of inflammation and still increasing at 48 hours of inflammation. This second wave of increased apoferritin synthesis was characterized by a simultaneous increase in the synthesis of haemopexin, an acute-phase reactant in rats, and total protein synthesis, as well as a drop in the synthesis of albumin, a protein whose synthesis and serum levels are known to decrease in inflammation. Increased apoferritin synthesis was also observed in mouse peritoneal macrophages by Birgegård and Caro (1984) following either intraperitoneal administration of thioglycolate broth or an intramuscular injection of turpentine. These authors found no measurable apoferritin synthesis in resident macrophages. These data conflict with a report by Alvarez-Hernandez, Felstein and Brock (1986), who found a decrease in apoferritin synthesis in thioglycolate-elicited mouse peritoneal macrophages compared to control, resident or *Corynebacterium parvum*-activated peritoneal macrophages. The thioglycolate-elicited macrophages also contained reduced concentrations of ferritin. However, following pulse labelling with ^{59}Fe-labelled transferrin–anti-transferrin immune complexes, thioglycolate-elicited macrophages released less iron than control cells. Similarly, McLaren et al. (1982) found less apoferritin synthesis in human peripheral blood monocytes from rheumatoid arthritis patients than in monocytes obtained from healthy donors, but iron release was not studied.

Konijn et al. (1981) used cell-free protein-synthesizing systems in order to study the mechanism of increased ferritin synthesis in inflammation. By using combinations of polysomes and cell sap factors from inflamed and control rats, it was shown that the changes in hepatic apoferritin, haemopexin and albumin synthesis induced by inflammation could be reproduced in cell-free protein-synthesizing systems. Liver polysomes and autologous cell sap factors obtained from inflamed rats synthesized more ferritin than controls as early as 6 hours after the intramuscular injection of turpentine. After 48 hours of inflammation, ferritin synthesis was still increasing (Table 6.2). When liver cell sap factors from inflamed animals were incubated with polyribosomes obtained from livers of normal rats and *vice versa*, it could be shown that at the early stages of turpentine-induced inflammation, cell sap factors were more active in ferritin synthesis, but at a later stage of turpentine-induced inflammation, polysomes too had an increased ferritin synthetic activity, in parallel with an increased capacity for total protein synthesis. The latter finding implied increased mRNA content encoding other acute-phase reactants, as evidenced by increased haemopexin synthesis (Table 6.3). These observations point to a possible translational control of the first wave of ferritin synthesis in inflammation, and both translational and transcriptional control at a later stage of inflammation. Similarly, liver polyribosomes (Konijn et al., 1981) or microsomes (Bratcher and Shetlar, 1974) from turpentine-treated rats, incubated with their homologous cell sap, incorporated more amino acids (Table 6.2) (Konijn et al., 1981), or glucosamine (Bratcher and Shetlar, 1974) into their proteins than normal controls. Picoletti et al. (1984) and Konijn et al. (1981) have shown the importance of cell sap in this increase.

TABLE 6.2 Total protein, apoferritin, haemopexin and albumin synthesis ([^{3}H]amino acid incorporation, cpm $\times$ 10^{-3} ml^{-1} incubation) by rat liver cell-free protein-synthesizing systems after induction of inflammation by intramuscular injection of turpentine. Adapted from Konijn et al. (1981) by permission of the *British Journal of Haematology*

Source of polysomes and cell sap	Total protein	Ferritin	Haemopexin	Albumin
Control	520	6.3	13.5	82.1
6 h inflammation	572	21.3	12.5	93.9
48 h inflammation	1293	45.1	84.0	61.2

TABLE 6.3 Total protein, ferritin, haemopexin and albumin synthesis ([^{3}H]leucine incorporation, cpm × 10^{-3} ml^{-1} incubation) by rat liver cell-free protein-synthesizing systems employing cell sap of livers from control rats and polyribosomes from inflamed rats (A), and cell sap from inflamed rats and polyribosomes from control rat livers (B). Adapted from Konijn et al. (1981) by permission of the British Journal of Haematology

Source of polysomes	Total protein	Ferritin	Haemopexin	Albumin
(A)				
Control	193	3.2	1.5	32.0
6 h inflammation	197	2.6	1.9	27.3
48 h inflammation	273	7.3	4.4	14.2
Source of cell sap				
(B)				
Control	193	3.2	1.5	32.0
6 h inflammation	217	4.0	0.7	36.5
48 h inflammation	231	7.1	4.2	28.8

More recently, Cajone and Bernelli-Zazzera (1985) demonstrated increased amounts of leucyl-tRNA in the liver cell sap of inflamed animals, which may have contributed to the increase in protein synthesis. Another possible factor may be an increase in initiation factor activity in inflamed cell sap. Eukaryotic initiation factor eIF-2 is effective in relieving competitive inhibition of rat liver apoferritin mRNA from competition from more effectively translated mRNAs (Kaempfer and Konijn, 1983; Konijn and Kaempfer, 1983).

Although an increased activity of cell sap factors is associated with both the early and late phases of increased apoferritin synthesis (Table 6.3), increased polysomal activity is associated only with the later phase. This may be caused by either increased transcription of ferritin mRNA, as is the case with other acute-phase reactants (Gehring et al., 1987; Northemann et al., 1983a, 1983b; Princen et al., 1981) concomitant with a decreased transcription of albumin mRNA (Gehring et al., 1987; Northemann et al., 1983b; Princen et al., 1981), and/or channelling of free protoplasmic ferritin messenger ribonucleoprotein to polysomes, analogous to the mechanism proposed by Zähringer, Baliga and Munro (1976) for increased apoferritin synthesis in rat liver polysomes following iron induction.

SERUM FERRITIN

Serum ferritin levels are increased in patients with inflammatory disease (Baynes et al., 1986; Birgegård et al., 1978, 1979; Birgegård, 1980), Hodgkin's disease (Eschar, Order and Katz, 1974), haematological malignancies (Hershko and Konijn, 1984; Matzner, Konijn and Hershko, 1980), solid tumours such as breast cancer (Jacobs et al., 1976; Marcus and Zinberg, 1975), neuroblastoma (Hann, Levy and Evans, 1980; Hann, Stahlhut and Evans, 1986), some gynaecological malignancies (Wurtz, Von Moers and Zippel, 1985), and even in acquired immune deficiency syndrome (Gupta, Imam and Licorish, 1986). The response of serum ferritin levels to inflammation was found to parallel the acute-phase plasma proteins, haptoglobin (Birgegård et al., 1978) and C-reactive protein (Baynes et al., 1986), suggesting again that serum ferritin behaves as an acute-phase reactant. However, the degree to which serum ferritin rises is influenced by the iron status of the patients (Baynes et al., 1986; Bentley and Williams, 1974). Thus, a highly significant correlation between serum ferritin concentration and the grade of stainable iron in the bone marrow (Bentley and Williams, 1974) and RBC ferritin (Montecucco et al., 1986) has been found in patients with inflammatory disease. Serum ferritin is probably a secretory protein. Worwood et al. (1979) and Cragg, Wagstaff and Worwood (1980) proved by concanavalin-A (Con-A) absorption that most of the circulating ferritin is glycosylated, as opposed to intracellular tissue ferritin, which is mostly non-glycosylated. Except for albumin and retinol-binding protein, the secretory proteins in the plasma are glycosylated. Thus, it is most likely that glycosylated ferritin is a secretory plasma protein and non-glycosylated ferritin is the intracellular iron-storage protein. Most of the ferritin is synthesized on free polyribosomes in the cell (Hicks, Drysdale and Munro, 1968; Konijn, Baliga and Munro, 1973); this is probably true in relation to intracellular ferritin. However, some ferritin is also synthesized on membrane-bound polyribosomes (Konijn, Baliga and Munro, 1973; Puro and Richter, 1971; Zähringer et al., 1977). Membrane-bound polyribosomes synthesize mainly secretory proteins (Siekevitz and Palade, 1960). Hence, it is conceivable that ferritin produced on membrane-bound polyribosomes is secreted into the circulation following its glycosylation in the Golgi complex. In spite of the increase in serum ferritin in inflammatory conditions, the ratio between glycosylated and non-glycosylated forms in sera from normal controls and in inflammation is constant (Birgegård, 1980). The same is true for the increase in serum ferritin in patients with neuroblastoma (Hann, Stahlhut and Evans, 1986). Thus, it is reasonable to assume that increased serum ferritin is not the result of leakage from cells, but mainly of increased synthesis and active secretion of ferritin from cells and tissues. This conclusion is drawn from the fact that the ratio between the glycosylated form of ferritin and the non-glycosylated form is much lower in tissues than in the serum (Cragg, Wagstaff and Worwood, 1980; Hann, Stahlhut and Evans, 1986; Worwood et al., 1979). This observation and the increase in tissue ferritin concentrations associated with inflammation (Konijn et al., 1981) indicate increased ferritin synthesis on both membrane-bound and free polyribosomes. Consequently, the mechanism of induction of ferritin synthesis in inflammation may be different from that of induction of ferritin synthesis by iron, which is mainly on free polyribosomes (Konijn, Baliga and Munro, 1973).

THE ROLE OF INTERLEUKIN-1

The remarkable similarity in the haematological and acute-phase responses to inflammation and chronic diseases in different organisms is related to the central role of cytokines, especially IL-1, in this response. IL-1 is a factor secreted mainly by stimulated mononuclear phagocytes, but also by other cells (Dinarello, 1984). IL-1 has multiple actions in the response of the organism to inflammation, and according to its activity it has been given a number of different names; endogenous pyrogen (EP) (Atkins and Wood, 1955), lymphocyte-activating factor (LAF) (Gery, Gershon and Waksman, 1972; Gery and Waksman, 1972) and leukocyte endogenous mediator (LEM) (Pekarek and Beisel, 1971; Pekarek, Wannemacher and Beisel, 1972; Pekarek, Powenda and Wannemacher, 1972) were initially believed to represent different molecules but were found to be the same, or a family of very similar compounds with a molecular mass between 13 and 16 kDa (Oppenheim et al., 1982). In 1979 the term interleukin-1 was coined (Aarden et al., 1979). The hypoferraemic response to inflammation was attributed to a factor known as LEM, which copurified with EP and LAF and was thought to be IL-1 (Bornstein, 1982), but could not be proven to be identical with it (see reviews by Lee (1983) and Dinarello (1984)). Evidence for the identity of the hypoferraemic (and hypozincaemic) factor of inflammation with IL-1 was circumstantial, showing that supernatants of activated mononuclear macrophages were able to lower serum iron and zinc levels (Klasing, 1984). Recently, definitive proof for the involvement of IL-1 *per se* in the hypoferraemic response to inflammation and other acute-phase responses was obtained by Westmacott et al. (1986), using recombinant human and murine IL-1. They observed a dose dependent response to IL-1 for both the increase in acute-phase plasma proteins and decrease in plasma iron concentration. As mentioned earlier, decreased serum iron concentrations in inflammation are attributed to increased apoferritin synthesis in RE and parenchymal cells. This newly synthesized apoferritin is responsible for the sequestration of iron in tissues (Konijn and Hershko, 1977). Klasing (1984) found comparable results with zinc. By injecting partly purified IL-1 or endotoxin into leghorn chicks, a decrease in serum zinc concentrations and an increase in hepatic metallothionein and zinc concentrations were found. Klasing (1984) proposed that the changes in zinc metabolism associated with inflammation, and mediated through

IL-1, are caused by sequestration of zinc in the liver, in a fashion similar to that suggested previously for the changes in iron metabolism (Konijn and Hershko, 1977).

Injection of IL-1 (Ramadori *et al.*, 1985) causes an increase in serum glycoproteins referred to as acute-phase reactants (Bratcher and Shetlar, 1974) synthesized in the liver. Addition of IL-1 or monocyte-conditioned medium to hepatocyte cultures (Dinarello, 1984; Hooper *et al.*, 1981; Koj *et al.*, 1984, 1985) or cultured hepatoma cells (Darlington, Wilson and Lachman, 1986) induces increased synthesis of acute-phase reactant proteins and reduced synthesis of plasma albumin. It has been demonstrated lately that the increase in acute-phase reactant proteins is, at least partly, under transcriptional control. Levels of mRNAs for acute-phase proteins are increased in inflammation. Thus, a 66-fold increase in translatable α-2-macroglobulin was detected in rat livers 18 hours after intramuscular injection of turpentine (Northemann *et al.*, 1983a). Recent experiments employing cDNA hybridization (Gehring *et al.*, 1987) showed a 214-fold increase of α-2-macroglobulin mRNA over control values 18 hours after intraperitoneal administration of complete Freund's adjuvant to male rats. However, the increase in transcription rate of the α-2-macroglobulin gene was less than three-fold in nuclei from inflamed rats, as compared to controls, indicating altered post-transcriptional processing in addition to increased transcription of the acute-phase protein mRNA. Intravenous injection of recombinant murine IL-1 into endotoxin-resistant C3H/HeJ mice induced a dose-dependent increase in the specific hepatic mRNAs for the acute-phase proteins serum amyloid A (SAA) and factor B as measured by Northern blot analysis, and a decrease in serum albumin mRNA (Ramadori *et al.*, 1985), a negative acute-phase reactant. It can be assumed that the changes in iron metabolism mediated by IL-1 action are caused by the induction of apoferritin synthesis simultaneously with the other acute-phase reactants. The parallel changes in the concentrations of some acute-phase reactants and ferritin in the plasma of patients with inflammatory diseases (Baynes *et al.*, 1986; Birgegård *et al.*, 1978) support this contention.

A scheme of the proposed events in the early phase of increased apoferritin synthesis in inflammation is given in Figure 6.4. As the increase in ferritin synthesis in the early phase of inflammation is caused by cell sap factors, it is most probably associated with increased activity of elongation factors and/or increased availability of apoferritin mRNA-specific tRNA. Increased initiation factor activity would result in increased polysomal activity, or relieve apoferritin mRNA from competition with stronger competing mRNAs (Kaempfer and Konijn, 1983; Konijn and Kaempfer, 1983). Since the ratio between the glycosylated and non-glycosylated plasma ferritin is not affected by the inflammatory disease (Birgegård, 1980), the synthesis of apoferritin appears to be augmented on both free

```
CYTOPLASM
                        Ferritin mRNA
             Initiation factors ◄────── IL-1
  Membrane bound polyribosomes ◄──  ╳  ──► Free polyribosomes
             │              ┌─────────────────────────────┐              │
             │              │ Elongation factors          │              │
             │              │ Ferritin mRNA specific tRNA │              │
             │              └─────────────────────────────┘              │
             ▼                                                           ▼
   Translation and
   initiation of glycosylation                                    Translation
             │                                                           │
             ▼                                                           ▼
   Intracellular apoferritin                              Intracellular apoferritin
             │
             ▼
   Addition of carbohydrate
   in golgi complex
             │
             ▼
   Packaging in secretory                                  Iron sequestration
   vesicles                                                         │
             │                                                      ▼
             │                                                Increased cell
   Secretion                                                 ferritin iron
```

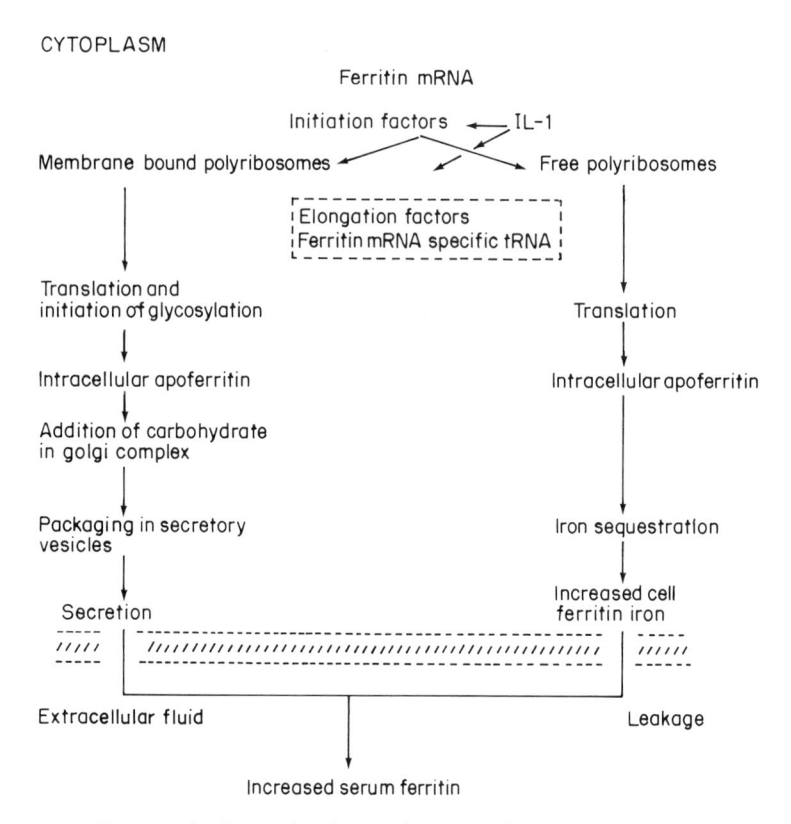

Figure 6.4 Proposed scheme for the mechanism of post-transcriptional regulation of apoferritin synthesis in inflammation, the increased intracellular ferritin iron and serum ferritin, and the role of IL-1

and bound polyribosomes. We may postulate for the first wave, and part of the second wave of increased apoferritin synthesis in inflammation the sequence of events described in Figure 6.4. The late wave of increased apoferritin synthesis is characterized by both increased polysomal and increased cell sap activity and can be explained by IL-1 affecting initiation factor activity (Figure 6.4) and/or increased transcription of apoferritin mRNA subunits (Figure 6.5). Thus IL-1 will cause an increase in the level of apoferritin mRNA in the cell. Normally, much of the apoferritin mRNA is located in the cytoplasm as untranslatable messenger ribonucleoprotein (Zähringer, Baliga and Munro, 1976) or 'repressed mRNP'. It is possible that IL-1 may cause derepression of apoferritin mRNP to translatable mRNA (Figure 6.5) which will then be transported from the cytoplasm to polyribosomes, resulting in increased apoferritin synthesis by polyribosomes, analogous to the mechanism proposed by Zähringer, Baliga and

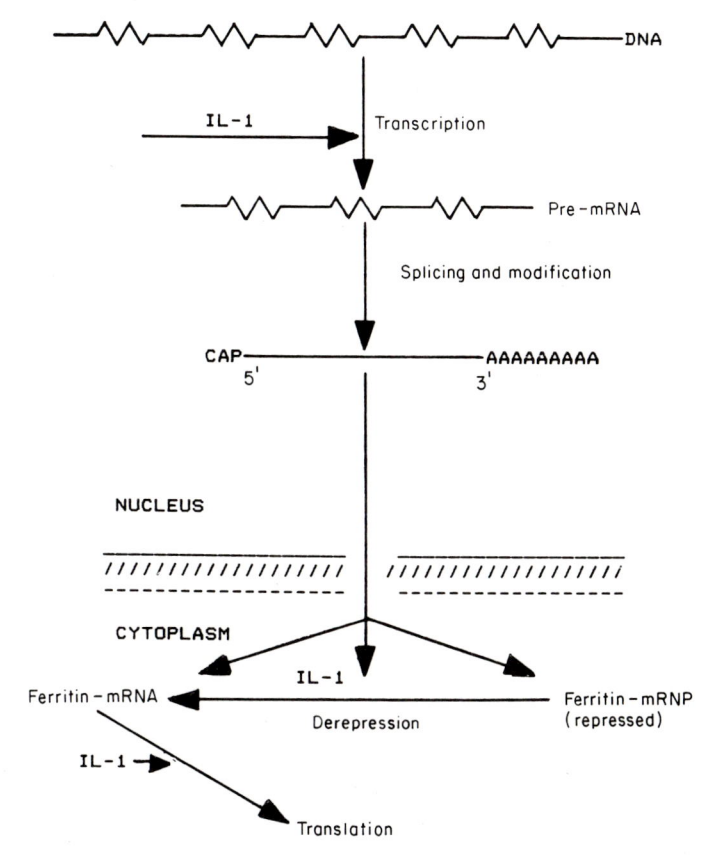

Figure 6.5 Proposed scheme for the mechanism of increased polyribosomal activity or ferritin mRNA availability in inflammation and the suggested role of IL-1

Munro (1976) for the action of iron on the induction of apoferritin synthesis. Increased apoferritin synthesis, in addition to increased apolactoferrin secretion from polymorphonuclear leukocytes due to degranulation caused by IL-1 (Klempner, Dinarello and Gallin, 1978) or complement component C5a (Webster et al., 1980) may explain the changes in iron metabolism along the lines proposed by Roeser (1980) (Figure 6.1): (a) Augmented apoferritin synthesis, followed by an accelerated entry of iron into the cell in the form of haemoglobin (due to shortened RBC survival), and as lactoferrin (following iron chelation at the site of inflammation or in the extracellular fluid by apolactoferrin secreted by activated polymorphonuclear leucocytes). (b) Lactoferrin releases its iron in the lysosomal system. Preformed apoferritin accelerates the diversion of the released iron into the preformed apoferritin, thus decreasing the 'labile' cellular iron pool. In

```
                    INFECTION, INJURY, MALIGNANCY
                                  │
                                  ↓
                             Inflammation
                                  │
                           C5a    │
                                  ↓
                    Mononuclear phagocyte cell activation
         ┌────────────────────────┘
         │
     IL-1 Release
         │           ┌──→ Blockade of iron release
         │   Macrophages ──→ Increased ferritin synthesis (?)
         │           └──→ Increased ferritin release   (?)
         │
         ├──→ Granulocytes ──→ Apolactoferrin release
         │
         │                    ──→ Increased ferritin synthesis
         ├──→ Liver           ──→ Blockade of iron release
         │                        Increased ferritin release
         │
         └──→ Intestine       ──→ Decreased iron absorption
```

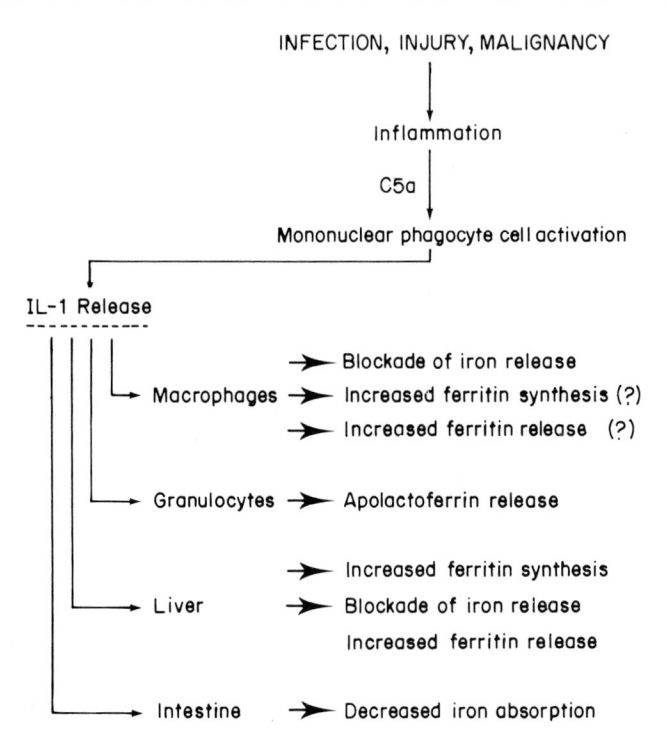

Figure 6.6 Proposed scheme for the effect of inflammation and IL-1 on iron metabolism in different target tissues

addition, lysosomal enzymes, discharged into the cell due to the destabilizing effect of intracellular mediators of inflammation on the lysosomal membrane, will cause enhanced formation of haemosiderin from ferritin with the net effect of making iron even less available to the labile cellular iron pool. The overall effect is therefore a decrease of the plasma iron pool, resulting in a reduction of iron available for erythropoiesis. By employing recombinant IL-1 it was recently shown that IL-1 *per se* is able to decrease serum iron in experimental animals (Westmacott *et al.*, 1986). However, its mechanism of action in the altered iron metabolism of inflammation is still obscure. Its effect on iron metabolism in inflammation is summarized in Figure 6.6. Taken together, these effects cause a reduction in available iron. The blockade of iron release and the resultant hypoferraemia is believed by some to be a host defence mechanism, withholding iron from pathogenic micro-organisms or tumour cells, representing a form of nutritional immunity (Kochan, 1973; Weinberg, 1975, 1978, 1986). However, the 'nutritional immunity' hypothesis is a subject of current controversy (Brock and Mainou-Fowler, 1986).

REFERENCES

Aarden, L. A., Brunner, T. K., Cerottini, J. C. et al., (1979). Revised nomenclature for antigen-nonspecific T-cell proliferation and helper factors, *J. Immunol.*, **123**, 2928–9.
Alexanian, R. (1972). Erythropoietin excretion in hemolytic anemia and in the hypoferremia of chronic disease, *Blood*, **40**, 946–51.
Alvarez-Hernandez, X., Felstein, M. V., and Brock, J. H. (1986). The relation between iron release, ferritin synthesis and intracellular iron distribution in mouse peritoneal macrophages. Evidence for a reduced level of metabolically available iron in elicited macrophages, *Biochem. Biophys. Acta*, **886**, 214–22.
Atkins, E., and Wood, W. B. Jr (1955). Studies on the pathogenesis of fever. II. Identification of an endogenous pyrogen in the bloodstream following the injection of typhoid vaccine, *J. Exp. Med.*, **102**, 449–616.
Bagicalupo, A., Podesta, M., Mingari, M., Morreta, L., Piagio, G., Van Lint, M., Durando, A., and Marmont, A. (1981). Generation of CFU-c/suppressor T-cells *in vitro*: An experimental model for immune-mediated marrow failure, *Blood*, **57**, 491–6.
Bailey, P. T., Abeles, F. B., Hauer, E. C., and Mapes, C. A. (1976). Intracerebroventricular administration of leukocytic endogenous mediators (LEM) in the rat, *Proc. Soc. Exp. Biol. Med.*, **153**, 419–23.
Baynes, R., Beswoda, W., Bothwell, T., Khan, Q., and Mansoor, N. (1986). The non-immune inflammatory response: serial changes in plasma iron, iron binding capacity, lactoferrin and C-reactive protein, *Scand. J. Clin. Lab. Invest.*, **46**, 695–704.
Bentley, D. P., and Williams, P. (1974). Serum ferritin concentrations as an index of storage iron in rheumatoid arthritis, *J. Clin. Pathol.*, **27**, 786–93.
Berglund, B., Hemmingsson, P., and Birgegård, G. (1987). Detection of autologous blood transfusions in cross-country skiers, *Int. J. Sports Med.*, **8**, 66–70.
Birgegård, G. (1980). The source of serum ferritin during infection. Studies with concanavalin A-Sepharose absorption, *Clin. Sci.*, **59**, 385–7.
Birgegård, G., and Caro, J. (1984). Increased ferritin synthesis and iron uptake in inflammatory mouse macrophages, *Scand. J. Haematol.*, **33**, 43–8.
Birgegård, G., Hällgren, R., and Caro, J. (1987). Serum erythropoietin in rheumatoid arthritis and other inflammatory arthritides: relationship to anaemia and the effect of anti-inflammatory treatment, *Br. J. Haematol.*, **65**, 479–83.
Birgegård, G., Hällgren, R., Killander, A., Stromberg, A., Venge, P., and Wide, L. (1978). Serum ferritin during infection. A longitudinal study, *Scand. J. Haematol.*, **21**, 333–40.
Birgegård G., Hällgren, R., Killander, A., Venge, P., and Wide, L. (1979). Serum ferritin during infection. A longitudinal study in renal transplant patients, *Acta Med. Scand.* **205**, 641–5.
Bornstein, D. L. (1982). Leukocytic pyrogen: A mediator of the acute phase reaction, *Ann. N.Y. Acad. Sci.*, **389**, 323–7.
Bratcher, S. C., and Shetlar, M. R. (1974). Glycoprotein biosynthesis in a rat liver microsome system following inflammation, *Am. J. Physiol.*, **227**, 1394–8.
Brock, J. H., and Mainou-Fowler, T. (1986). Iron and immunity, *Proc. Nutr. Soc.*, **45**, 305–15.
Broxmeyer, H. E., Bognacki, J., Dorner, M. H., and de Sousa, M. (1981). The identification of leukemia-associated inhibitory activity (LIA) as acidic isoferritins in the production of granulocytes and macrophages, *J. Exp. Med.*, **153**, 1426–44.

Broxmeyer, H. E., Lu, L., Bicknell, D. C., Williams, D. E., Cooper, S., Levi, S., Salfeld, J., and Arosio, P. (1986). The influence of purified recombinant human heavy subunit and light subunit ferritins on colony formation *in vitro* by granulocyte-macrophage and erythroid progenitor cells, *Blood*, **68**, 1257–63.

Cajone, F., and Bernelli-Zazzera, A. (1985). Soluble factors of protein synthesis in rat liver during the acute phase reaction, *Exp. Mol. Pathol.*, **43**, 56–63.

Cartwright, G. E., and Lee, G. R. (1971). The anaemia of chronic disorders, *Br. J. Haematol.*, **21**, 147–52.

Cavill, I., and Bentley, D. P. (1982). Erythropoiesis in the anaemia of rheumatoid arthritis, *Br. J. Haematol.*, **50**, 583–90.

Cavill, I., Ricketts, C., and Napier, J. A. F. (1977). Erythropoiesis in the anaemia of chronic disease, *Scand. J. Haematol.*, **19**, 509–12.

Cazzola, M., Arosio, P., Gobbi, P. G., Barosi, G., Bergamaschi, G., Dezza, L., Iacobello, C., and Ascari, E. (1983). Basic and acidic isoferritins in the serum of patients with Hodgkin's disease, *Eur. J. Cancer Clin. Oncol.*, **19**, 339–45.

Chandler, F. W. Jr, and Fletcher, O. J. Jr (1973). Effects of a transplantable lymphoid tumor (Olson) on erythropoiesis and erythroid survival, *Avian Dis.*, **17**, 737–42.

Chenoweth, D. E., and Hugli, T. E. (1980). Human C5a and C5a analogs as probes of the neutrophil C5a receptor, *Mol. Immunol.*, **17**, 151–61.

Chenoweth, D. E., Goodman, M. G., and Weigle, W. O. (1982). Demonstration of a specific receptor for human C5a anaphylatoxin on murine macrophages, *J. Exp. Med.*, **156**, 68–78.

Cotes, P. M., Brozovic, B., Mausel, M., and Samson, D. M. (1980). Radioimmunoassay of erythropoietin (Ep) in human serum: validation and application of an assay system, *Exp. Haematol.*, **8** (Supplement 8), 292–4.

Cox, R., Musial, T., and Gyde, O. H. B. (1986). Reduced erythropoietin levels as a cause of anaemia in patients with lung cancer, *Eur. J. Cancer Clin. Oncol.*, **22**, 511–14.

Craddock, P. R., Hammerschmidt, D., White, J. G., Dalmasso, A. P., and Jacob, H. S. (1977). Complement (C5a) induced granulocyte aggregation *in vitro*, *J. Clin. Invest.*, **60**, 260–4.

Cragg, S. J., Wagstaff, M., and Worwood, M. (1980). Sialic acid and the microheterogeneity of human serum ferritin, *Clin. Sci.*, **58**, 259–62.

Dainiak, N., Kulkarni, V., Howard, D., Kalmanti, M., Dewey, M. C., and Hoffman, R. (1983). Mechanism of abnormal erythropoiesis in malignancy, *Cancer*, **51**, 1101–6.

Darlington, G. J., Wilson, D. R., and Lachman, L. B. (1986). Monocyte conditioned medium, interleukin-1, and tumor necrosis factor *in vitro*, *J. Cell Biol.*, **103**, 787–93.

Dinant, H. J., and de Maat, C. E. M. (1978). Erythropoiesis and mean red cell life span in normal subjects and in patients with the anaemia of active rheumatoid arthritis, *Br. J. Haematol.*, **39**, 437–44.

Dinarello, C. A. (1984). Interleukin-1, *Rev. Infect. Dis.*, **6**, 51–95.

Doll, D. C., and Weiss, R. B. (1985). Neoplasia and the erythron, *J. Clin. Oncol.*, **3**, 429–45.

Dörner, M. H., Silverstone, A., Nishiya, K., de Sostoa, A., Munn, G., and de Sousa, M. (1980). Ferritin synthesis by human T-lymphocytes, *Science*, **209**, 1019–20.

Douglas, S. W., and Adamson, J. W. (1975). The anaemia of chronic disorders. Studies of marrow regulation and iron metabolism, *Blood*, **45**, 55–65.

Drysdale, J. W., and Munro, H. N. (1966). Regulation of synthesis and turnover of ferritin in rat liver, *J. Biol. Chem.*, **241**, 3630–7.

Elin, R. J., Wolff, S. M., and Finch, C. A. (1977). Effect of induced fever on serum iron and ferritin concentrations in man, *Blood*, **49**, 147–53.

Erslev, A. J., Caro, J., Miller, O., and Silver, R. (1980). Plasma erythropoietin in health and disease, *Ann. Clin. Lab. Sci.*, **10**, 250–9.

Eschar, Z., Order, S. E., and Katz, D. H. (1974). Ferritin: a Hodgkin's disease associated antigen, *Proc. Natl Acad. Sci. USA*, **71**, 3956–60.

Esparza, I., and Brock, J. H. (1981). Release of iron by resident and stimulated mouse peritoneal macrophages following ingestion and degradation of transferrin–antitransferrin immune complexes, *Br. J. Haematol.*, **49**, 603–14.

Fernandez, H. N., Henson, P. M., Otani, A., and Hugli, T. E. (1978). Chemotactic response to human C3a and C5a anaphylatoxins. I. Evaluation of C3a and C5a leukotaxis *in vitro* and under stimulated *in vivo* conditions,. *J. Immunol.*, **120**, 109–15.

Fibach, E., Konijn, A. M., and Rachmilewitz, E. A. (1985). Changes in cellular ferritin content during myeloid differentiation of human leukemic cell lines, *Am. J. Hematol.*, **18**, 143–51.

Fillet, G., Cook, J. D., and Finch, C. A. (1974). Storage iron kinetics VII. A biological model for reticuloendothelial iron transport, *J. Clin. Invest.*, **53**, 1527–33.

Freireich, E. J., Miller, A., Emerson, C. P., and Finch, S. C. (1957). Radioactive iron metabolism and erythrocyte survival. Studies of the mechanism of the anemia associated with rheumatoid arthritis, *J. Clin. Invest.*, **36**, 1043–58.

Gehring, M. R., Sheils, B. R., Northemann, W., de Bruin, M. H. L., Kan, C. C., Chain, A. C., Noonan, D. J., and Fey, G. H. (1987). Sequence of rat liver α-2-macroglobulin and acute phase control of its messenger RNA, *J. Biol. Chem.*, **262**, 446–54.

Gery, I., Gershon, R. K., and Waksman, B. H. (1972). Potentiation of the T-lymphocyte response to mitogens. I. The responding cell, *J. Exp. Med.*, **136**, 128–42.

Gery, I., and Waksman, B. H. (1972). Potentiation of the T-lymphocyte response to mitogens. II. The cellular source of potentiating mediator(s), *J. Exp. Med.*, **136**, 143–55.

Goodman, M. G., Chenoweth, D. E., and Weigle, W. O. (1982). Induction of interleukin-1 secretion and enhancement of humoral immunity by binding of human C5a to macrophage surface C5a receptors, *J. Exp. Med.*, **156**, 912–17.

Gorodetski, R., Fuks, Z., Peretz, T., and Ginsburg, H. (1985). Direct fluorometric determination of erythrocyte zinc and free protoporphyrins in whole blood, *J. Clin. Biochem.*, **18**, 362–86.

Gorodetski, R., Fuks, Z., Peretz, T., and Ginsburg, H. (1986). Elevation of erythrocyte zinc- and free protoporphyrins with metastatic spread in cancer patients, *Eur. J. Cancer Clin. Oncol.*, **22**, 1515–21.

Gupta, S., Imam, A., and Licorish, K. (1986). Serum ferritin in acquired immune deficiency syndrome, *J. Clin. Lab. Immunol.*, **20**, 11–13.

Gutinsky, A., and Van Dyke, K. (1963). Normal response to erythropoietin or hypoxia in rats made anemic with turpentine abscess, *Proc. Soc. Exp. Biol. Med.*, **112**, 75–8.

Hammond, D., Shore, N., and Movassaghi, N. (1968). Production, utilization and excretion of erythropoietin. I. Chronic anemias. II. Aplastic crisis. III. Erythropoietic effects of normal plasma, *Proc. N.Y. Acad. Sci.*, **149**, 516–27.

Hann, H. L., Levy, H. M., and Evans, A. E. (1980). Serum ferritin as a guide to therapy in neuroblastoma, *Cancer Res.*, **40**, 1411–13.

Hann, H. L., Stahlhut, M. W., and Evans, A. E. (1986). Source of increased ferritin in neuroblastoma, *J. Natl Cancer Inst.*, **76**, 1031–3.

Hansen, N. E., Karle, H., Andersen, V., Malmquist, J., and Hoff, G. E. (1976). Neutrophilic granulocytes in acute bacterial infection. Sequential studies on lysosome myeloperoxidase and lactoferrin, *Clin. Exp. Immunol.*, **26**, 463–8.

Hershko, C. (1977). Storage iron regulation. In E. B. Brown (ed.) *Progress in Haematology 10*, pp. 105–48, Grune and Stratton, New York, San Francisco, London.

Hershko, C., Cook, J. D., and Finch, C. A. (1974). Storage iron kinetics. VI. The effect of inflammation on iron exchange in the rat, *Br. J. Haematol.*, **28**, 67–75.

Hershko, C., and Konijn, A. M. (1984). Serum ferritin in hematological disorders. In A. Albertini, P. Arosio, E. Chiancone and J. W. Drysdale (eds) *Ferritin and Isoferritins as Biological Markers*, pp. 143–58, Elsevier Science Publishers, Amsterdam, New York, London.

Hicks, S. J., Drysdale, J. W., and Munro, H. N. (1968). Preferential synthesis of ferritin and albumin by different populations of liver polysomes, *Science*, **164**, 584–5.

Hoffman, R., Kopel, S., Hsu, S. D., Dainiak, N., and Zanjani, E. D. (1978). T-cell chronic lymphocytic leukemia: Presence in bone marrow and peripheral blood of cells that suppress erythropoiesis *in vitro*, *Blood*, **52**, 255–60.

Hooper, D. C., Steer, C. J., Dinarello, C. A., and Peacock, A. C. (1981). Haptoglobin and albumin synthesis in isolated rat hepatocytes. Response to potential mediators of the acute phase reaction, *Biochim. Biophys. Acta*, **653**, 118–29.

Hoy, T. G., and Jacobs, A. (1981). Ferritin polymers and the formation of haemosiderin, *Br. J. Haematol.*, **49**, 593–602.

Ito, M., Bognacki, J., Broxmeyer, H., de Sousa, M., and Hadden, J. W. (1983). Augmentation of human monocyte chemiluminescence by iron-saturated lactoferrin, *Int. J. Immunopharmacol.*, **5**, 359–64.

Jacobs, A. (1980). The pathology of iron overload. In A. Jacobs and M. Worwood (eds) *Iron in Biochemistry and Medicine II*, pp. 427–59, Academic Press, London and New York.

Jacobs, A., Jones, B., Rickets, C., Bulbrook, R. D., and Wang, D. Y. (1976). Serum ferritin concentrations in early breast cancer, *Br. J. Cancer*, **34**, 286–90.

Janossy, G., Tidman, N., Selby, W. S., Thomas, J. A., Granger, S., Kung, P. C., and Goldstein, G. (1980). Human T-lymphocytes of inducer and suppressor type occupy different micro-environments, *Nature*, **288**, 81–4.

Jelkman, W. (1982). Temporal pattern of erythropoietin titers in kidney tissues during hypoxic hypoxia, *Pflugers Arch.*, **393**, 88–91.

Kaempfer, R., and Konijn, A. M. (1983). Translational competition by mRNA species encoding albumin, haemopexin, ferritin and globin, *Eur. J. Biochem.*, **131**, 545–50.

Kaaba, S., Jacobs, A., Schreuder, W., Ting, W. C., and Smith, S. (1984). Pathogenesis of anaemia in untreated patients with disseminated bronchial cancer, *Br. J. Haematol.*, **56**, 675–6.

Kampschmidt, R. F., and Upchurch, H. F. (1962). Effects of bacterial endotoxin on plasma iron, *Proc. Soc. Exp. Biol. Med.*, **110**, 191–3.

Kampschmidt, R. F., and Upchurch, H. F. (1969). Lowering of plasma iron concentrations in the rat with leukocytic extracts, *Am. J. Physiol.*, **216**, 1287–91.

Karle, H. (1968). The site of abnormal erythrocyte destruction during experimental fever, *Br. J. Haematol.*, **15**, 475–85.

Karle, H. (1974). The pathogenesis of the anaemia of chronic disorders and the role of fever in erythrokinetics, *Scand. J. Haematol.*, **13**, 81–6.
Karle, H., and Hansen, N. E. (1970). Changes in the red cell membrane induced by a small rise in temperature, *Scand. J. Clin. Lab. Invest.*, **26**, 169–74.
Klasing, K. C. (1984). Effect of inflammatory agents and interleukin-1 on iron and zinc metabolism, *Am. J. Physiol.*, **247**, R901–4.
Klempner, M. S., Dinarello, C. A., and Gallin, J. I. (1978). Human leukocytic pyrogen induces release of specific granule contents from human neutrophils, *J. Clin. Invest.*, **61**, 1330–6.
Kochan, I. (1973). The role of iron in bacterial infections with special consideration of host-tubercle bacillus interaction, *Curr. Top. Microbiol. Immunol.*, **60**, 1–30.
Koj, A., Gauldie, J., Regoeczi, E., Sauder, D. N., and Sweeney, G. D. (1984). The acute phase response of cultured rat hepatocytes. System characterization and the effect of human cytokines, *Biochem. J.*, **224**, 505–14.
Koj, A., Gauldie, J., Sweeney, G. D., Regoeczi, E., and Sauder, D. N. (1985). A simple bioassay for monocyte-derived hepatocyte stimulating factor: increased synthesis of α-2-macroglobulin and reduced synthesis of albumin by cultured rat hepatocytes, *J. Immunol. Methods*, **76**, 317–28.
Konijn, A. M., and Hershko, C. (1977). Ferritin synthesis in inflammation. I. Pathogenesis of impaired iron release, *Br. J. Haematol.*, **37**, 7–16.
Konijn, A. M., and Kaempfer, R. (1983). Translational competition by mRNA species encoding ferritin, haemopexin, albumin and globin. In I. Urushizaki, P. Aisen, I. Listowsky and J. W. Drysdale (eds) *Structure and Function of Iron Storage and Transport Proteins*, pp. 97–103, Elsevier Science Publishers, Amsterdam.
Konijn, A. M., Baliga, B. S., and Munro, H. N. (1973). Synthesis of liver ferritin on free and membrane-bound polyribosomes of different sizes, *FEBS Lett.*, **37**, 249–52.
Konijn, A. M., Hershko, C., and Izak, G. (1979). Ferritin synthesis and iron uptake in developing erythroid cells, *Am. J. Hematol.*, **6**, 373–9.
Konijn, A. M., Carmel, N., Levy, R., and Hershko, C. (1981). Ferritin synthesis in inflammation. II. Mechanism of increased ferritin synthesis, *Br. J. Haematol.*, **49**, 361–70.
Lee, G. R. (1983). The anaemia of chronic disease, *Semin. Hematol.*, **20**, 61–80.
Letendre, E. D., and Holbein, B. E. (1983). Turnover in the transferrin pool during the hypoferremic phase of experimental *Neisseria meningitidis* infection in mice, *Infect. Immun.*, **39**, 50–9.
Linch, D. C. (1985). Activated suppressor T-cells and the role of interferon in aplastic anemia, *Immunology Today*, **6**, 155–6.
Lipschitz, D. A., Cook, J. D., and Finch, C. A. (1974). A clinical evaluation of serum ferritin as an index of iron stores, *N. Engl. J. Med.*, **290**, 213–16.
Lukens, J. N. (1973). Control of erythropoiesis in rats with adjuvant-induced chronic inflammation, *Blood*, **41**, 37–44.
Lynch, S. R., Lipschitz, D. A., Bothwell, T. H., and Charlton, R. W. (1974). Iron and the reticuloendothelial system. In A. Jacobs and M. Worwood (eds) *Iron in Biochemistry and Medicine I*, pp. 563–87, Academic Press, London.
Macdonald, R. A., MacSween, R. N. M., and Pechet, G. S. (1969). Iron metabolism by reticuloendothelial cells *in vitro*: Physical and chemical conditions, lipotrope deficiency, and acute inflammation, *Lab. Invest.*, **21**, 236–45.
Mahmood, T., Robinson, W. A., and Vautrin, R. (1977). Granulopoietic and erythropoietic activity in patients with anemias of iron deficiency and chronic disease, *Blood*, **50**, 449–55.
Mangan, K. F., Chikkappa, G., and Farley, P. C. (1982). T-Gamma (Tγ) cells

suppress growth of erythroid colony-forming units *in vitro* in the pure red cell aplasia of B-cell chronic lymphocytic leukemia, *J. Clin. Invest.*, **70**, 1148–56.

Mangan, K. F., Hartnett, M. E., Matis, S. A., Winkelstein, A., and Abo, T. (1984). Natural killer cells suppress human erythroid stem proliferation *in vitro*, *Blood*, **63**, 260–9.

Marchal, G., and Milon, G. (1981a). Decreased erythropoiesis: The origin of BCG induced anaemia in mice, *Br. J. Haematol.*, **48**, 551–60.

Marchal, G., and Milon, G. (1981b). Anémie et leukocytose induites par le BCG chez la souris: Nécessité de la présence de lymphocytes thymodépendants, *Ann. Immunol. Paris*, **132D**, 249–56.

Marchal, G., and Milon, G. (1986). Control of hemopoiesis in mice by sensitized L3T4+ Lyt2− lymphocytes during infection with Bacillus Calmette-Guerin, *Proc. Natl Acad. Sci. USA*, **83**, 3977–81.

Marcus, D. M., and Zinberg, N. (1975). Measurement of serum ferritin by radioimmunoassay: results in normal individuals and patients with breast cancer, *J. Natl Cancer Inst.*, **55**, 791–5.

Matzner, Y., and Brzezinski, A. (1984). A C5a inhibitor in peritoneal fluid, *J. Lab. Clin. Med.*, **103**, 227–35.

Matzner, Y., Konijn, A. M., and Hershko, C. (1980). Serum ferritin in hematologic malignancies, *Am. J. Hematol.*, **9**, 13–22.

Matzner, Y., Partridge, R. E. H., and Babior, B. M. (1983). A chemotactic inhibitor in synovial fluid, *Immunology*, **49**, 131–8.

Mclaren, G. D., Konijn, A. M., Bentley, D. P., and Jacobs, A. (1982). Iron uptake and ferritin synthesis by human peripheral blood monocytes incubated *in vitro* with a particulate suspension of radio iron. In P. Saltman and J. Hegenauer (eds) *The Biochemistry and Physiology of Iron*, pp. 605–9, Elsevier Biomedical, New York.

Mikolajew, M., Kuratowska, K., Kossakowska, Z., Placheska, M., and Kopec, M. (1969). Haematological changes in adjuvant disease in the rat. II. Iron metabolism and ^{51}-Cr erythrocyte survival, *Ann. Rheum. Dis.*, **28**, 172–8.

Milon, G., Lebastard, M., and Marchal, G. (1985). T-dependent production and activation of mononuclear phagocyte during murine BCG infection, *Immunol. Lett.*, **11**, 189–94.

Milon, G., and Marchal, G. (1981). Anémie induite par le BCG chez la souris: Nécessité de la presence de lymphocytes thymo-dépéndants, *Ann. Immunol. Paris*, **132C**, 21–8.

Montecucco, C., Carnevale, R., Cazzola, M., Longhi, M., Caporali, R., Goggi, P. L., and Cherie-Ligniere, E. L. (1986). Microcytic anaemia in rheumatoid arthritis. Relationship with activity and duration of the disease and iron status, *Haematologica*, **71**, 383–7.

Movassaghi, N., Shore, N. A., and Hammond, D. (1967). Serum and urinary levels of erythropoietin in iron deficient anemia, *Proc. Soc. Exp. Biol. Med.*, **126**, 615–18.

Nakao, S., Harada, M., Kondo, K., Odaka, K., Ueda, M., Matsue, K., Mori, T., and Hattori, K. (1984). Effect of activated lymphocytes on the regulation of hematopoiesis: Suppression of *in vitro* granulopoiesis by OKT8+Ia+ T-cells induced by alloantigen stimulation, *J. Immunol.*, **132**, 160–4.

Niitsu, Y., Goto, Y., Kohgo, Y., Adachi, C., Onodera, Y., and Urushizaki, I. (1980). Evaluation of heart isoferritin assay for diagnosis of cancer. In A. Albertini (ed.) *Radioimmunoassay of Hormones, Proteins and Enzymes*, pp. 256–66, Excerpta Medica, Amsterdam.

Niitsu, Y., Onodera, Y., Kohgo, Y., Goto, Y., Watanabe, N., and Urushizaki, I. (1984). Isoferritins in malignant diseases. In A. Albertini, P. Arosio, E. Chiancone

and J. Drysdale (eds) *Ferritins and Isoferritins as Biological Markers*, pp. 159–69, Elsevier Science Publishers, Amsterdam.
Nishisato, T., and Aisen, P. (1983). Interaction of transferrin with iron loaded macrophages. In I. Urushizaki, P. Aisen, I. Listowsky and J. W. Drysdale (eds) *Structure and Function of Iron Storage and Transport Proteins*, pp. 353–8, Elsevier Science Publishers, Amsterdam.
Northemann, W., Andus, T., Gross, V., and Heinrich, P. C. (1983a). Cell free synthesis of rat α-2-macroglobulin and induction of its mRNA during experimental inflammation, *Eur. J. Biochem.*, **137**, 257–62.
Northemann, W., Andus, T., Cross, V., Nagashima, M., Schreiber, G., and Heinrich, P. C. (1983b). Messenger RNA activities of four acute phase proteins during inflammation, *FEBS Lett.*, **161**, 319–22.
Noyes, W. D., Bothwell, T. H., and Finch, C. A. (1960). The role of the reticuloendothelial cell in iron metabolism, *Br. J. Haematol.*, **6**, 43–55.
O'Flaherty, J. T., Kreutzer, D. L., and Ward, P. A. (1977). Neutrophil aggregation and swelling induced by chemotactic agents, *J. Immunol.*, **119**, 232–9.
Oppenheim, J. J., Stadler, B. M., Siraganian, R. P., Mage, M., and Mathieson, B. (1982). Lymphokines: their role in lymphocyte responses. Properties of interleukin-1, *Fed. Proc.*, **41**, 257–62.
Pagé, M., Thériault, L., and Caron, M. (1979). Serum ferritin in the evaluation of leukemic patients and its synthesis in cell culture, *Protides Biol. Fluids*, **27**, 81–4.
Pekarek, R. S., and Beisel, W. R. (1971). Characterization of the endogenous mediator(s) of serum zinc and iron depression during infection and other stresses, *Proc. Soc. Exp. Biol. Med.*, **138**, 728–31.
Pekarek, R. S., Powenda, M. C., and Wannemacher, R. W. Jr (1972). The effect of leukocytic endogenous mediator (LEM) on serum copper and ceruloplasmin concentrations in the rat, *Proc. Soc. Exp. Biol. Med.*, **141**, 1029–31.
Pekarek, R. S., Wannemacher, R. W. Jr, and Beisel, W. R. (1972). The effect of leukocytic endogenous mediator (LEM) on the tissue distribution of zinc and iron, *Proc. Soc. Exp. Biol. Med.*, **140**, 685–8.
Pekarek, R. S., Wannemacher, R. W. Jr, Chappel, F. E. III, Powanda, M. C., and Beisel, W. R. (1972). Further characterization and species specificity of leukocytic endogenous mediator (LEM), *Proc. Soc. Exp. Biol. Med.*, **141**, 643–8.
Pelkonen, P., Swanljung, K., and Siimes, M. A. (1986). Ferritinemia as an indicator of systemic disease activity in children with systemic juvenile rheumatoid arthritis, *Acta Paediatr. Scand.*, **75**, 64–8.
Piccoletti, R., Alletti, M. G., Cajone, F., and Bernelli-Zazzera, A. (1984). The role of nuclei, polyribosomes and cytosol factors in the onset of the acute phase reaction in the liver cells, *Br. J. Exp. Pathol.*, **65**, 419–30.
Podesta, M., Frassoni, F., Van Lint, M., Piagio, G., Marmont, A., and Bacigalupo, A. (1982). Generation of CFU-c suppressor T-cells *in vitro*. II. Effect of PHA, PWM, and Con-A on bone marrow and peripheral blood lymphocytes from healthy donors, *Exp. Hematol.*, **10**, 256–62.
Princen, J. M. G., Nieuwenhuizen, W., Mol-Backx, G. P. B. M., and Yap, S. N. (1981). Direct evidence of transcriptional control of fibrinogen and albumin synthesis in rat liver during the acute phase response, *Biochem. Biophys. Res. Commun.*, **102**, 717–23.
Puro, D. G., and Richter, G. W. (1971). Ferritin synthesis by free and membrane bound polyribosomes of rat liver, *Proc. Soc. Exp. Biol. Med.*, **138**, 399–403.
Quastel, M. R., and Ross, J. F. (1966). The effect of acute inflammation on the

utilization and distribution of transferrin-bound and erythrocyte radio iron, *Blood*, **28**, 738–57.

Ramadori, G., Sipe, J. D., Dinarello, C. A., Mizel, S. B., and Cotten, H. R. (1985). Pretranslational modulationof acute phase hepatic protein synthesis by murine recombinant interleukin-1 (IL-1), *J. Exp. Med.*, **162**, 930–42.

Reid, C. D. L., Prouse, P. J., Baptista, L. C., Gumple, J. M., and Chanarin, I. (1984). The mechanism of the anaemia in rheumatoid arthritis: effects of bone marrow adherent cells and of serum on *in vitro* erythropoiesis, *Br. J. Haematol.*, **58**, 607–15.

Reissman, K. R., and Udupa, K. B. (1978). Effect of inflammation on erythroid precursors (BFU-e and CFU-e) in bone marrow and spleen of mice, *J. Lab. Clin. Med.*, **92**, 22–9.

Rigby, P. G., Strasser, H., Emmerson, C. P., Betts, A., and Friedell, G. H. (1962). Studies in the anemia of inflammatory states. I. Erythrocyte survival in dogs with acute and chronic turpentine abscess, *J. Lab. Clin. Med.*, **59**, 244–8.

Roeser, H. P. (1980). Iron metabolism in inflammation and malignant disease. In A. Jacobs and M. Worwood (eds) *Iron in Biochemistry and Medicine*, pp. 605–40. Academic Press, London.

Roodman, G. D., Horadam, V. M., and Wright, T. L. (1983). Inhibition of erythroid colony formation by autologous bone marrow adherent cells from patients with anemia of chronic disease, *Blood*, **62**, 406–12.

Sawatzki, G., Hoffmann, F., and Kubanek, B. (1983). The role of iron binding proteins, lactoferrin and transferrin, in *Salmonella typhimurium* infections in mice, In I. Urushizaki, P. Aisen, I. Listowsky and J. W. Drysdale (eds) *Structure and Function of Iron Storage and Transport Proteins*, pp. 435–9, Elsevier Science Publishers, Amsterdam.

Sawatzki, G., Hoffmann, F., and Kubanek, B. (1984). The role of lactoferrin in *Salmonella* infections in a mouse model, *European Iron Club Meeting* (Abstract), Rennes, France.

Schade, S. G., and Fried, W. (1976). Suppressive effect of endotoxin on erythropoietin responsive cells in mice, *Am. J. Physiol.*, **231**, 73–6.

Schooley, J. C., Kullgren, B., and Allison, A. C. (1987). Inhibition by interleukin-I of the action of erythropoietin on erythroid precursors and its possible role in the pathogenesis of hypoplastic anaemias, *Br. J. Haematol.*, **67**, 11–17.

Siekevitz, P., and Palade, G. E. (1960). A cytochemical study on the pancreas of the guinea pig. V. *In vivo* incorporation of leucine-1-C-14 into the chymotrypsinogen of various cell fractions, *J. Biophys. Biochem. Cytol.*, **7**, 619–30.

Van Miert, A. S. J. P. A. M., Van Duin, C. T. M., Verheyden, J. H. M., Schotman, A. J. H., and Nieuwenhuis, J. (1984). Fever and changes in plasma zinc and iron concentrations in the goat: The role of leukocytic pyrogen, *J. Comp. Pathol.*, **94**, 543–57.

Van Snick, J. L., Masson, P. L., and Heremans, J. F. (1974). The involvement of lactoferrin in the hyposideremia of acute inflammation, *J. Exp. Med.*, **140**, 1068–84.

Wallner, S. F., Kurnick, J. E., Vautrin, R. M., White, M. J., Chapman, R. G., and Ward, H. P. (1977). Levels of erythropoietin in patients with the anaemias of chronic diseases and liver failure, *Am. J. Hematol.*, **3**, 37–44.

Ward, H. P., Gordon, B., and Picket, J. C. (1969). Serum levels of erythropoietin in rheumatoid arthritis, *J. Lab. Clin. Med.*, **74**, 93–7.

Ward, H. P., Kurnick, J. E., and Pysarczyk, M. J. (1971). Serum levels of erythropoietin in anaemias associated with chronic infection, malignancy and primary hematologic disease, *J. Clin. Invest.*, **50**, 332–49.

Webster, R. O., Hong, S. R., Johnston, R. B. Jr, and Henson, P. M. (1980). Biological effects of the human complement fragments C5a and C5ades Arg on neutrophil function, *Immunopharmacology*, **2**, 201–19.

Weinberg, E. D. (1975). Nutritional immunity. Host attempt to withhold iron from microbial invaders, *J. Am. Med. Assoc.*, **231**, 39–41.

Weinberg, E. D. (1978). Iron and infection, *Microbiol. Rev.*, **42**, 45–66.

Weinberg, E. D. (1986). Iron, infection and neoplasia, *Clin. Physiol. Biochem.*, **4**, 50–60.

Weiss, D. J., and Krehbiel, J. D. (1983). Studies of the pathogenesis of anaemia of inflammation: Erythrocyte survival, *Am. J. Vet. Res.*, **14**, 1830–1.

Weiss, D. K., Krehbiel, J. D., and Lund, J. E. (1983). Studies on the pathogenesis of anaemia of inflammation: Mechanism of impaired erythropoiesis, *Am. J. Vet. Res.*, **44**, 1832–5.

Westmacott, D., Hawkes, J. E., Hill, R. P., Clarke, L. E., and Bloxham, D. P. (1986). Comparison of the effects of recombinant murine and human interleukin-1 *in vitro* and *in vivo*, *Lymphokine Res.*, **5** (Supplement 1), s87–91.

Worwood, M. (1979). Serum ferritin, *CRC Crit. Rev. Clin. Lab. Sci.*, **10**, 171–204.

Worwood, M., Cragg, S. J., Wagstaff, M., and Jacobs, A. (1979). Binding of human serum ferritin to Concanavalin A, *Clin. Sci.*, **56**, 83–7.

Wurz, H., Von Moers, F., and Zippel, H. H. (1985). Serum ferritin in patients with gynaecological cancer, *Protides Biol. Fluids*, **32**, 683–6.

Zähringer, J., Baliga, B. S., and Munro, H. N. (1976). Novel mechanisms for translational control in regulation of ferritin synthesis by iron, *Proc. Natl Acad. Sci. USA*, **73**, 857–61.

Zähringer, J., Baliga, B. S., Drake, R. L., and Munro, H. N. (1977). Distribution of ferritin mRNA and albumin between free and membrane bound rat liver polysomes, *Biochim. Biophys. Acta*, **474**, 234–44.

Zarrabi, M. H., Lysik, R., and Zucker, S. (1977). The anemia of chronic disorders: Studies of iron reutilization of the anaemia of experimental malignancy and chronic inflammation, *Br. J. Haematol.*, **35**, 647–58.

Zoumbos, N. C., Djue, J. Y., and Young, N. S. (1984). Interferon is the suppressor of hematopoiesis generated by stimulated lymphocytes *in vitro*, *J. Immunol.*, **133**, 769–74.

Zoumbos, N. C., Gascon, P., Djue, J. Y., Trost, S. R., and Young, N. S. (1985a). Circulating activated suppressor T-lymphocytes in aplastic anemia, *N. Engl. J. Med.*, **312**, 257–65.

Zoumbos, N. C., Gascon, P., Djue, J. Y., and Young, N. S. (1985b). Interferon is a mediator of hematopoietic suppression in aplastic anemia *in vitro* and possibly *in vivo*, *Proc. Natl Acad. Sci. USA*, **82**, 188–92.

Zucker, S. (1985). Anemia in cancer, *Cancer Invest.*, **3**, 249–60.

Zucker, S., Freidman, S., and Lysik, R. M. (1974). Bone marrow erythropoiesis in the anaemia of infection, inflammation and malignancy, *J. Clin. Invest.*, **53**, 1132–8.

Zucker, S., and Lysik, R. M. (1977). Cancer induced cytolysis of normal bone marrow cells, *Nature*, **265**, 736–7.

Zucker, S., Lysik, R. M., and Di Stefano, J. F. (1977). Pathogenesis of anemia in rats with Walker-256 carcinosarcoma, *J. Lab. Clin. Med.*, **90**, 502–11.

Zucker, S., Lysik, R. M., and Di Stefano, J. F. (1980). Cancer cell inhibition of erythropoiesis, *J. Lab. Clin. Med.*, **95**, 770–82.

Iron in Immunity, Cancer and Inflammation
Edited by M. de Sousa and J. H. Brock
© 1989 John Wiley & Sons Ltd

7
Iron and Joint Inflammation

F. J. Andrews*, D. R. Blake† and C. J. Morris†
*Department of Surgery, Monash University Medical School, Melbourne 3181, Australia
†Bone and Joint Research Unit, London Hospital Medical College, London E1 1AD, UK

IRON AND JOINT PATHOLOGY

Haemarthrosis

Iron and joint inflammation were first associated by Hochsletter in his description in 1674 of the arthritis 'associated with excessive bleeding' (Bulloch and Fildes, 1912). The clasical clinical description of haemophilic arthropathy was given by Konig (1892) and since then it has been recognized that recurrent intra-articular haemorrhages result in a florid, proliferative, inflammatory synovitis associated with erosive bone disease and destruction of cartilage (Key, 1932; Ghormley and Clegg, 1948; DePalma and Cotler, 1956; Rodnan et al., 1957; Mainardi et al., 1978). The distribution of the arthritis strongly suggests that mechanical factors are important. A recent review showed that between 53% and 95% of haemophiliacs have joint damage (Stein and Duthie, 1981), and as anticipated the synovial membrane is heavily iron-laden.

Early animal studies carried out by Key (1929) showed that a single injection of autologous blood into the knee of a rabbit produced a mild proliferation of the synovial lining cells and an infiltration of leukocytes and macrophages, which resolved within six days. Seven injections over a period of three weeks produced marked thickening of the synovium, with villus formation which persisted for at least one month. Wolf and Mankin (1965) confirmed these results and observed oedema, vascular dilatation, inflammatory cell infiltration and deposition of iron in the synovial lining cells of rabbits given twice-daily injections of homologous blood. These changes were followed by progressive fibrosis and scarring, but unlike in the human haemophilic joint, there was no cartilage damage. Ultrastructural studies of both human haemophilic (Roy and Ghadially, 1967) and rabbit haemarthritic synovia (Roy and Ghadially, 1966) revealed that erythrocytes within the joint space could pass between synovial cells, or were phagocytized by synovial macrophages. Further work on the rabbit synovium showed that iron was deposited in specialized lysosomes or siderosomes within the synovial macrophages, and that the associated inflammatory cell exudate and fibrosis persisted for as long as six months after cessation of blood injections (Richter, 1957; Roy and Ghadially, 1969).

Hoaglund (1967) also produced experimental haemarthrosis in the dog, using daily intra-articular injections of autologous blood for 12–18 weeks. Findings were similar to those in human haemophilic arthritis and included synovial pigmentation, fibrosis and cartilage damage. In a later study, loss of cartilage integrity associated with a reduction in glycosaminoglycan content and a consequent reduction in shear resistance was observed in dogs injected with autologous blood (Convery et al., 1976). It was concluded that cartilage damage was associated with persistence of blood within the joint and reflected a later stage in the inflammatory process.

Repeated intra-articular haemorrhages due to trauma have also been implicated in the aetiology of pigmented villonodular synovitis (PVNS) (Young and Hudacek, 1954; Myers, Masi and Feigenbaum, 1980). In a classic article, Jaffe, Lichtenstein and Sulvo (1941) described the gross pathological changes of the synovium, including nodular villus proliferation, heavy iron pigmentation and local bone erosion. Further studies reviewed by Docken (1979) have shown that the histopathology of PVNS is characterized by giant cells, haemosiderin, variable collagenization, lipid-laden cells and histiocyte infiltrate. PVNS occurs in two forms, a localized solitary lesion, frequently on the digits of the hand, or as an intra-articular nodule, usually at the knee. Diffuse PVNS occurs as a monoarticular arthritis with chronic swelling and stiffness. Laboratory data are normal except for a predominance of erythrocytes in the synovial fluid. Extravasated erythrocytes seen in PVNS biopsies are thought to be the source of iron and membrane-derived lipid (Schumacher et al., 1982). Singh, Grewal and Chakravarti (1969) produced PVNS-like lesions in the rhesus monkey given weekly intra-articular injections of autologous blood or iron dextran, and concluded that the iron moiety of the blood was the factor responsible for eliciting the characteristic synovial villus proliferation and erosive joint damage. These are both features of a variety of forms of inflammatory joint disease, but particularly rheumatoid arthritis (see below).

Iron overload

Excessive oral iron intake has been associated with arthropathy. Hiyeda (1939) suggested that an arthritis seen in Russia and Asia known as

Kaschin Beck's disease was due to excessive iron intake from drinking water. Youths (10–18 years) residing in endemic areas showed shortening of long bones and joint deformities. Swollen metacarpophalangeal and proximal interphalangeal joints (joints commonly involved in early rheumatoid disease) were most conspicuous, with other joints being involved later. The joints were mostly affected symmetrically. Exacerbations with increased swelling were seen in the early spring and autumn when the iron content of the water rose, whilst removal from such areas in childhood prevented these changes. Serum iron and tissue iron levels in the patients were found to be raised. Hiyeda (1939) also showed that rabbits fed on a high iron diet developed ulcerative lesions on the joint surface and cartilagenous and fibrous tissue changes when subjected to percussion apparatus and forced exercise for 30 minutes; control animals did not show joint lesions.

A further example of excessive iron intake resulting in iron overload is seen in the South African Bantu, who drink beer brewed in iron cooking pots. Isaacson and Bothwell (1981) reported significant amounts of iron in the synovial lining cells of 41 subjects, and Seftel *et al.* (1966) found radiological evidence of osteopenia, possibly associated with secondary ascorbic acid deficiency in Bantu patients. Wapnick *et al.* (1968) proposed that increased iron stores in the Bantu lead to irreversible oxidation of ascorbic acid, which may account for the deficiency.

The association of arthritis with hereditary haemochromatosis was first observed by Schumacher (1964). In a study of two haemochromatosis patients, he observed haemosiderin deposition in the synovial lining cells and significant X-ray changes. These results have been confirmed by further studies (Kra, Hollingsworth and Finch, 1965; Seffar, Fornaiser and Fox, 1977; Schumacher, 1982). Joint abnormalities are seen in approximately half the haemochromatosis patients, and particularly in those over 50 years old (Walker *et al.*, 1972). The most characteristic arthropathy appears to involve the second and third metacarpophalangeal joints and radiological changes include bone cysts, condensation of the subchondral plate, irregular erosion of articular cartilage and generalized chondrocalcinosis (Jensen, 1976). It is interesting that the arthritis is not improved by phlebotomy although iron is cleared from the synovium (Laborde *et al.*, 1977). This suggests that while iron deposition may be the primary aetiological factor, the inflammatory and destructive process may become self-perpetuating.

Animal models of systemic iron overload have also been associated with joint inflammation. Brighton, Bigley and Smolenski (1970) treated immature rabbits with intramuscular iron dextran and observed iron deposition in the articular cartilage and synovium which led to destruction of the cartilage matrix and chondrocyte death. More recent work by De Sousa *et al.* (1988) showed that intravenous administration of iron citrate to rats resulted in synovial thickening, hypervascularization and an increase in numbers of intrasynovial capillaries with mononuclear cell infiltration.

Rheumatoid disease

Basic disturbances in iron metabolism resulting from persistent inflammatory rheumatoid synovitis are well known (Cartwright, 1966) and lead to a fall in serum iron and haemoglobin levels and a sequestering of iron within the activated reticuloendothelial system to which the synovium contributes (see also Chapter 6). Although pathologists had long recognized that haemosiderin could occur in the rheumatoid synovial membrane (Collins, 1951), the fact that iron deposits were consistently present and frequently very extensive was not appreciated.

In view of these observations and the previously discussed proinflammatory role of iron in haemophilic and iron overload arthropathies, Muirden (1966) investigated further the iron deposition within rheumatoid synovia. He noted the presence of dense cytoplasmic bodies which were structurally comparable to, and associated with, lysosomes within type A macrophage-like cells. These bodies contained recognizable ferritin granules and were considered to arise from microbleeding into the joint. He based his proposals on previous experiments (Muirden, 1963; Ball, Chapman and Muirden, 1964) in which he had shown that intra-articular injection of ferritin or iron dextran into the knee joints of rabbits produced a distribution of cellular ferritin similar to that observed in rheumatoid patients. *In vitro* experiments (Muirden, Fraser and Clarris, 1967) showed that synovial cells in culture could synthesize ferritin in response to haemoglobin in the culture medium, suggesting that synovial iron deposition may be derived from the breakdown of erythrocytes *in vivo*.

In a subsequent paper, Muirden and Senator (1968) described the prominent deposition of haemosiderin within the subintimal zone of the synovium in 22/23 patients with rheumatoid disease. Chemical measurement of iron in the same patients mirrored these results, with significantly higher synovial tissue and synovial fluid concentrations in rheumatoid patients compared with normal controls (347 μg iron per g dry tissue compared with 15.2 μg g^{-1}) (Senator and Muirden, 1968).

A link between synovial iron deposits and the persistence of rheumatoid synovitis was proposed by Muirden (1970). He reported a highly significant relationship between the presence of anaemia due to rheumatoid disease and the histochemically detected synovial iron deposits, as well as a relationship between the duration of disease in the joint and the joint damage assessed by X-rays. He speculated that iron deposits arising from bleeding vascular granulation tissue in synovial villi and the sequestering of haem iron in the synovial macrophages had a cytotoxic effect on the joint tissue.

Within the last six years Muirden's proposals for the proinflammatory effect of iron deposits within the rheumatoid joint have been expanded (Blake *et al.*, 1981a). Synovial fluid ferritin levels have been found to be significantly higher than serum ferritin levels in rheumatoid patients and correlate negatively with haemoglobin levels, suggesting that synovial iron contributes to the rheumatoid anaemia (Blake and Bacon, 1980). Further studies have shown that synovial fluid ferritin levels correlate with more conventional indices of rheumatoid inflammation such as the Rose Waaler test, synovial fluid cell count and levels of circulating immune complexes (Blake and Bacon, 1981), perhaps suggesting a more direct relationship between synovial iron and inflammation.

In early rheumatoid patients the amount of synovial membrane ferritin has been significantly associated with the activity of disease at the time of biopsy, and the amount of Perls' (ferric) iron is associated with persistence of disease (Blake *et al.*, 1984). In a detailed ultrastructural study of a variety of synovitides (Morris *et al.*, 1985), iron deposits occurring as siderosomes were observed in the B (or fibroblast-like) cells of rheumatoid synovia. This was in contrast to some earlier studies which reported iron deposits within synovial A (macrophage-like) cells (Muirden, 1966; Ogilvie-Harris and Fornaiser, 1980). Morris *et al.* (1985) postulated that ferritin is initially phagocytized by the A cells, where it gives rise to cell damage and is liberated and taken up by the B cells in the more stable form of haemosiderin. Alternatively, inflammation or iron itself may cause a change of cellular function with a transition from an A (macrophage-like) to B (fibroblast-like) cell type morphology (Hamerman, 1970).

In spite of the toxic effects of iron on joint tissue, certain rheumatoid patients require iron therapy for genuine iron deficiency anaemia as opposed to the frequent anaemia associated with persistent inflammation. Both total dose intravenous iron dextran (Reddy and Lewis, 1969; Lloyd and Williams, 1970; Blake *et al.*, 1985a; Winyard *et al.*, 1987) and occasionally oral iron (Blake and Bacon, 1982) have been shown to exacerbate inflammatory synovitis. In the patients treated with iron dextran, exacerbation of synovitis tended to occur 24–48 hours post-infusion and only in joints previously inflamed. Resting the joints prior to and immediately after the infusion minimized this proinflammatory effect and it is of interest that there are no reports of iron dextran promoting inflammation at sites other than the joint.

In animal studies, intramuscular iron dextran has been found to increase the severity of adjuvant arthritis in the rat as assessed by joint score. Interestingly the effect was more pronounced in male rats, although the females had an overall greater severity of joint symptoms (Mowat and Garner, 1972). Uno *et al.* (1985) showed that 'ionic' iron increased fluid exudation and granulation tissue weight in the rat air pouch model of inflammatory synovitis. Autologous whole blood injected into an inflamed air pouch in rats has been shown to prolong a low-grade inflammatory air response. Isolation and testing of the individual blood components in this model showed that the haem-containing fractions alone were responsible for the proinflammatory effect (Yoshino et al., 1985). In recent studies Morris et al. (1987) observed a significant increase in the number of macrophages containing ferritin and ferric iron in rat inflammatory pouches injected with blood compared with controls. The presence of such iron deposits was associated with an increased proliferation of vascular and connective tissue elements, particularly during the chronic inflammatory phase.

Thus it appears that synovial iron deposition derived from systemic iron overload or microbleeding into the joint is associated with arthropathy or exacerbation of existing inflammation in man and animal models. In inflammatory joint disease either direct microbleeding into the inflamed synovial cavity or persistent inflammation concurrent with the redistribution anaemia leads to iron deposition within the inflamed synovium. This appears to result in an exacerbation of inflammatory synovitis and a progression of bone and cartilage damage, particularly if the joint is mobile.

IRON DEFICIENCY AND THE JOINT

Introduction

In view of the toxic effects of iron deposition in the inflamed joint, removal of the iron might be expected to reduce inflammation (see Chapter 17). Iron deficiency has traditionally been described as detrimental to host defences against disease (see Chapter 5). In recent reports, however, iron deficiency has been shown to protect against heart disease (Shaper and Jones, 1959; Sullivan, 1986), cancer (Martin, 1984), and bacterial and parasitic infections (Masawe, 1974; Harvey, Bell and Nesheim, 1985). This concept could be applied to rheumatoid disease. Epidemiological data show that the incidence of rheumatoid disease in females increases rapidly after the menopause (Lawrence, 1977) and that severe rheumatoid disease with systemic complications is rarely reported in underdeveloped rural populations where malnutritional and parasitic infections may lead to iron deficiency.

Nutritional iron deficiency

To investigate further the possible role of iron in inflammatory joint disease, we have studied the effect of nutritional iron deficiency in an animal model of joint inflammation. The model selected, adjuvant disease, is well documented and was first described by Pearson (1956) as a focal arthritis, synovitis and tendonitis in rats injected with Freund's complete adjuvant. There are also some similarities in joint pathology between adjuvant disease and rheumatoid disease (Pearson, 1963), including the deposition of iron within the inflamed synovium (Muirden and Peace, 1969). Subsequent reports have demonstrated the systemic nature of adjuvant disease, including local inflammation at the site of injection (Pearson and Wood, 1959), increases in levels of serum acute-phase reactants (Gralla and Wiseman, 1968) and characteristic pathological changes in the lymph nodes (Glenn and Gray, 1965), liver and spleen (Silverstein and Sokoloff, 1960).

We have shown (Andrews, Morris and Blake, 1987) that nutritional iron deficiency produced by feeding rats a diet containing 10 ppm iron, leading to a mild anaemia (haemoglobin 11.5 g/100 ml) and decreased hepatic iron levels, significantly reduced adjuvant joint inflammation assessed by clinical score, histology and radiography. However, iron deficiency had no effect on the systemic components of the disease, such as the acute-phase response, liver pathology, lymph node hyperplasia and local inflammatory response at the site of injection. Further studies showed that the same level of iron deficiency had no effect on the development of an acute inflammatory response to carrageenan, pyrophosphate or urate crystals in animal models of inflammation not involving the joint.

Iron chelation

A number of different experiments with the iron chelator desferrioxamine have produced similar results. At a dose of 100 mg kg^{-1} desferrioxamine markedly depressed the chronic inflammatory phase in the Glynn–Dumonde model of synovitis in the guinea-pig (Blake et al., 1983). However, lower doses had a proinflammatory effect. Desferrioxamine reduced the joint inflammation associated with adjuvant disease (at a dose of 100 or 200 mg kg^{-1}) but as with nutritional iron deficiency did not affect the systemic response (Andrews et al., 1987). In the rat allergic air pouch model of inflammation, desferrioxamine significantly reduced the chronic phase of the model but had a proinflammatory effect on the acute reaction (Yoshino, Blake and Bacon, 1984). Variations in response to low and high doses and the proinflammatory effect on acute inflammation may be related to the ability of desferrioxamine to chelate other trace metals (Hider, 1984).

Protective mechanisms of iron deficiency

The aetiology of adjuvant disease is not firmly established but is thought to involve immune mechanisms either in the development of disease

(Waksman, Pearson and Sharp, 1960) or as an exacerbatory influence (Billingham, 1983). Nutritional iron deficiency has been associated with a suppression of immune function (Dallman, Beutler and Finch, 1978). Iron-deficient patients are reported to have a decreased percentage of T lymphocytes (MacDougall et al., 1975), impaired incorporation of [^{3}H]thymidine by stimulated lymphocytes in culture (Joynson et al., 1972) and a depressed delayed hypersensitivity response (Swarup-Mitra and Sinha, 1984). Nutritionally iron-deficient rats have been reported to have impaired humoral (Kochanowski and Sherman, 1985a) and cell-mediated (Kochanowski and Sherman, 1985b) immunity. It may be, therefore, that iron deficiency protects against joint inflammation by inducing a generalized immune suppression. However, the modest level of iron deficiency produced in our experiments did not affect the development of hypersensitivity to oxazalone or thymidine incorporation by lymphocytes (Andrews, Morris and Blake, 1987).

Nutritional iron deficiency also affects neutrophil function. Iron-deficient neutrophils have been shown to be defective in the reduction of nitroblue tetrazolium dye, suggesting that the activity of the iron-containing enzyme NADPH oxidase is reduced (Moore and Humbert, 1984). This enzyme catalyses the formation of superoxide which leads ultimately to the production of other reactive oxygen species capable of damaging not only microorganisms but also under certain circumstances the host's own tissue (see below). In addition, the activity of myeloperoxidase, which contains iron and is also part of the important bactericidal system, may be adversely affected by iron deficiency (Mackler et al., 1984). We have shown that the polymorphonuclear leukocyte is the predominant cell type in the inflamed adjuvant joint and that nutritionally iron-deficient rats had fewer polymorphonuclear leukocytes within the joint tissue than control rats (Andrews, Morris and Blake, 1987). It may be that those polymorphonuclear leukocytes present in the iron-deficient rats also have a reduced capacity to produce reactive oxygen species in response to adjuvant.

In conclusion, iron deficiency induced by a low iron diet or chelation appears to have a significant anti-inflammatory effect on animal models of joint inflammation and synovitis. It is of interest that the effect appears to be most marked during the chronic inflammatory phase of these models, and in adjuvant disease iron deficiency is anti-inflammatory only to those components of the disease that involve the joint. To understand this peculiar 'joint specificity' we describe in the following section the potential mechanisms by which iron may exacerbate inflammation, with particular emphasis on iron-promoted oxidative damage.

BIOCHEMISTRY OF IRON RELATED TO JOINT DISEASE

Oxygen radicals and iron

The rheumatoid joint provides an ideal environment for the occurrence of iron-promoted tissue damage. The presence of inflammatory cells such as polymorphonuclear leukocytes in the synovial fluid and the macrophage-like A cells of the synovial membrane provides a putative source of oxygen radicals. Phagocytosis of immune complexes and cell debris is accompanied by the activation of the membrane-bound NADPH oxidase complex which will release superoxide (O_2^-) into the phagocyte vacuole and outside the cell (Babior, Kipnes and Curnutte, 1973). Biemond *et al.* (1986a) have demonstrated increased *in vitro* production of superoxide by stimulated polymorphonuclear leukocytes from rheumatoid patients compared with controls.

The superoxide radical is relatively inactive, particularly in aqueous solution. However, in the presence of transition metal ions the toxic hydroxyl radical (OH·) can be produced via the Fenton reaction, as shown below:

$$2O_2^- + 2H^+ \rightarrow H_2O_2 + O_2$$
$$H_2O_2 + Fe^{2+} \rightarrow OH\cdot + OH^- + Fe^{3+}$$

Free iron ions seldom exist *in vivo* but complexes of iron salts with phosphate esters, e.g. ATP, carbohydrates, organic acids, DNA or membrane lipids which may constitute small pools of 'transit' iron within cells (Jacobs, 1977), are effective at decomposing hydrogen peroxide (Floyd, 1981, Flitter, Rowley and Halliwell, 1983). Clearly, segregation of iron at the subcellular and macromolecular level is important for the integrity of cell structure and function.

In rheumatoid disease, low molecular weight iron complexes capable of participating in the formation of the hydroxyl radical have been demonstrated in the synovial fluid (Rowley *et al.*, 1984). Levels of iron complexes correlated with the activity of the arthritis as assessed by a clinical index of local inflammation and various laboratory parameters, suggesting an involvement in the disease process. At present the exact origin of the non-protein-bound iron complexes is uncertain. Tissue damage resulting in cell death may be accompanied by the release of non-protein-bound iron from the cell transit pool (Willson, 1977). The low synovial fluid pH found in rheumatoid joints (Etherington, Pugh and Silver, 1981) may facilitate the release of iron from transferrin assisted by the presence of ascorbic acid in the synovial fluid. The released iron can be kept in the reduced state by ascorbate or superoxide and may not easily rebind to transferrin.

At present there is dispute as to whether transferrin-bound iron can itself catalyse the Fenton reaction. The activity of transferrin-bound iron in promoting hydroxyl radical production has been reported as good (McCord and Day, 1978), moderate (Bannister *et al.*, 1982a), poor (Motohashi and Mori, 1983) and not detected (Maguire, Kellog and Packer, 1982). Similarly, Ambruso and Johnston (1981) reported that iron-loaded lactoferrin was an efficient catalyst of the Fenton reaction. These results were confirmed by Bannister *et al.* (1982b) using a different assay. However, Winterbourn (1983) pointed out artifacts in the assays used and came to the conclusion, supported by others (Gutteridge *et al.*, 1981; Baldwin, Jenny and Aisen, 1984; see also Chapter 10), that lactoferrin, if effective at all, is a poor catalyst compared with non-protein-bound iron. Rheumatoid synovial fluid contains increased levels of lactoferrin (Bennett and Skosey, 1977) and Halliwell, Gutteridge and Blake (1985) have proposed that lactoferrin, far from acting as a catalyst of hydroxyl radical formation, may at low synovial fluid pH actually bind iron and minimize damage. There have been claims that haemoglobin and methaemoglobin are also catalysts of the Fenton reaction (Bennatti *et al.*, 1983; Sadrzadeh *et al.*, 1985; Winterbourn, 1985). However, as with transferrin and lactoferrin, there is some controversy as to whether such reactions occur *in vivo* (Halliwell and Gutteridge, 1985).

Ferritin is often regarded as a safe storage form of iron, yet ferritin stimulates the formation of hydroxyl radicals from superoxide and hydrogen peroxide *in vitro* (Bannister, Bannister and Thornalley, 1984; Carlin and Djursater, 1984). The superoxide radical can mobilize iron from ferritin, leading to hydroxyl radical production (Williams, Lee and Cartwright, 1974; Biemond *et al.*, 1984a). This is of particular relevance to the rheumatoid joint, given the presence of ferritin deposits and a potential source of superoxide from infiltrating polymorphonuclear leukocytes. Biemond *et al.* (1986b) also showed that rheumatoid patients had significantly higher ferritin levels in the synovial fluid than controls, and moreover the iron content of ferritin in the rheumatoid patients was significantly elevated. Haemosiderin, which is believed to be formed from lysosomal degradation of ferritin (Fischbach *et al.*, 1971), can also promote hydroxyl radical production but is less effective than ferritin on a unit iron basis (O'Connell *et al.*, 1986). Conversion of stored ferritin into haemosiderin may thus be biologically advantageous (Halliwell and Gutteridge, 1985).

The rheumatoid synovial fluid also contains ascorbic acid, which as a reducing agent may reduce iron, allowing it to react with hydrogen peroxide to produce the hydroxyl radical (see Fenton reaction above) and form dehydroascorbate. Lunec and Blake (1985) have shown that rheumatoid synovial fluid ascorbic acid occurs mainly in the oxidized (dehydroascorbate) form (see above), possibly as a consequence of iron-dependent oxidation.

Lipid peroxidation, lysosomal enzymes and tissue damage

The hydroxyl radical is highly reactive and will react with a variety of biomolecules at or close to its site of formation. The methylene interrupted double bond of polyunsaturated fatty acids (predominantly distributed in the form of membrane lipids) is particularly susceptible to attack by the hydroxyl radical with the loss of a hydrogen atom. The remaining carbon radical rearranges and in the presence of oxygen initiates an autocatalytic reaction known as lipid peroxidation. Lipid peroxides are fairly stable molecules under physiological conditions but their decomposition is catalysed by all the iron complexes present *in vivo* that participate in the Fenton reaction (Halliwell and Gutteridge, 1985).

Iron dextran-exacerbated synovitis (see above) appears to be mediated via lipid peroxidation. After an infusion of iron dextran, serum and synovial fluid iron-binding capacity is saturated and low molecular weight iron chelates with the capacity to cause oxidative damage are present in both serum and synovial fluid. At this time lipid peroxidation products are present in the serum and synovial fluid, with levels falling as the exacerbation of synovitis subsides (Winyard *et al.*, 1987).

Lipid peroxidation may also contribute to tissue damage in rheumatoid patients not treated with iron dextran. Rowley *et al.* (1984) found that levels of non-protein-bound iron in rheumatoid synovial fluid correlated with the extent of lipid peroxidation measured by the thiobarbituric acid assay in rheumatoid synovial fluid. Lunec *et al.* (1981) have demonstrated free radical peroxidation products in 90% of rheumatoid synovial fluid samples, and levels were significantly higher in rheumatoid sera compared with healthy controls. It was of interest that levels of peroxidation products declined after treatment with anti-inflammatory drugs. Extensive lipid peroxidation in biological membranes causes loss of fluidity, falls in membrane potential, increased permeability to ions and eventual rupture leading to release of cell and organelle contents, e.g. lysosomal hydrolytic enzymes (Fong *et al.*, 1973). Diseased or damaged tissues show evidence of increased lipid peroxidation. Simple *in vitro* experiments demonstrate that dead or damaged tissues peroxidize more rapidly than living ones, presumably because of membrane disruption by lysosomal enzymes released from their storage sites (Halliwell, 1984).

There is considerable evidence to suggest that lysosomal enzymes play a role in the tissue damage associated with rheumatoid arthritis. High levels of neutral protease (Al Haik, Lewis and Struthers, 1984), collagenase (Harris *et al.*, 1970; Al Haik, Lewis and Struthers, 1984), elastaste (Al Haik, Lewis and Struthers, 1984; Gysen *et al.*, 1985) and cathepsin D (Poole, Hembry and Dingle, 1974) have been found in rheumatoid synovial fluid.

In one study the activity of the enzymes was shown to correlate with biochemical parameters such as C-reactive protein and erythrocyte sedimentation rate, consistent with the view that proteolytic activity and inflammation increase in parallel with each other (Al Haik, Lewis and Struthers, 1984). Both collagenase and elastase have been demonstrated histochemically at the site of cartilage erosion in the rheumatoid joint (Woolley, Crossley and Evans, 1977; Meninger *et al.*, 1980; Velvart *et al.*, 1981). Increased storage of iron within lysosomes of phagocytic cells in the rheumatoid joint may, as in the iron-overloaded liver, lead to an increase in lysosomal fragility (Peters, Selden and Seymour, 1977) and loss of latency of lysosomal enzymes (Peters and Seymour, 1976). Iron may labilize the lysosomal membrane by purely mechanical effects (Peters and Selden, 1982) or by iron-promoted oxygen radical reactions (Weir, Gibson and Peters, 1984). Okazaki *et al.* (1981) have also shown that ionic iron is taken up by rabbit synovial fibroblasts, accompanied by an increase in production of both latent collagenase and PGE_2. Concomitant addition of desferrioxamine prevented iron uptake and induction of collagenase and PGE_2. This observation has important implications in the rheumatoid joint, as not only is collagenase associated with tissue damage, but also PGE_2 has been shown to induce periosteal proliferation and bone resorption (Galasko and Bennett, 1976).

High levels of lysosomal enzymes in the inflamed joint may also reflect inactivity of enzyme inhibitors. Carp and Janoff (1980) showed that polymorphonuclear leukocytes stimulated *in vitro* released reactive oxygen species able to suppress the elastase inhibitor capacity of human serum by oxidative inactivation of the inhibitor molecule. Further evidence for the involvement of oxygen radical reactions in the inactivation of elastase inhibitor came from studies where superoxide dismutase (SOD) and catalase were found to partially protect elastase inhibitor activity. Pritchard (1984) showed that the ratio of enzyme to inhibitor was increased in rheumatoid synovial fluid as the erosive potential of the disease increased, and he also suggested that levels of enzyme may be even higher within the micro-environment of the eroded cartilage surface. Extracted proteinase inhibitor from inflammatory synovial fluid had the first 17 residues missing and was unable to form a complex with porcine pancreatic elastase. Sequence studies on this fraction indicated that two of the methionyl residues were oxidized (Wong and Travis, 1980).

Damage to proteins and other biomolecules

Proteins are important targets of iron-promoted oxygen radical reactions. Wolff and Dean (1986) have shown that in the presence of oxygen the hydroxyl radical can attack bovine serum albumin (BSA), with the loss or modification of the tryptophan residues, resulting in changes in conformation and degradation of the molecule. The degraded protein was also more susceptible to enzyme proteolysis. Degradation of BSA was inhibited by iron chelators and it was concluded that iron-catalysed oxygen radical reactions caused direct oxidation of residues crucial to the integrity of the protein.

Direct activation of UV-generated free radicals on the immunoglobulin G (IgG) molecule appears to significantly affect its biological properties (Wickens *et al.*, 1983). Damage to IgG appeared to be related to changes in cystine, tryptophan and other aromatic amino acids (Lunec, 1982) and can be detected by alterations in fluorescence characteristics. Further studies have shown that IgG altered by free radicals can stimulate the release of superoxide from normal human neutrophils (Lunec *et al.*, 1985). In the presence of excess altered IgG, further damage to IgG occurred, indicating a self-perpetuating system of oxygen radical damage. Measurement and isolation of altered IgG from *in vitro* systems and from fresh rheumatoid sera and synovial fluid by high-pressure liquid chromatography showed that identical complexes are present *in vivo*, all the complexes sharing the property of enhancing superoxide production from neutrophils (Lunec *et al.*, 1985). Alterations in IgG fluorescence properties have been shown to be inhibited by the iron chelator desferrioxamine, catalase and hydroxyl radical scavengers, emphasizing the importance of iron-promoted reactions in the formation of altered IgG (Lunec *et al.*, 1985).

Later work by Lunec *et al.* (1986a) showed that free radicals denatured IgG so that it was no longer reactive with anti-IgG antibody. This loss of reactivity may be due to changes in both the antibody combining region (Fab) of the molecule and the Fc portion (the area thought to contain the antigenic sites for rheumatoid factor binding). Concomitant with this change, free radicals also appeared either to induce new, or to expose previously hidden, antigenic sites in the molecule. Subsequently, the molecule may become a stimulus for the formation of the immune complexes, thereby promoting and amplifying tissue damage (Lunec *et al.*, 1985). Analysis of sera and synovial fluid from rheumatoid patients showed that as patients on conventional second line improved, the degree of fluorescence relative to the total amount of IgG decreased, corresponding to a lowering of immune complexes, measured as aggregates of IgG (Lunec *et al.*, 1985). In animal models, the addition of free radical-altered IgG to the rat allergic air pouch model has been shown to prolong the inflammatory response. Re-isolated IgG from the pouch exudates was increasingly fluorescent with time, suggesting self-perpetuating oxidative damage (Lunec *et al.*, 1986b). Taken together with the clinical studies, these results suggest that iron-promoted radical-induced damage to the IgG molecule may play an important role in the prolonging of the inflammatory response in rheumatoid arthritis.

There is evidence that the major constituents of cartilage are also susceptible to iron-promoted oxygen radical reactions. Greenwald, Moy and Lazarus (1976) showed that proteoglycans were decomposed by superoxide *in vitro*. Later, Greenwald and Moy (1979) observed that exposure of collagen to superoxide caused an inhibition of gelation, an effect abolished by the presence of SOD. In a study of cartilage biopsies from thirteen rheumatoid patients, cartilage proteoglycan was diminished or absent in many areas (Mitchell and Shepard, 1978). Fragmentation of collagen and phagocytosis of the fragments by chondrocytes was also noted.

A decrease in synovial fluid viscosity is one of the characteristic features of inflammatory joint disease and has been attributed to the depolymerization of hyaluronic acid. Several studies have implicated oxygen free radicals in the breakdown of hyaluronic acid. Greenwald and Moy (1980) observed a decrease in synovial fluid viscosity when fluid was exposed to superoxide generated either enzymatically or from stimulated neutrophils. The depolymerized hyaluronic acid also became more susceptible to further degradation by the enzyme β-N-acetyl glucosamidase.

The direct role of iron in the breakdown of hyaluronic acid was demonstrated by Wong *et al.* (1981), who observed that addition of Fe^{2+} to purified commercial hyaluronic acid caused depolymerization, an effect inhibited by catalase and hydroxyl radical scavengers but not by SOD. Further work showed that ascorbate was able to enhance depolymerization of hyaluronic acid by way of its ability to reduce Fe^{3+} to Fe^{2+} within the medium. Depolymerization was inhibited by the iron chelator desferrioxamine, catalase and hydroxyl radical scavengers. Niedermeier (1982) confirmed these results and showed that caeruloplasmin (a serum ferroxidase, see next section) inhibited ascorbate-metal catalysed depolymerization of hyaluronic acid, presumably by maintaining iron in the ferric state. Iron chelation using a range of chelators has also been shown to reduce hyaluronic acid degradation (Betts and Cleland, 1982).

It has been suggested that oxygen radicals are also responsible for the destruction of endothelial cells, induction of increased vascular permeability (Vapaatalo, 1986), and damage to DNA (Knuutila, 1984), and probably participate in many inflammatory stages and various single events.

Oxygen radical scavengers and antioxidants

In view of the toxic effects of iron-promoted oxygen radical reactions, levels of scavengers and protective molecules within the rheumatoid joint are crucial in the prevention of tissue damage. Reports of levels of SOD, catalase and glutathione are confusing. In an early study, Rister *et al.* (1978)

demonstrated significantly lower SOD activity in neutrophils of juvenile rheumatoid patients compared with controls, but glutathione peroxidase activity was unchanged. Later, Pasquier et al. (1984, 1985) showed that polymorphonuclear leukocytes of patients with rheumatoid arthritis contained only half the control level of manganese-containing SOD. Blake et al. (1981b) found no SOD in cell-free rheumatoid synovial fluid, whilst Igari et al. (1982) showed low concentrations in osteoarthritic synovial fluid but four times higher levels in rheumatoid synovial fluid. However they did not centrifuge the fluid to remove the cells. In a detailed study by Biemond et al. (1984b), levels of SOD were found to be low in rheumatoid synovial fluid and appeared insufficient to protect against reactive oxygen species. Glutathione peroxidase levels were slightly elevated and catalase levels were strongly elevated compared with controls.

Caeruloplasmin, an important antioxidant because of its ability to oxidize Fe^{2+}, was found to be raised in rheumatoid synovial fluid (Biemond et al.,1984). After removal of caeruloplasmin from serum or synovial fluid, 70% of the protective capacity disappeared and it was concluded that caeruloplasmin is an important protector against oxygen radical reactions. However, Winyard et al. (1984) have shown that the caeruloplasmin molecule itself is susceptible to oxygen radical damage. Exposure of human caeruloplasmin to a source of oxygen radicals decreased its ferroxidase and ascorbate oxidase activity and its ability to inhibit lipid peroxidation. Exposure to UV irradiation depressed the ability of caeruloplasmin to inhibit iron-catalysed hyaluronic acid degradation. In view of its susceptibility to oxygen radical damage, Winyard et al. (1984) suggested that this may result in the presence of catalytic non-protein-bound iron in the rheumatoid synovial fluid which will promote further oxidative damage.

Serum thiols are also important extracellular scavengers of peroxides (Koster, Biemond and Swaak, 1986). It has been reported that the number of free thiol groups in the sera of rheumatoid patients is depressed, the depression being associated with the activity of the disease (Haalaja, 1975). Munthe, Guldal and Jellum (1979) reported that levels of erythrocyte glutathione increased in patients with rheumatoid arthritis receiving treatment with penicillamine. However, other reports have disputed these results (Chirico et al., 1986; Mottonen et al., 1984).

Although ascorbic acid is an important reducing agent, at high concentrations it also has antioxidant properties. Lunec and Blake (1985) reported less reduced ascorbate and more dehydroascorbate in rheumatoid synovial fluid, and suggested that ascorbate may in some circumstances act as a hydroxyl radical scavenger in the rheumatoid synovial fluid.

The inflammation and tissue damage associated with rheumatoid arthritis is obviously derived from many different mechanisms, several of which appear to involve iron and oxygen radicals. The basic mechanisms outlined above do not easily explain the apparent joint-specific proinflammatory effects of iron dextran therapy nor the joint-selective anti-inflammatory effect of iron deficiency in adjuvant disease.

Ischaemia/reperfusion injury

Recently, considerable interest has been shown in the role of reactive oxygen species such as superoxide and hydrogen peroxide in mediating ischaemic tissue damage in a variety of different tissues (Weisiger, 1986; Parks and Bulkey, 1983; Burton, McCord and Ghai, 1984; Granger, Adkinson and Hollworth, 1985). It appears paradoxical that essentially oxidative processes are occuring within oxygen-depleted tissues. However, it is believed that oxidative tissue damage occurs following the ischaemic phase during the period of reperfusion of the tissues. Cellular metabolic changes occurring during the ischaemic phase may be responsible for the formation of reactive oxygen species during the reperfusion period.

McCord (1985) found that during ischaemia mitochondrial oxidative phosphorylation ceases and cellular ATP levels drop. Eventually cellular AMP levels rise and AMP is metabolized to hypoxanthine. Under normal conditions hypoxanthine is metabolized by the iron-dependent enzyme xanthine dehydrogenase to xanthine and then to uric acid. However, during ischaemia the normal xanthine dehydrogenase is converted to an oxidase by a calcium-dependent protease or by thiol group modification. Xanthine oxidase utilizes molecular oxygen instead of NAD^+ as its electron acceptor and catalyses the production of superoxide and hydrogen peroxide during the reperfusion period. Xanthine oxidase inhibitors have been shown to protect ischaemic tissues from oxidative damage during reperfusion (Owens et al., 1974; Nordstrom, Seeman and Hasselgren, 1985; Im et al., 1984).

As well as providing a source of superoxide, xanthine oxidase has been shown to mobilize iron from ferritin (Biemond et al., 1986c). Periods of ischaemia creating a reducing environment are also associated with a delocalization of cellular protein-bound iron to chemical species capable of catalysing hydroxyl radical production (White et al., 1985). *In vivo* support for these observations comes from experiments using post-ischaemic brain tissue from dogs which was found to contain low molecular weight iron chelates (Nayini et al., 1985). Babbs (1985) and Aust and White (1985) also showed that the iron chelator desferrioxamine reduced tissue damage following ischaemia resulting from cardiac arrest. These observations taken together suggest a role for iron in reperfusion injury.

Recent studies may link oxygen radical formation in the inflamed joint with periods of ischaemia. In one study, measurement of rheumatoid synovial fluid oxygen tension revealed that effusions with low PO_2 were associated with more severe histological changes (Falchuk, Goetzl and Kulka, 1970). Measurement of synovial fluid lactate, pH and PO_2 showed that effusions with the lowest PO_2 were associated with a high lactate concentration and a low pH, suggesting periods of anaerobic glycolysis by a hypoxic synovium (Treuhaft and McCarthy, 1971). A study into the effect of exercise on synovial fluid PO_2 showed a fall in PO_2 as a result of exercise in 3/4 patients (Lund-Olesen, 1970). The latter finding, we believe, might link with the important clinical observation that prolonged bed rest is beneficial to patients with synovitis, perhaps as a result of reducing PO_2 fluctuations.

Synovial fluid PO_2 is dependent upon the blood supply to the synovium, which has been shown to be influenced by the intra-articular pressure within the joint. Jayson and Dixon (1970a) found that patients with rheumatoid arthritis had significantly higher resting pressures within the joint than control subjects with a simulated effusion of the same volume of dextrose–sodium chloride. In the rheumatoid patients only fluctuations in intra-articular pressure synchronous with the arterial pulse were observed, suggesting that increased intra-articular pressure interfered with the synovial circulation (Jayson and Dixon, 1970b). In a further study it was demonstrated that pressures of up to 250 mmHg (well in excess of the capillary hydrostatic pressure) were produced during walking in the presence of a 20 ml effusion in the rheumatoid patients (Jayson and Dixon, 1970c).

In view of these observations we decided to investigate further the role of ischaemia, reperfusion, iron and free radical production in the inflamed joint. In a study of eleven rheumatoid patients and two osteoarthritic patients we have demonstrated that 2 minutes exercise of the inflamed knee resulted in a significant increase in intra-articular pressure during exercise that fell to normal levels at rest. In the rheumatoid patients measurement of synovial fluid PO_2 during this period showed a significant drop in PO_2 during exercise followed by a significant increase 5–10 minutes post-exercise. The osteoarthritic patients showed no significant alterations in synovial fluid PO_2. In one patient 'fluorescent IgG' levels were measured as an *in vivo* index of free radical damage and were found to rise in parallel with the increase in PO_2 immediately post-exercise (Andrews et al., 1986).

These results suggest that significant fluctuations in oxygen tension occur in the synovial fluid as a result of exercise of an inflamed joint, giving rise to a potentially ischaemic situation followed by reperfusion of the tissue post-exercise. The mechanisms surrounding such fluctuations are complex and will depend on any factor that influences the solubility and diffusion of oxygen through a fluid, such as the viscosity of the synovial fluid, the volume of the effusion, and pathological changes within the joint affecting both the blood supply and the extent of inflammatory granulation tissue. The transmission of increased pressures through fluid and tissues may affect oxygen concentrations in these areas. Exercise of the joint itself results in a redistribution of blood flow with an increase to the muscle and consequent decrease in flow to the joint tissue. Exercise of the joint may also give rise to an increase in oxygen consumption by the inflamed tissue and infiltrating cells. However, we and others have demonstrated no correlation between synovial fluid PO_2 and total leukocyte counts (Falchuk, Goetzl and Kulka, 1970; Treuhaft and McCarty, 1971; Andrews et al., 1986).

Although these mechanisms need further study, we have proposed that exercise of the inflamed rheumatoid joint results in an increase in intra-articular pressure sufficient to reduce the blood supply, leading to a period of ischaemia followed by reperfusion of the tissues at rest (Woodruff et al., 1986). Preliminary data on human synovial xanthine oxidase content indicate that the enzyme is present, albeit in low quantities (Allen et al., 1987). Xanthine oxidase may contribute to reperfusion injury by mobilizing iron from the ferritin deposits in the rheumatoid synovium (Muirden, 1966) and by direct production of superoxide leading to oxygen radical-induced tissue damage. This theory may go some way to explain the joint-specific effects of iron deficiency observed in adjuvant disease. Iron deficiency or chelation may protect the joint by reducing the levels of iron available to promote oxygen radical reactions, possibly in conjunction with decreasing the activity of the iron-dependent xanthine oxidase (Kelley and Amy, 1984).

IRON, LYMPHOCYTES AND THE JOINT

Lymphocyte proliferation and migration

The rheumatoid synovium, as well as containing quantities of iron and infiltrating polymorphonuclear leukocytes and mononuclear cells, also shows a profound infiltration of lymphocytes. Indeed Schumacher and Kitridou (1972) demonstrated that one of the earliest changes in the rheumatoid synovium is an infiltration of lymphocytes. The majority of the lymphocytes are T cells, many of which are activated. Perhaps the most convincing evidence of a role for lymphocytes in the pathogenesis of rheumatoid disease has come from lymphocyte depletion studies, where both thoracic duct drainage (Paulus et al., 1977) and lymphophoresis (Karsh et al., 1981) result in considerable clinical improvement. How might these observations relate to iron metabolism?

Lymphocytes have been shown to require iron for proliferation, and activated cells express the transferrin receptor on their surface (Larrick and Cresswell, 1979; Page-Faulk, Hsi and Stevens, 1980; Galbraith et al., 1980).

Lymphocyte proliferation will not proceed *in vitro* in the absence of iron (Brock, 1981). It seems probable that proliferation is inhibited because ribonucleotide reductase, the rate-controlling enzyme in DNA synthesis, is iron-dependent (Lederman *et al.*, 1984).

De Sousa (1978) suggested that the migration of circulating lymphocytes could be based on interaction with iron and iron-binding proteins. Although the idea that lymphocytes home to areas of high iron levels to saturate surface apotransferrin has been criticized (Salmon, 1986), the concept of iron-dependent lymphocyte proliferation and its role in disease has stimulated further research. In rheumatoid disease there is an anaemia, and serum iron levels may not be expected to support lymphocyte proliferation, whereas the inflamed joint contains substantial iron deposits. Salmon *et al.* (1985) showed that rheumatoid patients had greater numbers of transferrin receptor-bearing peripheral lymphocytes than normal controls and that the receptor-bearing population consisted mainly of CD4 (helper/inducer) cells rather than CD8 (suppressor/cytotoxic) cells, leading to a high CD4/CD8 ratio. This pattern was reflected in the rheumatoid synovium, suggesting that lymphocyte activation is extra-articular and that there is a close interaction between populations of lymphocytes in the synovium and in the periphery. Further studies on early rheumatoid patients showed that levels of transferrin receptor-bearing cells increased about the time of the initial flare, whereas later on in the disease high levels related to a worsening rather than a particular level of activity.

Salmon (1986) postulated that during disease flares activated transferrin receptor-bearing lymphocytes travelling through the highly vascular bed of the subsynovial stroma (which is the richest source of iron), may become localized in what is in effect the most favourable micro-environment to support proliferation. The theory may also explain the joint-specific anti-inflammatory effects of iron deficiency seen in adjuvant disease. Roberts and Davies (1987) have also postulated that the exacerbation of synovitis seen in rheumatoid patients given intravenous iron dextran may be related to an increase in lymphocyte proliferation in the synovial membrane.

Lymphocytes and oxygen radicals

Reactive oxygen species, besides having a role in tissue damage, may also affect the function of lymphocytes within the inflamed joint. Allan *et al.* (1986) have shown that UV irradiation of lymphocytes in culture resulted in a dose-dependent killing of cells. Both catalase and desferrioxamine had a significant protective effect, suggesting hydroxyl radical-mediated killing via hydrogen peroxide intermediates. Fluorescent staining of viable cells indicated that T cells were most susceptible to oxidant killing and that CD8+ cells were particularly susceptible at low levels of radicals. Significant loss of CD4+ cells occurred with increasing levels of radicals and a small viable population of B cells remained even at high oxidant stress. Allan *et al.* (1986) proposed that oxygen radicals may be involved in modulating the immunological responses associated with rheumatoid disease and that depletion of lymphocyte subpopulations may play a role in determining the overall immunological status of the synovium.

CONCLUSION

Iron clearly has an important role in inflammatory joint disease, either through its ability to enhance oxidative damage or through its effects on lymphocyte function and possibly trafficking. Such basic mechanisms are thought relevant to the role of iron in inflammation generally and do not explain why either iron overload or iron deficiency have apparent pro- or anti-inflammatory effects that are joint-selective. It appears strange that in haemophilia it is the joint that is a target for a prolonged inflammatory response when bleeding occurs in many other tissues, and that iron dextran therapy promotes a synovitis but is not reported to exacerbate inflammation in other sites. Similarly, why does mild nutritional iron deficiency in a complex inflammatory model such as adjuvant disease lead to an anti-inflammatory effect in the joints but not influence other inflammatory sites? In an attempt to answer these questions, which we believe have a fundamental bearing on the problem of why inflammation in joints tends to be so persistent and destructive, we draw on observations made by others on the effects of iron in ischaemic/reperfusion injury.

The inflamed and mobile joint, with its propensity to generate intermittent high pressures and subsequent tissue hypoxia, seems to be a target for recurrent episodes of iron-promoted ischaemia/reperfusion injury. Such a hypothesis might provide a rationale for the clinical benefits of rest in inflammatory disease and explain the peculiar clinical observation that patients with 'a stroke' do not develop inflammatory joint disease in the paralysed limb (Thompson and Bywaters, 1962). An understanding of the complex mechanisms by which ischaemia may lead to a decompartmentalization of iron, which is then capable of inducing oxidative damage when the ischaemic episode settles, may lead to novel therapeutic approaches to inflammatory joint problems. It is clear, however, that iron chelation (with desferrioxamine) is not in itself a therapeutic option in inflammatory synovitis due to its neurophthalmic toxicity (Blake *et al.*, 1985b; Polson *et al.*, 1986) (see also Chapter 17). However, with the development of new iron chelators and a greater understanding of the role of iron in joint inflammation, therapeutic strategies built around some of the ideas discussed may be possible (see Chapter 17).

REFERENCES

Al Haik, N., Lewis, D. A., and Struthers, G. (1984). Neutral protease, collagenase and elastase activities in synovial fluid from arthritic patients, *Agents Actions*, **15**, 436–46.

Allan, I. M., Lunec, J., Salmon, M., and Bacon, P. A. (1986). Selective lymphocyte killing by reactive oxygen species, *Agents Actions*, **19**, 351–2.

Allen, R. E., Outhwaite, J. M., Morris, C. J., and Blake, D. R. (1987). Xanthine oxido-reductase is present in human synovium, *Ann. Rheum. Dis.*, **46**, 843–5.

Ambruso, D. R., and Johnston, R. B. (1981). Lactoferrin enhances hydroxyl radical production by human neutrophils, neutrophil particulate fractions and an enzymatic generating system, *J. Clin. Invest.*, **67**, 352–60.

Andrews, F. J., Morris, C. J., and Blake, D. R. (1987). The effect of nutritional iron deficiency on acute and chronic inflammation, *Ann. Rheum. Dis.*, **46**, 859–65.

Andrews, F. J., Blake, D. R., Freeman, J., Woodruff, T., Salt, P., Morris, C. J., and Lunec, J. (1986). Free radicals and reperfusion injury in the inflamed joint. In A. J. G. Swaak and J. F. Koster (eds) *Free Radicals and Arthritic Diseases*, pp. 167–78, Eurage, Rijswijk.

Andrews, F. J., Morris, C. J., Kondratowicz, G., and Blake, D. R. (1987). Effect of iron chelation on inflammatory joint disease, *Ann. Rheum. Dis.*, **46**, 327–33.

Aust, S. D., and White, B. C. (1985). Iron chelation prevents tissue injury following ischaemia, *Adv. Free Radical Biol. Med.*, **1**, 1–17.

Babbs, C. F. (1985). Role of iron ions in the genesis of reperfusion injury following successful cardiopulmonary resuscitation: Preliminary data and a biochemical hypothesis, *Ann. Emerg. Med.*, **14**, 777–83.

Babior, B. M., Kipnes, R. S., and Curnutte, J. T. (1973). Biological defense mechanism. The production of superoxide, a potent bactericidal agent, *J. Clin. Invest.*, **52**, 741–4.

Baldwin, A., Jenny, E. R., and Aisen, P. (1984). The effect of human serum transferrin and milk lactoferrin on hydroxyl radical formation from superoxide and hydrogen peroxide, *J. Biol. Chem.*, **259**, 13391–4.

Ball, J., Chapman, J. A., and Muirden, K. D. (1964). The uptake of iron in rabbit synovial tissue following intra-articular injection of iron dextran, *J. Cell Biol.*, **22**, 354–64.

Bannister, J. V., Bellarite, P., Davoli, A., Thornalley, P. J., and Rossi, F. (1982a). The generation of hydroxyl radicals following superoxide production by neutrophil NADPH oxidase, *FEBS Lett.*, **150**, 300–2.

Bannister, J. V., Bannister, W. H., Hill, H. A. O., and Thornalley, P. J. (1982b). Enhanced production of hydroxyl radicals by the xanthine–xanthine oxidase system in the presence of lactoferrin, *Biochim. Biophys. Acta*, **715**, 116–20.

Bannister, J. V., Bannister, W. H., and Thornalley, P. J. (1984). The effect of ferritin iron loading on hydroxyl radical production, *Life Chem. Rep.*, Supplement 2, 64–74.

Benatti, U., Morelli, A., Guida, L., and DeFiora, A. (1983). The production of activated oxygen species by an interaction of methaemoglobin with ascorbate, *Biochem. Biophys. Res. Commun.*, **111**, 980–7.

Bennett, R. M., and Skosey, J. L. (1977). Lactoferrin and lysozyme levels in synovial fluid, *Arthritis Rheum.*, **20**, 84–90.

Bennett, R. M., Hughes, G. R. V., Bywaters, E. G. L., and Holt, P. J. L. (1972). Studies of a popliteal synovial fistula, *Ann. Rheum. Dis.*, **31**, 482–9.

Bennett, R. M., Williams, E. D., Lewis, S. M., and Holt, P. J. L. (1973). Synovial iron deposition in rheumatoid arthritis, *Arthritis Rheum.*, **16**, 295–303.

Betts, W. H., and Cleland, L. G. (1982). Effect of metal chelators and antiinflammatory drugs on the degradation of hyaluronic acid, *Arthritis Rheum.*, **25**, 1469–76.

Biemond, P., Van Eijk, H. G., Swaak, A. J. G., and Koster, J. F. (1984a). Iron mobilisation from ferritin by superoxide derived from stimulated polymorphonuclear leukocytes. Possible mechanism in inflammation diseases, *J. Clin. Invest.*, **73**, 1576–9.

Biemond, P., Swaak, A. J. G., and Koster, J. F. (1984b). Protective factors against oxygen free radicals and hydrogen peroxide in rheumatoid arthritis synovial fluid, *Arthritis Rheum.*, **27**, 760–5.

Biemond, P., Swaak, A. J. G., Penders, J. M. A., Beindorff, C. M., and Koster, J. F. (1986a). Superoxide production by polymorphonuclear leukocytes in rheumatoid arthritis and osteoarthritis: In vivo inhibition by the anti-rheumatic drug piroxicam due to interference with the activation of the NADPH-oxidase, *Ann. Rheum. Dis.*, **45**, 249–55.

Biemond, P., Swaak, A. J. G., van Eijk, H. G., and Koster, J. F. (1986b). Intraarticular ferritin bound iron in rheumatoid arthritis. A factor that increases oxygen radical induced tissue destruction, *Arthritis Rheum.*, **29**, 1187–93.

Biemond, P., Swaak, A. J. G., Beindorff, C. F., and Koster, J. F. (1986c). On the superoxide-dependent and independent mechanism of iron mobilisation from ferritin by xanthine oxidase. Its implications for oxygen free radical induced tissue destruction during ischaemia and inflammation, *Biochem. J.*, **239**, 169–73.

Billingham, M. E. J. (1983). Models of arthritis and the search for antiarthritic drugs, *Pharmacol. Ther.*, **21**, 389–428.

Blake, D. R., and Bacon, P. A. (1980). Synovial fluid ferritin in rheumatoid arthritis, *Br. Med. J.*, **281**, 715–16.

Blake, D. R., and Bacon, P. A. (1981). Synovial fluid ferritin in rheumatoid arthritis: an index or cause of inflammation? *Br. Med. J.*, **282**, 189.

Blake, D. R., and Bacon, P. A. (1982). Effect of oral iron on rheumatoid patients, *Lancet*, **i**, 623.

Blake, D. R., Hall, N. D., Bacon, P. A., Dieppe, P. A., Halliwell, B., and Gutteridge, J. M. C. (1981a). The importance of iron in rheumatoid disease, *Lancet*, **ii**, 1142–4.

Blake, D. R., Hall, N. D., Treby, D. A., Halliwell, B., and Gutteridge, J. M. C. (1981b). Protection against superoxide and hydrogen peroxide in synovial fluid, *Clin. Sci.*, **61**, 483–6.

Blake, D. R., Hall, N. D., Bacon, P. A., Halliwell, B., and Gutteridge, J. M. C. (1983). The effect of a specific iron chelating agent on animal models of inflammation, *Ann. Rheum. Dis.*, **42**, 89–93.

Blake, D. R., Gallagher, P., Potter, A., Bell, M., and Bacon, P. A. (1984). The effect of synovial iron on the progression of rheumatoid disease. A histological assessment of patients with early rheumatoid synovitis, *Arthritis Rheum.*, **26**, 495–501.

Blake, D. R., Lunec, J., Ahern, M., Ring, E. F. J., Bradfield, J., and Gutteridge, J. M. C. (1985a). The effect of intravenous iron dextran on rheumatoid synovitis, *Ann. Rheum. Dis.*, **44**, 183–8.

Blake, D. R., Winyard, P., Lunec, J., Williams, A., Good, P. A., Crewes, S. J., Gutteridge, J. M. C., Rowley, D., Halliwell, B., Cornish, A., and Hider, R. C. (1985b). Cerebral and ocular toxicity induced by desferrioxamine, *Q. J. Med.*, **219**, 344–55.

Brighton, C. T., Bigley, E. C., and Smolenski, B. I. (1970). Iron induced arthritis in immature rabbits, *Arthritis Rheum.*, **13**, 849–57.

Brock, J. H. (1981). The effect of iron and transferrin on the response of serum free cultures of mouse lymphocytes to concanavalin A and lipopolysaccharide, *Immunology*, **43**, 387–92.

Bulloch, W., and Fildes, P. (1912). Haemophilia. In *Treasury of Human Inheritance*. Vol. 1, Section XIVa, pp. 169–354, Dulau and Co., London.

Burton, K. P., McCord, J. M., and Ghai, B. (1984). Myocardial alterations due to free radical generation, *Am. J. Physiol.*, **246**, H776–83.

Carlin, G., and Djursater, R. (1984). Xanthine oxidase induced depolymerisation of hyaluronic acid in the presence of ferritin, *FEBS Lett.*, **177**, 27–30.

Carp, H., and Janoff, A. (1980). Phagocyte derived oxidants suppress the elastase inhibitory capacity of proteinase inhibitor in vitro. *J. Clin. Invest.*, **66**, 987–95.

Cartwright, G. E. (1966). The anaemia of chronic disorders, *Semin. Hematol.*, **3**, 351–75.

Chirico, S., Andrews, D., Lunec, J., Arthur, V., Woodruff, T., McCleary, S., and Blake, D. (1986). Do glutathione levels predict a clinical response in RA patients? *Br. J. Rheumatol.*, **25**, 109.

Collins, D. H. (1951). Haemosiderosis and haemochromatosis of synovial tissue, *J. Bone Joint Surg.*, **33B**, 436–41.

Convery, F. R., Woo, S. L.-Y., Akeson, W. H., Amiel, D., and Malcolm, L. L. (1976). Experimental haemarthrosis in the knee of the mature canine, *Arthritis Rheum.*, **19**, 59–67.

Dallman, P. R., Beutler, E., and Finch, C. A. (1978). Effects of iron deficiency exclusive of anaemia, *Br. J. Haematol.*, **40**, 179–84.

DePalma, A. F., and Cotler, J. M. (1956). Hemophilic arthropathy, *Arch. Surg.*, **72**, 247–50.

De Sousa, M. (1981). *Lymphocyte Circulation: Experimental and Clinical Aspects*, pp. 197–217, Wiley, Chichester.

De Sousa, M., Denysius-Trentham, R., Garcia, F. M., DaSilva, M. T., and Trentham, D. (1988). Activation of the rat synovium by iron, *Arthritis Rheum.*, **31** 653–61.

Docken, W. P. (1979). Pigmented villonodular synovitis: A review with illustrative case reports, *Semin. Arthritis Rheum.*, **9**, 1–22.

Etherington, D. J., Pugh, G., and Silver, I. A. (1981). Collagen degradation in experimental inflammatory lesions: studies on the role of the macrophage, *Acta Biol. Med. Germ.*, **40**, 1625–31.

Falchuk, K. H., Goetzl, E. J., and Kulka, I. P. (1970). Respiratory gases of synovial fluids, *Am. J. Med.*, **49**, 223–31.

Fischbach, F. A., Gregory, D. W., Harrison, P. M., Hoy, T. G., and Williams, J. M. (1971). Structure of haemosiderin and its relationship to ferritin, *J. Ultrastruct. Res.*, **37**, 495–503.

Flitter, W., Rowley, D. A., and Halliwell, B. (1983). Superoxide dependent formation of hydroxyl radicals in the presence of iron salts, *FEBS Lett.*, **158**, 310–12.

Floyd, R. A. (1981). DNA-ferrous iron catalysed hydroxyl free radical formation from hydrogen peroxide, *Biochem. Biophys. Res. Commun.*, **99**, 1209–15.

Fong, K. L., McCay, P. B., Poyer, J. L., Keele, B. B., and Misra, H. (1973). Evidence that peroxidation of lysosomal membranes is initiated by hydroxyl free radicals produced during flavin enzyme activity, *J. Biol. Chem.*, **248**, 7792–6.

Galasko, C. S. B., and Bennett, A. (1976). Relationships of bone destruction in skeletal metastases to osteoclast activation and prostaglandins, *Nature*, **263**, 508–10.

Galbraith, G. M. P., Galbraith, R. M., Temple, A., and Page-Faulk, W. (1980).

Demonstration of transferrin receptors on human placental trophoblast, *Blood*, **55**, 240–2.
Ghormley, R. K., and Clegg, R. S. (1948). Bone and joint changes in haemophilia, *J. Bone Joint Surg.*, **30A**, 589–600.
Glenn, E. M., and Gray, J. (1965). Adjuvant induced polyarthritis in rats: biologic and histologic background, *Am. J. Vet. Res.*, **26**, 1180–94.
Gralla, E. J., and Wiseman, E. H. (1968). The adjuvant arthritic rat inflammatory parameters during the development and regression of gross lesions, *Proc. Soc. Exp. Biol. Med.*, **128**, 493–5.
Granger, D. N., Adkinson, D., and Hollwarth, M. E. (1985). Role of oxygen free radicals in ischaemia–reperfusion injury to the liver, *Gastroenterology*, **88**, 1662.
Greenwald, R. A., and Moy, W. W. (1979). Inhibition of collagen gelation by action of the superoxide radical, *Arthritis Rheum.*, **22**, 251–9.
Greenwald, R. A., and Moy, W. W. (1980). Effect of oxygen derived free radicals on hyaluronic acid, *Arthritis Rheum.*, **23**, 455–63.
Greenwald, R. A., Moy, W. W., and Lazarus, D. (1976). Degradation of cartilage proteoglycans and collagen by the superoxide radical, *Arthritis Rheum.*, **19**, 799.
Gutteridge, J. M. C., Patterson, S. K., Segal, A. W., and Halliwell, B. (1981). Inhibition of lipid peroxidation by the iron binding protein lactoferrin, *Biochem. J.*, **199**, 259–61.
Gysen, P., Malaise, M., Gaspar, S., and Franchimont, P. (1985). Measurement of proteoglycans, elastase, collagenase and protein in synovial fluid in inflammatory and degenerative arthropathies, *Clin. Rheumatol.*, **41**, 39–50.
Haalaja, M. (1975). Evaluation of the activity of rheumatoid arthritis. A comparative study on clinical symptoms and laboratory tests with special reference to serum and sulphydryl groups, *Scand. J. Rheumatol.*, **4**, 3–54.
Halliwell, B. (1984). Oxygen radicals: A common sense look at their nature and medical importance. *Med. Biol.*, **62**, 71–7.
Halliwell, B., and Gutteridge, J. M. C. (1985). The importance of free radicals and catalytic ions in human disease, *Mol. Aspects Med.*, **8**, 89–193.
Halliwell, B., Gutteridge, J. M. C., and Blake, D. (1985). Metal ions and oxygen radical reactions in human inflammatory joint disease, *Philos. Trans. R. Soc. Lond. (Biol.).* **311**, 659–71.
Hamerman, D. (1970). Synovial joints. Aspects of structure and function. In S. Balaz (ed.) *Chemistry and Molecular Biology of the Intracellular Matrix*, pp. 1259–72, Academic Press, London.
Harris, E. D., Evanson, J. M., DiBona, D. R., and Krane, S. M. (1970). Collagenase and rheumatoid arthritis, *Arthritis Rheum.*, **13**, 83–94.
Harvey, P. W. J., Bell, R. G., and Nesheim, M. C. (1985). Iron deficiency protects inbred mice against infection with *Plasmodium chabaudi*, *Infec. Immun.*, **50**, 932–4.
Hider, R. C. (1984). Siderophore mediated absorption of iron, *Structure and Bonding*, **58**, 26–87.
Hiyeda, K. (1939). The cause of Kaschin Beck's disease, *Jpn. J. Med. Sci.*, **4**, 91–106.
Hoaglund, F. T. (1967). Experimental haemarthrosis. The response of canine knees to injection of autologous blood, *J. Bone Joint Surg.*, **49A**, 285–98.
Igari, T., Kaneda, H., Horiuchi, S., and Ono, S. (1982). A remarkable increase of superoxide dismutase activity in synovial fluid of patients with rheumatoid arthritis, *Clin. Orthop.*, **162**, 282–7.
Im, M. J., Shen, W. H., Pak, C. J., Manson, P. N., Bulkey, G. B., and Hoopes, J. E. (1984). Effect of allopurinol on the survival on the hyperemic island skin flaps, *Plast. Reconstr. Surg.*, **73**, 276–8.

Isaacson, C., and Bothwell, T. H. (1981). Synovial iron deposits in black subjects with iron overload, *Arch. Pathol. Lab. Med.*, **105**, 487–9.
Jacobs, A. (1977). Iron overload—clinical and pathological aspects, *Semin. Hematol.*, **14**, 89–113.
Jaffe, A., Lichtenstein, L., and Sulvo, C. J. (1941). Pigmented villonodular synovitis, bursitis and tenosynovitis, *Arch. Pathol.*, **31**, 731–65.
Jayson, M. I. V., and Dixon, A. St. J. (1970a). Intra-articular pressure in rheumatoid arthritis of the knee. I. Pressure changes during passive joint distention, *Ann. Rheum. Dis.*, **29**, 261–5.
Jayson, M. I. V., and Dixon, A. St. J. (1970b). Intra-articular pressure in rheumatoid arthritis of the knee. II. Effect of intra-articular pressure on blood circulation to the synovium, *Ann. Rheum. Dis.*, **29**, 266–8.
Jayson, M. I. V., and Dixon, A. St. J. (1970c). Intra-articular pressure in rheumatoid arthritis of the knee. III. Pressure changes during joint use, *Ann. Rheum. Dis.*, **29**, 401–8.
Jensen, P. S. (1976). Haemochromatosis: a disease often silent but not invisible, *Am. J. Roentgenol.*, **126**, 343–51.
Joynson, D. H. M., Jacobs, A., Murray-Walker, D., and Dolby, A. E. (1972). Defect of cell mediated immunity in patients with iron deficiency anaemia, *Lancet*, **ii**, 1058–9.
Karsh, J., Klippel, J. H., Plotz, P. H., Decker J. L., Wright, D. G., and Flye, M. W. (1981). Lymphophoresis in rheumatoid arthritis, *Arthritis Rheum.*, **24**, 867–73.
Kelley, M. K., and Amy, N. K. (1984). Effect of molybdenum deficient and low iron diets on xanthine oxidase activity and iron status in rats, *J. Nutr.*, **114**, 1652–9.
Key, J. A. (1929). Experimental arthritis. The reaction of joints to mild irritants, *J. Bone Joint Surg.*, **11**, 705–8.
Key, J. A. (1932). Haemophilic arthritis, *Ann. Surg.*, **95**, 198–225.
Knuutila, S. (1984). Role of free radicals in genetic damage (mutation), *Med. Biol.*, **62**, 110–14.
Kochanowski, B. A., and Sherman, A. R. (1985a). Decreased antibody formation in iron deficient rat pups: effect of iron repletion, *Am. J. Clin. Nutr.*, **41**, 278–84.
Kochanowski, B. A., and Sherman, A. R. (1985b). Cellular growth in iron deficient rats: effect of pre- and post-weaning iron repletion, *J. Nutr.*, **115**, 279–87.
Konig, F. (1892). Die gelenkerkrankungen bei blutern mit besonderer berucksichtiging der diagnose, *Samml. Klin. Vort. Chir.*, **11**, 233–42.
Koster, J. F., Biemond, P., and Swaak, A. J. G. (1986). Intra-cellular and extra-cellular sulphydryl levels in rheumatoid arthritis, *Ann. Rheum. Dis.*, **45**, 44–6.
Kra, S. J., Hollingsworth, J. W., and Finch, S. C. (1965). Arthritis with synovial iron deposition in a patient with haemochromatosis, *N. Engl. J. Med.*, **272**, 1268–71.
Laborde, J. M., Green, D. L., Askari, A. D., and Muir, A. (1977). Arthritis in haemochromatosis. A case report, *J. Bone Joint Surg.*, **59**, 1103.
Larrick, J. W., and Cresswell, P. (1979). Transferrin receptors on B and T lymphoblastoid cell lines, *Biochim. Biophys. Acta*, **583**, 483–90.
Lawrence, J. S. (1977). Rheumatoid arthritis. In *Rheumatism in Populations*, pp. 156–271, William Heinemann, London.
Lederman, H. M., Cohen, A., Lee, J. W. W., Freedman, M. H., and Gelfand, E. W. (1984). Desferrioxamine: a reversible S-phase inhibitor of human lymphocyte proliferation, *Blood*, **64**, 748–53.
Lloyd, K. N., and Williams, P. (1970). Reactions to total dose infusion of iron dextran in rheumatoid arthritis, *Br. Med. J.*, **2**, 323–5.

Lund-Olesen, K. (1970). Oxygen tensions in synovial fluids, *Arthritis Rheum.*, **13**, 769–76.

Lunec, J. (1982). Fluorescence: A marker of the free radical damage induced in human gamma globulin, *Biochem. Soc. Trans.*, **10**, 21.

Lunec, J., and Blake, D. R. (1985). Determination of dehydroascorbic acid and ascorbic acid in serum and synovial fluid of patients with rheumatoid arthritis, *Free Radical Res. Commun.*, **1**, 31–41.

Lunec, J., Halloran, S. P., White, A. G., and Dormandy, T. L. (1981). Free radical oxidation (peroxidation) products in serum and synovial fluid in rheumatoid arthritis, *J. Rheumatol.*, **8**, 233–45.

Lunec, J., Blake, D. R., McCleary, S. J., Brailsford, S., and Bacon, P. A. (1985). Self perpetuating mechanisms of immunoglobulin G aggregation in rheumatoid inflammation, *J. Clin. Invest.*, **76**, 2084–90.

Lunec, J., Wakefield, A., Brailsford, S., and Blake, D. R. (1986a). Free radical altered IgG and its interaction with rheumatoid factor. In C. Rice Evans (ed.) *Free Radicals, Cell Damage and Disease*, pp. 241–61. Richelieu Press, London.

Lunec, J., Brailsford, S., Hewitt, S. D., Morris, C. J., and Blake, D. R. (1986b). Free radicals: are they possible mediators of IgG denaturation and immune complex formation in RA. *Int. J. Immunotherapy*, **11**, 6442–6.

MacDougall, L. G., Anderson, R., McNab, G. M., and Katz, J. (1975). The immune response in iron deficient children: impaired cellular defence mechanisms with altered humoral components, *J. Pediatr.*, **86**, 833–43.

Mackler, B., Person, R., Ochs, H., and Finch, C. A. (1984). Iron deficiency in the rat: effects on neutrophil activation and metabolism, *Pediatr. Res.*, **18**, 549–51.

Maguire, J. T., Kellog, E. W., and Packer, L. (1982). Protection against free radical formation by protein bound iron, *Toxicol. Lett.*, **14**, 27–34.

Mainardi, C. L., Levine, P. H., Werb, Z., and Harris, E. D. (1978). Proliferative synovitis in haemophilia, *Arthritis Rheum.*, **21**, 137–44.

Martin, W. (1984). Do we get too much iron? *Med. Hypotheses*, **13**, 119–21.

Masawe, A. E. J. (1974). Infections in iron deficiency and other types of anaemia in the tropics, *Lancet*, **ii**, 314–17.

McCord, J. M. (1985). Oxygen derived free radicals in post ischaemic tissue injury, *N. Engl. J. Med.*, **312**, 159–63.

McCord, J. M., and Day, E. D. (1978). Superoxide dependent production of hydroxyl radical catalysed by iron-EDTA complex, *FEBS Lett.*, **86**, 139–42.

Meninger, H., Putzier, R., Mohr, W., Wessinghage, D., and Tillman, K. (1980). Granulocyte elastase at the site of cartilage erosion by rheumatoid synovial tissue, *Z. Rheumatol.*, **39**, 145–56.

Mitchell, N. S., and Shepard, N. (1978). Changes in proteoglycan and collagen in cartilage in rheumatoid arthritis, *J. Bone Joint Surg.*, **60A**, 349–54.

Moore, L. L., and Humbert, J. R. (1984). Neutrophil bacterial dysfunction towards oxidant radical-sensitive micro-organisms during experimental iron deficiency, *Pediatr. Res.*, **18**, 684–6.

Morris, C. J., Blake, D. R., Wainwright, A. C., and Steven, M. M. (1985). The relationship between iron deposits and tissue damage in the synovium—an ultrastructural study, *Ann. Rheum. Dis.*, **45**, 21–6.

Morris, C. J., Blake, D. R., Hewitt, S. D., and Lunec, J. (1987). Macrophage ferritin and iron deposition in the rat air pouch model of inflammatory synovitis, *Ann. Rheum. Dis.*, **46**, 334–8.

Motohashi, N., and Mori, I. (1983). Superoxide dependent formation of hydroxyl radical catalysed by transferrin, *FEBS Lett.*, **157**, 197–9.

Mottonen, T., Hannoren, P., Seppala, O., Alfthan, G., and Oka, M. (1984). Glutathione and selenium in RA, *Clin. Rheum.*, **3**, 195–200.
Mowat, A. G., and Garner, R. W. (1972). Influence of iron dextran on adjuvant arthritis in the rat, *Ann. Rheum. Dis.*, **31**, 339–43.
Muirden, K. D. (1963). An electron microscope study of the uptake of ferritin by the synovial membrane, *Arthritis Rheum.*, **6**, 289.
Muirden, K. D. (1966). Ferritin in synovial cells in patients with rheumatoid arthritis, *Ann. Rheum. Dis.*, **25**, 387–401.
Muirden, K. D. (1970). The anaemia of rheumatoid arthritis: The significance of iron deposits in the synovial membrane, *Aust. Ann. Med.*, **2**, 97–104.
Muirden, K. D., and Peace, G. (1969). Light and electron microscope studies in carrageenan, adjuvant and tuberculin induced arthritis, *Ann. Rheum. Dis.*, **28**, 392–401.
Muirden, K. D., and Senator, G. B. (1968). Iron in the synovial membrane in rheumatoid arthritis and other joint diseases, *Ann. Rheum. Dis.*, **27**, 38–47.
Muirden, K. D., Fraser, J. R. E., and Clarris, B. (1967). Ferritin formation by synovial cells exposed to haemoglobin in vitro, *Ann. Rheum. Dis.*, **26**, 251–9.
Munthe, E., Guldal, G., and Jellun, E. (1979). Increased intracellular glutathione deriving penicillamine treatment for rheumatoid arthritis, *Lancet*, **ii**, 1126–7.
Myers, B. W., Masi, A. T., and Feigenbaum, S. L. (1980). Pigmented villonodular synovitis and tenosynovitis. A clinical epidemiological study of 166 cases and literature review, *Medicine*, **59**, 223–38.
Nayini, N. R., White, B. C., Aust, S. D., Huang, R. R., Indrieri, R. J., Evans, A. T., Bialek, H., Jacobs, W., and Komara, J. (1985). Post resuscitation iron delocalisation and malondialdehyde production in the brain following cardiac arrest, *J. Free Radical Biol. Med.*, **1**, 111–16.
Niedermeier, N. (1982). The effect of caeruloplasmin and iron on the ascorbic acid induced depolymerisation of hyaluronic acid. In J. R. J. Sorenson (ed.) *Inflammatory Diseases and Copper*, pp. 223–9, Humana Press, New Jersey.
Nordstrom, G., Seeman, T., and Hasselgren, P. O. (1985). Beneficial effect of allopurinol in liver ischaemia, *Surgery*, **97**, 679–83.
O'Connell, M. J., Halliwell, B., Moorhouse, C. P., Aruoma, O. I., Baum, H., and Peters, T. J. (1986). Formation of hydroxyl radicals in the presence of ferritin and haemosiderin. Is haemosiderin formation a biological protective mechanism? *Biochem. J.*, **234**, 727–31.
Ogilvie-Harris, D. J., and Fornaiser, V. L. (1980). Synovial iron deposition in osteoarthritis and rheumatoid arthritis, *J. Rheumatol.*, **7**, 30–6.
Okazaki, I., Brinckerhoff, C. E., Sinclair, J. F., Sinclair, P. R., Bonkowsky, H. L., and Harris, E. D. (1981). Iron increases collagenase production by rabbit synovial fibroblasts, *J. Lab. Clin. Med.*, **97**, 396–402.
Owens, M. L., Lazarus, H. M., Wolcott, M. W., Maxwell, J. G., and Taylor, B. (1974). Allopurinol and hypoxanthine pretreatment of canine kidney donors, *Transplantation*, **17**, 424–7.
Page-Faulk, W., Hsi, B. L., and Stevens P. J. (1980). Transferrin and transferrin receptors in carcinoma of the breast, *Lancet*, **ii**, 390–2.
Parks, D. A., and Bulkey, D. N. (1983). Role of oxygen derived free radicals in digestive tract diseases, *Surgery*, **94**, 415–22.
Pasquier, C., Mach, P. S., Raichvarg, D., Sarfati, G., Amor, B., and Delbarre, F. (1984). Manganese containing superoxide dismutase deficiency in polymorphonuclear leukocytes of adults with rheumatoid arthritis, *Inflammation*, **8**, 27–32.
Pasquier, C., Laossadi, S., Sarfati, G., Raichvarg, D., and Amor, B. (1985). Super-

oxide dismutase in polymorphonuclear leukocytes from patients with ankylosing spondylitis or rheumatoid arthritis, *Clin. Exp. Rheum.*, **3**, 123–6.

Paulus, H. E., Machleder, H. I., Levine, S., Yu, D. T. Y., and MacDonald, N. S. (1977). Lymphocyte involvement in rheumatoid arthritis, *Arthritis Rheum.*, **20**, 1249–62.

Pearson, C. M. (1956). Development of arthritis, periarthritis and periostitis in rats given adjuvant, *Proc. Soc. Exp. Biol. Med.*, **91**, 95–101.

Pearson, C. M. (1963). Experimental joint disease. Observations on adjuvant induced arthritis, *J. Chronic Dis.*, **16**, 863–74.

Pearson, C. M., and Wood, F. D. (1959). Studies of polyarthritis and other lesions induced in rats by injection of mycobacteria adjuvant. I. General, clinical and pathologic characteristics and some modifying factors, *Arthritis Rheum.*, **2**, 440–59.

Peters, T. J., and Selden, C. (1982). Hepatotoxicity due to chronic iron overload: the role of lysosomes and haemosiderin. In D. J. Wetherall (ed.) *Advances in Red Cell Biology*, pp. 71–81, Raven Press, New York.

Peters, T. J., and Seymour, C. A. (1976). Acid hydrolase activities and lysosomal integrity in liver biopsies from patients with iron overload, *Clin. Sci. Mol. Med.*, **50**, 75–8.

Peters, T. J., Selden, A. C., and Seymour, C. A. (1977). Lysosomal disruption in the pathogenesis of primary and secondary haemochromatosis. *Ciba Found. Symp.*, **51**, 317–29.

Polson, R. J., Jawad, A. S. M., Bomford, A., Berry, H., and Williams, R. (1986). Treatment of rheumatoid arthritis with desferrioxamine, *Q. J. Med.*, **61**, 1153–8.

Poole, A. R., Hembry, R. M., and Dingle, J. T. (1974). Cathepsin D in cartilage: The immunohistochemical demonstration of extracellular enzyme in normal and pathological conditions, *J. Cell. Sci.*, **14**, 139–61.

Pritchard, M. H. (1984). Synovial protease/inhibitor ratios in erosive and non-erosive arthropathies, *Ann. Rheum. Dis.*, **43**, 50–5.

Reddy, P. S., and Lewis, M. (1969). The adverse effect of intravenous iron dextran in rheumatoid arthritis, *Arthritis Rheum.*, **12**, 454–7.

Richter, G. W. (1957). A study of haemosiderosis with the aid of electron microscopy, *J. Exp. Med.*, **106**, 203–17.

Rister, M., Bauermeister, K., Gravert, U., and Gladtke, E. (1978). Superoxide dismutase deficiency in rheumatoid arthritis, *Lancet*, **i**, 1094.

Roberts, D., and Davies, J. (1987). Exacerbation of rheumatoid synovitis by iron dextran infusion, *Lancet*, **i**, 391.

Rodnan, G. P., Lewis, J. H., Warren, J. E., and Brower, T. D. (1957). Haemophilic arthritis, *Bull. Rheum. Dis.*, **8**, 137–8.

Rowley, D., Gutteridge, J. M. C., Blake, D. R., Farr, M., and Halliwell, B. (1984). Lipid peroxidation in rheumatoid arthritis: thiobarbituric acid reactive material and catalytic iron salts in synovial fluid from rheumatoid arthritis, *Clin. Sci.*, **66**, 691–5.

Roy, S., and Ghadially, F. N. (1966). Pathology of experimental haemarthrosis, *Ann. Rheum. Dis.*, **26**, 402–15.

Roy, S., and Ghadially, F. N. (1967). Ultrastructure of synovial membrane in human haemarthrosis, *J. Bone Joint Surg.*, **49A**, 1636–46.

Roy, S., and Ghadially, F. N. (1969). Synovial membrane in experimentally produced haemarthrosis, *Ann. Rheum. Dis.*, **28**, 402–13.

Sadrzadeh, S. M. H., Graf, E., Panter, S. S., Hallaway, P. E., and Eaton, J. W. (1985). Haemoglobin. A biologic Fenton reagent, *J. Biol. Chem.*, **259**, 14354–6.

Salmon, M. (1986). Transferrin receptor bearing cells in rheumatoid arthritis and an in vitro model of lymphocyte activation, Ph.D. Thesis, University of Birmingham.
Salmon, M., Bacon, P. A., Symmons, D. P. M., and Blann, A. D. (1985). Transferrin receptor bearing cells in the peripheral blood of patients with rheumatoid arthritis, *Clin. Exp. Immunol.*, **62**, 346-52.
Schumacher, H. R. (1964). Haemochromatosis and arthritis, *Arthritis Rheum.*, **7**, 41-50.
Schumacher, H. R. (1982). Articular cartilage in the degenerative arthropathy of haemochromatosis, *Arthritis Rheum.*, **25**, 1460-8.
Schumacher, H. R., and Kitridou, R. C. (1972). Synovitis of recent onset: a clinicopathologic study during the first month of disease, *Arthritis Rheum.*, **15**, 465-84.
Schumacher, H. R., Lotke, P., Athreya, B., and Rothfuss, S. (1982). Pigmented villonodular synovitis: Light and electron microscope studies, *Semin. Arthritis Rheum.*, **12**, 32-43.
Seffar, M., Fornaiser, V. L., and Fox, I. H. (1977). Arthropathy as the major clinical indicator of occult iron storage disease, *J. Am. Med. Assoc.*, **238**, 1825-8.
Seftel, H. C., Malkin, C., Schmaman, A., Abraham, S. C., Lynch, S. R., Charlton, R. W., and Bothwell, T. H. (1966). Osteoporosis, scurvy and siderosis in Johannesburg Bantu, *Br. Med. J.*, **1**, 642.
Senator, G. B., and Muirden, K. D. (1968). Concentration of iron in synovial membrane, synovial fluid and serum in rheumatoid arthritis and other joint diseases, *Ann. Rheum. Dis.*, **27**, 49-54.
Shaper, A. G., and Jones, K. W. (1959). Serum cholesterol, diet and coronary heart disease in Africans and Asians in Uganda, *Lancet*, **ii**, 534-7.
Silverstein, E., and Sokoloff, L. (1958). Periarthritis in rats with Freund's adjuvant, *Arthritis Rheum.*, **3**, 485-95.
Singh, R., Grewal, D. S., and Chakravarti, R. N. (1969). Experimental production of pigmented villonodular synovitis in the knee and ankle joints of rhesus monkeys, *J. Pathol.*, **98**, 137-42.
Stein, H., and Duthie, R. B. (1981). The pathogenesis of chronic haemophilic arthropathy, *J. Bone Joint Surg.*, **63B**, 601-9.
Sullivan, J. L. (1986). Sex, iron and heart disease, *Lancet*, **ii**, 1162.
Swarup-Mitra, S., and Sinha, A. K. (1984). Cell mediated immunity in nutritional anaemia, *Indian J. Med. Res.*, **79**, 354-62.
Thompson, M., and Bywaters, E. G. L. (1962). Unilateral rheumatoid arthritis following hemiplegia, *Ann. Rheum. Dis.*, **21**, 370-7.
Treuhaft, P. S., and McCarty, D. J. (1971). Synovial fluid pH, lactate, oxygen and carbon dioxide partial pressure in various joint disease, *Arthritis Rheum.*, **14**, 475-84.
Uno, S., Nishimura, T., Furuya, E., Shimokobe, H., and Nishikaze, O. (1985). Action of ionic iron in carrageenin induced inflammation, *Int. J. Tissue React.*, **7**, 21-6.
Vapaatalo, H. (1986). Free radicals and anti-inflammatory drugs, *Med. Biol.*, **64**, 1-7.
Velvart, M., Fehr, K., Baici, A., Saumermajer, G., Knopfel, M., Cancer, M., Salgam, P., and Boni, A. (1981). Degradation in vivo of articular cartilage in rheumatoid arthritis by leukocyte elastase from polymorphonuclear leukocytes, *Rheumatol. Int.*, **1**, 121-30.
Waksman, B. H., Pearson, C. M., and Sharp, J. T. (1960). Studies of arthritis and other lesions induced in rats by injection of mycobacterial adjuvant. II. Evidence

that the disease is a disseminated immunologic response to exogenous antigen, *J. Immunol.*, **85**, 403–17.
Walker, R. J., Dymock, I. W., Ansell, I. D., Hamilton, E. B. D., and Williams, R. (1972). Synovial biopsy in haemochromatosis arthropathy: histological findings and iron deposition in relation to total body iron overload, *Ann. Rheum. Dis.*, **31**, 98–102.
Wapnick, A. A., Lynch, S. R., Krawitz, P., Seftel, H. C., Charlton, R. W., and Bothwell, T. H. (1968). Effects of iron overload on ascorbic acid metabolism, *Br. Med. J.*, **3**, 704–7.
Weir, M. P., Gibson, J. F., and Peters, T. J. (1984). Haemosiderin and tissue damage, *Cell Biochem. Funct.*, **2**, 186–94.
Weisiger, R. A. (1986). Oxygen radicals and ischaemic tissue injury, *Gastroenterology*, **90**, 494–6.
White, B. C., Krause, G. S., Aust, S. D., and Eysler, G. E. (1985). Post ischaemic tissue injury by iron mediated free radical lipid peroxidation, *Ann. Emerg. Med.*, **14**, 804–9.
Wickens, D. G., Norden, A. G., Lunec, J., and Dormandy, T. L. (1983). Fluorescence changes in human gamma globulin induced free radical activity, *Biochim. Biophys. Acta*, **742**, 607–16.
Williams, D. M., Lee, G. R., and Cartwright, G. E. (1974). The role of superoxide anion radical in the reduction of ferritin iron by xanthine oxidase, *J. Clin. Invest.*, **53**, 665–7.
Williams, R. (1972). Synovial biopsy in haemochromatosis arthropathy: histological findings and iron deposition in relation to total body iron overload, *Ann. Rheum. Dis.*, **31**, 98–102.
Willson, R. L. (1977). Iron, zinc, free radicals and oxygen in tissue disorders and cancer control, *Ciba Found. Symp.*, **51**, 331–54.
Winterbourn, C. C. (1983). Lactoferrin catalysed hydroxyl radical production, *Biochem. J.*, **210**, 15–19.
Winterbourn, C. C. (1985). Free radical and oxidative reaction of haemoglobin, *Environ. Health Perspect.*, **64**, 321–30.
Winyard, P. G., Lunec, J., Brailsford, S., and Blake, D. (1984). Action of free radical generating systems upon the biological and immunological properties of caeruloplasmin, *Int. J. Biochem.*, **16**, 1273–8.
Winyard, P. G., Blake, D. R., Chirico, S., Gutteridge, J. M. C., and Lunec, J. (1987). Mechanism of exacerbation of rheumatoid synovitis by total dose infusion of iron dextran: In vivo demonstration of iron promoted oxidant stress, *Lancet*, **i**, 69–72.
Wolf, C. R., and Mankin, H. J. (1965). The effect of experimental haemarthrosis on articular cartilage of rabbit knee joints, *J. Bone Joint Surg.*, **47A**, 1203–10.
Wolff, S. P., and Dean, R. T. (1986). Fragmentation of proteins by free radicals and its effect on their susceptibility to enzyme hydrolysis, *Biochem. J.*, **234**, 399–403.
Wong, P. S., and Travis, J. (1980). Isolation and properties of oxidised proteinase inhibitor from human rheumatoid synovial fluid, *Biochim. Biophys. Res. Commun.*, **96**, 1449–54.
Wong, S. F., Halliwell, B., Richmond, R., and Skowroneck, W. R. (1981). The role of superoxide and hydroxyl radicals in the degradation of hyaluronic acid induced by metal ions and by ascorbic acid, *J. Inorg. Biochem.*, **14**, 127–34.
Woodruff, T., Blake, D. R., Freeman, J., Andrews, F. J., Salt, P., and Lunec, J. (1986). Is chronic synovitis an example of reperfusion injury?, *Ann. Rheum. Dis.*, **45**, 608–11.
Woolley, D. E., Crossley, M. J., and Evans, J. M. (1977). Collagenase at sites of cartilage erosion in the rheumatoid joint, *Arthritis Rheum.*, **20**, 1231–9.

Yoshino, S., Blake, D. R., and Bacon, P. A. (1984). The effect of desferrioxamine on antigen induced inflammation in the rat air pouch, *J. Pharm. Pharmacol.*, **36**, 543–5.

Yoshino, S., Blake, D. R., Hewitt, S., Morris, C., and Bacon, P. A. (1985). Effect of blood on the activity and persistence of antigen induced inflammation in the rat air pouch, *Ann. Rheum. Dis.*, **44**, 485–91.

Young, J. M., and Hudacek, A. C. (1954). Experimental production of pigmented villonodular synovitis in dogs, *Am. J. Pathol.*, **30**, 799–812.

Iron in Immunity, Cancer and Inflammation
Edited by M. De Sousa and J. H. Brock
© 1989 John Wiley & Sons Ltd.

8
Inflammation and Parasitic Disease

I. A. Clark* and G. Chaudhri†
*Zoology Department and †John Curtin School of Medical Research,
Australian National University, Canberra, ACT 2601, Australia

INTRODUCTION

Examples of the interconnection between iron and inflammatory processes are becoming increasingly frequent. The field of mediators in inflammation is itself enlarging and becoming more complex with the availability of the recombinant cytokines and the possibility of the 'fine tuning' of their functions and interactions. The effector arm of the inflammatory response is mainly mediated by molecules released from phagocytic cells. These include lysosomal enzymes, free oxygen radicals, prostanoids, tumour necrosis factor, interleukin-1 and platelet-activating factor. This chapter reviews their actions and interrelationships in this context and also the current evidence that these mediators, in particular tumour necrosis factor, may be important in the pathogenesis of parasitic disease.

Malaria is cited as an example of the disease caused by systemic release of these mediators, and granulomas that form during schistosomiasis as an example of the effects of their persistent local release. Further details of the contribution of iron to some of the processes cited in this chapter are to be found in Chapters 6 and 7.

The changes that occur during inflammation are complex, and inevitably a brief review such as this cannot be comprehensive, but will be biased towards the authors' experience and interests. References to other reviews will point the reader in the directions given less attention.

The first half of this chapter reviews some important mediators of inflammation in a general sense, stressing the way in which they interact, reinforcing or inhibiting each other. We concentrate on the effects of lymphokines and monokines (the soluble products of lymphocytes and monocytes–macrophages, respectively) rather than how they are induced.

Since blood vessels are central to inflammation, the effects of these mediators on endothelial cells, and the vasculature in general, receive close attention. Likewise, we discuss the complex interactions between the immune system and inflammation. In some circumstances the inflammatory response can be usefully viewed as a crude (though none-the-less useful) forerunner of a specific immune response, whereas in others it seems that the immune system directs inflammatory processes as one of its effector arms, as if trusting that the parasite will be eliminated before the host is irreparably injured.

The rest of the chapter applies these principles to parasitic diseases. The pathology of various acute systemic parasitic infections can be remarkably similar, irrespective of whether protozoa, bacteria or viruses are involved. The key seems to be whether systemic macrophage activation occurs. Indeed, Maegraith made the similarities of malaria and certain systemic bacterial infections the central theme of his monograph (Maegraith, 1948), and influenza continues to be diagnostically confused with imported malaria in First World countries (Brown, 1986).

THE MEDIATORS OF INFLAMMATION

At the microscopic level, leukocytic accumulation is the hallmark of inflammation. While these leukocytes can at times be phagocytic, they function largely through secreting various molecules, some of which are involved in iron binding (see Chapter 5). This section of the chapter will be devoted to the secretions of phagocytic cells, which can conveniently be termed the mediators of inflammation, and concentrates on recent developments in those mediators that initiate events leading to tissue damage. A comprehensive list of the currently known secretions of macrophages is found in Nathan (1987). For a wider background in the processes of inflammation the reader is directed to Larsen and Hensen (1983), a review that particularly covers vascular permeability and leukocyte chemotaxis, and to Moore and Weiss (1985), who give a comprehensive account of the role of the complement and Hageman factor systems.

Lysosomal enzymes

Until a few years ago lysosomal enzymes (previously thought to restrict their activity to within the lysosomal vacuole, but realized subsequently also to be released extracellularly) dominated the literature on tissue damage in inflammation. The individual enzymes operate at characteristic points across the pH range, and the neutral proteases (including elastases, collagenases and cathepsins) have been favoured candidates because they do not need the low pH of the lysosomal vacuole before they can act extracellularly. These concepts have been reviewed by Wintroub (1982). More recent experiments have questioned the importance (of proteases *in vivo*) in this context: immune complexes induce macrophages to secrete lysosomal enzymes *in vitro* (Cardella, Davies and Allison, 1974), yet vascular damage after immune complex deposition is as high in mice congenitally deficient in leukocytic protease activity as in normal animals (Johnson *et al.*, 1979), and antiproteases have little effect on neutrophil-induced lung injury (Fantone and Ward, 1982).

The extent and duration of the extracellular activity of proteolytic enzymes is normally limited by protease inhibitors present in serum. Interaction of these inhibitors and free oxygen radicals has been extensively studied, and there is ample evidence that free oxygen radicals (or in functional terms, oxidant stress) released by phagocytes can inactivate α_1-protease inhibitor (Carp and Janoff, 1979, 1980), as well as cause tissue injury in their own right (see below and Chapter 7). This would lead to synergy between these two systems of cell-mediated tissue damage by allowing proteases to maintain effective extracellular concentrations for longer periods. Enhanced release of superoxide from macrophages after they have been exposed to proteolytic enzymes (Speer *et al.*, 1983) affords a further opportunity for synergy.

Free oxygen radicals

Details of the chemical nature of free radicals, and why oxygen is prone to form them, are outside the scope of this chapter. Halliwell and Gutteridge (1984) and Slater (1984) provide clear reviews on their formation and how they cause tissue injury, and we have recently reviewed them in the context of parasitic disease (Clark, Hunt and Cowden, 1986). Slater (1987) gives a useful cautionary tale of the dangers of misinterpreting secondary radical formation as the cause of tissue damage. What is important from an inflammation perspective is that suitably triggered neutrophils and mononuclear phagocytes will, through the NADPH oxidase complex on their surfaces, reduce oxygen to superoxide (O_2^-), and release this superoxide into their surroundings. This soon converts to hydrogen peroxide with subsequent reduction to more harmful species depending largely on the availability of transition metals (mainly iron) in a suitable form (Halliwell and Gutteridge, 1984). Other factors that determine whether tissue damage occurs are the rate of superoxide generation, local concentrations of antioxidant enzymes (chiefly superoxide dismutase and catalase), the state of the glutathione redox system, and the availability of the various endogenous radical scavengers (Fantone and Ward, 1982).

As noted later, a further degree of complexity is now emerging, with these radicals, and the lipid peroxidation products they generate, regulating the production of other inflammatory mediators (e.g. prostaglandins) as well as having direct effects themselves.

Prostanoids

The term prostanoids conveniently describes the prostaglandins, thromboxanes and leukotrienes produced when arachidonic acid, which is freed from phospholipids by phospholipase A_2, is metabolized. Prostanoids are produced and released by many types of cells, including macrophages, other leukocytes, endothelium and parenchymal cells. Moore and Weiss (1985) give a succinct account of the biochemical pathways involved. Prostaglandins were first described over 50 years ago, but it took 35 years for them to be thought of as mediators of inflammation (Willis, 1970). All of the now-known prostaglandins (e.g. PGD_2, PGE_2, PGF_2 and PGI_2, or prostacyclin), as well as thromboxane A_2 and the various leukotrienes, are now prominent in the literature on inflammation (Davies *et al.*, 1984). In recent years it has been realized that their chief role in this context may not be to mediate inflammation directly, but to enhance or otherwise regulate the effects of other mediators. This is not to deny certain apparently direct effects, such as the potent vasoconstrictive and platelet-aggregating properties of thromboxane A_2 (Hamberg, Svensson and Samuelson, 1975), and the opposite effects of prostacyclin (Jarman *et al.*, 1979). Nevertheless, understanding their interactions with other mediators, such as free oxygen radicals and tumour necrosis factor, is evidently central to appreciating their role in inflammation.

Tumour necrosis factor

Tumour necrosis factor (TNF), a polypeptide of 17,000 molecular weight is released predominantly from mononuclear phagocytes, but also, in lesser amounts, from mast cells, some T lymphocytes, and certain tumour cells. This list will presumably be extended. It is sometimes called TNFα to distinguish it from TNFβ—the term used to refer to lymphotoxin (LT). LT is secreted by activated T lymphocytes, and shares some, but by no means all, of the functions of TNF. The two molecules have about 35% homology, and compete for the same receptor. Because recombinant (r) LT is not as readily available as rTNF, its activities are not yet as well explored as are those of TNF, but it has the potential to be an important mediator of inflammation. LT, and its relationship to TNF, have been reviewed by Gardner *et al.* (1987).

TNF was first described by Carswell *et al.* (1975) as an undefined functional entity with anti-tumour activity. Some years ago we (Clark, 1978; Clark *et al.*, 1981) and others (Taverne, Dockrell and Playfair, 1981) proposed its involvement in malaria. Since then, the advent of recombinant TNF has led to rapid advances. TNF has been shown to be identical to cachectin (Beutler *et al.*, 1985a), a monokine recognized for its capacity to cause hypertriglyceridaemia and cachexia (Hotez *et al.*, 1984) by suppressing the activity of lipoprotein lipase (Beutler *et al.*, 1985b). As well as killing tumour cells, TNF influences many biological functions. At low concentrations it acts as an immunological cytokine, influencing, for instance, the expression of class I and class II histocompatibility antigens on some human tumour cells (Collins *et al.*, 1986; Pfizenmaier *et al.*, 1987). It also has activities as diverse as upregulating receptors for epidermal growth factor on fibroblasts (Palombella *et al.*, 1987), causing secretion of platelet-derived growth factor from vascular endothelial cells (Hajjar *et al.*, 1987) and inducing macrophages, neutrophils and endothelial cells to synthesize and secrete platelet-activating factor (Camussi *et al.*, 1987). In addition, TNF causes endothelial cells to express procoagulant activity (Nawroth and Stern, 1986), be more easily adhered to by leukocytes (Gamble *et al.*, 1985), secrete interleukin-1 (Nawroth *et al.*, 1986), and change their shape in ways consistent with increased permeability of the endothelium (Stolpen *et al.*, 1986).

As well as possessing these and many other *in vitro*-defined cytokine activities (Nathan, 1987), the evidence now points to TNF being a major mediator of acute illness, as we proposed earlier in a malarial context (Clark, 1978, 1982; Clark *et al.*, 1981). Investigations into its role in endotoxicity are well advanced, with reports of antibody to TNF protecting mice *in vivo* against endotoxin (Beutler, Milsark and Cerami, 1985) and baboons against a large injection of *E. coli* (Tracey *et al.*, 1987b). These results are consistent with the outcome of a recent study in Norway, which reported correlation between serum levels of TNF and fatal outcome in human meningococcal septicaemia, a condition believed to be triggered by bacterial endotoxin (Waage, Halstensen and Espevik, 1987). Beutler and Cerami (1987) have written a comprehensive review that stresses these aspects of TNF.

Interleukin-1

The term interleukin-1 (IL-1) was coined (Aarden *et al.*, 1979) as a synonym for lymphocyte-activating factor (LAF), a monokine originally described for its capacity to enhance mitogen-driven lymphocyte proliferation, but by then also known to possess several other functions. It is now recognized that IL-1 can be assigned to at least two distinct cytokines, termed IL-1α and IL-1β, produced by a diverse array of cell types, though predominantly by mononuclear phagocytes. Even though these two molecules have only about 25% homology, they bind to the same receptor (Matsushima et al., 1986).

The functions now attributed to IL-1 include many previously ascribed to monokines with other names, such as endogenous pyrogen and serum amyloid A inducer: in short, IL-1 has become an umbrella term for a wide range of functions affecting such unrelated organs as muscle, cartilage, bone, brain, and liver, as well as leukocytes. In this respect it is rivalled only by TNF, and is quite unlike most other cytokines termed interleukin-2, -3 etc., which seem to be single molecules with few functions and a narrow range of target cells.

IL-1 is interesting from an inflammation viewpoint mainly because it can cause neutrophils to aggregate and adhere, along with monocytes, to endothelium (Bevilacqua et al., 1985), and degranulate. It also increases secretion of free oxygen radicals, PGE_2 and thromboxane from various cells, and induces endothelial cells to express procoagulant activity and synthesize platelet-activating factor. References to the plethora of functions of IL-1, indicating those it shares with TNF, are given by Nathan (1987) and Le and Vilček (1987), while Dinarello (1985) gives a more detailed account of IL-1 itself. IL-1 probably contributes to the anaemia of inflammatory disease, as discussed in Chapter 6.

Platelet-activating factor

Platelet-activating factor (PAF), or acetyl glyceryl ether phosphorylcholine (AGEPC), is a low molecular weight phospholipid. Discovered through its effects on platelets (Benveniste, Henson and Cockrane, 1972), it was soon shown to have multiple effects, and to be generated by leukocytes, platelets, and vascular endothelial cells (Braquet et al., 1987). Knowledge of its functions expanded rapidly once synthetic preparations became available (Godfroid et al., 1980), and it is now considered to be one of the main inflammatory mediators. In brief, it aggregates platelets (causing them to sequester in tissues, leading to a functional thrombocytopenia), causes hypotension and a large increase in plasma thromboxane (Lefer, Muller and Smith, 1984), activates neutrophils, increases vascular permeability and also has a range of other, as yet partially explored, functions (reviewed by Braquet et al., 1987; Camussi et al., 1987). The similarities between the effects of PAF infusion and experimental endotoxicity were first noticed by Bessin et al. (1983), and others soon demonstrated that various PAF antagonists protect animals against the lethal effects of endotoxin (Terashita et al., 1985; Doebber et al., 1985; Casals-Stenzel, 1987). Since antibody to TNF also protects against endotoxicity, it is not surprising (indeed, it had been predicted: see Tracey et al. (1986)) that TNF is a very effective inducer of PAF synthesis and release (Camussi *et al.*, 1987). The information is an important step forward in understanding effector mechanisms in inflammation. As discussed below, it throws light on, for example, those aspects of free radical-induced pathology that seem intimately associated with TNF.

INTERACTIONS BETWEEN MEDIATORS

While these mediators are individually interesting, studying any one of them in detail eventually becomes an empty exercise without taking their interactions into account. The picture is not complete, but what will eventually emerge, on current evidence, is an interwoven pattern of inhibition, enhancement, synergy, duplication and dependency. Unless this is understood, opportunities for developing therapeutic interventions will be missed.

As had been noted above, there are several routes for synergy between proteases and free oxygen radicals, one being inactivation, by radical species, of protease inhibitors present in plasma (Carp and Janoff, 1979; Cohen, 1979). Another is the increased readiness of macrophages, after exposure to proteases, to release superoxide (Speer *et al.*, 1983).

Free radicals and prostanoids also have many close links. Egan, Paxton and Kuehl (1976) first argued that radical species were formed, and had an essential role, during the metabolism of arachidonic acid by cyclooxygenase, and others (Hemler and Lands, 1980) demonstrated that the activity of this enzyme is amplified by lipid peroxides formed by radical-induced oxidant stress on lipids. The general theme of their subsequent work (reviewed by Warso and Lands, 1983) has been that low-level oxidant stress is inherent in this pathway, and that the lipid peroxides so formed are key regulators of prostaglandin and thromboxane synthesis. More direct experiments, using stimulators of the leukocytic respiratory burst or small quantities of hydrogen peroxide, appear to have confirmed this relationship (Marshall and Lands, 1986). These links have been put to practical use by the group in Richmond, Virginia, who have, in a variety of circumstances, controlled prostaglandin-induced increase in cerebral vascular permeability by using superoxide dismutase and catalase (e.g. Kontos *et al.*, 1980, 1985; Wei *et al.*, 1986). Control of free iron by agents such as desferrioxamine is yet to be investigated in these circumstances.

A less direct set of arguments exists for involvement of free radicals in the lipoxygenase pathway that leads to leukotriene production. Certain well-known inhibitors of this enzyme are also efficient free radical scavengers (e.g. butylated hydroxyanisole; Billah, Bryant and Siegel (1985)), and

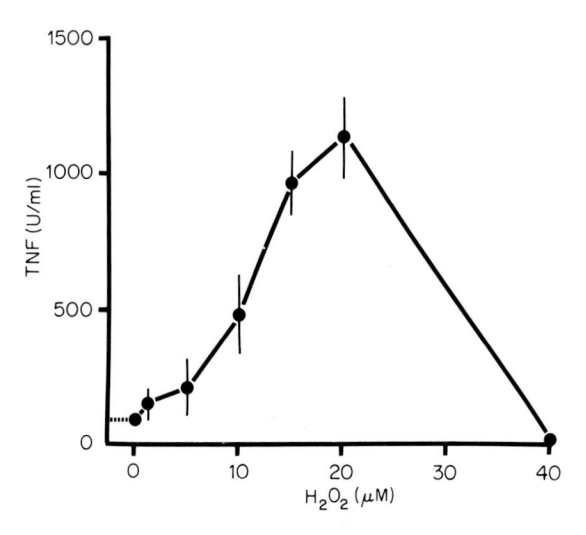

Figure 8.1 The effect of oxidant stress (H_2O_2) on TNF production. Peritoneal exudate cells were harvested from male CBA mice and cultured at 10^6 cells ml^{-1} in Dulbecco's Modified Eagle's medium supplemented with 10% heat-inactivated fetal calf serum. These cells were suboptimally stimulated with 1 μg ml^{-1} lipopolysaccharide in the presence of various concentrations of H_2O_2, as indicated. The cultures were incubated at 37°C and 5% CO_2 atmosphere. Supernatants were then collected at 20 h and TNF quantitated by a bioassay using actinomycin-sensitized WEHI-164 cells, essentially as described by Espevik and Nissen-Meyer (1986). Human rTNF from Chiron (10^7 units ml^{-1}) was used as control. Data represent mean ± SEM of duplicates from three separate experiments

conjugated dienes, which are formed when free radicals react with lipids, are generated along this pathway (reviewed by Kuhn et al., 1986).

There is ample evidence that TNF increases the readiness of leukocytes to release superoxide (Klebanoff et al., 1986), but no information is available on whether free radical-induced oxidant stress increases the capacity of macrophages to release TNF. Were this so it would explain certain parallels in the pathology induced by oxidant stress and by TNF. Accordingly, we examined the effect of added oxidant stress (in the form of hydrogen peroxide) on *in vitro* TNF production. We also generated TNF in the presence of butylated hydroxyanisole (BHA), a free radical scavenger, or desferrioxamine, an iron chelator, both of these being treatments that reduce oxidant stress. As shown, adding oxidant stress significantly increased TNF release (Figure 8.1), whereas reducing it inhibited TNF secretion in a dose-dependent manner (Figure 8.2). Thus oxidant stress may amplify TNF-induced pathology, with free radicals from TNF-exposed leukocytes causing a further increase in TNF secretion. At the same time, TNF would act as an amplifying loop for oxidant stress.

Inflammation and Parasitic Disease

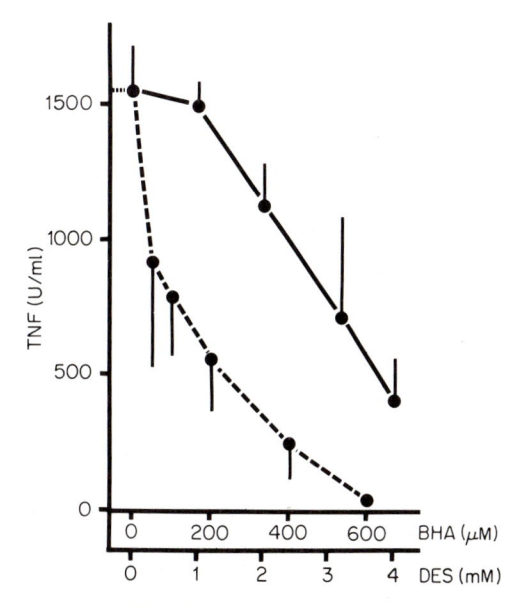

Figure 8.2 The effect of (●--●) butylated hydroxyanisole (BHA) and (●—●) desferrioxamine (DES) on TNF production. Peritoneal exudate cells were harvested and cultured as described in Figure 8.1. These cells, in contrast, were optimally stimulated with 10 μg ml^{-1} lipopolysaccharide in the presence or absence of various concentrations of either BHA or DES, as indicated. Supernatants were collected at 20 h and TNF quantitated as for Figure 8.1. Data represent mean ± SEM of duplicates from three separate experiments

As noted earlier, it has recently been reported that TNF stimulates leukocytes and endothelial cells to synthesize and release PAF (Camussi et al., 1987). This throws a new light on many of the *in vivo* changes now attributed to TNF. PAF can cause hypotension, increased plasma thromboxane levels, thrombocytopenia, neutrophil adherence and neutrophil priming (references given in Camussi et al. (1987) and Braquet et al. (1987)), and may well be the reason why these events occur after injection of TNF. The pathogenesis of other changes brought on by TNF, such as altered body temperature, hypoglycaemia and diarrhoea, evidently involves products of the cyclooxygenase pathway, since in the rat inhibitors of this enzyme (indomethacin and ibuprofen) will prevent these perturbations (Kettelhut, Fiers and Goldberg, 1987) and yet do not antagonize PAF (Hwang et al., 1984). The relationship is further complicated by the observation that one of the cyclooxygenase products, PGE$_2$, stimulates TNF production at low doses (0.1–10 ng ml^{-1}), and inhibits production, in a dose-dependent fashion, above 10 ng ml^{-1} (Renz et al., 1987). From these examples it can be seen that free oxygen radicals, TNF, PAF and products of the cyclooxygenase pathway form an interacting network, and that tinkering with one part of the system can have unexpected results unless the broader pattern is appreciated. Nor should the lipoxygenase pathway of arachidonate metabolism be neglected, for its products can increase PAF formation by enhancing expression of phospholipase A_2 (Billah, Bryant and Siegel, 1985).

These mediators of inflammation are also greatly influenced by the immune system. For example, interferon-γ (IFN-γ), a product of activated T cells, can increase gene transcription for TNF and IL-1 (Collart *et al.*, 1986), and increase expression of TNF receptors (Ruggiero *et al.*, 1986). These observations probably explain, at least in part, why IFN-γ enhances the toxicity of TNF (Tribble *et al.*, 1987). IL-2, another product of activated T cells, also enhances release of TNF (Nedwin *et al.*, 1985), as well as IL-1α and IL-1β (Numerof *et al.*, 1987) from human peripheral blood mononuclear cells.

In its turn, the immune system is greatly influenced by TNF. In 1984 it became evident that a major function of IFN-γ was to enhance expression of class I major histocompatibility complex (MHC) antigens, the cell surface structures on target cells recognized by cytotoxic T lymphocytes (Wong *et al.*, 1984). This was found to occur on a wide range of cell types. Class II MHC antigens, normally present only on antigen-presenting cells, were also induced on certain cells by IFN-γ (Wong *et al.*, 1984). What is surprising is the role TNF can play in this immunoregulatory function of IFN-γ. When added alone, TNF will increase cell surface expression of class I MHC antigens (Collins *et al.*, 1986), and in the presence of IFN-γ it greatly enhances expression of both class I and class II antigens (Pfizenmaier *et al.*, 1987).

SOME ROLES OF INFLAMMATION IN PARASITIC DISEASE

While systemic and localized inflammatory changes lead to very different outcomes, similar principles are involved at the effector level. Malaria is probably the most dramatic example of the involvement of systemic inflammation in a parasitic disease.

Malaria

On the face of it, malaria is an unlikely disease: a protozoan parasite that is restricted to erythrocytes (the liver forms are not associated with illness or tissue injury) and often so rare at the onset of illness that diagnosis can be a real problem, causes systemic organ pathology that can be life-threatening. The presence of this parasite also alters carbohydrate and fat metabolism and causes headaches, fever, nausea and muscle pains. In falciparum malaria, with its more rapid parasite multiplication, this illness can progress to a syndrome of multi-organ failure, compounded by parasitized erythrocytes adhering to vascular endothelium. When this occurs in cerebral blood vessels, cerebral malaria ensues.

Four decades ago Maegraith (1948), in his monograph on the pathogenesis of malaria, noted that 'the circulatory phenomena of malaria are in many ways so similar to those of acute general inflammation that it would not be surprising if similar substances (to those generated in acute inflammation) were produced . . .'. How does this prediction stand up to scrutiny in the light of present-day knowledge of the effects of inflammation? Remarkably well, we suggest. TNF is now recognized as a key mediator of inflammation, and when administered to cancer patients produces side-effects that are very similar to clinical malaria. These read like a textbook on human malaria, and include fever, rigors, headache, myalgia, nausea with vomiting, hypotension and thrombocytopenia (Spriggs *et al.*, 1987). The pathological changes seen when larger doses are given to rats (Tracey *et al.*, 1986) or dogs (Tracey *et al.*, 1987a) include hypoglycaemia, hypertriglyceridaemia, elevated blood lactate, diarrhoea, acute renal tubular necrosis, neutrophil accumulations in pulmonary vasculature, and hypotension. All of these occur in human falciparum malaria, as recently reviewed by Phillips and Warrell (1986) and Warrell (1987).

One experimental approach is to see how closely the pathology produced by injecting recombinant TNF compares, in the same species, to the tissue damage and metabolic disturbances seen in severe malaria. We have recently reported, using *P. vinckei* infections in mice as our model, that the pathology is the same in each case. This includes pulmonary neutrophil margination, liver damage, hypoglycaemia and high serum lactate (Clark *et al.*, 1987a) and dyserythropoiesis, erythrophagocytosis and abortion (Clark and Chaudhri, 1988). Furthermore, TNF, in nanogram quantities per ml, was present in serum at the parasite density at which these changes begin to occur in undisturbed infections (Clark and Chaudhri, 1987). Several groups (Scuderi *et al.*, 1986; Teppo and Maury, 1987; Van der Meer *et al.*, 1988) have now reported detecting TNF in serum from clinical cases of malaria. In addition, Bate, Taverne and Playfair (1988) have recently demonstrated (as earlier predicted by Clark (1978)) that some component of the malaria parasite triggers release of TNF from macrophages.

An obvious next step is to see if antibody to mouse TNF inhibits the onset of pathology as the disease progresses. At present, only one group working in this general area has had access to sufficient antibody for *in vivo* use, and they reported recently that a single dose almost entirely prevented *P. berghei*-induced cerebral malaria in the mouse (Grau *et al.*, 1987).

The emerging central role of TNF in malarial illness may explain malarial tolerance, a phenomenon commonly seen, after repeated attacks of malaria, in children in hyperendemic areas (Hill, Cambournac and Simoes, 1943).

Such individuals are evidently quite healthy, yet may harbour parasite loads 1000 times greater than those seen in previously unexposed individuals who are distinctly ill. When one combines the old observation that several weeks of untreated clinical malaria endows human subjects with tolerance to endotoxin (Rubenstein *et al.*, 1965) and the new finding (Galanos and Freudenberg, 1987) that endotoxin and TNF cross-tolerize, it seems likely that the people in the 1965 study were tolerant to TNF as well as endotoxin. Malaria-tolerant children are, we suggest, a field example of the same phenomenon, and hence show no fever, malaise or other changes despite heavy parasite loads.

We have stressed the possible role of TNF above the other mediators of inflammation simply because this is where the evidence is coming from at present. But IFN-γ (which, as we have noted, enhances TNF toxicity, and along with TNF induces surface expression of MHC antigens) has been detected in serum of patients with falciparum malaria (Rhodes-Feuillete *et al.*, 1985), so the interactions described *in vitro* presumably occur *in vivo* also. We have found, for instance, that malaria-infected mice receiving parenteral rIFN-γ have much more TNF in their serum than do infected controls (Chaudhri and Clark, unpublished data) and that athymic mice (which lack the capacity to make IFN-γ, a T cell product) have much less tissue damage in terminal malaria (Clark and Clouston, 1980). Likewise, PAF is unexplored in this context, but the newly recognized capacity of TNF to stimulate its generation and release (Camussi *et al.*, 1987), viewed alongside its known properties, implies that the contribution of PAF to the hypotension, increased endothelial permeability, thrombocytopenia and neutrophil adherence of both malaria and TNF toxicity needs assessing. Similarly, the complete picture will not emerge until the *in vivo* contribution of free oxygen radicals, both in enhancing TNF release and being generated by TNF-primed leukocytes, is examined closely. The only relevant observations so far reported are that incorporating 0.75% butylated hydroxyanisole or 0.5% ethoxyquine (both free radical scavengers used commercially in food preservation) into the diet of mice infected with ANKA strain of *P. berghei* inhibits development of pathology in cerebral vessels (Clark *et al.*, 1987b) in the same way, and to the same extent, as does antibody to TNF (Grau *et al.*, 1987). We have recently reviewed the arguments for a direct influence of free radicals in malarial pathology (Clark, Hunt and Cowden, 1986).

Granuloma formation in parasitic disease

Local inflammatory responses are not usually fatal in the short term, so the tissue changes they induce have the chance to develop to a more chronic state, with fibroblast accumulation, and hence formation of granulomas. From the effector aspect, however, the processes may not be very different from what is seen in systemic inflammation, as in malaria.

Schistosomiasis provides a particularly good example. Destruction and remodelling of connective tissue in inflammatory reactions has long been attributed to local production of proteolytic enzymes, a process reportedly under the control of PGE_2 (Baracos et al., 1983). Macrophages from the granulomas that form around the eggs of Schistosoma mansoni are evidently kept in a continuous state of activation, since they secrete superoxide, PGE_2, $PGF_{2\alpha}$ and products of the lipoxygenase pathway without exogenous stimulus (Chensue et al., 1983). This group has also provided evidence that oxygen radicals are required for continued growth of pulmonary granulomas in schistosomiasis, since treatment with vitamin E, superoxide dismutase or catalase inhibited their development (Chensue et al., 1984). BHA or a superoxide-scavenging copper salt produced the same result (Feldman et al., 1985).

There seems to be no report yet of IL-1 or TNF release from the macrophages in schistosome granulomas, but production of both by alveolar macrophages is enhanced in pulmonary sarcoidosis (Hunninghake, 1984; Bachwich et al., 1986), where similar lesions occur. Both of these monokines stimulate collagenase synthesis (Dayer et al., 1979) and fibroblast proliferation (Schmidt et al., 1982; Sugarman et al., 1985), two processes central to granuloma growth.

While Mycobacterium spp. are, by convention, not within the ambit of parasitology (though parasites they certainly are), it is relevant here to note newer work on the secretory properties of activated macrophages in the presence of Mycobacterium tuberculosis. Rook et al. (1987) have found that these cells very effectively secrete TNF when triggered by this organism in the absence of endotoxin and the more virulent the organism the more TNF is produced. Doubtless this approach will soon be tried with schistosome granulomas.

In these ways these interacting monokines and lymphokines appear to enhance and consolidate the granulomas that form in various examples of local inflammation, including parasitic diseases such as schistosomiasis. While this response may have evolved to wall off the pathogen and protect the host from further invasion, in practice it is the granulomas themselves, by their position and size, that are the chief clinical concern in schistosomiasis. Thus, whether the inflammatory mediators are released systemically (malaria) or locally (schistosomiasis) determines the nature of the disease: in malaria the host may die through the acute toxicity of these mediators, and in schistosomiasis from the secondary effects of their local release. Yet in each of these superficially very different diseases it can be argued that the cause of death was ultimately the same—the mediators of inflammation causing immunopathology.

REFERENCES

Aarden, L. A., Brunner, T. K., Cerottini, J.-C. et al. (1979). Revised nomenclature for antigen-nonspecific T cell proliferation and helper factors, *J. Immunol.*, **123**, 2928–9.
Bachwich, P. R., Lynch, J. P., Larrick, J., Spengler, M., and Kunkel, S. L. (1986). Tumor necrosis factor production by human sarcoid alveolar macrophages, *Am. J. Pathol.*, **125**, 421–5.
Baracos, V., Rodemann, H. P., Dinarello, C. A., and Goldberg, A. L. (1983). Stimulation of muscle protein degradation and prostaglandin E_2 release by leukocytic pyrogen (interleukin-1): a mechanism for the increased degradation of muscle proteins during fever, *N. Engl. J. Med.*, **308**, 553–8.
Bate, C. A. W., Taverne, J., and Playfair, J. H. L. (1988). Malaria parasites induce tumour necrosis factor production by macrophages, *Immunology*, **64**, 227–31.
Benveniste, J., Henson, P. M., and Cockrane, C. G. (1972). Leukocyte-dependent histamine release from rabbit platelets: the role of IgE, basophils, and a platelet-activating factor, *J. Exp. Med.*, **136**, 1356–77.
Bessin, P., Bonnet, J., Apffel, P., Soulard, C., Desgrou, L., Pelassi, I., and Benveniste, J. (1983). Acute circulatory shock caused by platelet-activating factor (PAF-acether) in dogs, *Eur. J. Pharmacol.*, **86**, 403–13.
Beutler, B. and Cerami, A. (1987). Cachectin: more than just a tumor necrosis factor. *N. Engl. J. Med.*, **316**, 379–85.
Beutler, B., Milsark, I. W., and Cerami, A. (1985). Passive immunization against cachectin/tumor necrosis factor protects mice from lethal effects of endotoxin, *Science*, **229**, 869–71.
Beutler, B., Greenwald, D., Hulmes, J. D., Chang, M., Pan, Y. E., Mathison, J., Ulevich, R., and Cerami, A. (1985a). Identity of tumor necrosis factor and the macrophage-secreted factor cachectin, *Nature*, **316**, 552–4.
Beutler, B., Mahoney, J., Le Trang, N., Pekala, P., and Cerami, A. (1985b). Purification of cachectin, a lipoprotein lipase-suppressing hormone secreted by endotoxin-induced RAW 264.7 cells, *J. Exp. Med.*, **161**, 984–95.
Bevilacqua, M. P., Pober, J. S., Wheeler, M. E., Cotran, R. S., and Gimbrone, M. A. (1985). Interleukin 1 acts on cultured human vascular endothelium to increase the adhesion of polymorphonuclear leukocytes, monocytes and related cell lines, *J. Clin. Invest.*, **76**, 2003–11.
Billah, M. M., Bryant, R. W., and Siegel, M. I. (1985). Lipoxygenase products of arachidonic acid modulate biosynthesis of platelet-activating factor by human neutrophils via phospholipase A_2, *J. Biol. Chem.*, **260**, 6899–906.
Braquet, P., Touqui, L., Shen, T. Y., and Vargaftig, B. B. (1987). Perspectives in platelet-activating factor research, *Pharmacol. Rev.*, **39**, 97–145.
Brown, G. V. (1986). Chemoprophylaxis of malaria, *Med. J. Aust.*, **144**, 696–702.
Camussi, G., Bussolino, F., Salvidio, G., and Baglioni, C. (1987). Tumor necrosis factor/cachectin stimulates peritoneal macrophages, polymorphonuclear neutrophils and vascular endothelial cells to synthesize and release platelet-activating factor, *J. Exp. Med.*, **166**, 1390–404.
Cardella, C. J., Davies, P., and Allison, A. C. (1974). Immune complexes induce selective release of lysosomal hydrolases from macrophages, *Nature*, **247**, 46–8.
Carp, H., and Janoff, A. (1979). In vitro suppression of serum elastase-inhibitory capacity by reactive oxygen species generated by phagocytosing polymorphonuclear phagocytes, *J. Clin. Invest.*, **63**, 793–7.

Carp, H., and Janoff, A. (1980). Potential mediator of inflammation. Phagocyte-derived oxidants suppress the elastase-inhibitory capacity of alpha$_1$-protease inhibitor *in vitro*, *J. Clin. Invest.*, **66**, 987–95.

Carswell, E. A., Old, L. J., Kassel, R. L., Green, S., Fiore, N., and Williamson, B. (1975). An endotoxin-induced serum factor that causes necrosis of tumors, *Proc. Natl Acad. Sci. USA*, **72**, 3666–70.

Casals-Stenzel, J. (1987). Protective effect of WEB 2086, a novel antagonist of platelet-activating factor, in endotoxin shock, *Eur. J. Pharmacol.*, **135**, 117–22.

Chensue, S. W., Kunkel, S. L., Higashi, G. I., Ward, P. A., and Boros, D. L. (1983). Production of superoxide anion, prostaglandins, and hydroxyeicosatetraenoic acids by macrophages from hypersensitivity-type (*Schistosoma mansoni* egg) and foreign body-type granulomas, *Infect. Immun.*, **42**, 1116–25.

Chensue, S. W., Quinlan, L., Higashi, G. I., and Kunkel, S. L. (1984). Role of oxygen reactive species in *Schistosoma mansoni* egg-induced granulomatous inflammation, *Biochem. Biophys. Res. Commun.*, **122**, 184–90.

Clark, I. A. (1978). Does endotoxin cause both the disease and parasite death in acute malaria and babesiosis? *Lancet*, **i**, 75–7.

Clark, I. A. (1982). Suggested importance of monokines in pathophysiology of endotoxin shock and malaria, *Klin. Wochenschr.*, **60**, 756–8.

Clark, I. A., and Chaudhri, G. (1988). Roles of TNF in malaria. In B. Bonavida and H. Kirchner (eds) *Tumor Necrosis Factor/Cachectin and Related Cytokines, pp. 240–5,* , September 14–18, Karger, Basel.

Clark, I. A., and Clouston, W. M. (1980). Effects of endotoxin on the histology of intact and athymic mice infected with *Plasmodium vinckei petteri*, *J. Pathol.*, **131**, 221–34.

Clark, I. A., Hunt, N. H., and Cowden, W. B. (1986). Oxygen-derived free radicals in the pathogenesis of parasitic disease, *Adv. Parasitol.*, **25**, 1–44.

Clark, I. A., Virelizier, J.-L., Carswell, E. A., and Wood, P. R. (1981). Possible importance of macrophage-derived mediators in acute malaria, *Infect. Immun.*, **32**, 1058–66.

Clark, I. A., Cowden, W. B., Butcher, G. A., and Hunt, N. H. (1987a). Possible roles of tumor necrosis factor in the pathology of malaria, *Am. J. Pathol.*, **129**, 192–7.

Clark, I. A., Chaudhri, G., Thumwood, C. M., Hunt, N. H., and Cowden, W. B. (1987b). Free radicals in malarial immunopathology. In C. Rice-Evans (ed.) *Free Radicals, Oxidant Stress and Drug Action*, pp. 237–55, Richelieu Press, London.

Cohen, A. B. (1979). The effect of *in vivo* and *in vitro* oxidative damage to purified α_1-antitrypsin and to the enzyme-inhibiting activity of plasma, *Am. Rev. Resp. Dis.*, **119**, 953–60.

Collart, M. A., Belin, D., Vassali, J.-D., De Kassado, S., and Varsalli, P. (1986). γ-interferon enhances macrophage transcription of the tumor necrosis factor/cachectin, interleukin 1, and urokinase genes, which are controlled by short-lived suppressors, *J. Exp. Med.*, **164**, 2113–18.

Collins, T., Lapierre, L. A., Fiers, W., Strominger, J. L., and Pober, J. S. (1986). Recombinant human tumor necrosis factor increases mRNA levels and surface expression of HLA-A,B antigens in vascular endothelial cells and dermal fibroblast *in vitro*, *Proc. Natl Acad. Sci. USA*, **83**, 446–50.

Davies, P., Bailey, P. J., Goldenberg, M. M., and Ford-Hutchinson, A. W. (1984). The role of arachidonic acid oxygenation products in pain and inflammation, *Ann. Rev. Immunol.*, **2**, 335–57.

Dayer, J.-M., Beutler, B., and Cerami, A. (1978). Cachectin/tumor necrosis factor stimulates collagenase and prostaglandin E$_2$ production by human synovial cells and dermal fibroblasts, *J. Exp. Med.*, **162**, 2163–8.

Dayer, J.-M., Breard, J., Chess, L., and Krane, S. M. (1979). Participation of monocyte-macrophages and lymphocytes in the production of a factor that stimulates collagenase and prostaglandin release by rheumatoid synovial cells, *J. Clin. Invest.*, **64**, 1386–92.

Dinarello, C. A. (1985). An update on human interleukin-1: from molecular biology to clinical relevance, *J. Clin. Immunol.*, **5**, 287–94.

Doebber, T. W., Wu, M. S., Robbins, J. C., Choy, B. M., Chang, M. N., and Shen, T. Y. (1985). Platelet activating factor (PAF) involvement in endotoxin-induced hypotension in rats. Studies with PAF-receptor antagonist kadsurenone, *Biochem. Biophys. Res. Commun.*, **29**, 799–808.

Egan, R. W., Paxton, J., and Kuehl, F. A. (1976). Mechanism for irreversible self-deactivation of prostaglandin synthetase, *J. Biol. Chem.*, **251**, 7329–35.

Espevik, T., and Nissen-Meyer, J. (1986). A highly sensitive cell line, WEHI 164 clone 13, for measuring cytotoxic factor/tumour necrosis factor from human monocytes, *J. Immunol. Methods*, **95**, 99–105.

Fantone, J. C., and Ward, P. A. (1982). Role of oxygen-derived free radicals and metabolites in leukocyte-dependent inflammatory reactions, *Am. J. Pathol.*, **107**, 397–418.

Feldman, G. M., Naples, J. M., Seed, J. L., and Beuding, E. (1985). Effects of anethole dithiolthione and 2(3)-tert-butyl-4-hydroxyanisole on schistosome granuloma formation, *Parasite Immunol.*, **7**, 567–73.

Galanos, C., and Freudenberg, M. (1987). Tumor necrosis factor (TNF), a mediator of endotoxin lethality, *Immunobiology*, **175**, 13.

Gamble, J. R., Harlan, J. M., Klebanoff, S. J., and Vades, M. A. (1985). Stimulation of the adherence of neutrophils to umbilical vein endothelium by human recombinant tumor necrosis factor, *Proc. Natl Acad. Sci. USA*, **82**, 8667–71.

Gardner, S. M., Mack, B. A., Hilgers, J., Huppi, K. E., and Roeder, W. D. (1987). Mouse lymphotoxin and tumor necrosis factor: structural analysis of the cloned genes, physical linkage, and chromosomal position, *J. Immunol.*, **139**, 476–83.

Godfroid, J. J., Heymans, F., Michel, E., Redeuilh, C., Steiner, C., and Benveniste, J. (1980). Platelet activating factor (PAF-acether): total synthesis of 1-*O*-octadecyl 2-*O*-acetyl *sn*-glycero-3-phosphorylcholine, *FEBS Lett.*, **116**, 161–4.

Grau, G. E., Fajardo, L. F., Piquet, P.-F., Allet, B., Lambert, P.-H and Vassali, P. (1987). Tumor necrosis factor (cachectin) as an essential mediator in murine cerebral malaria, *Science*, **237**, 1210–12.

Hajjar, K. A., Hajjar, D. P., Silverstein, R. L., and Nachman, R. L. (1987). Tumor necrosis factor-mediated release of platelet-derived growth factor from cultured endothelial cells, *J. Exp. Med.*, **166**, 235–45.

Halliwell, B., and Gutteridge, J. M. C. (1984). Oxygen toxicity, oxygen radicals, transition metals and disease, *Biochem. J.*, **219**, 1–4.

Hamberg, M., Svensson, J., and Samuelson, B. (1975). A new group of biologically active compounds derived from prostaglandin endoperoxides, *Proc. Natl Acad. Sci. USA*, **72**, 2994–8.

Hemler, M. E., and Lands, W. E. M. (1980). Evidence for a peroxide-initiated free radical mechanism of prostaglandin biosynthesis, *J. Biol. Chem.*, **255**, 6253–61.

Hill, R. B., Cambournac, F. J. C., and Simoes, M. P. (1943). Observations on the course of malaria in children in an endemic region, *Am. J. Trop. Med. Hyg.*, **23**, 147–62.

Hotez, P. J., Le Trang, N., Fairlamb, A. H., and Cerami, A. (1984). Lipoprotein lipase suppression in 3T3-L1 cells by a haemoprotozoan-induced mediator from peritoneal exudate cells, *Parasite Immunol.*, **6**, 203–9.

Hunninghake, G. W. (1984). Release of interleukin-1 by alveolar macrophages of patients with active pulmonary sarcoidosis, *Am. Rev. Resp. Dis.*, **129**, 569–72.

Hwang, S. B., Cheak, M. J., Lee, C. S. C., and Shen, T. Y. (1984). Effects of nonsteroid antiinflammatory drugs on the specific binding of platelet activating factor to membrane preparations of rabbit platelets, *Thromb. Res.*, **34**, 519–31.

Jarman, D. A., Du Boulay, G. H., Kendall, B., and Boullin, D. J. (1979). Responses of baboon cerebral and extracerebral arteries to prostacyclin and prostaglandin endoperoxide *in vitro* and *in vivo*, *J. Neurol. Neurosurg. Psychiatry*, **42**, 677–86.

Johnson, K. J., Varani, J., Oliver, J., and Ward, P. A. (1979). Immunologic vasculitis in beige mice with deficiency of leukocyte neutral protease, *J. Immunol.*, **122**, 1807–11.

Kettelhut, I. C., Fiers, W., and Goldberg, A. L. (1987). The toxic effects of tumor necrosis factor *in vivo* and their prevention by cyclooxygenase inhibitors, *Proc. Natl Acad. Sci, USA*, **84**, 4273–7.

Klebanoff, S. J., Vadas, M. A., Harlan, J. M., Sparks, L. H., Gamble, J. R., Agosti, J. M., and Waltersdorph, A. M. (1986). Stimulation of neutrophils by tumor necrosis factor, *J. Immunol.*, **136**, 4420–5.

Kontos, H. A., Wei, E. P., Povlishock, J. T., Dietrich, W. D., Magiera, C. J., and Ellis, E. F. (1980). Cerebral arteriolar damage by arachidonic acid and prostaglandin G_2, *Science*, **209**, 1242–5.

Kontos, H. A., Wei, E. P., Ellis, E. F., Jenkins, L. W., Povlishock, J. T., Rowe, G. T., and Hess, M. L. (1985). Appearance of superoxide anion radical in cerebral extracellular space during increased prostaglandin synthesis in cats, *Circ. Res.*, **57**, 142–51.

Kuhn, H., Salzmann-Reinhart, U., Ludwig, P., Ponicke, K., Schewe, T., and Rapoport, S. (1986). The stoichiometry of oxygen uptake and conjugated diene formation during the dioxygenation of linoleic acid by the pure reticulocyte lipoxygenase. Evidence for aerobic hydroperoxidase activity, *Biochim. Biophys. Acta.* **867**, 187–93.

Larson, G. L., and Hensen, P. M. (1983). Mediators of inflammation, *Ann. Rev. Immunol.*, **1**, 335–59.

Le, J., and Vilcek, J. (1987). Tumor necrosis factor and interleukin-1: cytokines with multiple overlapping biological activities, *Lab. Invest.*, **56**, 234–48.

Lefer, A. M., Muller, H. F., and Smith, J. B. (1984). Pathophysiological mechanisms of sudden death induced by platelet-activating factor, *Br. J. Pharmacol.*, **83**, 125–30.

Maegraith, B. (1948). *Pathological Processes in Malaria and Blackwater Fever*, Blackwell, Oxford.

Marshall, P. J., and Lands, W. E. M. (1986). *In vitro* formation of activators for prostaglandin synthesis by neutrophils and macrophages from humans and guinea pigs, *J. Lab. Clin. Med.*, **108**, 525–34.

Matsushima, K., Akahoshi, T., Yamada, M., Furutani, Y., and Oppenheim, J. J. (1986). Properties of a specific interleukin-1 (IL-1) receptor on human Epstein-Barr virus-transformed B lymphocytes: identity of the receptor for IL-1-α and IL-1-β, *J. Immunol.*, **136**, 4496–502.

Moore, T. L., and Weiss, T. D. (1985). Mediators of inflammation, *Semin. Arthritis Rheum.*, **14**, 247–62.

Nathan, C. F. (1987). Secretory products of macrophages, *J. Clin. Invest.*, **79**, 319–26.

Nawroth, P. P., and Stern, D. M. (1986). Modulation of endothelial cell hemostatic properties by tumor necrosis factor, *J. Exp. Med.*, **163**, 740–5.

Nawroth, P. P., Bank, I., Handley, D., Cassimeris, J., Chess, L., and Stern, D. (1986). Tumor necrosis factor/cachectin interacts with endothelial cell receptors to induce release of interleukin 1, *J. Exp. Med.*, **163**, 1363–75.

Nedwin, G. E., Svedersky, L. P., Bringman, T. S., Palladino, M. A., and Goeddel, D. V. (1985). Effect of interleukin-2, interferon and mitogens on the production of tumor necrosis factors α and β, *J. Immunol.*, **135**, 2492–7.

Numerof, R. P., Dinarello, C. A., Endres, S., Lonnemann, G., Van der Mer, J. W. M., and Mier, J. W. (1987). Interleukin 2 (IL-2) stimulates the production of interleukin 1β (IL-1β), interleukin 1α (IL-1α), and tumor necrosis factor α (TNF-α) from human peripheral blood mononuclear cells (PBMC), *Immunobiology*, **175**, 117.

Palombella, V. J., Yamashiro, D. J., Maxfield, F. R., Decker, S. J., and Vilcek, J. (1987). Tumor necrosis factor increases the number of epidermal growth factor receptors on human fibroblasts. *J. Biol. Chem.*, **262**, 1950–4.

Pfizenmaier, K., Scheurich, P., Schluter, C., and Kronke, M. (1987). Tumor necrosis factor enhances HLA-A, B, C and HLA-DR gene expression in human tumor cells, *J. Immunol.*, **138**, 975–80.

Phillips, R. E., and Warrell, D. A. (1986). The pathophysiology of severe falciparum malaria, *Parasitol. Today*, **2**, 271–82.

Renz, H., Nain, M., Gong, J.-H., and Gemsa, D. (1987). Prostaglandin E_2 (PGE$_2$) dose-dependently stimulates or suppresses tumor necrosis factor-α (TNF-α) production, *Immunobiology*, **175**, 135.

Rhodes-Feuillette, A., Bellosguardo, M., Druilhe, P., Ballet, J. J., Chousterman, S., Canivet, M., and Périès, J. (1985). The interferon compartment of the immune response in human malaria. II. Presence of serum interferon-gamma following the acute attack, *J. Interferon Res.*, **5**, 169–78.

Rook, G. A. W., Taverne, J., Leveton, C., and Steele, J. (1987). The role of gamma-interferon, vitamin D$_3$ metabolites and tumour necrosis factor in the pathogenesis of tuberculosis, *Immunology*, **62**, 229–34.

Rubenstein, M., Mulholland, J. H., Jeffrey, G. M., and Wolff, S. M. (1965). Malaria-induced endotoxin tolerance, *Proc. Soc. Exp. Biol. Med.*, **118**, 283–7.

Ruggierrio, V., Tavernier, J., Fiers, W., and Baglioni, C. (1986). Induction of the synthesis of tumor necrosis factor receptors by interferon-γ, *J. Immunol.*, **136**, 2445–50.

Schmidt, J. A., Mizel, S. B., Cohen, D., and Green, I. (1982). Interleukin-1, a potent regulator of fibroblast proliferation, *J. Immunol.*, **128**, 2177–82.

Scuderi, P., Sterling, K. E., Lam, K. S., Finley, P. R., Ryan, K. J., Ray, C. G., Petersen, F., Slyman, D. J. and Salmon, S. E. (1986). Raised serum levels of tumour necrosis factor in parasitic infections, *Lancet*, **ii**, 1364–5.

Slater, T. F. (1984). Free radical mechanisms in tissue injury, *Biochem. J.*, **222**, 1–15.

Slater, T. F. (1987). Free radical, and tissue injury: fact and fiction, *Br. J. Cancer*, **55** (supplement VIII), 5–10.

Speer, C. P., Pabst, M. J., Hedegaard, H. B., Rest, R. F., and Johnston, R. B. (1983). Human neutrophil elastase and cathepsin G prime human monocyte-derived macrophages for increased oxidative metabolism, *J. Reticuloendothel. Soc.*, **34**, 189.

Spriggs, D. R., Sherman, M. L., Frei, E., and Kufe, D. W. (1987). Clinical studies with tumour necrosis factor, *Ciba Found. Symp.*, **131**, 206–27.

Stolpen, A. H., Guinan, E. C., Fiers, W., and Pober, J. S. (1986). Recombinant tumor necrosis factor and immune interferon act singly or in combination to reorganize human vascular endothelial cell monolayers, *Am. J. Pathol.*, **123**, 16–24.

Sugarman, B. J., Aggarwal, B. B., Hass, P. E., Figari, I. S., Palladino, M. A., and Shepard, H. M. (1985). Recombinant h.TNF-α: effects on proliferation of normal and transformed cells *in vitro*. *Science*, **230**, 943–5.

Taverne, J., Dockrell, H. M., and Playfair, J. H. L. (1981). Endotoxin-induced serum factor kills malaria parasites *in vitro*, *Infect. Immun.*, **33**, 83–9.

Teppo, A.-M., and Maury, C. P. J. (1987). Radioimmunoassay of tumor necrosis factor in serum, *Clin. Chem.*, **33**, 2024–7.

Terashita, Z., Imura, Y., Nishikawe, K., and Sumida, S. (1985). Is platelet-activating factor (PAF) a mediator of endotoxin shock? *Eur. J. Pharmacol.*, **109**, 257–61.

Tracey, K. J., Beutler, B., Lowry, S. F., Merryweather, J., Wolpe, S., Milsark, I. W., Hariri, R. J., Fahey, T. J., Zentella, A., Albert, J. D., Shires, G. T., and Cerami, A. (1986). Shock and tissue injury induced by recombinant human cachectin, *Science*, **234**, 470–4.

Tracey, K. J., Lowry, S. F., Fahey, T. J., Albert, J. D., Fong, Y., Hesse, D., Beutler, B., Manogue, K. R., Calvano, S., Wei, H., Cerami, A., and Shires, G. T. (1987a). Cachectin/tumor necrosis factor induces lethal shock and stress hormone response in the dog, *Surg. Gynecol. Obstet.*, **164**, 415–22.

Tracey, K. J. Fong, Y., Hesse, D. G., Manogue, K. R., Lee, A. T., Kuo, G. C., Lowry, S. F., and Cerami, A. (1987b). Anti-cachectin/TNF monoclonal antibodies prevent septic shock during lethal bacteraemia, *Nature*, **330**, 662–4.

Tribble, H., Schneider, M., Bowersox, O., and Talmadge, J. E. (1987). Combination immunotherapy with RH TNF and RM IFN G: increased therapy and toxicity, *Fed. Proc.*, **46**, 561.

Van der Meer, J. W. M., Enders, S., Lonnemann, G., Cannon, J. G., Ikejima, T., Okusawa, S., Gelfand, J. A., and Dinarello, C. A. (1988). Concentrations of immunoreactive human tumor necrosis factor alpha produced in human mononuclear cells *in vitro*, *J. Leukocyte Biol.*, **43**, 216–23.

Waage, A., Hallstensen, A., and Espevik, T. (1987). Association between tumour necrosis factor in serum and fatal outcome in patients with meningococcal disease, *Lancet*, **1**, 355–7.

Warrell, D. A. (1987). Pathophysiology of severe falciparum malaria in man, *Parasitology*, **94**, S53–76.

Warso, M. A., and Lands, W. E. M. (1983). Lipid peroxidation in relation to prostacyclin and thromboxane physiology and pathophysiology, *Br. Med. Bull.*, **39**, 277–80.

Wei, E. P., Ellison, M. D., Kontos, H. A., and Povlishock, J. T. (1986). O_2 radicals in arachidonate-induced increased blood–brain barrier permeability to proteins, *Am. J. Physiol.*, **251**, H693–9.

Wintroub, B. U. (1982). Neutrophil-dependent generation of biologically active peptides. In G. Weissman (ed.) *Advances in Inflammation Research*, pp. 131–45, Raven, New York.

Willis, A. L. (1970). Identification of prostaglandin E_2 in rat inflammatory exudate, *Pharmacol. Res. Commun.*, **2**, 297–304.

Wong, G. H. W., Clark-Lewis, I., Harris, A. W., and Schrader, J. W. (1984). Effect of cloned interferon-γ on expression of H-2 and Ia antigens on cell lines of hemopoietic, lymphoid, epithelial, fibroblastic and neuronal origin, *Eur. J. Immunol.*, **14**, 52–6.

Part III

Iron and Haematopoiesis

Iron in Immunity, Cancer and Inflammation
Edited by M. de Sousa and J. H. Brock
© 1989 John Wiley & Sons Ltd.

9
Iron-binding Proteins and the Regulation of Hematopoietic Cell Proliferation/Differentiation

Hal E. Broxmeyer

Departments of Medicine (Hematology/Oncology), Microbiology and Immunology, The Walther Oncology Center, Indiana University School of Medicine, Indianapolis, IN 46223, USA

INTRODUCTION

The proliferation and differentiation of blood cells is a dynamic process, tightly controlled under normal conditions by stimulating, enhancing and suppressing biomolecule–cell interactions, which are aberrant during disease (Broxmeyer and Moore, 1978; Broxmeyer, 1982b, 1982c). Networks of cell–cell and biomolecule–cell feedback systems have been uncovered based on studies of hematopoietic cells in culture (Broxmeyer and Moore, 1978; Broxmeyer and Williams, 1987, 1988; Broxmeyer, 1982b, 1982c, 1983, 1986a). More recent studies *in vivo* using animal model studies and phase I/II clinical trials in humans have suggested that some of the regulatory systems uncovered *in vitro* may be relevant to blood cell regulation *in vivo* (Broxmeyer and Williams, 1987; Broxmeyer and Vadhan-Raj, 1989). Recent reviews have described our knowledge of these control systems. The present review focuses on three metal-binding proteins, acidic ferritin, lactoferrin, and transferrin, in the context of myeloid blood cell regulation.

The production of myeloid blood cells—erythrocytes, granulocytes, monocytes–macrophages, and platelets—simplistically involves the proliferation and differentiation of early immature stem and progenitor cells and their regulation by accessory cells and the biomolecules released from these accessory cells. The pipeline hierarchy of proliferation and differentiation (Broxmeyer and Moore, 1978; Broxmeyer and Williams, 1987; Broxmeyer, 1982b, 1982c, 1983, 1986a) starts with pluripotential hematopoietic stem cells. These cells are not morphologically recognizable, have extensive self-renewal or self-maintenance capacity, and can differentiate towards any of the myeloid lineages. The stem cells then give rise to progenitor cells, also not capable of being recognized morphologically. Progenitor cells have little or no self-renewal capacity and multipotential progenitors give rise to more lineage restricted progenitors. These latter cells move into the morphologically recognizable proliferating precursor cell compartments such as the proerythroblasts, myeloblasts, promonocytes, and megakaryocytes, which then give rise to the end-stage functionally mature circulating myeloid blood cells. Hematopoietic stem and progenitor cells can be recognized *in vitro* by the progeny they form as colonies in semi-solid culture medium when the appropriate growth molecules are supplied (Broxmeyer and Moore, 1978; Broxmeyer and Williams, 1987; Broxmeyer, 1982b, 1982c, 1983, 1986a; Williams, Lu and Broxmeyer, 1987). Most of the studies involving the influence of iron-binding proteins on blood cell production are based on *in vitro* assays that detect multipotential (CFU-GEMM, colony-forming unit granulocyte, erythroid, macrophage megakaryocyte), erythroid (BFU-E, burst-forming unit erythroid), granulocyte–macrophage (CFU-GM), granulocyte (CFU-G), and macrophage (CFU-M) progenitor cells. The stimulating molecules involved in colony formation for these progenitors include: interleukin-3 (IL-3, also termed multi-colony-stimulating factor), granulocyte–macrophage colony-stimulating factor (GM-CSF), granulocyte (G)-CSF, macrophage (M)-CSF, also termed CSF-1, and other molecules such as erythropoietin (Epo), interleukin-1 (IL-1, now considered to be equivalent to hemopoietin-1) and interleukin-4 (IL-4, also called B cell growth factor 1). The purification, gene expression, production and action of these and other relevant molecules have been described elsewhere (Broxmeyer, 1986a; Broxmeyer and Williams, 1988).

The three metal-binding proteins will be described separately, but it will become apparent that in some cases the production and action of each is related.

ACIDIC FERRITIN

Ferritin is an iron-storage protein with 24 subunits. The structure, iron-binding functions, and molecular biology of ferritin are discussed in detail in Chapters 3 and 4. Isotypes of ferritin exist and are composed of varying proportions of heavy (H) subunits, with molecular weights of approximately 21 000, and light (L) subunits, with molecular weights of approximately 19 000. The more acidic isoferritins (AIF) are composed of a greater proportion of H to L subunits. In this chapter, evidence for the role of AIF as a suppressor molecule of myelopoiesis will be reviewed in detail.

AIF was identified as a leukemia-associated inhibitory activity (LIA) (Bognacki, Broxmeyer and Lobue, 1981; Broxmeyer *et al.*, 1981) that suppressed colony formation *in vitro* of CFU-GM, BFU-E and CFU-GEMM from the marrows of normal donors (Broxmeyer *et al.*, 1981; Lu *et al.*, 1983), but had little or no effect on hematopoietic progenitors in marrow and blood of patients with non-remission acute leukemia, accelerated phases of chronic leukemia, myelodysplasia and other hematological disorders (Broxmeyer and Moore, 1978; Broxmeyer *et al.*, 1978, 1979a, 1987b; Auerback *et al.*, 1982). This activity was later found in the bone marrow and blood of normal donors (Broxmeyer *et al.*, 1982). The identification of LIA as AIF was based, in part, on the use of purified preparations of natural AIF and the capacity of both polyclonal and monoclonal antibodies, which recognize AIF, to inactivate the suppressive effects *in vitro* of AIF (Broxmeyer *et al.*, 1981, 1984a, 1984b). This identification was questioned by one group (Sala, Worwood and Jacobs, 1986), but substantiated by a number of other groups, including ourselves (Broxmeyer, 1986b; Taetle, 1981; Pelus, 1982; Dezza *et al.*, 1986; Moore *et al.*, 1986; Cukrova *et al.*, 1986; Bhalla *et al.*, 1986), and more recent studies using pure recombinant human H chain ferritin have solidified the *in vitro* myelopoietic suppressive activities associated with AIF (Broxmeyer, 1986b; Broxmeyer *et al.*, 1988; Dezza *et al.*, 1988).

AIF, but not basic isoferritin, suppresses colony formation by hematopoietic progenitors *in vitro* by acting on the progenitors while they are in the DNA synthesis (S)-phase of the cell cycle (Broxmeyer *et al.*, 1978b, 1981; Lu *et al.*, 1983). The S-phase action of AIF has been associated with the presence on the progenitors of a high-density distribution of major histocompatibility complex (MHC) class II antigens such as HLA-DR on human cells and I-A and I-E/C on mouse cells (Pelus, 1982; Broxmeyer, 1982a, 1982d; Lu, Pelus and Broxmeyer, 1984). Although the association between MHC class II antigens and the action of AIF is tight, definitive evidence that MHC class II antigens are directly involved in the action of AIF is lacking. AIF does not appear to have to contain iron in order to act (Broxmeyer *et al.*, 1981), although a role for iron in the action of AIF cannot be ruled out. Because progenitor cells are present as approximately 1 per 1000 nucleated marrow cells, evidence that AIF was acting directly on the progenitors was circumstantial and based on the fact that T lymphocytes and monocytes, two accessory cell compartments, were not needed for the activity of AIF. Murine CFU-GM have recently been purified such that up to 99% of the cells in an isolated marrow population were CFU-GM (Williams *et al.*, 1987b) and human CFU-GM, BFU-E and CFU-GEMM have been purified such that up to one of two cells in the isolated normal adult marrow were hematopoietic progenitors (Lu *et al.*, 1987b). The suppressive effect of pure recombinant human H subunit ferritin on colony formation by these purified murine (Williams, Cooper and Broxmeyer, 1988) and human (Lu and Broxmeyer, unpublished observations) cells was at least as great as that noted when unseparated nucleated marrow cells were used, demonstrating that AIF does have direct suppressive activity on the progenitors.

The suppressive activity of AIF is enhanced when normal human and murine bone marrow cells are cultured in the presence of, respectively, low concentrations of human or murine interferon-γ (Broxmeyer *et al.*, 1987b). The interactions involved in this synergistic activity are not known but may involve direct effects on the progenitors and/or indirect effects on accessory cells.

Our original report suggested that the inhibitory activity of natural AIF was associated with a glycosylated AIF molecule (Broxmeyer *et al.*, 1981), a result that was consistent with a later report by others (Dezza *et al.*, 1986). However, the use of non-glycosylated recombinant AIF, expressed from *E. coli*, demonstrated that glycosylation of AIF is certainly not an absolute prerequisite for functional activity (Broxmeyer *et al.*, 1986b). The recombinant AIF was active against human cells to concentrations as low as 10^{-10}–10^{-11} M (Broxmeyer *et al.*, 1986b). These are higher concentrations than we reported originally with our purified preparation of natural AIF (Broxmeyer *et al.*, 1981). It is possible that glycosylation may enhance the suppressive activity of AIF, and the eventual expression of recombinant human AIF from eukaryotic cells, which could allow for glycosylation, rather than from prokaryotic cells, which have been used and which do not allow for glycosylation, may help to determine this. It is also possible that greater activity may reside in a ferritin molecule containing mainly H subunits but with some L subunits, something we have noted previously using natural ferritin (Broxmeyer *et al.*, 1984a). Putting together ferritin molecules composed of differing proportions of H and L subunits may resolve this, and this is probably possible through recombinant technology. Another possibility, which we do not favor at present, could be that the natural AIF was acting in synergism with a small amount of another contaminating protein, a phenomenon noted with other molecules (Broxmeyer, 1986a; Broxmeyer and Williams, 1988) and described above for AIF.

AIF has also been found to increase the number of mature cells in colonies deriving from CFU-GM, an effect not apparent when AIF was pretreated with anti-AIF or when basic ferritin was used in place of AIF (Guimarães *et al.*, 1988). These results suggested that the inhibitory effect of AIF on the proliferation of CFU-GM might at least in part be mediated by a stimulus for differentiation of progenitors. In this context, AIF did not suppress differentiation of mouse myeloid leukemic M1 cells (Okabe-Kado et al., 1983).

The cells from patients with leukemia originally found to contain and release AIF were characterized as belonging to the third population of lymphoid-like cells which were neither T nor B but which had Fc receptors (Broxmeyer et al., 1979b). The cells were non-adherent, non-phagocytic, of low density (<1.070 g cm^{-3}), slowly sedimenting (2–6 mm h^{-1}) and present in the sheep red blood cell rosetting populations which were E$^-$, EAC$^-$, Ig$^-$ and EA$^+$. They appeared to be negative for MHC class II antigens. After the AIF activity was found in normal cells, the population of such cells was characterized as being of the mononuclear phagocytic lineage, monocytes and macrophages (Broxmeyer et al., 1982). These adherent low-density cells were found to express a high-density distribution of MHC class II antigens (Lu et al., 1985; Broxmeyer et al., 1983b). Thus, the human cells in normal donors and in patients with leukemia which contained and released this material were slightly different phenotypically, a fact verified using cells from normal mice and from mice infected with the polycythemia-inducing strain of the Friend virus complex (Lu et al., 1985). The differences may only reflect the same cells at different stages of maturation, namely promonocytes in leukemia versus monocytes–macrophages in normals.

The release of AIF from normal human monocytes is modulated by cell–cell interactions and by molecule–cell interactions. T cell subsets modulate release of AIF from monocytes by an MHC class II genetically restricted interaction (Broxmeyer et al., 1983b, 1984b). Thus, T helper (T4) cells induce and enhance the release of AIF from monocytes, and T suppressor (T8) cells suppress this release. It would appear that the T4 induction/enhancement and T8 suppression of AIF release is mediated respectively by interferon-γ and interferon-α (Broxmeyer et al., 1983c). Other molecules which suppress AIF release from monocytes are lactoferrin (Broxmeyer et al., 1985b; Broxmeyer, 1982e) and prostaglandin E (Broxmeyer, 1982e), and other factors which induce/enhance release of AIF are CSF-1 (Broxmeyer et al., 1985b) and prostaglandin F (Broxmeyer, 1982e). The CSF-1 induction of AIF release is not mimicked by the other CSFs, including IL-3, GM-CSF or G-CSF. These modulating molecules may all have to be taken into consideration when discussing the relevance of AIF *in vivo*. AIF has been detected in long-term *in vitro* cultures of murine bone marrow cells (Oblon, Broxmeyer and Vellis, 1983), a system which is probably the closest to what is actually occurring *in vivo* in terms of cell interactions. Various established myeloid leukemia cell lines, including HL-60, synthesize, contain and release AIF (Broxmeyer et al., 1982; Dörner et al., 1983). Of interest is that differentiation of HL-60 cells by an agent such as dimethylsulfoxide is associated with loss of AIF inhibitory activity

(Dörner et al., 1983). This could be of relevance since increased levels of AIF are associated with cells from patients with leukemia (Broxmeyer et al., 1978b), and AIF suppresses normal progenitor cell proliferation but not proliferation of cells from patients with leukemia (Broxmeyer et al., 1978a, 1978b, 1979a, 1987b; Auerback et al., 1982), thereby giving a potential proliferative growth advantage to the leukemia cells.

The non-responsiveness *in vitro* of primary cells from patients with leukemia, as well as the non-responsiveness of established cell lines, such as U937 and HL-60, to the suppressive effects of AIF, can be reversed by natural molecules such as prostaglandin E and interferon-γ (Pelus, 1982; Lu, Pelus and Broxmeyer, 1984; Broxmeyer et al., 1986c, 1986d; Piacibello, Rubin and Broxmeyer, 1986; Pelus et al., 1983). It is possible that such molecules might be able to modify the potential selective growth advantage of leukemia cells by making the leukemia cells responsive to AIF. Additionally, supraphysiological concentrations of the naturally occurring nucleoside deoxycytidine reverse the suppressive effect of AIF on CFU-GM *in vitro* (Bhalla et al., 1986), and preferentially protect normal versus leukemic myeloid progenitor cells from cytosine arabinoside-mediated cytotoxicity (Bhalla et al., 1987).

The above *in vitro* studies suggest that AIF may be relevant physiologically as well as pathologically. Further evidence for the physiological relevance of AIF derives from studies in which AIF has been administered to mice with assessment of subsequent hematological events. Human AIF is active *in vitro* against mouse marrow cells, although the activity is less than that noted on human cells (Broxmeyer et al., 1982). Inoculation of purified natural human AIF into mice undergoing rebound myelopoiesis during recovery from sublethal dosages of cyclophosphamide partially suppressed the numbers of CFU-GM, BFU-E and CFU-GEMM per femur and completely suppressed the cycling rates of these progenitors (Broxmeyer et al., 1984b). Cyclophosphamide-pretreated mice were used, since no inhibitory activity was detected in the marrow, spleen and blood of such mice, allowing for enhanced capability of detecting the effects of an exogenously administered candidate suppressor molecule. However, since it has been reported that levels of AIF are very low or not detectable in normal human sera (Cazzola et al., 1985), a fact possibly related to the presence in sera of molecules that bind AIF (Cazzola et al., 1985; Covell and Worwood, 1984; Bellotti et al., 1987), purified recombinant human heavy chain ferritin (rhHF) was assessed *in vivo* in mice for effects on numbers of CFU-GM, BFU-E and CFU-GEMM per femur and spleen, and on the proliferation of these hematopoietic progenitors, as assessed by the high specific activity [^{3}H]thymidine kill technique *in vitro* (Broxmeyer et al., 1987d, 1988). Mice were given one injection i.v. of sterile pyrogen-free saline or 100, 10 or 1 μg rhHF and sacrificed after varying time periods.

rhHF significantly decreased cycling rates and absolute numbers of marrow and splenic hematopoietic progenitors, and marrow and blood nucleated cellularity. These effects were apparent in BDF_1, C3H/Hej and DBA/2 mice and were dose-dependent, time-related and reversible. Suppressive effects were noted within 3 hours for progenitor cell cycling, within 24 hours for progenitor cell numbers and within 48 hours for circulating neutrophils. Additionally, hematopoietic progenitor cells in DBA/2 mice infected with the polycythemia-inducing strain of the Friend virus complex were insensitive to the *in vivo* administration of rhHF. These suppressive effects were not duplicated with light-chain (basic) ferritin or with 1–100 µg bacterial lipopolysaccharide. The results suggested that purified rhHF has a suppressive effect on hematopoietic progenitors *in vivo* in mice, consistent with its suppressive effect *in vitro* on cycling human and murine hematopoietic progenitors. Since rhHF suppresses CFU–GM from normal donors but not from patients with leukemia *in vitro*, acidic ferritin may be useful as a candidate adjunct molecule during chemotherapy.

Although the mechanisms of action of AIF in relationship to suppression of hematopoietic cell proliferation are not yet clear, it has been suggested that transferrin can block the inhibitory effect of AIF on erythroid (BFU-E) progenitors (Nocka, Ottman and Pelus, 1986). Whether iron itself is involved in the AIF-mediated suppression is not known, but the action may involve specific receptors for AIF, similar to those reported on established myeloid cells (Covell and Cook, 1988; Covell *et al.*, 1987; Fargion *et al.*, 1988). It is clear that cells need iron to proliferate, and the iron chelator, deferoxamine, has a suppressive effect on hematopoietic cells (Lederman *et al.*, 1984; Kaplinski *et al.*, 1987; Nocka and Pelus, 1988), including granulocyte–macrophage and erythroid progenitors (Nocka and Pelus, 1988). The latter effect is cell-cycle specific (Nocka and Pelus, 1988). AIF bonds iron rapidly (Wagstaff, Worwood and Jacobs, 1978) and this may be how it works. Of potential interest here is that deferoxamine has shown clinical efficacy in an infant with acute leukemia (Estrov *et al.*, 1987), although there is no evidence that this is mediated through effects on AIF production or action.

LACTOFERRIN

Lactoferrin (Lf) is a metal-binding glycoprotein synthesized in early cells of the neutrophilic blood series, starting with promyelocytes, and is found in the secondary granules of these cells. Its structure and molecular biology are described elsewhere in this volume (see Chapters 3 and 4).

A number of functions have been proposed for Lf (see Chapter 10). In particular, a role in the regulation of myelopoiesis has been described by several different groups of investigators (Bagby *et al.*, 1981, 1983; Bagby,

McCall and Bergstrom, 1983b; Fletcher and Willars, 1986; Brown et al., 1986; Yung and Moore, 1982; Wang et al., 1985) following our original observations (Broxmeyer et al., 1978c; Zucali, Broxmeyer and Ulatowski, 1979; Pelus et al., 1979; Broxmeyer et. al., 1980a), and will be the focus of this section. Lf was identified as a colony-inhibiting activity (CIA) derived from neutrophilic granulocytes which decreased the production/release from monocytes–macrophages of GM-CSF (Broxmeyer, Moore and Ralph, 1976; Broxmeyer et al., 1978c; Mendelsohn et al., 1978). It was subsequently shown to decrease the production/release from monocytes–macrophages of a monokine or monokines which then trigger other cells, such as T lymphocytes, fibroblasts and endothelial cells, to release GM-CSF and/or other myeloid-stimulating factors (Bagby et al., 1981, 1983; Bagby, McCall and Layman, 1983). The monokine stimulating the release of stimulating factors from fibroblasts and endothelial cells has been identified as IL-1 (Zucali et al., 1986, 1987a; Bagby et al., 1986), a fact now substantiated by numerous groups (Fibbe et al., 1986; Louvaug et al., 1986; Segal et al., 1987; Sieff, Tsai and Faller, 1987). This suggested that Lf might mediate its effects through suppression of IL-1 production, and some evidence for this has now been reported (Zucali et al., 1987b) and confirmed by radioimmuno-assay of IL-1 beta (Zucali and Broxmeyer, unpublished observations) and gene expression of IL-1 beta (Harrington and Broxmeyer, unpublished observations) in monocytes treated with Lf. Suppression by Lf of IL-1 production has further ramifications, because IL-1 has been identified as hemopoietin-1 (Mochizuki et al., 1987), which is involved as a synergistic activity associated with proliferation of early hematopoietic stem cells (Bartelmez and Stanley, 1985; Stanley et al., 1986), and IL-1 has numerous immunologically associated activities, including triggering the release from T cells of IL-2, a T cell growth factor (Dinarello, 1984). In this context it is also relevant that Lf inhibits the mixed lymphocyte reaction by suppressing the production and release of transferable factors (Slater and Fletcher, 1987; see also Chapter 10). The presence of MHC class II antigens (HLA-DR and IA, IE/C) on monocytes–macrophages has been associated with the suppressive activity of Lf (Broxmeyer, 1979; Broxmeyer et al., 1983a, 1983b), which further links Lf with immunological cell interactions.

A monoclonal antibody was developed that recognized and neutralized Lf (Sledge et al., 1986) and this was used to demonstrate that the suppressive effects of Lf and extracts of mature neutrophils were due to the Lf itself. This Lf antibody was used (Broxmeyer et al., 1986a) to affinity-purify Lf from milk and mature neutrophils, and establish an immunoradiometric assay for Lf, and helped to further substantiate the findings of others that milk and neutrophil Lf are similar biochemically and functionally (Masson, Heremans and Schonne, 1969; Moguilevsky, Retegui and Masson, 1985).

An active form of Lf was found in a subpopulation of polymorphonuclear neutrophils that contained receptors recognized by rabbit IgG antibody coated sheep erythrocytes (Broxmeyer *et al.*, 1980d, 1983a). It was the iron-saturated Lf, but not apo (iron-depleted) Lf, that was suppressive, and other metals such as copper or zinc did not replace iron in this capacity (Broxmeyer *et al.*, 1978c, 1980a). The iron probably placed Lf into a conformational form necessary for optimal receptor binding. In terms of functional activity of Lf, agents such as bacterial lipopolysaccharide (LPS), lithium, testosterone, and estradiol can abrogate the action of Lf, but this depends on the relative concentrations of these agents to Lf (Broxmeyer *et al.*, 1978c, 1980a). The responsive cells appear to be subpopulations of monocytes and macrophages (Steinman *et al.*, 1982; Broxmeyer *et al.*, 1983a, 1986; Broxmeyer and Platzer, 1984; Broxmeyer, 1979; Pelus *et al.*, 1981) that have a relatively higher density distribution of MHC class II antigen than the other mononuclear phagocytes (Broxmeyer, 1979; Broxmeyer *et al.*, 1983a; Broxmeyer and Platzer, 1984), although, as with the acidic ferritin-responsive cells, it is not clear yet whether the MHC class II antigens themselves play a role in the action of Lf. A possibility exists that the bacteriostatic and myelosuppressive functions of Lf may be intimately related (Broxmeyer *et al.*, 1980c). Bacteria and their products, e.g. LPS, enhance myelopoiesis (Broxmeyer *et al.*, 1974). Lf is relatively iron-unsaturated in the neutrophilic granulocyte. Thus, apo-Lf, by removing iron from the surrounding environment after its release from neutrophils, could prevent bacteria from proliferating. This might remove a positive stimulus for myelopoietic cell growth. The now iron-saturated Lf would be in a form allowing for binding to specific receptors on its target cell and thus decrease the release from these cells of GM-CSF and/or IL-1, thereby further dampening myelopoiesis. It is relevant to note here that strong evidence now implicates CSF and IL-1 in the regulations of myelopoiesis *in vivo*, as well as *in vitro* (Broxmeyer, 1986a; Broxmeyer and Williams, 1987, 1988). Lf has been shown to bind to DNA (Bennet and Davis, 1982) and to cell membrane DNA (Bennett *et al.*, 1983; Bennett, Merritt and Gabor, 1986), which could suggest a possible role for cell membrane DNA and Lf in the receptor-binding process and subsequent Lf-mediated activity.

Lf-deficient neutrophils have been noted in cells from patients with leukemias and other related hematopoietic disorders (Odelberg and Olofsson, 1976; Olofsson, Olsson and Venge, 1977; Rausch *et al.*, 1978; Scholfield, Stone and Stuart, 1983; Miyauchi *et al.*, 1983; Rabe *et al.*, 1983; Brown, Rickard and Kronenberg, 1985), and abnormalities in Lf interactions have been detected with cells from such patients (Broxmeyer, Baker and Galbraith 1976; Broxmeyer, Mendelson and Moore, 1977; Broxmeyer *et al.*, 1983). Neutrophilic granulocytes from patients with leukemia contain low or non-detectable levels of active forms of Lf, even when Lf is detected in appreciable amounts. Affinity purification of Lf using a monoclonal anti-Lf antibody has now confirmed our original observations using crude extracts of neutrophils from patients with chronic myelogenous leukemia (CML), by demonstrating that purified CML neutrophil Lf is either inactive or is much less active than normal neutrophil Lf as a suppressor molecule for release of growth factors from normal human monocytes (Broxmeyer and Bicknell, unpublished observations), although the biochemical basis for the differences in activity between Lf derived from normal cells and that from cells of patients with leukemia is not known. In addition to low levels of Lf or relatively inactive Lf, the growth factors produced by monocytes from patients with leukemia are less sensitive to Lf suppression than are similar cells from normal donors. This double or triple defect is especially obvious during CML, a disease associated with granulocyte, monocyte and erythroid hyperplasia, and is consistent with the manifestations of this disease. A similar multiple defect in Lf interactions has been studied in a pediatric patient with neutrophilia of unknown etiology (Broxmeyer et al., 1984b) and these defects are also consistent with disease manifestations. The facts that acidic ferritin has been associated with the potential for a growth advantage of leukemia cells in patients with leukemia (Broxmeyer et al., 1978a, 1987b; Broxmeyer and Williams, 1988; Auerback et al., 1982), Lf decreases acidic ferritin release *in vitro* (Broxmeyer et al., 1985b; Broxmeyer, 1982e) and inactive Lf is associated with increased levels of acidic ferritin during leukemia (Broxmeyer et al., 1978b), relate abnormal Lf interactions in such patients to disease progression. The insensitivity of leukemia cells to the suppressive actions of Lf has been investigated using established myeloid cell lines, and of potential relevance is the fact that these cell lines can be induced by interferon-γ into a state of responsiveness to Lf (Broxmeyer et al., 1986c, 1986d; Piacibello, Rubin and Broxmeyer, 1986; Berman, Rubin and Broxmeyer, 1986).

There is a very small group of patients whose neutrophilic granulocytes are deficient in specific granules and Lf, and who do not manifest a peripheral blood hyperplasia of the granulocytic and monocytic series (Boxer et al., 1982), and patients with neutropenias of various etiologies have neutrophils that are deficient in Lf activity *in vitro* (Broxmeyer et al., 1980b). This might, in the absence of any other information, suggest that Lf is not physiologically relevant since absence of Lf, a suppressor of the release of growth factors, was not associated with neutrophilia, but was rather associated in these patients with either normal blood counts or a neutropenia. It is very clear now that networks of biomolecule–cell and cell–cell interactions are involved in the complex regulation of myelopoiesis (Broxmeyer and Moore, 1978; Broxmeyer and Williams, 1988; Broxmeyer, 1982b, 1982c, 1983, 1986a) and the physiological relevance of any one molecule must be considered in the context of other interrelated molecules and cells. In terms of the Lf-deficient patients with normal blood counts, we have had the opportunity to study (Broxmeyer *et al.*, 1985a) such a rare patient, who has been reported by others (Boxer *et al.*, 1982). While we confirmed, using our immunoradiometric assay for Lf, that the neutrophil and serum levels of Lf in this patient were low, they were not completely absent. The Lf from this patient's neutrophils was found to be active as a suppressor molecule, in contrast to the Lf obtained from patients with CML, mentioned above to be inactive, and this patient's mononuclear blood cells were as responsive as normal cells to the suppressive influence of Lf from this donor and from normal milk, again in contrast to the insensitivity of 'leukemia' cells to Lf. Of particular interest was that this patient's monocytes contained much higher concentrations of acidic ferritins than did normal monocytes, a fact consistent with *in vitro* studies showing that Lf decreases monocyte content and release of acidic ferritin, and with the lowered levels of Lf in this patient. Since acidic ferritin suppresses production of hematopoietic progenitors directly, rather than by an indirect mechanism of action on accessory cells, which is how Lf acts, it is possible to consider that increased levels of acidic ferritin compensated for decreased levels of Lf in the maintenance of the patient's normal blood cell levels, especially on top of the finding that the low levels of Lf found in this patient's neutrophils were functionally as active as that from normal neutrophils and could thus still decrease growth factor production. In terms of the Lf-deficient patients with neutropenia, we have identified another, as yet uncharacterized, suppressive molecule in such patients which is associated with the neutropenia (Broxmeyer *et al.*, 1980b). The above information suggests that when all known possible cell interactions are taken into account, the available information on Lf is still consistent with a physiologically relevant role for Lf as a regulator of myelopoiesis and as a molecule potentially involved in the progressive nature of leukemia when Lf–cell interactions are aberrant.

The potential physiological relevance of Lf is further supported by the action of purified human Lf, active against mouse cells *in vitro*, and on myelopoiesis in mice (Broxmeyer *et al.*, 1978c, 1987e; Broxmeyer, 1978; Gentile and Broxmeyer, 1983). Administration of Lf to mice results in a myelosuppressive effect similar to that noted *in vitro*; serum levels of CSF in these mice are reduced by up to 90% and the cycling rates and absolute numbers of CFU-GM, BFU-E and CFU-GMM in the marrow and spleen of these mice are reduced. Of interest is that while Lf partially decreases release of CSF from mononuclear cells *in vitro* (Broxmeyer *et al.*, 1978c) and partially reduces absolute numbers of hematopoietic progenitor cells per organ in mice (Broxmeyer *et al.*, 1978c, 1987e; Broxmeyer, 1978; Gentile and Broxmeyer, 1983), the cycling status (percentage of cells in S-phase) of the progenitors is completely suppressed such that these cells are reversibly placed into a slowly or non-cycling state (Gentile and Broxmeyer, 1983;

Broxmeyer et al., 1987e). At the concentrations of Lf used in those studies, effects of Lf on nucleated marrow cellularity were not consistent and no effects were noted on circulating blood cell levels (Gentile and Broxmeyer, 1987; Poppas, Faith and Bierman, 1986). The multilineage suppressive effects of Lf *in vivo* may relate to possible suppressive effects on IL-1 production which triggers accessory cells to release stimulating factors active on multilineage cells. The suppressive effects of Lf *in vivo* can be counterbalanced by the administration to mice *in vivo* of purified growth factors such as IL-3, GM-CSF, CSF-1 and G-CSF (Broxmeyer et al., 1987a, 1987c; Williams et al., 1987a).

The potential therapeutic usefulness of Lf in the treatment of leukemia has been described elsewhere (Broxmeyer, 1985). In this context, Lf has a protective effect on mice inoculated with the polycythemia-inducing strain of the murine Friend virus complex (Lu et al., 1987a; Chen, Lu and Broxmeyer, 1987). This effect may relate to the capacity of Lf to decrease cycling rates of the hematopoietic progenitors (Broxmeyer et al., 1987e), making cells less sensitive to viral infection. The susceptibility of Friend virus-sensitive mice to virus infection is increased by administration to these mice of IL-3 (Hangoc et al., 1987), probably relating to the increased progenitor cell proliferation induced by IL-3 in mice (Broxmeyer et al., 1987a, 1987c; Williams et al., 1987a), and this effect is counterbalanced by Lf (Hangoc et al., 1987), suggesting that Lf may be doing more in these mice than just suppressing release of growth factors. The Lf itself does not inactivate virus replication directly (Lu et al., 1987a), but may be influencing cells to inactivate the virus, or prevent viral replication. For Lf to be effective against infection with the Friend virus, the Lf has to be administered shortly before or shortly after virus inoculation. This may be due to cells in these mice becoming insensitive to the effects of Lf with time after virus infection (Lu et al., 1985). The ability of interferon-γ to induce sensitivity of leukemia cell lines *in vitro* to Lf (Broxmeyer et al., 1986c, 1986d; Piacibello, Rubin and Broxmeyer, 1986; Berman, Rubin and Broxmeyer, 1986) suggests that this or a related cytokine may be useful in enhancing the functional activity of Lf in mice after disease progression begins. If this occurs, it would be of interest to determine if Lf could influence replication of other viruses by a cell-mediated action, alone or in combination with other biomolecules.

TRANSFERRIN

Transferrin (Tf) is a metal-binding glycoprotein, similar to Lf biochemically, but antigenically distinct, whose main function is iron transport (see Chapter 3). Although Tf has a well-defined function in cell growth (see

Chapter 12), it has also been implicated as a suppressor molecule of the release of colony-stimulating activities from a helper phenotype subset of T lymphocytes (Broxmeyer, Lu and Bognacki, 1983; Lu et al., 1986), and a stimulating molecule of the release of colony-stimulating activities from adherent mononuclear blood cells (Taetle and Honeysett, 1986). The suppressive effects of Tf on growth factor release from mitogen-activated T lymphocytes requires that the molecule be saturated with iron, although zinc can replace iron to a small degree (Broxmeyer, Lu and Bognacki, 1983), and this effect is blocked by monoclonal antibodies for the Tf receptor, which block Tf binding (Broxmeyer, Lu and Bognacki, 1983), for MHC class II antigen, and for the human melanoma-associated antigen, p97 (Broxmeyer et al., 1985c). Consistent with this suppressive effect is evidence that Tf exerts suppressive activity *in vivo* on myelopoiesis when administered to mice, and this activity appears to be mediated mainly in the spleen, a lymphoid organ (Gentile and Broxmeyer, 1983). It is of interest also in this context that $CD8^+$ lymphocytes can control human immunodeficiency virus (HIV) infection *in vitro* by suppressing virus replication (Walker et al., 1986), and it is this subset of T lymphocytes that contain and release the Tf-like activity, capable of being inactivated with a monoclonal antibody to Tf, that suppresses CSF release from the $CD4^+(T4^+)$ population of T lymphocytes (Broxmeyer, Lu and Bognacki, 1983; Lu et al., 1986). It is intriguing to speculate on a possible relationship between Tf and suppression of HIV replication, but without any experimental evidence it is entirely optimistic speculation at this time.

CONCLUDING THOUGHTS

Myeloid blood cell production is controlled by networks of cell–cell and biomolecule–cell interactions. The iron-binding proteins acidic ferritin, lactoferrin and transferrin have been implicated in some of these networks as mentioned above. These molecules have been shown to each have many functional activities, which may or may not be associated with the roles that at least ferritins and transferrin have in relationship to iron metabolism and iron transport. The various functional activities described for each molecule itself may not be mutually exclusive and the close association of the three iron-binding molecules suggests that one molecule can and does influence the production and action of the other molecules, even if the effects are distantly mediated. While the physiological relevance of these molecules in the regulation of myelopoiesis is not yet definitively established, abnormalities in their interactions during disease may be associated with disease progression, e.g. leukemia and myeloproliferative disorders, and it is possible that intervention in such biomolecule–cell interactions, possibly through the use of these molecules, may help to slow disease progression. In fact, it may be such clinical trials that will help to establish the relevance of these molecules to myelopoietic regulation *in vivo*.

ACKNOWLEDGEMENTS

These studies were supported by Public Health Service grants CA 36464 and CA 36740 from the National Cancer Institute.

REFERENCES

Auerback, A. D., Weiner, M. A., Warburton, D., Yeboa, K., Lu, L., and Broxmeyer, H. E. (1982). Acute myeloid leukemia as the first hematologic manifestation of Fanconi anemia, *Am. J. Hematol.*, **12**, 289–300.

Bagby, G. C., McCall, E., Bergstrom, K. A., and Burger, D. (1983a). A monokine regulates colony-stimulating activity production by vascular endothelial cells, *Blood*, **62**, 663–8.

Bagby, G. C., McCall, E., and Layman, D. L. (1983b). Regulation of colony-stimulating activity production. Interaction of fibroblasts, mononuclear phagocytes and lactoferrin, *J. Clin. Invest.*, **71**, 340–4.

Bagby, G. C., Rigas, V. D., Bennett, R. M., Vandenbark, A. A., and Garewal, H. S. (1981). Interaction of lactoferrin, monocytes, and T lymphocyte subsets in the regulation of steady-state granulopoiesis *in vitro*, *J. Clin. Invest.*, **68**, 56–63.

Bagby, G. C., Dinarello, C. A., Wallace, P., Wagner, C., Hefeneider, S., and McCall, E. (1986). Interleukin 1 stimulates granulocyte macrophage colony-stimulating activity release by vascular endothelial cells, *J. Clin. Invest.*, **78**, 1316–23.

Bartelmez, S. H., and Stanley, E. R. (1985). Synergism between hemopoietic growth factors (HGFs) detected by their effects on cells bearing receptors for a lineage specific HGF: Assay of hemopoietin-1, *J. Cell. Physiol.*, **122**, 370–8.

Bellotti, V., Arosio, P., Cazzola, M., Cozzi, A., Levi, S., Meloni, F., and Zappone, E. (1987). Characteristics of a ferritin-binding protein present in human serum, *Br. J. Haematol.*, **65**, 489–93.

Bennett, R. M., and Davis, J. (1982). Lactoferrin interacts with deoxyribonucleic acid: a preferential reactivity with double stranded DNA and dissociation of DNA–anti-DNA complexes, *J. Lab. Clin. Med.*, **99**, 127–38.

Bennett, R. M., Merritt, M. M., and Gabor, G. (1986). Lactoferrin binds to neutrophilic membrane DNA, *Br. J. Haematol.*, **63**, 105–17.

Bennett, R. M., Davis, J., Campbell, S., and Portnoff, S. (1983). Lactoferrin binds to cell membrane DNA. Association of surface DNA with an enriched population of B cells and monocytes, *J. Clin. Invest.*, **71**, 611–18.

Berman, E., Rubin, B. Y., and Broxmeyer, H. E. (1986). Regulation of the proliferation of the established human monoblast cell line, U937, at the single cell level, *Cancer Res.*, **46**, 3309–12.

Bhalla, K., Cole, J., MacLaughlin, W., Baker, M., Arlin, Z., Graham, G., and Grant, S. (1986). Deoxycytidine stimulates the *in vitro* growth of normal CFU-GM and

reverses the negative regulatory effects of acidic isoferritin and prostaglandin E_1, *Blood*, **68**, 1136–41.
Bhalla, K., MacLaughlin, W., Cole, J., Arlin, Z., Baker, M., Graham, G., and Grant, S. (1987). Deoxycytidine preferentially protects normal versus leukemic myeloid progenitor cells from cytosine arabinose-mediated cytotoxicity, *Blood*, **70**, 568–71.
Bognacki, J., Broxmeyer, H. E., and Lobue, J. (1981). Isolation and biochemical characterization of leukemia associated inhibitory activity that suppresses colony and cluster formation of cells, *Biochim. Biophys. Acta*, **672**, 176–90.
Boxer, L. A., Coates, T. D., Haak, R. A., Wolach, J. B., Hoffstein, S., and Baehner, R. L. (1982). Lactoferrin deficiency associated with altered granulocyte function, *N. Engl. J. Med.*, **307**, 404–10.
Breton-Gorius, J., Mason, D. Y., Buriot, D., Vilde, J. L., and Griscelli, C. (1980). Lactoferrin deficiency as a consequence of a lack of specific granules in neutrophils from a patient with recurrent infections, *Am. J. Pathol.*, **99**, 413–28.
Brown, R. D., Rickard, K. A., and Kronenberg, H. (1985). Lactoferrin in the myeloproliferative disorders: a search for granulopoietic regulator defects, *Br. J. Haematol.*, **59**, 617–26.
Brown, R. D., Yuen, E., Rickard, K. A., Vincent, P. C., Young, G. M., and Kronenberg, H. (1986). Plasma lactoferrin in patients with neutropenia, *Blut*, **52**, 289–95.
Broxmeyer, H. E. (1978). In vivo inhibition of mouse granulopoiesis by cell-free activity derived from human polymorphonuclear neutrophils, *Blood*, **51**, 889–901.
Broxmeyer, H. E. (1979). Lactoferrin acts in Ia-like antigen positive subpopulations of human monocytes to inhibit production of colony stimulatory activity *in vitro*, *J. Clin. Invest.*, **64**, 1717–20.
Broxmeyer, H. E. (1982a). Detection of Ia-antigens for I-A and I-E/C subregions on mouse granulocyte–macrophage progenitor cells during DNA synthesis: Association with the action of acidic isoferritins *in vitro*, *J. Immunol.*, **129**, 1002–7.
Broxmeyer, H. E. (1982b). Granulopoiesis. In S. Trubowitz and S. Davis (eds) *The Human Bone Marrow*, pp. 145–208, CRC Press Inc., Florida.
Broxmeyer, H. E. (1982c). Hematopoietic stem cells, In S. Trubowitz and S. Davis (eds) *The Human Bone Marrow*, pp. 77–123, CRC Press Inc., Florida.
Broxmeyer, H. E. (1982d). Relationship of cell-cycle expression of Ia-like antigenic determinants on normal and leukemia human granulocyte–macrophage progenitor cells to regulation *in vitro* by acidic isoferritins, *J. Clin. Invest.*, **69**, 632–42.
Broxmeyer, H. E. (1982e). The production and/or release of acidic isoferritin-inhibitory activity (AFIA) from an Ia-antigen[+]-, Mac-1[+]- subpopulation of human monocytes is influenced by lactoferrin (LF) and products of monocytes and subpopulations of human T-lymphocytes *in vitro*, *Exp. Hematol.*, **10** (supplement), 23 (abstract).
Broxmeyer, H. E. (1983). Colony assays of hematopoietic progenitor cells and correlations to clinical situations, *CRC Crit. Rev. Oncol./Hematol.*, **1**, 227–57.
Broxmeyer, H. E. (1985). Potential therapeutic usefulness of lactoferrin in leukemia, *Nestle Research News 1984/1985*, pp. 93–99, Nestec LDA, Nestle Products Technical Assistance, Switzerland.
Broxmeyer, H. E. (1986a). Biomolecule–cell interactions and the regulation of myelopoiesis, *Int. J. Cell Cloning*, **4**, 378–405.
Broxmeyer, H. E. (1986b). Comments on article of Sala *et al.*, *Blood*, **68**, 794.
Broxmeyer, H. E., Baker, F., and Galbraith, P. R. (1976). In vitro regulation of granulopoiesis in human leukemia: Application of an assay for colony inhibiting cells, *Blood*, **47**, 389–402.

Broxmeyer, H. E., Lu, L., and Bognacki, J. (1983). Transferrin, derived from OKT8-positive subpopulation of T-lymphocytes, suppresses the production of granulocyte–macrophage colony stimulatory factors from mitogen-activated T-lymphocytes, *Blood*, **62**, 37–50.

Broxmeyer, H. E., Mendelson, N., and Moore, M. A. S. (1977). Abnormal granulocyte feedback regulation of colony forming and colony stimulating activity-producing cells from patients with chronic myelogenous leukemia, *Leuk. Res.*, **1**, 3–12.

Broxmeyer, H. E., and Moore, M. A. S. (1978). Communication between white cells and the abnormalities of this in leukemia, *Biochim. Biophys. Acta.*, **516**, 129–66.

Broxmeyer, H. E., Moore, M. A. S., and Ralph, P. (1976). Cell-free granulocyte colony inhibiting activity derived from human polymorphonuclear neutrophils, *Exp. Hematol.*, **5**, 87–102.

Broxmeyer, H. E., and Platzer, E. (1984). Lactoferrin acts on I-A and I-E/C antigen-positive subpopulations of mouse peritoneal macrophages in the absence of T-lymphocytes and other cell types to inhibit production of granulocyte–macrophage colony stimulatory factors *in vitro*, *J. Immunol.*, **133**, 306–14.

Broxmeyer, H. E., and Vadhan-Raj, S. (1989). Preclinical and clinical studies with the hematopoietic colony-stimulating factors and related interleukins. *Immunol. Res.* (in press).

Broxmeyer, H. E., and Williams, D. E. (1987). Actions of hematopoietic colony stimulating factors *in vivo*, *Pathol. Immunopathol. Res.*, **6**, 207–20.

Broxmeyer, H. E., and Williams, D. E. (1988). The production of myeloid blood cells and their regulation during health and disease. *CRC Crit. Rev. Oncol./Hematol*, **8**, 173–226.

Broxmeyer, H. E., VanZant, G., Zucali, J. R., LoBue, J., and Gordon, A. S. (1974). Mechanisms of leukocyte production and release. XII. A comparative assay of the leukocytosis-inducing factor (LIF) and the colony stimulating factor (CSF), *Proc. Soc. Exp. Biol. Med.*, **145**, 1262–7.

Broxmeyer, H. E., Grossbard, E. R., Jacobsen, N., and Moore, M. A. S. (1978a). Evidence for a proliferative advantage of human leukemic colony forming cells (CFU-c) *in vitro*, *J. Natl Cancer Inst.*, **60**, 513–21.

Broxmeyer, H. E., Jacobsen, N., Kurland, J., Mendelsohn, N., and Moore, M. A. S. (1978b). *In vitro* suppression of normal granulocyte stem cells by inhibitory activity derived from leukemic cells, *J. Natl Cancer Inst.*, **60**, 497–511.

Broxmeyer, H. E., Smithyman, A., Eger, R. R., Meyers, P. A., and de Sousa, M. (1978c). Identification of lactoferrin as the granulocyte-derived inhibitor of colony stimulating activity (CSA)-production, *J. Exp. Med.*, **148**, 1052–67.

Broxmeyer, H. E., Grossbard, E., Jacobsen, N., and Moore, M. A. S. (1979a). Persistence of leukemia inhibitory activity during remission of acute leukemia, *N. Engl. J. Med.*, **301**, 346–51.

Broxmeyer, H. E., Ralph, P., Margolis, V. B., Nakoinz, I., Meyers, P., Kapoor, N., and Moore, M. A. S. (1979b). Characteristics of bone marrow and blood cells in human leukemia inhibitory activity (LIA), *Leuk. Res.*, **3**, 193–203.

Broxmeyer, H. E., de Sousa, M., Smithyman, A., Ralph, P., Hamilton, J., Kurland, J. I., and Bognacki, J. (1980a). Specificity and modulation of the action of the lactoferrin, a negative feedback regulator of myelopoiesis, *Blood*, **55**, 324–33.

Broxmeyer, H. E., Pahwa, R., Jacobsen, N., Pelus, L. M., Ralph, P., Meyers, P. A., and Kapoor, M. (1980b). Specific inhibitory activity against granulocyte-progenitor cells produced by non-T-lymphocytes from patients with neutropenia, *Exp. Hematol.*, **8**, 278–97.

Broxmeyer, H. E., Pelus, L. M., Ralph, P., Bognacki, J., Moore, M. A. S., and de Sousa, M. (1980c). Regulation of myelopoiesis: Inhibitors of production and action of granulocyte–macrophage colony-stimulatory factors. In *Microbiology 1980*, pp. 108–14, ASM Publication, Washington D.C.

Broxmeyer, H. E., Ralph, P., Bognacki, J., Kincade, P., and de Sousa, M. (1980d). A subpopulation of human polymorphonuclear neutrophils contains an active form of lactoferrin capable of inhibiting production of granulocyte–macrophage colony stimulating activities by human monocytes, *J. Immunol.*, **125**, 903–9.

Broxmeyer, H. E., Bognacki, J., Dörner, M. H., and de Sousa, M. (1981). The identification of leukemia-associated inhibitory activity (LIA) as acidic isoferritins: A regulatory role for acidic isoferritins in the production of granulocytes and macrophages, *J. Exp. Med.*, **153**, 1426–44.

Broxmeyer, H. E., Bognacki, J., Ralph, P., Dörner, M. H., Lu, L., and Castro-Malaspina, H. (1982). Monocyte–macrophage derived acidic isoferritins: Normal feedback regulators of granulocyte–macrophage progenitor cells, *Blood*, **60**, 595–607.

Broxmeyer, H. E., Gentile, P., Bognacki, J., and Ralph, P. (1983a). Lactoferrin, transferrin and acidic isoferritins: Regulatory molecules with potential therapeutic value in leukemia, *Blood Cells*, **9**, 83–105.

Broxmeyer, H. E., Juliano, L., Lu, L., Platzer, E., and Dupont, B. (1983b). HLA-DR human histocompatibility leukocyte antigens—restricted lymphocyte–monocyte interactions in the release from monocytes of acidic isoferritins that suppress hematopoietic progenitor cells, *J. Clin. Invest.*, **73**, 939–53.

Broxmeyer, H. E., Rubin, B. Y., Juliano, L., Platzer, E., and Lu, L. (1983c). The HLA-DR restricted action of T-lymphocyte subsets on modulation of release of acidic isoferritin-inhibitory activity from monocytes is mediated by alpha and gamma interferon, interleukin-1, and transferrin, *Blood*, **62** (supplement), 131a (abstract).

Broxmeyer, H. E., Gentile, P., Listowsky, I., Cavanna, F., Feickert, H. J., Dörner, M. H., Ruggeri, G., Cazzola, M., and Cooper, S. (1984a). Acidic isoferritins in the regulation of hematopoiesis *in vitro* and *in vivo*. In A. Albertini, P. Arosio, E. Chiacone and J. Drysdale (eds) *Ferritins and Isoferritins as Biochemical Markers*, pp. 97–111, Elsevier Science Publishers, Amsterdam.

Broxmeyer, H. E., Gentile, P., Cooper, S., Lu, L., Juliano, L., Piacibello, W., Meyers, P. A., and Cavanna, F. (1984b). Functional activities of acidic isoferritins and lactoferrin *in vitro* and *in vivo*, *Blood Cells*, **10**, 379–426.

Broxmeyer, H. E., Bicknell, D. C., Cooper, S., Sledge, G., McGuire, W. A., and Coates, T. D. (1985a). Lactoferrin- and acidic isoferritin–cell interactions in a patient with lactoferrin deficiency, *Blood*, **66** (supplement 1), 77a.

Broxmeyer, H. E., Juliano, L., Waheed, A., and Shadduck, R. K. (1985b). Release from mouse macrophages of acidic isoferritins that suppress hematopoietic progenitor cells is induced by purified L-cell colony stimulating factors and suppressed by human lactoferrin, *J. Immunol.*, **135**, 3224–31.

Broxmeyer, H. E., Lu, L., Bicknell, D. C., Sledge, G. W., Williams, D., Dippold, W. G., Hangoc, G., McGuire, W., Coates, T., and Cooper, S. (1985c). The interacting roles of lactoferrin, transferrin and acidic isoferritins in the regulation of myelopoiesis *in vitro* and *in vivo*, In G. Spik, J. Montreuil, R. R. Crichton and J. Mazurier (eds) *Proteins of Iron Metabolism*, pp. 209–20, Elsevier Science Publishers, Amsterdam.

Broxmeyer, H. E., Bicknell, D. C., Gillis, S., Harris, E. L., Pelus, L. M., and Sledge, G. W. Jr. (1986a). Lactoferrin affinity purification from human milk and polymorphonuclear neutrophils using monoclonal antibody (II 2 C) to human lactoferrin, development of an immunoradiometric assay using II 2 C and receptor binding characteristics, *Blood Cells*, **11**, 429–46.

Broxmeyer, H. E., Lu, L., Bicknell, D. C., Williams, D. E., Cooper, S., Levi, S., Salfeld, J., and Arosio, P. (1986b). The influence of purified recombinant human acidic and basic isoferritins on colony formation *in vitro* by granulocyte–macrophage and erythroid progenitor cells, *Blood*, **68**, 1257–63.

Broxmeyer, H. E., Piacibello, W., Juliano, L., Platzer, E., Berman, E., and Rubin, B. Y. (1986c). Gamma interferon induces colony forming cells of the human monoblast cell line U937 to respond to inhibition by lactoferrin, transferrin and acidic isoferritins, *Exp. Hematol.*, **14**, 35–43.

Broxmeyer, H. E., Rubin, B. Y., Berman, E., Juliano, L., Lu, L., Hast, L. J., Cooper, S., and Singer, J. W. (1986d). Activities derived from established human myeloid cell lines reverse the suppression of cell line colony formation by lactoferrin and transferrin, *Exp. Hematol.*, **14**, 51–9.

Broxmeyer, H. E., Williams, D. E., Hangoc, G., Cooper, S., Gillis, S., Shadduck, R. K., and Bicknell, D. C. (1987a). Synergistic myelopoietic actions *in vivo* of combinations of purified natural murine colony stimulating factor-1, recombinant murine interleukin-3, and recombinant murine granulocyte–macrophage colony stimulating factor administered to mice, *Proc. Natl Acad. Sci. USA*, **84**, 3871–5.

Broxmeyer, H. E., Williams, D. E., Lu, L., Vadhan, S., Cooper, S., Bicknell, D. C., Ralph, P., Gutterman, J., and Tricot, G. (1987b). Biomolecules associated with suppression of myelopoiesis in normal conditions and during myeloid leukemia and other related disorders. In A. Najman, M. Guigon, N. C. Gorin, and J. Y. Mary (eds) *Inhibitory Factors in the Regulation of Hematopoiesis*, pp. 139–47, John Libbey Eurotext Limited, France.

Broxmeyer, H. E., Williams, D. E., Cooper, S., Shadduck, R. K., Gillis, S., Waheed, A., Urdal, D. L., and Bicknell, D. C. (1987c). The comparative effects *in vivo* of recombinant murine interleukin-3, natural murine colony stimulating factor-1 and recombinant murine granulocyte–macrophage colony stimulating factor on myelopoiesis in mice, *J. Clin. Invest.*, **79**, 721–30.

Broxmeyer, H. E., Williams, D. E., Cooper, S., Hangoc, G., Levi, S., and Arosio, P. (1987d). Suppressive effects *in vivo* of purified recombinant human H-chain (acidic) ferritin on hematopoietic progenitor cells in mice, *Blood*, **70**, 168a (abstract).

Broxmeyer, H. E., Williams, D. E., Hangoc, G., Cooper, S., Gentile, P., Shen, R.-N., Ralph, P., Gillis, S., and Bicknell, D. C. (1987e). The opposing actions *in vivo* on murine myelopoiesis of purified preparations of lactoferrin and the colony stimulating factors, *Blood Cells*, **13**, 31–48.

Broxmeyer, H. E., Williams, D. E., Geissler, K., Hangoc, G., Cooper, S., Bicknell, D. C., Levi, S., and Arosio, P. (1989). Suppressive effects *in vivo* of purified recombinant human H-subunit (acidic) ferritin on murine myelopoiesis. *Blood*, **73**, 64–9.

Cazzola, M., Arosio, P., Bellotti, V., Bergamaschi, G., Dezza, L., Iacobello, C., and Ruggeri, G. (1985). Use of a monoclonal antibody against heart ferritin for evaluating acidic ferritin concentration in human serum, *Br. J. Haematol.*, **61**, 445–53.

Chen, L. T., Lu, L., and Broxmeyer, H. E. (1987). Effects of purified iron-saturated human lactoferrin on spleen morphology in mice infected with Friend virus complex, *Am. J. Pathol.*, **126**, 285–92.

Covell, A. M., and Cook, J. D. (1988). Interaction of acidic isoferritins with human promyelocytic HL-60 cells, *Br. H. Haematol.*, **69**, 559–63.
Covell, A. M., and Worwood, M. (1984). Isoferritins in plasma. In A. Albertini, P. Arosio, E. Chiancone, and J. Drysdale (eds) *Ferritins and Isoferritins as Biochemical Markers*, p. 49. Elsevier, Amsterdam.
Covell, A. M., Einsphar, D. E., Skikne, B. S., and Cook, J. D. (1987). Specific binding of acidic isoferritins to erythroleukemia K562 cells, *J. Lab. Clin. Med.*, **110**, 784–90.
Cukrova, V., Hrkal, Z., Koprivova, H., and Neuwirt, J. (1986). Identification of leukemia cell-derived inhibitory activity (LIA) in conditioned media from human myeloid leukemia cell line ML-2, *Blut*, **52**, 51–8.
Dezza, L., Cazzola, M., Piacibello, W., Arosio, P., and Aglietta, M. (1986). Effect of acidic and basic isoferritins on the *in vitro* growth of human granulocyte–monocyte progenitors, *Blood*, **67**, 789–95.
Dezza, L., Cazzola, M., Bergamaschi, G., Carlo Stella, C., Pedrazzoli, P., and Recalde, H. R. (1988). Effects of recombinant human H-subunit and L-subunit ferritins on *in vitro* growth of human granulocyte–monocyte progenitors, *Br. J. Haematol.*, **68**, 367–72.
Dinarello, C. A. (1984). Interleukin 1, *Rev. Infect. Dis.*, **6**, 51–95.
Dörner, M. H., Broxmeyer, H. E., Silverstone, A., and Andreeff, M. (1983). Biosynthesis of ferritin subunits from different cell lines of HL-60 human promyelocytic leukemia cells and the release of acidic isoferritin-inhibitory acitivity against normal granulocyte–macrophage progenitor cells, *Br. J. Haematol.*, **55**, 47–58.
Estrov, Z., Tawa, A., Wang, X-H., Dube, I. D., Sulh, H., Cohen, A., Gelfand, E. W., and Freedman, M. H. (1987). *In vitro* and *in vivo* effects of deferoxamine in neonatal acute leukemia, *Blood*, **69**, 757–61.
Fargion, S., Arosio, P., Fracanzani, A. L., Cislaghi, V., Levi, S., Cozzi, A., Piperno, A., and Fiorelli, G. (1988). Characteristics and expression of binding sites specific for ferritin H-chain on human cell lines, *Blood*, **71**, 753–7.
Fibbe, W. E., van Damme, J., Billiau, A., Voogt, P. J., Dunkerken, N., Kluck, P. M. C., and Falkenburg, J. H. F. (1986). Interleukin 1 (22 K factor) induces release of granulocyte–macrophage colony-stimulating activity from human mononuclear phagocyte, *Blood*, **68**, 1316–21.
Fletcher, J., and Willars, J. (1986). The role of lactoferrin released by phagocytosing neutrophils in the regulation of colony-stimulating activity production by human mononuclear cells, *Blood Cells*, **11**, 447–54.
Gentile, P., and Broxmeyer, H. E. (1983). Suppression of mouse myelopoiesis by administration of human lactoferrin *in vivo* and the comparative action of human transferrin, *Blood*, **61**, 982–93.
Gentile, P., and Broxmeyer, H. E. (1987). *In vivo* action of lactoferrin, *Am. J. Hematol.*, **24**, 457–8.
Guimarães, J. E. T. E., Berney, J. J., Broxmeyer, H. E., Hoffbrand, A. V., and Francis, G. E. (1988). Acidic isoferritin stimulates differentiation of normal granulomonocytic progenitors, *Leukemia*, **2**, 466–71.
Hangoc, G., Lu, L., Ollif, A., Hu, W., Bicknell, D. C., Williams, D. E., Gillis, S., and Broxmeyer, H. E. (1987). Modulation of Friend virus infectivity in mice by purified human lactoferrin and purified recombinant murine interleukin-3, *Leukemia*, **1**, 762–4.
Kaplinsky, C., Estrov, Z., Freedman, M. H., Gelfand, E. W., and Cohen, A. (1987).

Effect of deferoxamine on DNA synthesis, DNA repair, cell proliferation, and differentiation of HL-60 cells, *Leukemia*, **1**, 437–41.

Lederman, H. M., Cohen, A., Lee, J. W. W., Freedman, M. H., and Gelfand, E. W. (1984). Deferoxamine: A reversible S-phase inhibitor of human lymphocyte proliferation, *Blood*, **64**, 748–53.

Louvaug, D., Pelus, L. M., Nordlie, E. M., Boyum, A., and Moore, M. A. S. (1986). Monocyte conditioned medium and interleukin 1 induce granulocyte–macrophage colony-stimulating factor production in the adherent cell layer of murine bone marrow cultures, *Exp. Hematol.*, **14**, 1037–42.

Lu, L., Pelus, L. M., and Broxmeyer, H. E. (1984). Modulation of expression of Ia-antigens and the proliferation of human erythroid (BFU-E) and multipotential (CFU-GEMM) progenitor cells by prostaglandin E, *Exp. Hematol.*, **12**, 741–8.

Lu, L., Broxmeyer, H. E., Meyers, P. A., Moore, M. A. S., and Thaler, H. T. (1983). Association of cell cycle expression of Ia-like antigenic determinants on normal human multipotential (CFU-GEMM) and erythroid (BFU-E) progenitor cells with regulation *in vitro* by acidic isoferritins, *Blood*, **61**, 250–6.

Lu, L., Broxmeyer, H. E., Moore, M. A. S., Sheridan, A. P., and Gentile, P. (1985). Abnormalities in myelopoietic regulatory interactions with acidic isoferritins and lactoferrin in mice infected with Friend virus complex: associations with altered expression of Ia-antigens on effector and responding cells, *Blood*, **65**, 91–9.

Lu, L., Bicknell, D. C., Piacibello, W., and Broxmeyer, H. E. (1986). Purified human transferrin and 'transferrin' released from sorted T8$^+$ lymphocytes suppress release of granulocyte–macrophage colony stimulating factors from sorted T4$^+$ lymphocytes stimulated by phytohemagglutinin, *Exp. Hematol.*, **14**, 955–62.

Lu, L., Hangoc, G., Chen, L. T., Shen, N. R., Oliff, A., and Broxmeyer, H. E. (1987a). The protective influence of lactoferrin on mice infected with the polycythemia inducing strain of the Friend virus complex, *Cancer Res.*, **47**, 4184–8.

Lu, L., Walker, D., Broxmeyer, H. E., Hoffman, R., Hu, W., and Walker, E. (1987b). Characterization of adult human marrow hematopoietic progenitors highly enriched by two-color sorting with My10 and major histocompatibility (MHC) class II monoclonal antibodies, *J. Immunol.*, **139**, 1823–9.

Masson, P. L., Heremans, J. F., and Schonne, E. (1969). Lactoferrin, an iron-binding protein in neutrophilic leukocytes, *J. Exp. Med.*, **130**, 643–58.

Mendelsohn, N., Eger, R. R., Broxmeyer, H. E., and Moore, M. A. S. (1978). Isolation of a granulocyte inhibiting activity derived from human polymorphonuclear neutrophils, *Biochim. Biophys. Acta*, **533**, 238–42.

Miyauchi, J., Watanabe, Y., Enomoto, Y., and Takeuchi, K. (1983). Lactoferrin-deficient neutrophil polymorphonuclear leukocytes in leukemias: a semiquantitative and ultrastructural cytochemical study, *J. Clin. Pathol.*, **36**, 1397–405.

Mochizuki, D. Y., Eisenman, J. R., Conlon, P. J., Larsen, A. D., and Tushinski, R. J. (1987). Interleukin 1 regulates hematopoietic activity, a role previously ascribed to hemopoietin 1, *Proc. Natl. Acad. Sci. USA*, **84**, 5267–71.

Moguilevsky, N., Retegui, L. A., and Masson, P. L. (1985). Comparison of human lactoferrins from milk and neutrophilic leukocytes. Relative molecular mass, isoelectric point, iron-binding properties and uptake by the liver, *Biochem. J.*, **229**, 353–9.

Moore, R. N., Joshi, J. G., Pitruzzello, F. J., Horohov, D. W., and Rouse, B. T. (1986). Characterization of a two-signal-dependent Ia$^+$ mononuclear phagocyte progenitor subpopulation that is sensitive to inhibition by ferritin, *J. Immunol.*, **136**, 1605–11.

Nocka, K., and Pelus, L. M. (1988). Cell cycle specific effects of deferoxamine on human and murine hematopoietic progenitor cells, *Cancer Res.*, **48**, 3571–5.

Nocka, K., Ottman, O., and Pelus, L. M. (1986). Antagonistic action of acidic isoferritin and iron saturated transferrin on the enhancement of human erythroid progenitor cells by prostaglandin E, *Exp. Hematol.*, **14**, 475 (abstract).

Oblon, D. J., Broxmeyer, H. E., and Vellis, K. (1983). Acidic isoferritin-inhibitory activity: A normal granulopoietic regulator within long term mouse bone marrow cultures, *Leuk. Res.*, **7**, 581–90.

Odelberg, H., and Olofsson, I. (1976). Primary and secondary granule contents and bactericidal capacity in acute leukemia, *Blood Cells*, **2**, 543–51.

Okabe-Kado, J., Hayashi, M., Honma, Y., Hozumi, M., and Broxmeyer, H. E. (1983). Acidic isoferritins do not suppress differentiation of mouse myeloid leukemic M1 cells, *Leuk. Res.*, **7**, 811–15.

Olofsson, T., Olsson, I., and Venge, P. (1977). Myeloperoxidase and lactoferrin of blood neutrophils and plasma in chronic granulocytic leukemia, *Scand. J. Haematol.*, **18**, 113–20.

Pelus, L. M. (1982). Association between colony forming units granulocyte–macrophage expression of Ia-like (HLA-DR) antigen and control of granulocyte and macrophage production. A new role for prostaglandin E, *J. Clin. Invest.*, **70**, 568–78.

Pelus, L. M., Broxmeyer, H. E., Kurland, J. I., and Moore, M. A. S. (1979). Regulation of macrophage and granulocyte proliferation: specificities of prostaglandin E and lactoferrin, *J. Exp. Med.*, **150**, 277–92.

Pelus, L. M., Broxmeyer, H. E., de Sousa, M., and Moore, M. A. S. (1981). Heterogeneity among resident murine peritoneal macrophages: Separation and functional characterization of monocytoid cells producing granulocyte–macrophage colony stimulating factor (GM-CSF), and responding to regulation by lactoferrin, *J. Immunol.*, **126**, 1016–21.

Pelus, L. M., Gold, E., Saletan, S., and Coleman, M. (1983). Restoration of responsiveness of chronic myeloid leukemia granulocyte–macrophage colony forming cells to growth regulation *in vitro* following preincubation with prostaglandin E, *Blood*, **62**, 158–65.

Piacibello, W., Rubin, B. Y., and Broxmeyer, H. E. (1986). Prostaglandin E counteracts modulation of the gamma interferon induction of Ia antigens on U937 cells and induction of responsiveness of U937 colony forming cells to suppression by lactoferrin, transferrin, acidic isoferritins and prostaglandin E, *Exp. Hematol.*, **14**, 44–50.

Poppas, A., Faith, M. R., and Bierman, H. R. (1986). In vivo study of lactoferrin and murine rebound myelopoiesis, *Am. J. Hematol.*, **22**, 1–8.

Rabe, K., Rehpenning, W., Winkler, K., Heinisch, B., Krause, U., Soltau, H., and Neth, R. (1983). Persistent deficiency of myeloperoxidase and lactoferrin in granulopoietic cells of patients with acute leukemia. In R. Neth, R. C. Gallo, M. F. Greaves, M. A. S. Moore and K. Winkler (eds) *Modern Trends in Human Leukemia V*, pp. 362–5, Springer-Verlag, Berlin.

Rausch, P. G., Pryzwansky, K. B., Spitznagel, J. K., and Herion, J. C. (1978). Immuno-cytochemical identification of abnormal polymorphonuclear neutrophils in patients with leukemia, *Blood Cells*, **4**, 369–76.

Sala, G., Worwood, M., and Jacobs, A. (1986). The effect of isoferritins on granulopoiesis, *Blood*, **67**, 436–43.

Schofield, K. P., Stone, P. C. W., and Stuart, J. (1983). Quantitative cytochemistry of blood neutrophils in acute myeloid leukemia, *Br. J. Haematol.*, **54**, 261–8.

Segal, G. M., McCall, E., Stueve, T., and Bagby, G. C. Jr (1987). Interleukin 1 stimulates endothelial cells to release multilineage human colony-stimulating activity, *J. Immunol*, **138**, 1772–8.

Sieff, C. A., Tsai, S., and Faller, D. V. (1987). Interleukin 1 induces cultured human endothelial cell production of granulocyte–macrophage colony-stimulating factor, *J. Clin. Invest.*, **79**, 48–51.

Slater, K., and Fletcher, J. (1987). Lactoferrin derived from neutrophils inhibits the mixed lymphocyte reaction, *Blood*, **69**, 1328–33.

Sledge, G. W. Jr, Bicknell, D. C., Harris, E. L., Zeggarra, G., and Broxmeyer, H. E. (1986). Monoclonal antibody (II2C) to human lactoferrin inactivates the myelopoietic suppressive effect of human lactoferrin *in vitro*, *Exp. Hematol.*, **14**, 333–7.

Stanley, E. R., Bartocci, A., Patinkin, D., Rosendaal, M., and Bradley, T. R. (1986). Regulation of very primitive multipotent hemopoietic cells by hemopoietin-1, *Cell*, **45**, 667–74.

Steinman, G., Broxmeyer, H. E., DeHarven, E., and Moore, M. A. S. (1982). Immunoelectron microscopic tracing of lactoferrin, a regulator of myelopoiesis into a subpopulation of human peripheral blood monocytes, *Br. J. Haematol.*, **50**, 75–84.

Taetle, R. (1981). Acidic isoferritins (leukemia-associated inhibitory activity) fail to inhibit blast proliferation in acute myelogenous leukemia, *Blood*, **58**, 653–7.

Taetle, R., and Honeysett, J. M. (1986). Transferrin modulation of colony stimulating factor elaboration by adherent blood and bone marrow cells, *Br. J. Haematol.*, **62**, 163–70.

Wagstaff, M., Worwood, M., and Jacobs, A. (1978). Properties of human tissue isoferritins, *Biochem. J.*, **173**, 969–77.

Walker, C. M., Moody, D. J., Stites, D. P., and Levy, J. A. (1986). CD8[+] lymphocytes can control HIV infection *in vitro* by suppressing virus replication, *Science*, **234**, 1563–6.

Wang, S.-Y., Castro-Malaspina, H., Lu, L., and Moore, M. A. S. (1985). Biological characterization of a granulopoietic enhancing activity derived from cultured human lipid-containing macrophages, *Blood*, **65**, 1181–90.

Williams, D. E., Cooper, S., and Broxmeyer, H. E. (1988). The effects of hematopoietic suppressor molecules on the *in vitro* proliferation of purified murine granulocyte–macrophage progenitor cells (CFU-CM), *Cancer Res.*, **48**, 1548–50.

Williams, D. E., Lu, L., and Broxmeyer, H. E. (1987). Characterization of hematopoietic stem and progenitor cells, *Immunological Res.*, **6**, 294–304.

Williams, D. E., Hangoc, G., Cooper, S., Boswell, H. S., Shadduck, R. K., Gillis, S., Waheed, A., Urdal, D., and Broxmeyer, H. E. (1987a). The *in vivo* effects of purified recombinant IL-3 and purified natural CSF-1 on murine high proliferative potential colony forming cell: Demonstration of *in vivo* synergism, *Blood*, **70**, 401–3.

Williams, D. E., Straneva, J. E., Shen, R. N., and Broxmeyer, H. E. (1987b). Purification of murine bone marrow-derived granulocyte–macrophage colony-forming cells and partial characterization of their growth and regulation *in vitro*, *Exp. Hematol.*, **15**, 243–50.

Yung, Y. P., and Moore, M. A. S. (1982). Long term in vitro culture of murine mast cells. III. Discrimination of mast cell growth factor and granulocyte CSF, *J. Immunol.*, **129**, 1256–61.

Zucali, J. R., Broxmeyer, H. E., and Ulatowski, J. A. (1979). Specificity of lactoferrin as an inhibitor of granulocyte–macrophage colony-stimulating activity production from fetal mouse liver cells, *Blood*, **54**, 951–4.

Zucali, J. R., Dinarello, C. A., Oblon, D. J., Gross, M. A., Anderson, L., and Weiner, R. S. (1986). Interleukin 1 stimulates fibroblasts to produce granulocyte–macrophage colony-stimulating activity and prostaglandin E_2, *J. Clin. Invest.*, **77**, 1857–63.

Zucali, J. R., Broxmeyer, H. E., Dinarello, C. A., Gross, M. A., and Weiner, R. S. (1987a). Regulation of early human hematopoietic (BFU-E and CFU-GEMM) progenitor cells *in vitro* by interleukin 1-induced fibroblast conditioned medium, *Blood*, **69**, 33–7.

Zucali, J. R., Levy, D. A., Broxmeyer, H. E., and Morse, C. A. (1987b). Lactoferrin acts on human monocytes to inhibit production of interleukin 1 and the ability of monocyte-conditioned medium to induce fibroblasts to produce granulocyte–macrophage colony stimulating factors, *Blood*, **70**, 191a (abstract).

10
Iron, the Iron-binding Proteins and Bone Marrow Cell Differentiation

J. Fletcher
Department of Haematology, City Hospital, Nottingham, UK

INTRODUCTION

Iron-binding proteins are usually considered in relation to their obvious functions. Transferrin is the plasma transport protein of iron, ferritin is the iron-storage protein and lactoferrin is responsible for nonspecific resistance to infection by limiting the availability of iron required for the growth of potential pathogens in milk and other body fluids. These functions (see Chapter 3) are fundamentally important but it is becoming increasingly apparent that the same proteins may have regulatory functions. De Sousa (1978) suggested that, since iron-binding proteins are synthesized and secreted by lymphoid cells, they may have a role in regulating the recirculation of these cells. Broxmeyer *et al.* (1983) have suggested that all three proteins may affect the growth of progenitor cells in the marrow and that defects of this regulatory function may contribute to the uncontrolled marrow proliferation of leukaemia (see Chapter 9). Clearly, an understanding of these mechanisms is potentially very important but it remains a controversial area of research with inconsistency of results between different investigators and lack of convincing evidence of physiological importance.

LACTOFERRIN AND MYELOPOIESIS

It has long been known that mature polymorphonuclear granulocytes release a factor (or factors), which inhibits the proliferation of granulocyte progenitor cells *in vitro* (Paran, Ichikawa and Sachs, 1969; Baker, Broxmeyer and Galbraith, 1975; Herman, Golde and Cline, 1978). Broxmeyer *et al.* (1978a) identified at least one of these factors as lactoferrin, an iron-binding protein related to transferrin, but with different physicochemical properties and functions (see Chapters 3 and 4). They showed that medium conditioned by neutrophils, or extracts of neutrophils obtained by freezing and thawing, partially inhibited granulocyte–macrophage colony-stimulating factor (GM-CSF) production from mononuclear cells. The inhibitory activity was reproduced by purified lactoferrin and blocked by specific antibody. The extent of iron saturation of the lactoferrin molecule was critical and for iron-saturated lactoferrin an effect was demonstrated even at extraordinarily low concentrations down to 10^{-17} M. Another unusual feature of the data was the isoelectric point, pH 6.5, of both the purified lactoferrin and neutrophil-derived inhibitory activity, as the isoelectric point of highly purified lactoferrin is pH 8.7 (Moguilevsky, Retegui and Masson, 1985). At the time, these findings were looked upon with some scepticism, particularly because it is difficult to envisage a regulatory function for lactoferrin at concentrations which are several orders of magnitude lower than the normal concentration in plasma (Burgess and Metcalf, 1980). However, other investigators have subsequently confirmed Broxmeyer's observations. Bagby *et al.* (1981) took the trouble to remove bovine lactoferrin from fetal calf serum in their culture system and were able to show inhibition of GM-CSF production by purified iron-saturated lactoferrin down to 10^{-17} M. Philip, Standen and Fletcher (1982) showed that neutrophils, during phagocytosis, rapidly release an inhibitor of GM-CSF production in a way consistent with release of lactoferrin from the secondary granules. However, two groups have reported their inability to reproduce the effects of lactoferrin. Winton *et al.* (1981), using murine lactoferrin on murine cells, failed to show an action of lactoferrin. Stryckmans *et al.* (1984) attempted to reproduce the conditions used by Broxmeyer and to answer his criticisms of Winton's technique but still failed to show an effect. More recently, Fletcher and Willars (1986) confirmed both Broxmeyer's and Bagby's results by showing that the inhibitory effect of products of phagocytizing neutrophils on GM-CSF production from mononuclear cells was proportional to its lactoferrin content, and the action of both pure lactoferrin and neutrophil products was abrogated by specific antibody. They emphasized the importance of close cell contact by showing that a relatively high concentration of mononuclear cells, 5×10^6 ml^{-1}, or crowding of cells, is necessary to allow the inhibitory effect of lactoferrin on GM-CSF production. This may well provide the explanation for the failure of both Winton *et al.* (1981) and Stryckmans *et al.* (1984), as both of these groups used mononuclear cells at concentrations of 10^6 ml^{-1} or less spread in the bottom of plastic dishes and these are exactly the conditions which Fletcher and Willars (1986) found to be ineffective.

Another area of controversy is whether lactoferrin is acting directly on

GM-CSF production by monocytes and macrophages or indirectly on a monokine responsible for GM-CSF production from T lymphocytes and other tissues. Broxmeyer's group, using both human and murine monocytes and macrophages, has shown that the effect of lactoferrin persists when lymphocytes have been rigorously removed by adherence, rosetting, and the use of monoclonal antibodies together with complement lysis (Broxmeyer, 1979; Broxmeyer and Platzer, 1984). These data contrast with those of Bagby et al. (1981), who were unable to show an effect of lactoferrin when monocytes were separated from lymphocytes. Bagby's group have subsequently shown that lactoferrin acts indirectly by inhibiting a monokine which is responsible for the release of GM-CSF from T lymphocytes, fibroblasts and vascular endothelial cells (Bagby et al., 1981, 1983; Bagby, McCall and Layman, 1983). Their concept is that if GM-CSF is a biologically relevant regulator of haemopoiesis then its production from a variety of cell sources must also be regulated. Bagby et al. (1986) have recently identified the monokine released from monocytes and controlling GM-CSF production as interleukin-1 (IL-1), which implies, although it has not been confirmed, that lactoferrin inhibits IL-1 production from monocytes and macrophages. Support for this concept has recently come from Seiff, Tsai and Faller (1987), who failed to find mRNA for GM-CSF in monocytes but were able to show that stimulated monocytes release IL-1 and another monokine, tumour necrosis factor (TNF), which induce mRNA for GM-CSF in fibroblasts and endothelial cells. Since IL-1 and TNF are also potent activators of neutrophils (Klempner, Dinarello and Gallin, 1978; Larrick et al., 1987), it is possible to envisage a complex interaction between neutrophils, monocytes and tissues releasing GM-CSF (Figure 10.1), particularly as GM-CSF also activates both neutrophils and monocytes (Weisbart et al., 1985; Moore et al., 1980).

The idea that lactoferrin, released from neutrophils, is acting indirectly, suggests that its effects will not be confined to GM-CSF. A scheme of growth factor release by T lymphocytes indicates that it should also inhibit IL-2 production and factors controlling B cell growth and differentiation (Figure 10.2). Slater and Fletcher (1987a) showed that lactoferrin inhibited uridine uptake, a measure of transcription, by allogeneic mixed lymphocyte cultures. This effect was only seen when the cells were crowded together in round-bottomed wells and not when they were spread in flat-bottomed wells. It was associated with a reduction in release into the medium of a soluble factor subsequently identified as IL-2 (Slater and Fletcher, 1987b). They were able to show this effect both with products of phagocytizing neutrophils and with lactoferrin purified from these products by absorption on to a monoclonal antibody column. Duncan and McArthur (1981) have described inhibition by lactoferrin of the primary antibody response of murine cells to T lymphocyte-dependent and

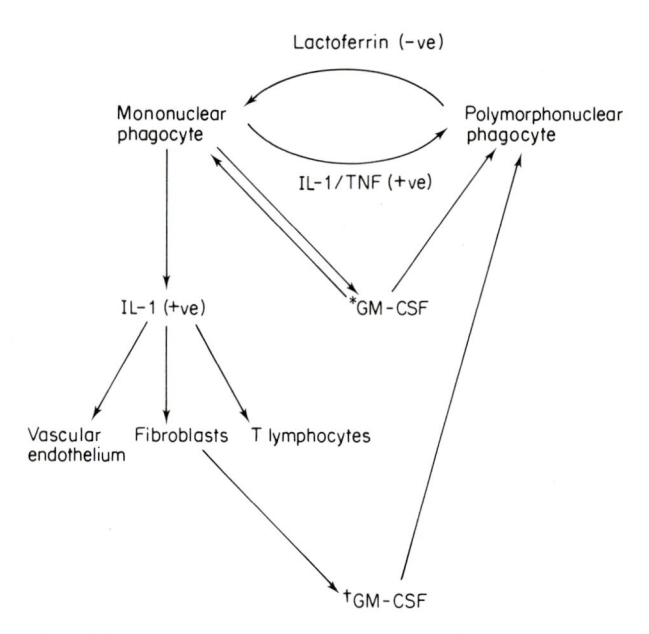

Figure 10.1 Possible interactions between mononuclear and polymorphonuclear phagocytes. *According to Broxmeyer and Platzer (1984); †According to Bagby et al. (1981)

-independent antigens and suggested that this is due to an effect on macrophages. Thus there is experimental evidence to support the suggestion that lactoferrin will have widespread effects upon growth factors elaborated by lymphocytes in the presence of mononuclear phagocytes. Furthermore, Broxmeyer et al. (1987) have reported an inhibitory effect of lactoferrin on growth factor production by a number of different haemopoietic cell lines in which GM-CSF is not involved.

All those who have successfully demonstrated an effect of lactoferrin agree that GM-CSF production by mononuclear cells is only partially inhibited, usually by about 50%, which implies that some sources of GM-CSF are not affected. Broxmeyer has shown that the inhibitory action of lactoferrin requires an Ia antigen-positive subpopulation of murine peritoneal macrophages or the equivalent antigenic determinants (HLA-DR) on human monocytes (Broxmeyer, 1979; Broxmeyer and Platzer, 1984). Treatment of the cells with monoclonal antibody against HLA-DR blocks the inhibitory actions of lactoferrin without the antibody affecting GM-CSF production. The data suggest a close relationship between major histocompatibility complex (MHC) class 2 (HLA-DR) antigens and the action of lactoferrin. This is in keeping with the data of Fletcher and Willars (1986), and Slater and Fletcher (1987b), showing that lactoferrin inhibits the

Iron and Bone Marrow Cell Differentiation

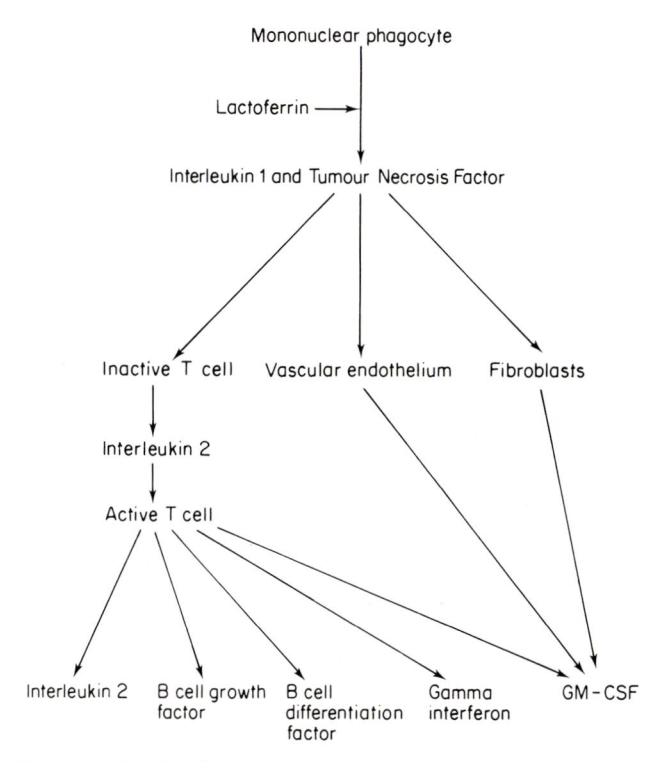

Figure 10.2 Cytokines which might be affected by lactoferrin

production of growth factors (GM-CSF and IL-2) which depends upon cell–cell interaction; this is a known function of histocompatibility antigens. It may be that lactoferrin interferes with the function of these MHC antigens and simply blocks cell–cell interaction by a mechanism not requiring binding at a separate specific receptor. This would be in keeping with the data showing that only a short exposure to lactoferrin at the beginning of cell culture is necessary to obtain an inhibitory effect (Broxmeyer and Platzer, 1984).

IRON SATURATION OF LACTOFERRIN—ACTIVE AND INACTIVE FORMS OF THE MOLECULE

Iron-free or apolactoferrin lacks inhibitory activity both for GM-CSF production and in mixed lymphocyte cultures (Broxmeyer *et al.*, 1978); Slater and Fletcher, 1987a). 'Native' lactoferrin, thought to be about 8% saturated with iron (Bullen, 1981), and lactoferrin released from phagocytizing neutrophils, are active at dilutions of 10^{-11} and 10^{-12} M. Iron-saturated lactoferrin shows inhibitory activity, at least against GM-CSF production, at concentrations as low as 10^{-16} and 10^{-17} M (Broxmeyer et al., 1978a; Bagby et al., 1981). At these very low concentrations of iron-saturated lactoferrin there can be very few molecules of protein per cell and it is difficult to see how lactoferrin is acting if it depends upon binding at specific cellular receptors. Both Broxmeyer et al. (1978a) and Bagby et al. (1981) have reported results with lactoferrin which was iron-saturated by addition of an excess of iron salt and followed by removal of unbound iron by dialysis and passage through an ion-exchange column. However, it is known that great care has to be taken when iron is added to either lactoferrin or transferrin and it requires the presence of an excess of a low molecular weight chelator, such as citrate or nitrolotriacetate, to prevent hydrolysis, polymerization and nonspecific binding of iron (Bates and Schlabach, 1973). The inhibitory effect of very low concentrations of iron-saturated lactoferrin could be due to nonspecific surface-bound iron acting as a catalyst in reactions such as the Haber–Weiss reaction which produce toxic oxygen radicals, particularly the highly active hydroxyl radical:

$$\frac{[O_2^- + Fe^{3+} \rightarrow O_2 + Fe^{2+}]}{[H_2O_2 + Fe^{2+} \rightarrow OH\cdot + OH^- + Fe^{3+}]}$$
$$\text{net } [O_2^- + H_2O_2 \rightarrow OH\cdot + OH^- + O_2]$$

Superoxide (O_2^-) and hydrogen peroxide (H_2O_2) are products of activated polymorphonuclear and mononuclear phagocytes. The involvement of lactoferrin in such reactions is controversial as it is not clear whether iron bound at the physiological site can catalyse such reactions or whether physiological binding prevents the reaction. Ambruso and Johnston (1981) showed that lactoferrin saturated by various techniques, including that used by Broxmeyer, enhanced production of hydroxyl radicals, while iron-poor lactoferrin (apparently not completely depleted of iron) either had no effect or inhibited hydroxyl radical production. Lactoferrin, either by binding at specific sites or because it is highly cationic and binds specifically to membranes (Hekman, 1971), would focus any toxic oxygen species on to cell surfaces. On the other hand, Gutteridge et al. (1981), using lipid peroxidation as an indicator of hydroxyl radical activity, showed that lactoferrin, 20% saturated with iron, inhibited the reaction but the iron-saturated protein had no effect. Since it is unlikely that lactoferrin ever occurs completely saturated under physiological conditions, the data of Gutteridge et al. are the more convincing, and would suggest that one of the functions of unsaturated lactoferrin is to dampen these potentially toxic reactions.

Although there are almost no data on the iron saturation of lactoferrin within neutrophils, it is usually considered to be iron-free, whereas both the pink colour when lactoferrin from activated neutrophils is retained on an antibody column and its inhibitory activity on GM-CSF production suggest that when actively released it carries iron. This raises the intriguing possibility that lactoferrin released passively by cell death is iron-free and inactive, while lactoferrin released by activation of neutrophils acquires iron and, with it, biological activity. It is sometimes assumed that lactoferrin will remove iron from transferrin because its binding constant is higher. However, this is pH-dependent, and at physiological pH the avidity of transferrin for iron is enormous, resulting in no movement of iron to lactoferrin in plasma. In the presence of phagocytizing neutrophils there is also no detectable movement of iron from transferrin to lactoferrin (Fletcher, unpublished observations). An alternative source of iron is ferritin. Superoxide anions generated by the neutrophil's respiratory burst, and involved in microbial killing, can certainly mobilize iron from ferritin (Biemond et al., 1984), but it is not known whether neutrophil ferritin is available at the sites of superoxide release. It is just possible that ferritin could also be available from ingested micro-organisms. However, there is experimental evidence to support the suggestion that products of the neutrophil's respiratory burst are involved in production of biologically active lactoferrin, as addition of superoxide dismutase to phagocytizing neutrophils prevents release of inhibitory activity (Fletcher and Willars, unpublished observations). Broxmeyer et al. (1980) have also emphasized the importance of metabolically active neutrophils in the release of biologically active lactoferrin. They separated neutrophils according to the presence of Fc receptors into more and less metabolically active populations. The more active cells contained and released inhibitory activity, in contrast to the less active. Both neutrophil populations contained lactoferrin and the results might have been due to the metabolically active cells releasing lactoferrin under conditions in which it would acquire iron. However, addition of iron to fully saturate lactoferrin did not produce inhibitory activity in extracts of metabolically less active cells. The data certainly emphasize that biologically active lactoferrin comes from metabolically active neutrophils capable of mounting an oxidative burst, and there is a precedent for such a mechanism, as Aune and Pierce (1981) have described an inhibitor of lymphocyte proliferation secreted by T lymphocytes which requires activation by hydrogen peroxide. To understand the role of iron in the biological activity of lactoferrin requires more data about the iron saturation of lactoferrin in neutrophil secondary granules, of lactoferrin released by phagocytizing neutrophils, and of circulating plasma lactoferrin. The iron saturation of the high plasma lactoferrin concentrations characteristic of myeloproliferative disorders, which is presumably biologically inactive, should be compared with that of the high levels generated during inflammatory conditions, which is presumably biologically active.

The problem of active and inactive forms of lactoferrin is important when considering its possible physiological role, particularly in the presence of concentrations in the plasma which appear to be higher than the minimal concentrations showing inhibitory activity *in vitro*. Concentrations around 10^{-9} M have been reported (Bennett and Mohla, 1976) but these may be overestimates, as care has to be taken to avoid degranulation of neutrophils and release of secondary granule proteins during venesection. Use of heparin as an anticoagulant does not prevent activation of complement to produce active components which, in the presence of calcium, cause neutrophil degranulation. When blood is taken carefully into EDTA in the cold and separated immediately, plasma lactoferrin concentrations may be as low as 10^{-11} M (Broxmeyer *et al.*, 1983), although this has been disputed (Baynes *et al.*, 1986b). However, even 10^{-11} M is still within the concentration range that exhibits inhibitory activity *in vitro*.

LACTOFERRIN INTERACTION WITH CELL SURFACES

As already discussed, the inhibitory effect of lactoferrin on production of GM-CSF and other growth factors involves interaction with mononuclear cells. There is certainly evidence from other sources to substantiate attachment of lactoferrin to the surface of mononucler phagocytes *in vitro*. Van Snick and Masson (1976) showed the binding of human lactoferrin to mouse peritoneal macrophages, with the subsequent ingestion and digestion of lactoferrin and the transfer of its iron into ferritin (Van Snick, Markowitz and Masson, 1977). Nishiya and Horwitz (1982) showed enhancement of monocyte natural killer activity by both saturated and unsaturated lactoferrin. However, both of these groups used high concentrations of lactoferrin (10^{-6}–10^{-8} M), at which it may polymerize (Bagby *et al.*, 1982), and this could explain its uptake by, and activation of, mononuclear phagocytes, and does not necessarily indicate a more specific interaction dependent upon receptors. Stryckmans *et al.* (1984), using very gentle methods for the separation of mononuclear cells, were unable to show binding of lactoferrin. However, a number of claims have been made for specific binding sites on mononuclear phagocytes, B lymphocytes and neutrophils (Bennett and Davies, 1981; Boxer *et al.*, 1982b). These binding sites are claimed to be specific on the grounds that they are saturable, binding of radioactively labelled lactoferrin can be blocked by an excess of unlabelled protein, and Scatchard analysis gives a linear relationship compatible with a homogeneous population. There is equal binding of both human breast milk and neutrophil lactoferrin with about 10^7 sites per blood monocyte and a dissociation constant of 4×10^{-7} M (Birgens, Hansen and Karle, 1983). However, one of the well-recognized features of lactoferrin is that it tends to stick to surfaces and to other proteins because it is strongly cationic (Hekman, 1971). Recent work indicates that the liver reticuloendothelial system and isolated alveolar macrophages possess a common binding site for lactoferrin and certain other strongly cationic proteins such as pancreatic elastase (Campbell, 1982; Retegui et al., 1984). A candidate for this common cell surface receptor is DNA, as binding of lactoferrin to mononuclear cells and neutrophils is considerably reduced by their prior exposure to DNase (Bennett, Merritt and Gabor, 1986). The presence of DNA on the surface of phagocytic cells *in vitro* may be an artefact arising from DNA having been released by damaged cells. However, it remains possible that a specific double-stranded DNA within the cell surface is the physiological receptor, although it will be very difficult to prove conclusively, as there also appears to be a specific receptor for DNA (Bennett, Merritt and Gabor, 1986).

LACTOFERRIN AND CHRONIC MYELOID LEUKAEMIA

Broxmeyer, Mendelsohn and Moore (1977) reported that neutrophils from patients with chronic myeloid leukaemia (CML) lacked inhibitory activity against GM-CSF production from normal mononuclear cells. They obtained their inhibitory activity by disrupting neutrophils by freezing and thawing, and attributed its deficiency to a quantitative reduction of lactoferrin in CML compared with normal neutrophils as reported by others (Olofsson, Olsson and Venge, 1977). More recently, Broxmeyer *et al.* (1983) have claimed that the almost complete lack of inhibitory activity in neutrophils from many patients with CML is out of proportion to the quantitative reduction of lactoferrin and therefore suggest that CML neutrophil lactoferrin is qualitatively abnormal. The work of Fletcher and colleagues extends Broxmeyer's observations and suggests that the abnormality of CML neutrophils may provide the key to understanding the difference between active and inactive forms of lactoferrin.

Philip, Standen and Fletcher (1981, 1982) reported that phagocytizing but not resting neutrophils normally release an inhibitor of GM-CSF production by mononuclear cells. Neutrophils from patients with CML were found to contain the inhibitor but there was a failure to release significant amounts during phagocytosis. The amount of inhibitor was the same in extracts of normal and CML neutrophils disrupted by sonication. Normal neutrophils released about half their inhibitory activity during phagocytosis while CML neutrophils released approximately 2%, so that there was a 30-fold difference in inhibitory activity released by leukaemic cells compared with normal. As expected from these results, the amount of lactoferrin in both CML and normal neutrophils was the same but, surprisingly, the amount released during phagocytosis was also the same and failure of secondary granule release did not explain the failure to release inhibitory activity. Indeed, during phagocytosis there was no difference in the quantity or kinetics of secondary granule protein release when polymorphonuclear cells and band forms from Philadelphia-positive CML patients in the chronic phase of their disease were compared with normal (Maallem, Sheppard and Fletcher, 1982). However, CML neutrophils are metabolically abnormal. There is cytochemical evidence of a failure of the primary granules to discharge their content of lysozyme, hydrolases, proteinases and myeloperoxidase into the phagocytic vacuole (El-Maallem and Fletcher, 1976). There is also a quantitative deficiency in hydrogen peroxide formation while superoxide production appears to be normal (El Maallem and Fletcher, 1979; Rule, Knights and Fletcher, 1986). Thus it seems that lactoferrin with inhibitory activity for GM-CSF production requires 'activation' by interaction with products of the primary granule which may be involved in generation of hydrogen peroxide from superoxide.

It is an attractive idea that CML, characterized by continued inappropriate bone marrow proliferation, is due to a failure of circulating CML cells to release the normal feedback inhibitor of granulopoeisis. However, any hypothesis about the pathogenesis of CML must take into account recent evidence about the Philadelphia chromosome which is produced by a reciprocal translocation between chromosomes 9 and 22, resulting in the transfer of the abl cellular oncogene from chromosome 9 on to the bcr gene of chromosome 22. The result is an abnormal mRNA which is the fused transcript of the two genes and itself appears to transcribe a protein with phosphorylating activity and is therefore likely to be involved in stimulus–secretion coupling (Shtivelman *et al.*, 1985). This is not incompatible with defective primary granule fusion with the phagocytic vacuole as discussed above, but this is simply speculation.

In their original paper, Broxmeyer, Mendelsohn and Moore (1977) not only drew attention to lack of inhibitory activity in CML neutrophil extracts but also suggested that leukaemic mononuclear target cells lacked sensitivity to the inhibitor. Broxmeyer *et al.* (1983) have subsequently suggested that lack of sensitivity would be due to lack of expression of histocompatibility antigens. Unfortunately, the original data are difficult to interpret, as normal neutrophil extracts were simply added to CML mononuclear cells suspended in agar, and changes in numbers of spontaneous clusters and colonies taken to indicate changes in GM-CSF production. Inhibitory activity may be missed if there is already excess GM-CSF present, and the experiments need repeating using a system in which CML mononuclear cells condition medium so that GM-CSF production can be measured in the presence and absence of inhibitor. Even this may not give a clear answer, as it is notoriously difficult to separate CML mononuclear cells from other leukaemic myeloid cells with similar density. Up to the present, no other group has repeated the observations of Broxmeyer, Mendelsohn and Moore (1977).

IN VIVO EVIDENCE FOR THE IMPORTANCE OF LACTOFERRIN AS A PHYSIOLOGICAL REGULATOR

In animals

Following the report (Broxmeyer, Moore and Ralph, 1977) that neutrophil extracts obtained by freezing and thawing inhibit GM-CSF production by mononuclear cells *in vitro*, Broxmeyer (1978) injected similar extracts of human polymorphonuclear granulocytes into the peritoneal cavity of mice. These neutrophil extracts had no effect on normal mice, but when mice were treated with cyclophosphamide to deplete them of mature neutrophils, and therefore of the cells containing inhibitory activity, there was a significant effect. Three daily injections of neutrophil extracts after cyclophosphamide treatment produced a significant reduction in GM-CSF production and in granulocyte–macrophage colony-forming units (CFU-GM) in the marrow from animals sacrificed at 3 days. Extracts of CML neutrophils had no effect and were used as negative controls. No data were given on the influence of the human neutrophil extracts on the speed of recovery of granulocytes in the peripheral blood.

After identification of lactoferrin as the active principle in neutrophil extracts, Gentile and Broxmeyer (1983) reported similar experiments in which human lactoferrin was injected intravenously into cyclophosphamide-treated mice. Daily injection of iron-saturated lactoferrin produced a reduction in the total number of CFU-GM and in the proportion in S-phase, and in total nucleated cells in the femoral marrow of animals sacrificed 7 days after the cyclophosphamide injection. This effect could be produced with a total dose of iron-saturated lactoferrin ranging from 300 to 10^{-4} µg and persisted for up to 14 days after the injections had ceased. Apolactoferrin was as effective as iron-saturated lactoferrin. Furthermore, unlike neutrophil extracts, iron-saturated lactoferrin produced a reduction in the number of CFU-GM and mature granulocytes in the marrow of normal mice. As before, the observations were made on marrow *ex vivo* without direct information about the speed of marrow recovery from the cyclophosphamide treatment.

It is difficult to assess the physiological significance of results obtained by injecting human neutrophil extracts or lactoferrin into mice. Certainly, human lactoferrin suppresses GM-CSF production from mouse peritoneal macrophages *in vitro*, apparently in the same way as it suppresses GM-CSF production from human mononuclear cells (Broxmeyer and Platzer, 1984). Nevertheless, the human protein is antigenically distinct from murine lactoferrin, and in the experiments of Gentile and Broxmeyer (1983) it must be interacting as an antigen with the mouse immune system. The observation that apolactoferrin is as effective as iron-saturated lactoferrin *in vivo* but not *in vitro* may mean that the mechanism of lactoferrin action in these experiments is not the same as its *in vitro* action because it is difficult to see how injected human apolactoferrin would acquire iron in the presence of an excess of murine transferrin at physiological pH. There are no reports in the literature of attempts to repeat these experiments and no other data from animal experiments which shed light on the possible role of lactoferrin in control of haemopoiesis.

In humans

Inevitably there is only circumstantial evidence about the role of lactoferrin in the control of haemopoiesis in human subjects.

The concentration of plasma lactoferrin apparently results from a dynamic equilibrium established between its release from neutrophils and its rapid uptake by the reticuloendothelial system, particularly in the liver (Bennett and Kokocinski, 1979). Studies in a patient with no circulating neutrophils who received a bone marrow graft revealed that the clearance of lactoferrin followed an exponential pattern and had an initial half-time of 2.2 hours (Baynes *et al.*, 1986a). The study of patients with cyclic neutropenia or recovering from bone marrow transplantation provides no evidence that lactoferrin acts as a feedback inhibitor of granulopoiesis in these situations (Brown *et al.*, 1986).

There is a quantitative relationship between plasma lactoferrin concentration and neutrophil count and neutrophil turnover. In uninfected patients it indicates the total blood granulocyte pool, and the lactoferrin to neutrophil ratio indicates the degree of granulocyte margination and sequestration in the spleen. In infected patients neutrophils are stimulated to discharge their secondary granule proteins, and raised levels of plasma lactoferrin are detectable (Hansen *et al.*, 1976). It is in this situation that lactoferrin may be acting as a feedback regulator, as during infection and inflammation the marrow will be driven by factors such as endotoxin to increase granulocyte output, but as the infection is overcome, so marrow activity must be reduced back to a maintenance level. In myeloproliferative disorders there are also high levels of secondary granule proteins, reflecting the total granulocyte pool (Olofsson, Olsson and Venge, 1977), and here there is *in vitro* evidence that lactoferrin is in its biologically inactive form because of metabolically defective but otherwise mature circulating granulocytes (Philip, Standen and Fletcher, 1981). However, there are other conditions with metabolically abnormal granulocytes, particularly chronic granulomatous disease, in which there is an inherited inability to mount a respiratory burst and produce the oxygen radicals which appear to be necessary to activate lactoferrin but which is not associated with uncontrolled myeloproliferation. There are also reports of patients with neutrophils lacking secondary granules who did not suffer with inappropriate marrow proliferation; however, the neutrophil defect was not confined to lack of lactoferrin (Breton-Gorius *et al.*, 1980; Gallin *et al.*, 1982; Boxer *et al.*, 1982a).

Conclusion

There is an increasing body of evidence that lactoferrin released from stimulated neutrophils interacts with mononuclear cells *in vitro* to inhibit the production or release of a number of growth factors. Consequently, lactoferrin may be an important local regulator of inflammation. Its role in control of bone marrow proliferation and differentiation is not clear. However, there must be a link between the function of mature neutrophils at sites of inflammation and production of fresh neutrophils by the marrow to explain the neutrophil leukocytosis and increased marrow activity followed by a return to the normal steady state as the inflammatory reaction succeeds. Lactoferrin is a likely candidate for this link.

TRANSFERRIN

In their original observations on lactoferrin, Broxmeyer *et al.* (1978a) used transferrin as a control due to its lack of activity against GM-CSF production both *in vitro* and *in vivo*. Consequently, the report of Broxmeyer, Lu and Bognacki (1983) that transferrin also suppresses GM-CSF production was rather surprising. They showed that both 'native' unsaturated and iron-saturated transferrin at concentrations as low as 10^{-11} M inhibited GM-CSF production from separated T lymphocytes stimulated with either phytohaemagglutinin or concanavalin A. The T lymphocytes were further separated by fluorescence cell sorting, using monoclonal antibodies, into the inducer T4+ and suppressor T8+ subsets, and the effect of transferrin was found to be on the stimulated inducer T4+ cells. Finally, medium conditioned by suppressor T8+ cells was found to inhibit GM-CSF production by inducer T4+ cells and this activity could be blocked by both polyclonal and monoclonal antibody to transferrin (Lu et al., 1986). Gentile and Broxmeyer (1983) injected iron-saturated human transferrin into mice recovering from cyclophosphamide-induced suppression of myelopoiesis and found little effect on the bone marrow but a reduction in splenic cellularity and CFU-GM content.

These data are very difficult to understand, as transferrin is a required growth factor for lymphocytes, and transformed lymphocytes express the transferrin receptor. The *in vitro* experiments were all conducted in the presence of fetal calf serum, which contains a large amount of bovine transferrin, far more than the minimal concentration of human transferrin inhibiting GM-CSF production. Human transferrin may be more effective than bovine for human cells, as Taetle and Honeysett (1986) report that human transferrin (10^{-6}–10^{-7} M) enhances GM-CSF production from human peripheral blood and bone marrow mononuclear cells in the presence of fetal calf serum. Nevertheless, there is no doubt that bovine transferrin can support human lymphocyte cell growth and therefore binds with, and delivers iron to, the cells via their transferrin receptors. Lum et al. (1986) have demonstrated mRNA for transferrin in inducer T4+ peripheral blood lymphocytes but not in suppressor T8+ cells. Their data suggest that transferrin may be an autocrine growth factor both produced and required by inducer T4+ proliferating lymphocytes, and while it is possible that transferrin might promote proliferation at the same time as reducing GM-CSF production, this seems unlikely as proliferation is associated with the production of other growth factors, including IL-2. In their experiments, Broxmeyer and his colleagues used human transferrin saturated with iron *in vitro*, and it is already known, at least for mouse cells, that T cell transformation is optimal when the iron saturation of transferrin is 30–70%, and above this, transformation is markedly reduced (Brock, 1981). Furthermore, if addition of iron salts to transferrin *in vitro* leaves iron attached to the protein away from the physiological binding site, then the affinity of transferrin for its receptor, which is expressed on mitogen-stimulated T4+ lymphocytes, will concentrate this iron first on to the surface of the cell and then within the cell as the receptor–transferrin complex is internalized. This may contribute to a toxic effect particularly directed at T4+ cells even at low concentrations of iron-saturated transferrin. There remains the observation that medium conditioned by suppressor T8+ lymphocytes contains a factor which inhibits GM-CSF production by stimulated inducer T4+lymphocytes and that this inhibitory factor can be blocked by a specific antibody against transferrin. Since suppressor T8+ lymphocytes do not appear to synthesize transferrin, the data might suggest that the suppressive factor released by these cells shares an epitope with transferrin. However, such interesting speculation must be treated with considerable caution, as the experimental data show that incubating mononuclear cells in the presence of antibody to transferrin did not in fact increase GM-CSF production (Broxmeyer, Lu and Bognacki, 1983).

FERRITIN

One of the characteristics of leukaemia is the overgrowth of normal bone marrow by the leukaemic clone. Co-culture experiments suggest that the leukaemic cells actively suppress normal progenitor cells (Morris, McNeill and Bridges, 1975). Two high molecular weight inhibitors have been identified from leukaemic blasts, named, confusingly, leukaemia associated inhibitor (LAI) and leukaemia cell-derived inhibitory activity (LIA). Both of these factors have been shown to suppress growth of normal progenitor cells in the S-phase but cells from patients with acute and chronic myeloid leukaemia are in general resistant, so providing an explanation for the proliferative advantage of leukaemic cells and failure of normal granulopoiesis. While both factors appear to act in the same way and both have apparent molecular weights of greater than 500000, it is suggested that they are, in fact, different. LAI has been characterized as a subunit of a larger protein and appears to be a glycoprotein present in the peripheral cell membrane (Olofsson and Olsson, 1980a, 1980b). LIA, on the other hand, is claimed to be acidic isoferritin and has been renamed acidic isoferritin inhibitory activity or AIFIA.

LIA was originally obtained in crude extracts of cells from patients suffering from a variety of malignant conditions, including acute and chronic myeloid and lymphatic leukaemia, myelodysplasia and involvement of the bone marrow by high-grade non-Hodgkin's lymphoma. In spite of these disparate sources it appears to have a uniform action of inhibiting CFU in S-phase and, unlike lactoferrin, does not affect colony-stimulating activity production. Extracts from normal haematopoietic cells did not contain inhibitory activity (Broxmeyer *et al.*, 1978b). Progenitor cells from the same variety of conditions and from patients with acute leukaemia in remission were resistant to the action of LIA (Broxmeyer *et al.*, 1978a). The evidence that LIA is acidic isoferritin included the finding of LIA in preparations of ferritin from various sources, demonstration that LIA is composed almost entirely of acidic isoferritin by immunoassay, inactivation of inhibitory activity by antisera which appear to be specific for acidic isoferritin, and the correspondence of molecular weight (550 000) and p*I* value (4.7). LIA also showed features of a glycoprotein, as it bound to concanavalin A-sepharose and was eluted by α-methyl mannose. One striking finding was the titration of the inhibitory activity of partially purified acidic isoferritin, which was active down to concentrations of only

10^{-17} or 10^{-18} M. Activity did not depend upon iron binding (Broxmeyer et al., 1981). The finding of acidic isoferritin inhibitory activity in normal heart, spleen, liver and placenta suggested that it might be involved in normal regulation of granulopoiesis as well as being associated with leukaemia. By the use of antisera against acidic isoferritin, inhibitory activity was demonstrated in medium conditioned by cells of the mononuclear phagocyte lineage (Broxmeyer et al., 1982). The amount of acidic isoferritin inhibitory activity produced by the monocyte–macrophage cells is increased by stimulatory agents, including CSF. Since the production of CSF is inhibited by lactoferrin, there appears to be an inverse relationship between the two inhibitors. Lactoferrin reduces CSF production, which has the secondary effect of reducing acidic isoferritin production (Broxmeyer et al., 1985). The production of acidic isoferritin inhibitory activity from monocytes is also modulated by T lymphocyte subpopulations; the suppressor T8+ subset suppresses AIFIA activity, and the inducer T4+ subset enhances release of this activity. Furthermore this modulation appears to be restricted genetically by HLA-DR antigens (Broxmeyer et al., 1984a). MHC class 2 antigens are also important on the target progenitor cells, as it is during S-phase of the cell cycle that CFU-GM express Ia-like antigens and it is the cells expressing these antigens that are sensitive to regulation by acidic isoferritin (Broxmeyer, 1982). This may provide the explanation for the lack of sensitivity of leukaemic progenitor cells to the action of acidic isoferritin, as the density of these antigens on the cell surface may be insufficient (Piacibello, Rubin and Broxmeyer, 1986). Finally the *in vivo* importance of acidic isoferritin has been suggested by its dampening effect upon rebound myelopoiesis when injected in microgram quantities into mice recovering from sublethal doses of cyclophosphamide in the same way as previously described for lactoferrin and transferrin (Broxmeyer et al., 1984b).

There has been, however, some criticism of the data published by Broxmeyer and his colleagues over the last few years. There is no doubt that crude extracts of leukaemic cells contain large molecular weight inhibitors of normal progenitor cells, and leukaemic progenitor cells are relatively resistant to their action (Olofsson and Olsson, 1980a; Taetle, 1981; Stryckmans et al., 1984). The doubt centres around the role of acidic isoferritins and whether these can function as normal regulators of haemopoiesis. Jacobs (1983) pointed out that Broxmeyer's description of acidic isoferritin appeared to include characteristics of both the H subunit-rich tissue ferritins and the glycosylated plasma ferritin. Jacobs and his colleagues tried to reproduce Broxmeyer's results using purified well-characterized isoferritins, but were unable to obtain consistent inhibitory activity with heart (acidic), spleen (basic), or serum (glycosylated) isoferritins on CFU-GM colony formation *in vitro* (Sala, Worwood and Jacobs,

1986). Using crude cell extracts and conditioned medium, inhibitory activity could not be related to the presence of acidic isoferritins nor could inhibitory activity be blocked by a monoclonal antibody to acidic isoferritins. Re-examination of preparations of 'acidic isoferritin' from the spleen of a patient with chronic myeloid leukaemia and from a normal heart, which had previously shown potent inhibitory activity, revealed that they contained very much less ferritin than previously claimed, and the ferritin was not predominantly the acidic form (Sala, Worwood and Jacobs, 1986). On the other hand, Dezza *et al*. (1986) have confirmed that some preparations of ferritin enriched for glycosylated acidic isoferritins do inhibit growth of normal CFU-GM (see Chapter 9).

The present position seems to be that the leukaemic cells and cells of the monocyte–macrophage lineage release high molecular weight glycoproteins *in vitro* which inhibit growth of normal myelopoietic progenitor cells in the S-phase of the cell cycle, possibly by interaction with Ia-like antigens. Whether this has any physiological significance is not clear, nor is the possible role of acidic isoferritin, particularly as normal progenitor cells themselves release significant quantities of acidic isoferritins when cultured *in vitro* (Sala, Worwood and Jacobs, 1986).

REFERENCES

Ambruso, D. R., and Johnston, R. B. (1981). Lactoferrin enhances hydroxyl radical production by human neutrophils, neutrophil particulate fractions and an enzymatic generating system, *J. Clin. Invest.*, **67**, 352–60.

Aune, T. M., and Pierce, C. W. (1981). Conversion of soluble immune response suppressor to macrophage-derived suppressor factor by peroxide, *Proc. Natl Acad. Sci. USA*, **78**, 5099–103.

Bagby, G. C. Jr, McCall, E., and Layman, D. L. (1983). Regulation of colony stimulating activity production. Interactions of fibroblasts, mononuclear phagocytes and lactoferrin, *J. Clin. Invest.*, **71**, 340–4.

Bagby, G. C. Jr, Rigas, V. D., Bennett, R. M., Vandenbark, A. A., and Garewal, H. S. (1981). Interaction of lactoferrin, monocytes and T-lymphocyte subsets in the regulation of steady state granulopoiesis in vitro, *J. Clin. Invest.*, **68**, 56–63.

Bagby, G. C. Jr, Bennett, R. M., Wilkinson, B., and Davis, J. (1982). Feedback regulation of granulopoiesis: Polymerisation of lactoferrin abrogates its ability to inhibit CSA production, *Blood*, **60**, 108–12.

Bagby, G. C. Jr, McCall, E., Bergstrom, K. A., and Burger, D. (1983). A monokine regulates colony-stimulating activity production by vascular endothelial cells, *Blood*, **62**, 662–8.

Bagby, G. C. Jr, Dinarello, C. A., Wallace, P., Wagner, C., Hefeneider, S., and McCall, E. (1986). Interleukin 1 stimulates granulocyte macrophage colony-stimulating activity release by vascular endothelial cells, *J. Clin. Invest.*, **78**, 1316–23.

Baker, F. L., Broxmeyer, H. E., and Galbraith, P. R. (1975). Control of granulopoiesis in man. III. Inhibition of colony formation by dense leukocytes, *J. Cell. Physiol.*, **86**, 337–42.

Bates, G. W., and Schlabach, M. R. (1973). The reaction of ferric salts with transferrin, *J. Biol. Chem.*, **248**, 3228–32.

Baynes, R. D., Bezwoda, W. R., Khan, Q., and Mansoor, N. (1986a). Relationship of plasma lactoferrin content to neutrophil regeneration and bone marrow infusion. *Scand. J. Haematol.*, **36**, 79–84.

Baynes, R. D., Bezwoda, W. R., Khan, Q., and Mansoor, N. (1986b). Plasma lactoferrin content: differential effect of steroid administration and infective illnesses: lack of effect of ambient temperature at which specimens are collected, *Scand. J. Haematol.*, **37**, 353–9.

Bennett, R. M., and Davis, J. (1981). Lactoferrin binding to human peripheral blood cells: an interaction with a B-enriched population of lymphocytes and a subpopulation of adherent mononuclear cells, *J. Immunol.*, **127**, 1211–16.

Bennett, R. M., and Kokocinski, T. (1979). Lactoferrin turnover in man, *Clin. Sci.*, **57**, 453–60.

Bennett, R. M., Merritt, M. M., and Gabor, G. (1986). Lactoferrin binds to neutrophilic membrane DNA, *Br. J. Haematol.*, **63**, 105–17.

Bennett, R. M., and Mohla, C. (1976). A solid phase radioimmunoassay for the measurement of lactoferrin in human plasma: variations with age, sex and disease, *J. Lab. Clin. Med.*, **88**, 156–66.

Biemond, P., Van Eijk, H. G., Swaak, J. G., and Koster, J. F. (1984). Iron mobilisation from ferritin by superoxide derived from stimulated polymorphonuclear leucocytes, *J. Clin. Invest.*, **73**, 1576–9.

Birgens, H. S., Hansen, N. E., and Karle, H. (1983). Receptor binding of lactoferrin by human monocytes, *Br. J. Haematol.*, **54**, 383–91.

Boxer, L. A., Coates, T. D., Haak, R. A., Wolach, J. B., Hoffstein, S., and Baehner, R. L. (1982a). Lactoferrin deficiency associated with altered granulocyte function, *N. Engl. J. Med.*, **307**, 404–10.

Boxer, L. A., Haak, R. A., Yang, H. H., Wolack, J. B., Whitcomb, J. A., Butterick, C. J., and Baehner, R. L. (1982b). Membrane bound lactoferrin alters surface properties of polymorphonuclear leukocytes, *J. Clin. Invest.*, **70**, 1047–9.

Breton-Gorius, J., Mason, D. Y., Buriot, D., Vilde, J. L., and Griscelli, C. (1980). Lactoferrin deficiency as a consequence of a lack of specific granules in neutrophils from a patient with recurrent infections, *Am. J. Pathol.*, **99**, 413–28.

Brock, J. H. (1981). The effect of iron and transferrin on the response of serum-free cultures of mouse lymphocytes to concanavalin A and lipopolysaccharide, *Immunology*, **43**, 387–92.

Brown, R. D., Yuen, E., Rickard, K. A., Vincent, P. C., Young G., and Kronenberg, H. (1986). Plasma lactoferrin in patients with neutropenia, *Blut*, **52**, 289–95.

Broxmeyer, H. E. (1978). Inhibition in vivo of mouse granulopoiesis by cell-free activity derived from human polymorphonuclear neutrophils, *Blood*, **51**, 889–901.

Broxmeyer, H. E. (1979). Lactoferrin acts on Ia-like antigen positive subpopulations of human monocytes to inhibit production of colony stimulatory activity in vitro, *J. Clin. Invest.*, **64**, 1717–24.

Broxmeyer, H. E. (1982). Relationship of cell-cycle expression of Ia-like antigenic determinants on normal and leukaemic human granulocyte–macrophage progenitor cells to regulation by acidic isoferritins, *J. Clin. Invest.*, **69**, 632–42.

Broxmeyer, H. E., Lu, L., and Bognacki, J. (1983). Transferrin derived from OKT8+ subpopulation of T lymphocytes suppresses the production of granulocyte macrophage colony stimulating factors from mitogen-activated T lymphocytes, *Blood*, **62**, 37–50.

Broxmeyer, H. E., Mendelsohn, N., and Moore, M. A. S. (1977). Abnormal granulocyte feedback regulation of colony forming and colony stimulatory activity—producing cells from patients with chronic myelogenous leukaemia, *Leuk. Res.*, **1**, 3–12.

Broxmeyer, H. E., Moore, M. A. S., and Ralph, P. (1977). Cell-free granulocyte colony inhibitory activity derived from human polymorphonuclear neutrophils, *Exp. Hematol.*, **5**, 87–102.

Broxmeyer, H. E., and Platzer, E. (1984). Lactoferrin acts on I-A and I-E/C antigen[+] subpopulations of mouse peritoneal macrophages in the absence of T lymphocytes and other cell types to inhibit production of granulocyte–macrophage colony stimulatory factors in vitro, *J. Immunol.*, **133**, 306–14.

Broxmeyer, H. E., Smithyman, A., Eger, R. R., Meyers, P. A., and de Sousa, M. (1978a). Identification of lactoferrin as the granulocyte-derived inhibitor of colony-stimulatory activity production, *J. Exp. Med.*, **148**, 1052–67.

Broxmeyer, H. E., Jacobsen, N., Kurland, J., Mendelsohn, N., and Moore, M. A. S. (1978b). 'In vitro' suppression of normal granulocytic stem cells by inhibitory activity derived from human leukaemia cells, *J. Natl Cancer Inst.*, **60**, 497–511.

Broxmeyer, H. E., Grossbard, E., Jacobsen, N., and Moore, M. A. S. (1978c). Evidence for a proliferative advantage of human leukaemia colony-forming cells in vitro, *J. Natl Cancer Inst.*, **60**, 513–21.

Broxmeyer, H. E., Ralph, P., Bognacki, J., Kincade, P. W., and de Sousa, M. (1980). A subpopulation of human polymorphonuclear neutrophils contains an active form of lactoferrin capable of binding to human monocytes and inhibiting production of granulocyte–macrophage colony stimulatory activities, *J. Immunol.*, **125**, 903–9.

Broxmeyer, H. E., Bognacki, J., Dörner, M. H., and de Sousa, M. (1981). Identification of leukaemia-associated inhibitory activity as acidic isoferritins, *J. Exp. Med.*, **153**, 1426–44.

Broxmeyer, H. E., Bognacki, J., Ralph, P., Dörner, M. H., Lu, L., and Castro-Malaspina, H. (1982). Monocyte–macrophage derived acidic isoferritins. Normal feedback regulation of granulocyte–macrophage progenitor cells in vitro, *Blood*, **60**, 595–607.

Broxmeyer, H. E., Gentile, P., Bognacki, J., and Ralph, P. (1983). Lactoferrin, transferrin and acidic isoferritins: Regulatory molecules with potential therapeutic value in leukaemia, *Blood Cells*, **9**, 83–105.

Broxmeyer, H. E., Juliano, L., Lu, L., Platzer, E., and Dupont, B. (1984). HLA-DR Human histocompatibility leukocyte antigens—restricted lymphocyte–monocyte interactions in the release from monocytes of acidic isoferritins that suppress haematopoietic progenitor cells, *J. Clin. Invest.*, **73**, 939–53.

Broxmeyer, H. E., Gentile, P., Cooper, S., Lu, L., Juliano, L., Piacibello, W., Meyers, P. A., and Cavanna, F. (1984b). Functional activities of isoferritins and lactoferrin 'in vitro' and 'in vivo', *Blood Cells*, **10**, 397–426.

Broxmeyer, H. E., Juliano, L., Waheed, A., and Shadduck, R. K. (1985). Release from mouse macrophages of acidic isoferritins that suppress haematopoietic progenitor cells is induced by purified L cell colony stimulating factor and suppressed by human lactoferrin, *J. Immunol.*, **135**, 3224–31.

Broxmeyer, H. E., Rubin, B. Y., Berman, E., Juliano, L., Lu, L., Hast, L. J., Cooper, S., and Singer, J. W. (1987). Activities derived from established human myeloid cell lines reverse the suppression of cell line colony formation by lactoferrin and transferrin, *Exp. Hematol.*, **14**, 51–9.

Bullen, J. J. (1981). The significance of iron in infection. *Rev. Infect. Dis.*, **3**, 1127–40.

Burgess, A. W., and Metcalf, D. (1980). The nature and action of granulocyte–macrophage colony stimulating factors, *Blood*, **56**, 947–58.

Campbell, E. J. (1982). Human leucocyte elastase, cathepsin G and lactoferrin: family of neutrophil granule glycoproteins that bind to an alveolar macrophage receptor, *Proc. Natl Acad. Sci. USA*, **79**, 6941–5.

De Sousa, M. (1978). Lymphoid cell positioning: a new proposal for the mechanism of control of lymphoid cell migration, *Symp. Soc. Exp. Biol.*, **32**, 393–409.

Dezza, L., Cazzola, M., Piacibello, W., Arosio, P., Levi, S., and Aglietta, M. (1986). Effect of acidic and basic isoferritins on *in vitro* growth of human granulocyte–monocyte progenitors, *Blood*, **67**, 789–95.

Duncan, R. L., and McArthur, W. P. (1981). Lactoferrin-mediated modulation of mononuclear cell activities. Suppression of murine in-vitro primary antibody response, *Cell. Immunol.*, **63**, 308–20.

El-Maallem, H., and Fletcher, J. (1976). Defective neutrophil function in chronic granulocytic leukaemia, *Br. J. Haematol.*, **34**, 95–103.

El-Maallem, H., and Fletcher, J. (1979). Defective hydrogen peroxide production in chronic granulocytic leukaemia neutrophils, *Br. J. Haematol.*, **41**, 49–55.

Fletcher, J., and Willars, J. (1986). The role of lactoferrin released by phagocytosing neutrophils in the regulation of colony stimulating activity production by human mononuclear cells, *Blood Cells*, **11**, 447–54.

Gallin, J. I., Fletcher, M. P., Seligmann, B. E., Hoffstein, S., Cehrs, K., and Mounessa, N. (1982). Human neutrophil-specific granule deficiency: A model to assess the role of neutrophil-specific granules in the evaluation of the inflammatory response, *Blood*, **59**, 1317–29.

Gentile, P., and Broxmeyer, H. E. (1983). Suppression of mouse myelopoiesis by administration of human lactoferrin in vivo and the comparative action of human transferrin, *Blood*, **61**, 982–93.

Gutteridge, J. M. C., Paterson, S. K., Segal, A. W., and Halliwell, B. (1981). Inhibition of lipid peroxidation by the iron-binding protein lactoferrin, *Biochem. J.*, **199**, 259–61.

Hansen, N. E., Karle, H., Andersen, V., Malmquist, J., and Hoff, G. E. (1976). Neutrophilic granulocytes in acute bacterial infection. Sequential studies on lysozyme, myeloperoxidase and lactoferrin, *Clin. Exp. Immunol.*, **26**, 463–8.

Hekman, A. (1971). Association of lactoferrin with other proteins as demonstrated by changes in electrophoretic mobility, *Biochim. Biophys. Acta*, **251**, 380–5.

Herman, S. P., Golde, D. W., and Cline, M. J. (1978). Neutrophil products that inhibit cell proliferation: relation to granulocyte 'Chalone', *Blood*, **51**, 207–19.

Jacobs, A. (1983). Do acidic isoferritins regulate haemopoiesis? *Br. J. Haematol.*, **55**, 199–202.

Klempner, M. S., Dinarello, C. A., and Gallin, J. I. (1978). Human leukocyte pyrogen induces release of specific granule contents from human neutrophils, *J. Clin. Invest.*, **61**, 1330–6.

Larrick, J. W., Graham, D., Toy, K., Lin, L. S., Senyk, G., and Findly, B. M. (1987). Recombinant tumour necrosis factor causes activation of human granulocytes, *Blood*, **69**, 640–4.

Lu, L., Bicknell, D. C., Piacibello, W., and Broxmeyer, H. E. (1986). Purified human transferrin and 'transferrin' released from sorted T8+ lymphocytes suppress release of granulocyte–macrophage colony stimulatory factors from sorted T4+ lymphocytes stimulated by phytohaemagglutinin, *Exp. Hematol.*, **14**, 955–62.

Lum, J. B., Infante, A. J., Makker, D. M., Yang, F., and Bowman, B. H. (1986). Transferrin synthesis by inducer T lymphocytes, *J. Clin. Invest.*, **77**, 841–9.

Maallem, H., Sheppard, K., and Fletcher, J. (1982). The discharge of primary and secondary granules during immune phagocytosis by normal and chronic granulocytic leukaemia polymorphonuclear neutrophils, *Br. J. Haematol.*, **51**, 201–8.

Moguilevsky, N., Retegui, L. A., and Masson, P. L. (1985). Comparison of human lactoferrins from milk and neutrophilic leucocytes, *Biochem. J.*, **229**, 353–9.

Moore, R. N., Oppenheim, J. S., Farrar, J. J., Carter, C. S., Waheed, A., and Shadduck, R. K. (1980). Production of lymphocyte-activating factor (interleukin 1) by macrophages activated with colony stimulating factors, *J. Immunol.*, **125**, 1302–5.

Morris, T. C., McNeill, T. A., and Bridges, J. M. (1975). Inhibition of normal 'in vitro' colony-forming cells from leukaemic patients, *Br. J. Cancer*, **31**, 641–7.

Nishiya, K., and Horwitz, P. A. (1982). Contrasting effects of lactoferrin on human lymphocyte and monocyte natural killer activity and antibody-dependent cell-mediated cytotoxicity, *J. Immunol.*, **129**, 2519–23.

Olofsson, T., and Olsson, I. (1980a). Suppression of normal granulopoiesis 'in vitro' by a leukaemia-associated inhibitor (LAI) of acute and chronic leukaemia, *Blood*, **55**, 975–82.

Olofsson, T., and Olsson, I. (1980b). Biochemical characterisation of leukaemia associated inhibitor (LAI) suppressing normal granulopoiesis 'in vitro', *Blood*, **55**, 983–91.

Olofsson, T., Olsson, I., and Venge, P. (1977). Myeloperoxidase and lactoferrin of blood neutrophils and plasma in chronic granulocytic leukaemia, *Scand. J. Haematol.*, **18**, 113–20.

Paran, M., Ichikawa, Y., and Sachs, L. (1969). Feedback inhibition of the development of macrophage and granulocyte colonies. II. Inhibition by granulocytes, *Proc. Natl Acad. Sci. USA*, **62**, 81–7.

Philip, M. A., Standen, G., and Fletcher, J. (1981). Failure of chronic-granulocytic-leukaemia leucocytes to release an inhibitor of granulopoiesis, *Lancet*, **i**, 866–8.

Philip, M. A., Standen, G., and Fletcher, J. (1982). Phagocytosing neutrophils rapidly release a factor which inhibits granulopoiesis in vitro, *Acta Haematol.*, **67**, 20–26.

Piacibello, W., Rubin, B. Y., and Broxmeyer, H. E. (1986). Prostaglandin E counteracts the gamma interferon induction of major histocompatibility complex class 2 antigens on U937 colony-forming cells to suppression by lactoferrin, transferrin, acidic isoferritins and prostaglandin E, *Exp. Hematol.*, **14**, 44–50.

Retegui, L. A., Moguilevsky, N., Castracane, C. F., and Masson, P. L. (1984). Uptake of lactoferrin by the liver. 1. Role of the reticuloendothelial system as indicated by blockade experiments, *Lab. Invest.*, **50**, 323–8.

Rule, S. A. J., Knights, S. G., and Fletcher, J. (1986). Defective release of hydrogen peroxide and myeloperoxidase by chronic granulocytic leukaemia neutrophils, *Eur. J. Clin. Invest.*, **16**, 49.

Sala, G., Worwood, M., and Jacobs, A. (1986). The effect of isoferritins on granulopoiesis, *Blood*, **67**, 436–43.

Seiff, C. A., Tsai, S., and Faller, D. V. (1987). Interleukin-1 induces cultured human endothelial cell production of granulocyte–macrophage colony stimulatory factor, *J. Clin. Invest.*, **79**, 48–51.

Shtivelman, E., Lifshitz, B., Gale, R. P., and Canaani, E. (1985). Fused transcript of abl and bcr genes in chronic myelogenous leukaemia, *Nature*, **315**, 550–4.

Slater, K., and Fletcher, J. (1987a). Lactoferrin derived from neutrophils inhibits the mixed lymphocyte reaction, *Blood*, **69**, 1328–33.

Slater, K., and Fletcher, J. (1987b). Lactoferrin inhibits interleukin-2 production in mixed lymphocyte culture. In A. Najman, M. Guigon *et al.* (eds) *The Inhibitors of Haematopoiesis*, Vol. 162, pp. 67–8, Colloque Inserm/John Libby Eurotext Ltd.

Stryckmans, P., Delforge, A., Amson, R. B., Prieels, J. P., Telerman, A., Bieva, C., Deschuyteneer, M., and Ronge-Collard, E. (1984). Lactoferrin: No evidence for its role in regulation of C.S.A. production by human lymphocytes and monocytes, *Blood Cells*, **10**, 369–95.

Taetle, R. (1981). Acidic isoferritins (leukaemia asociated inhibitory activity) fail to inhibit blast proliferation in acute myelogenous leukaemia, *Blood*, **58**, 653–7.

Taetle, R., and Honeysett, J. M. (1986). Transferrin modulation of colony stimulating factor elaboration by adherent blood and bone marrow cells, *Br. J. Haematol.*, **62**, 163–70.

Van Snick, J. L., Markowitz, B., and Masson, P. L. (1977). The ingestion and digestion of human lactoferrin by mouse peritoneal macrophages and the transfer of its iron into ferritin, *J. Exp. Med.*, **146**, 817–27.

Van Snick, J. L., and Masson, P. L. (1976). The binding of human lactoferrin to mouse peritoneal cells, *J. Exp. Med.*, **144**, 1568–80.

Weisbart, R. H., Golde, D. W., Clark, S. C., Wong, G. G., and Gasson, J. C. (1985). Human granulocyte–macrophage colony-stimulatory factor is a neutrophil activator, *Nature*, **314**, 361–3.

Winton, E. F., Kinkade, J. M., Vogler, W. R., Parker, M. B., and Barnes, K. C. (1981). In vitro studies of lactoferrin and granulopoiesis, *Blood*, **57**, 574–8.

Part IV

The Immunology of Iron Overload

Iron in Immunity, Cancer and Inflammation
Edited by M. de Sousa and J. H. Brock
© 1989 John Wiley & Sons Ltd.

11

The Immunology of Iron Overload

Maria de Sousa
Abel Salazar Institute for the Biomedical Sciences, Oporto, Portugal

INTRODUCTION

Interest in the study of immunological function in clinical conditions of iron overload appears to have developed first from the early observation of an increased susceptibility to infections in splenectomized patients with iron overload due to thalassaemia major (Caroline *et al.*, 1969) and, later, from the demonstration that *in vitro* iron had a modulating effect on the expression of some human lymphoid cell surface markers (de Sousa and Nishiya, 1978; Nishiya *et al.*, 1980) and immunological functions (Keown and Descamps, 1978; Bryan *et al.*, 1981) and that, in the mouse, it influenced lymphocyte distribution (de Sousa, 1978). Studies motivated by the interest in infection focused on macrophages and polymorphonuclear neutrophils (PMNs) (Khan *et al.*, 1977; van Asbeck *et al.*, 1982, 1984; Khalifa *et al.*, 1983; Martino *et al.*, 1984; Flament *et al.*, 1986; Ballart *et al.*, 1986); studies motivated by the recognition of the immunoregulatory actions of iron concentrated on the quantification of lymphoid cell sets (Kapadia *et al.*, 1980; Guglielmo *et al.*, 1984; Bryan *et al.*, 1984; Ballart *et al.*, 1986; Grady *et al.*, 1985; Akbar *et al.*, 1985; Goicoa *et al.*, 1986; Dwyer *et al.*, 1987; Pardalos *et al.*, 1987) and on different immunological functions, namely, mitogen responses (Munn *et al.*, 1981; Dwyer *et al.*, 1987), B cell differentiation (Akbar *et al.*, 1985; Nualart *et al.*, 1987), natural killer (NK) activity (Neri *et al.*, 1984; Akbar *et al.*, 1986, 1988) and the mixed lymphocyte reaction (MLR) (Dwyer *et al.*, 1987).

Although the majority of the studies cited above have been done with peripheral blood cells from patients with β-thalassaemia, a few have been carried out in idiopathic haemochromatosis, in haemodialysis patients and in experimental animal models of iron overload (Good *et al.*, 1987; de Sousa *et al.*, 1988). From the results of the *in vivo* studies and the results of many of the experiments done *in vitro* (reviewed in Chapter 5), a consensus can perhaps be reached concerning the delineation of an 'immunology of iron overload'; some uncertainties remain, however, which will be discussed.

NATURAL KILLER ACTIVITY

The observation of diminished NK activity has been reported in patients with β-thalassaemia major (Neri *et al.*, 1984; Goicoa *et al.*, 1986; Akbar *et al.*, 1986, 1988). This observation has been attributed to an effect of iron overload, because in one study it was shown that pretreatment of effector but not of target cells with desferrioxamine resulted in the recovery of NK activity of the patients' cells (Akbar *et al.*, 1986). Moreover, unpublished data of Cunningham-Rundles and her coworkers, following up the changes in NK activity of peripheral blood cells from patients receiving an intravenous infusion of desferrioxamine at various times before and after the infusion, also indicate that in some cases the iron-chelating therapy results in recovery of NK activity *in vivo*. In a study of NK activity in patients with idiopathic haemochromatosis, Good, Powell and Halliday (1988) could not find any alteration of that function, nor could they reproduce *in vitro* an inhibitory action of iron, concluding that the diminished NK activity reported by others in β-thalassaemia is probably a result of the effect of the multiple blood transfusions received by these patients (Kaplan *et al.*, 1984).

CELL SURFACE ANTIGENS

Thermostable E-rosette-forming lymphocytes in idiopathic haemochromatosis (IH)

In a study of IH patients, Bryan *et al.* (1984) reported that the numbers of peripheral blood lymphocytes making thermostable erythrocyte rosettes were significantly higher than that seen in controls. A value was considered significantly increased if it was greater than two standard deviations above the mean percentage control value (22%). Applying this criterion, 81% of the patients studied had abnormally high numbers of thermostable E-rosettes. Analysis of other cell surface markers, immunoglobulin levels and mitogen responses to phytohaemagglutinin (PHA), concanavalin A and pokeweed mitogen (PWM) all seemed to be normal. We have recently re-examined the question of the thermostable E-rosette-forming cell in IH patients and have failed to confirm the earlier results of Bryan *et al*. In a study of sixteen patients the average percentage of this type of cell was indeed high (54.9 ± 9.7) but not different from the control population studied (55.3 ± 8.8) (Reimão, Porto and de Sousa, unpublished data).

Circulating T6+ cells in patients with β-thalassaemia intermedia

One other abnormality observed in patients with iron overload uncomplicated by multiple blood transfusions has been reported by Guglielmo and coworkers in a study of fourteen patients with thalassaemia intermedia (Guglielmo et al., 1984). In addition to the finding of the 'consensus abnormality' (see below) of low percentages of T4+ cells, they have noted significantly higher proportions of circulating T6+ cells (5–15%) in the patient group than in the control group, where T6+ cells were almost absent. In vitro incubation of peripheral blood mononuclear cells from the patients with a crude thymic extract for 48 hours resulted in the return to the normal representation of the different T cell differentiation antigens, i.e. increase in the percentage of T4+ cells and absence of T6+ lymphocytes. These observations led the authors to conclude that in thalassaemia intermedia there may be a thymus-dependent anomaly of T cell maturation. This conclusion and the interesting observations upon which it is based have not been followed up by other groups.

Diminished proportions of T4+ lymphocytes

Our early study of T lymphoid cell subsets, which was done at a time when monoclonal antibodies against T cell surface differentiation antigens were not yet widely available, reported for the first time the finding of abnormal proportions of T cell subsets in patients with thalassaemia intermedia (Kapadia et al., 1980). The most consistent observation relating iron overload and lymphoid cell subsets concerns the finding of abnormally low numbers and functionally defective T4+ cells. This finding has been reported in thalassaemia intermedia (Guglielmo et al., 1984), in thalassaemia major (Grady et al., 1985; Dwyer et al., 1987; Pardalos et al., 1987) and in vitro (Bryan, Leech and Bozelka, 1986). In addition, ferric citrate has been shown to diminish the cloning efficiency of human memory T4+ lymphocytes (Good et al., 1986); spleen cells from iron-overloaded mice seem to lack precursor L3T4+ cells and fail to generate an allospecific cytotoxic response in the absence of interleukin-2 (Good et al., 1987).

Further evidence for the presence of a defective T helper cell population in thalassaemia major derives from a study of the cellular components involved in the defective generation of immunoglobulin-producing cells in culture in response to stimulation by PWM (Nualart et al., 1987). Comparing co-cultures of patients' T cells and control non-T cells, Nualart et al.

(1987) provided evidence indicating that the impaired response was attributable to a defective T helper cell population and not to the non-T cell population.

In an immunocytochemical study of the changes in rat synovium T cell subsets following a transient iron overload provoked by a single intravenous injection of ferric citrate (which caused a transient increase in the transferrin saturation above 100%), we found a relatively higher increase in the ingress of W3/25+ than OX8+ cells in the synovium at 24 hours after the injection (de Sousa *et al.*, 1988). This transient overload contrasts with the marked tissue overload provoked in Good's experiments in the mouse, in which the animals received three intraperitoneal injections of iron dextran over 2 weeks or had 0.5% carbonyl iron added to their diet for a period of 3–4 weeks (Good *et al.*, 1987). Nevertheless, the transient overload experiments illustrate and reinforce the apparent 'specific' response of the helper inducer T cell set to changes in serum iron concentration. The mechanism whereby this could occur remains unclear. The demonstration by Lum *et al.* (1986) that activated T4+ and not T8+ cells synthesize transferrin may provide a speculative basis for designing further experiments to clarify the apparent particular sensitivity of the T4+ subset to iron.

Increased proportions of T8+ cells

Increases in the numbers of T8+ cells have been reported in patients with thalassaemia major, whether splenectomized or not (Grady *et al.*, 1985; Dwyer *et al.*, 1987). Statistically significant correlations were observed between the increasing number of blood transfusions received and the proportions of T8+ cells (Grady *et al.*, 1985). It is therefore difficult to be sure that iron overload alone is responsible for this result. Dwyer *et al.*, in a careful statistical analysis of all the variables involved, i.e. age, splenectomy, number of transfusions and amount of desferrioxamine received, observed a negative correlation between the amount of desferrioxamine received and the numbers of T8+ cells present (Dwyer *et al.*, 1987). This observation thus constitutes an indirect piece of evidence in favour of iron overload influencing expansion of the T8+ cell population *in vivo*.

MITOGEN RESPONSES

Studies of the peripheral blood mononuclear blood cell responses to nonspecific mitogens have been done in patients with β-thalassaemia intermedia and β-thalassaemia major. Decreased responses to PHA were reported in the thalassaemia intermedia patients with iron levels of

> 200 μg dl^{-1} and serum ferritins > 600 ng ml^{-1} (Munn *et al.*, 1981) and in the thalassaemia major group (Dwyer *et al.*, 1987). Pretreatment of responding cells from normal donors with ferric citrate *in vitro* led to variable results, depending on the mitogen and dose of mitogen used (Munn *et al.*, 1981); inhibition was observed with the lowest doses of PHA (1.5 μg ml^{-1} and 3 μg ml^{-1}), enhancement with the highest doses of concanavalin A (29 μg ml^{-1} and 57 μg ml^{-1}) and no effect with all doses of PWM tested. Unaltered responses to PWM were also seen in the thalassaemia intermedia patients, regardless of serum iron or serum ferritin levels (Munn *et al.*, 1981). The response to *C. albicans* antigens was tested in patients with β-thalassaemia major and found to correlate negatively with serum ferritin levels (Dwyer *et al.*, 1987).

HLA, THE MIXED LYMPHOCYTE REACTION AND FERRITIN SECRETION

Studies of the MLR in iron overload *in vivo* have been done in homozygote β-thalassaemia patients (Dwyer *et al.*, 1987); earlier, Keown and Descamps (1978) and Bryan *et al.* (1981) examined the effect of addition of ferric salts to MLR cultures of normal peripheral blood mononuclear cells. Both in thalassaemia major patients and *in vitro*, a diminished MLR was observed. In the *in vitro* studies, we were able to demonstrate that: (a) pretreatment of the effector, but not of the target, cells was necessary for the inhibitory effect to be observed; (b) there was an individual variation which could be related to the HLA-A locus. Thus, HLA-A2 donors appeared to be less sensitive to the inhibitory action of iron than non-HLA-A2 donors (Bryan *et al.*, 1981).

The observation that the individual variation in sensitivity to the inhibitory action of iron on the MLR could be related to HLA phenotype led us to consider whether a variation in ferritin secretion observed with PHA-activated peripheral blood mononuclear cells in the presence of ferric citrate could also be associated with HLA phenotype (de Sousa *et al.*, 1982). Studies of ferritin secretion measured by a modified indirect haemolytic plaque assay (Gronowicz, Coutinho and Melchers, 1976) of PHA-stimulated peripheral blood mononuclear cells from HLA phenotyped normal blood donors led to the demonstration that HLA-A3 subjects produced a smaller number of haemolytic plaques than non-HLA-A3 subjects (Martins da Silva *et al.*, 1982; Pollack *et al.*, 1983), signifying that control of ferritin secretion by activated cells seems to be associated with the major histocompatibility complex (MHC). The fact that low ferritin secretion after activation seemed to be controlled by the HLA-A locus and related particularly to the antigen A3, known to be the antigen most frequently represented in IH (Simon et al., 1987; see below), raised the question whether these observations could have some relevance to the understanding of the behaviour of the macrophage system in IH.

THE MACROPHAGE IN IDIOPATHIC HAEMOCHROMATOSIS

IH is an autosomal hereditary disease transmitted recessively, characterized by a failure of the still unknown mechanism(s) regulating the absorption of iron. As a consequence of this failure, serum and tissue iron overload develop, reflected biochemically in high serum iron and ferritin levels, transferrin saturation in some cases exceeding 100%, with demonstrable non-transferrin-bound serum iron and circulating low molecular weight iron complexes (Batey et al., 1980; Gutteridge et al., 1985). Clinically, the manifestations of the disease reflect the abnormal accumulation of iron in the liver (cirrhosis), pancreas (diabetes), heart, joints (arthropathies), skin (abnormal pigmentation), etc. (Sheldon, 1935; Jacobs, 1977; Powell, Bassett and Halliday, 1980). An important advance leading to the early detection of family cases came with the demonstration that the frequency of the HLA antigen A3 is significantly higher in IH patients than in controls (Simon et al., 1976) and that certain HLA haplotypes are more frequent in the disease group, namely, A3B7, A3B14, A11B35 and A11B5 (see Simon et al. (1987) for review). IH provides an almost exclusive 'experimental' model of iron overload, uncomplicated, from the immunological point of view, by the effects of multiple blood transfusion or splenectomy seen in β-thalassaemia. This raised the expectation that the observations made in transfusional iron overload thought to be attributable to iron would also be found in IH. Although sporadically there have been case reports of infection associated with IH iron overload (Abbott, Galloway and Cunningham, 1985; van Asbeck et al., 1982), in general infections do not constitute major clinical problems in this disease. As reviewed in the next section, the association of infection with iron overload seems to pass through the demonstrable presence of intracellular iron in PMNs and macrophages. Rather surprisingly, and in marked contrast to the heavy parenchymal iron overload, the amount of demonstrable intracellular iron in the macrophages in IH is minimal, until the late stages of the disease (Ross et al., 1975; Valberg et al., 1975; Brink et al., 1976).

This dichotomy between parenchymal iron overload and iron 'sparing' of the reticuloendothelial system is perhaps most striking in the liver, where heavy iron deposits are seen in the parenchymal cells and only 'inconspicuous' amounts of iron are seen in the Kupffer cells (Ross et al., 1975). The evidence indicating that the absence of demonstrable iron in macrophages is in itself abnormal can be derived from comparative studies of IH patients and patients subjected to a diet containing excessive quantities of absorbable iron (Brink et al., 1976). In a comparative study of South African black subjects and IH haemochromatosis patients, Brink et al. examined non-haem iron concentrations in bone marrow and liver. In the subjects with a dietary iron overload, statistically significant correlations were observed between the amounts of non-haem iron in both organs ($r = +0.84$, $p = 0.001$, $n = 66$); in the eight IH cases, however, higher amounts of iron were consistently measured in the liver than in the bone marrow or spleen (Brink et al., 1976). One other disease in which tissue iron overload due to dietary high iron intake has been documented is Kaschin–Beck's disease. This disease was described in remote communities of nine provinces of Manchoukuo (Hiyeda, 1939) in patients found among farmers, hunters and woodcutters, who drank well water unusually rich in iron (> 0.3 mg l^{-1}). The description of the pathology of this disease and its illustration provide clear evidence that there were substantial amounts of iron present in the splenic macrophages (Figure 5 from Hiyeda (1939)). Thus the absence of demonstrable iron in IH macrophages can be viewed as evidence of some underlying metabolic abnormality. Studies of ferritin synthesis by IH macrophages have failed to demonstrate any abnormality in the synthesis of this protein (Jacobs and Summers, 1981; Bassett, Halliday and Powell, 1982).

Fillet and Marsaglia (1975) in a study of the release of erythrocyte iron to plasma transferrin after tracing ^{59}Fe heat-damaged erythrocytes, did observe an iron-release kinetic pattern in nine IH patients with significant iron-binding capacity and normal iron stores, similar to that seen in iron deficiency. More recently, Saab et al. (1986), comparing monocyte ferritin content in controls, thalassaemia patients and IH patients, observed that in four IH patients the mean ferritin content (50 fg cell^{-1}), although higher than that seen in controls ($n = 18$, 26.7 fg cell^{-1}), was much lower than those seen in thalassaemia major patients with comparable serum ferritin levels (375 fg cell^{-1}). Discrepancies between results of various studies are not exclusive to ferritin metabolism; a normal uptake of transferrin iron of monocytes was reported by one group (Sizemore and Bassett, 1984) and expression of abnormally high numbers of transferrin receptors by others (Bjorn-Rasmussen et al., 1985), indicating, above all, that a great deal more work seems to be needed in this area.

PHAGOCYTIC CELLS IN OTHER SITUATIONS OF IRON OVERLOAD

While the macrophage in IH continues to elude scrutiny by those interested in defining significant functional interactions between the metabolism of iron and the lymphomyeloid system, studies of PMNs and macrophages in other clinical situations of iron overload have yielded more predictable results.

Impairment of phagocytosis has been observed in haemodialysis patients with iron overload related to multiple blood transfusions (Waterlot et al., 1985; Flament et al., 1986). Phagocytosis is accompanied by an activation of oxidative metabolism resulting in the production of the superoxide anion and hydrogen peroxide. In a study of superoxide anion release by PMNs from haemodialysis patients, Flament et al. (1986) found that without stimulation of PMNs there were no significant differences observed between patient and control cells. After stimulation with opsonized zymosan, however, PMNs from patients with ferritin levels higher than 1000 ng ml^{-1} produced significantly less superoxide anion than patients with lower levels of circulating serum ferritin (Flament et al., 1986). Diminished superoxide anion production has also been reported in patients with β-thalassaemia major when the PMNs were stimulated with zymosan (Martino et al., 1984). Resting neutrophils or neutrophils stimulated with phorbol myristate acetate (PMA) from the same patients had a significantly higher superoxide anion generation than controls. Further differences between resting neutrophils and neutrophils stimulated with PMA or zymosan were noted when the correlations between serum ferritin levels and superoxide anion production were analysed. A positive correlation between serum ferritin levels and superoxide anion production was only observed with resting PMNs (Martino et al., 1984).

In another study of PMN function in β-thalassaemia major, Cantinieaux et al. (1987) examined NBT reduction, heated yeast phagocytosis, E. coli phagocytosis, E. coli killing and intracellular PMN iron by the Perl's reaction. On average, 13% of PMNs were Perl's positive in the patient group. All phagocytosis tests were impaired in comparison with the control PMNs; there were no significant differences, however, between the reduction of NBT and the killing rate in the two groups. In this study, the effect of incubation of normal PMNs with thalassaemic serum was also investigated. After incubation of normal PMNs with thalassaemic serum, 9% of the cells became Perl's positive and an impairment of phagocytosis was observed (Cantinieaux et al., 1987).

In a separate study of the phagocytic capacity and lytic ability of peripheral blood monocytes from thalassaemia major patients to phagocytize and kill *Candida pseudotropicalis*, no abnormality of the phagocytic activity was found (Ballart et al., 1986). The patients' monocytes showed, however, a decreased lytic ability which was significantly lower than that observed with control monocytes. In this study a significant inverse correlation was noted between lytic activity and serum ferritin levels (Ballart et al., 1986).

In a study of phagocytosis of cells from patients with iron overload, Van

Asbeck *et al.* observed diminished phagocytosis of *S. aureus* by macrophages but not by PMNs (Van Asbeck *et al.*, 1982, 1984b).

CONCLUDING REMARKS

In general, the studies of immunological function in patients with iron overload represent a counterpart *in vivo* to the observations made in experiments examining the effect of iron salts on immunological functions and lymphoid cell markers *in vitro*. Some of the reported discrepancies between results in the natural killer studies and monocyte phagocytosis are probably the reflection of the different patient groups studied; other differences, observed by the same investigators in one group of patients, i.e. differences in superoxide anion generation after zymosan or PMA stimulation and differences in the proportions of distinct T cell subsets and lymphoid cell functions, provide additional evidence for considering iron as an important immunoregulator (Bryan, Leech and Bozelka, 1986).

ACKNOWLEDGEMENTS

I thank my colleague Coralia Vicente for her generous help in the final preparation of the text.

REFERENCES

Abbot, M., Galloway, A., and Cunningham, J. L. (1985). Haemochromatosis presenting with a double yersinia infection, *J. Infect.*, **13**, 143–5.

Akbar, A. N., Giardina, P. J., Hilgartner, M. W., and Grady, R. W. (1985). Immunological abnormalities in thalassemia major. I. A transfusion-related increase in circulating cytoplasmic immunoglobulin-positive cells, *Clin. Exp. Immunol.*, **62**, 397–404.

Akbar, A. N., Fitzgerald-Bocarsly, P. A., de Sousa, M., Giardina, P. J., Hilgartner, M. W., and Grady, R. W. (1986). Decreased natural killer activity in thalassemia major: a possible consequence of iron overload, *J. Immunol.*, **136**, 1635–40.

Akbar, A. N., Fitzgerald-Bocarsly, P. A., Giardina, P. J., Hilgartner, M. W., and Grady, R. W. (1987). Modulation of the defective natural killer activity seen in thalassaemia major with desferrioxamine and α-interferon, *Clin. Exp. Immunol.*, **70**, 345–53.

Ballart, I. J., Estevez, M. E., Sen, L., Diez, R. A., Giuntoli, J., de Miani, S. A., and Penalver, J. (1986). Progressive dysfunction of monocytes associated with iron overload and age in patients with thalassemia major, *Blood*, **67**, 105–9.

Bassett, M. L., Halliday, J. W., and Powell, L. W. (1982). Ferritin synthesis in peripheral blood monocytes in idiopathic hemochromatosis, *J. Lab. Clin. Med.*, **100**, 137–45.

Batey, R. G., Lai Chung Fong, P., Shamir, S., and Sherlock, S. (1980). A nontransferrin bound serum iron in idiopathic hemochromatosis, *Dig. Dis. Sci.*, **25**, 340–6.
Bjorn-Rasmussen, E., Hageman, J., van Den Dungen, P., Prowit-Ksiazek, A., and Biberfeld, P. (1985). Transferrin receptors on circulating monocytes in hereditary hemochromatosis, *Scand. J. Haematol.*, **34**, 308–11.
Brink, B., Disler, P., Lynch, S., Jacobs, P., Charlton, R., and Bothwell, T. (1979). Patterns of iron storage in dietary iron overload and idiopathic hemochromatosis, *J. Lab. Clin. Med.*, **88**, 725–31.
Bryan, C. F., Leech, S. H., and Bozelka, B. (1986). The immunoregulatory nature of iron. II. Lymphocyte surface marker expression. *J. Leuk. Biol.*, **40**, 589–600.
Bryan, C. F., Nishiya, K., Pollack, M. S., Dupont, B., and de Sousa, M. (1981). Differential inhibition of the MLR by iron: association with HLA phenotype, *Immunogenetics*, **12**, 129–40.
Bryan, C. F., Leech, S. H., Dugos, R., Edwards, C. Q., Kushner, J. P., Skolnick, M. H., Bozelka, B., Linn, J. C., and Gaumer, R. (1984). Thermostable erythrocyte rosette-forming lymphocytes in hereditary hemochromatosis. I. Identification in peripheral blood, *J. Clin. Immunol.*, **4**, 134–42.
Cantinieaux, B., Hariga, C., Ferster, A., De Maertelaere, E., Toppet, M., and Fondu, P. (1987). Neutrophil dysfunctions in thalassemia major: the role of iron overload, *Eur. J. Haematol.*, **39**, 28–34.
Caroline, L., Kozinn, P. J., Feldman, F., and Stiefel, F. H. (1969). Infection and iron overload in thalassemia, *Ann. N.Y. Acad. Sci.*, **165**, 148–55.
de Sousa, M. (1978). Lymphoid cell positioning: New proposal for the mechanism of control of lymphoid cell migration, *Symp. Soc. Exp. Biol.*, **32**, 393–410.
de Sousa, M., and Nishiya, K. (1978). Inhibition of E-rosette formation by two iron salts, *Cell. Immunol.*, **38**, 203–8.
de Sousa, M., Martins da Silva, B., Dörner, M., Munn, G., Nishiya, K., Grady, R., and Silverstone, A. (1982). Iron and the lymphomyeloid system: rationale for considering iron as a target for 'immune surveillance'. In P. Saltman and J. Hegenauer (eds) *The Biochemistry and Physiology of Iron*, pp. 687–98, Elsevier Biomedical, Amsterdam.
de Sousa, M., Dynesius-Trentham, R. Mota-Garcia, F., Teixeira da Silva, M., and Trentham, D. E. (1988). Activation of the rat synovium by iron. *Arthritis Rheum.*, **31**, 653–661.
Dwyer, J., Wood, C., McNamara, J., Williams, A., Andiman, W., Rink, L., O'Connor, T., and Pearson, H. (1987). Abnormalities in the immune system of children with beta-thalassemia, *Clin. Exp. Immunol.*, **63**, 621–9.
Fillet, G., and Marsaglia, G. (1975). Idiopathic hemochromatosis (IH) abnormality in RBC transport of iron by the reticuloendothelial system (RES), *Blood*, **46**, 1007.
Flament, J., Goldman, M., Waterlot, Y., Dupont, E., Wybran, J., and Vanherweghem, J. L. (1986). Impairment of phagocyte oxidative metabolism in hemodialysed patients with iron overload, *Clin. Nephrol.*, **25**, 227–30.
Goicoa, M. A., Estevez, M. E., Ballart, I. J., Diez, R. A., Penalver, J. A., de Miani, S. A., and Sen, L. (1986). Impairment of natural killer function in carriers and patients with thalassemia major, *Nouv. Rev. Fr. Hematol.*, **28**, 57–9.
Good, M. F., Powell, L. W., and Halliday, J. W. (1988). Iron status and cellular immune competence, *Blood Rev.*, **2**, 43–9.
Good, M. F., Chapman, D. E., Powell, L. W., and Halliday, J. W. (1986). The effect of iron (Fe) on the cloning efficiency of human memory T4+ lymphocytes, *Clin. Exp. Immunol.*, **66**, 340–7.

Good, M. F., Chapman, D. E., Powell, L. W., and Halliday, J. W. (1987). The effect of experimental iron overload on splenic T cell function: analysis using cloning techniques, *Clin. Exp. Immunol.*, **68**, 375–83.

Grady, R. W., Akbar, A., Giardina, P. J., Hilgartner, M. W., and de Sousa, M. (1985). Disproportionate lymphoid cell subsets in thalassemia major: the relative contributions of transfusion and splenectomy, *Br. J. Haematol.*, **72**, 361–7.

Gronowicz, E., Coutinho, A., and Melchers, F. (1979). A plaque assay for all cells secreting Ig of a given type or class, *Eur. J. Immunol.*, **6**, 588–90.

Guglielmo, P., Cunsolo, F., Lombardo, T., Sortino, G., Giustolisi, R., Cacciola, E., and Cacciola, E. (1984). T subset abnormalities in thalassemia intermedia: possible evidence of a thymus functional deficiency, *Acta Haematol.*, **72**, 361–7.

Gutteridge, J. M. C., Rowley, D. A., Griffiths, E., and Halliwell, B. (1985). Low-molecular weight iron complexes and oxygen radical reactions in idiopathic hemochromatosis, *Clin. Sci.*, **68**, 463–7.

Hiyeda, K. (1939). The cause of Kaschin–Beck's disease, *Jap. J. Med. Sci.*, **4**, 91–106.

Jacobs, A. (1977). Iron overload—clinical and pathologic aspects, *Semin. Hematol.*, **14**, 89–113.

Jacobs, A., and Summers, M. R. (1981). Iron uptake and ferritin synthesis by peripheral blood leucocytes in patients with primary idiopathic haemochromatosis, *Br. J. Haematol.*, **49**, 647–52.

Kapadia, A., de Sousa, M., Markenson, A., Miller, D., Good, R. A., and Gupta, S. (1980). Lymphoid cell sets and serum immunoglobulins in patients with thalassemia intermedia: relationship to serum iron and splenectomy, *Br. J. Haematol.*, **45**, 405–16.

Kaplan, J., Samaik, S., Gitlin, J., and Lusher, J. (1984). Diminished helper/suppressor lymphocyte ratios and natural killer activity in recipients of repeated blood transfusions, *Blood*, **64**, 308–10.

Keown, P., and Descamps, D. (1978). Suppression de la réaction lymphocytaire mixte par des globules rouges autologues et leurs constituants: une hypothèse nouvelle sur l'effet apparemment tolérogène des transfusions sanguines en transplantation, *C. R. Acad. Sci. Paris (Série D)*, **287**, 749–52.

Khalifa, A. S., Fattah, S. A., Maged, Z., Sabry, F., and Mohamed, H. A. (1983). Immunoglobulin levels, opsonic activity and phagocytic power in Egyptian thalassemic children, *Acta Haematol.*, **69**, 136–9.

Khan, A., Chuck-Kwan, L., Wolff, J. A., Chang, H., Khan, P., and Evans, H. (1977). Defects of neutrophil chemotaxis and random migration in thalassemia major, *Pediatrics*, **60**, 349–51.

Lum, J. B., Infante, A. J., Makker, D. M., Yang, F., and Bowman, B. H. (1986). Transferrin synthesis by inducer T lymphocytes, *J. Clin. Invest.*, **77**, 841–9.

Martino, M., Rossi, M. E., Resti, M., Vullo, C., and Vierucci, A. (1984). Changes in superoxide anion production in neutrophils from multitransfused B-thalassemia patients: correlation with ferritin levels and liver damage, *Acta Haematol.*, **71**, 289–98.

Martins da Silva, B., Pollack, M. S., Dupont, B., and de Sousa, M. (1982). A study of ferritin secretion by human peripheral blood mononuclear cells in HLA-typed donors. In P. Saltman and J. Hegenauer (eds) *The Biochemistry and Physiology of Iron*, pp. 733–8, Elsevier Biomedical, Amsterdam.

Munn, C. G., Markenson, A. L., Kapadia, A., and de Sousa, M. (1981). Impaired T cell mitogen responses in some patients with thalassemia intermedia, *Thymus*, **3**, 119–28.

Neri, A., Brugiatelli, M., Iacopino, P., and Callea, F. (1984). Natural killer cell activity and T cell subpopulations in thalassemia major, *Acta Haematol.*, **71**, 263-9.

Nishiya, K., de Sousa, M., Tsoi, E., Bognacki, J. J., and de Harven, E. (1980). Regulation of expression of a human lymphoid cell surface marker by iron, *Cell. Immunol.*, **53**, 71-9.

Nualart, P., Estevez, M. E., Ballart, I. J., de Miani, S. A., Penalver, J., and Sen, L. (1987). Effect of alpha interferon on the altered T-B cell immunoregulation in patients with thalassemia major, *Am. J. Hematol.*, **24**, 151-9.

Pardalos, G., Kannakoudi-Tsakalidis, F., Malaka-Zafirin, M., Tsantali, H., and Papaevangelou, G. (1987). Iron-related disturbances of cell mediated immunity in multitransfused children with thalassemia major, *Clin. Exp. Immunol.*, **68**, 138-45.

Pollack, M. S., da Silva, B. M., Moshief, D., Dupont, B., and de Sousa, M. (1983). Ferritin secretion by human mononuclear cells: association with HLA phenotype, *Clin. Immunol. Immunopathol.*, **27**, 124-34.

Powell, L. W., Bassett, M. L., and Halliday, J. W. (1980). Haemochromatosis 1980 update, *Gastroenterology*, **78**, 374-81.

Ross, C. E., Muir, W. A., Ng, A. B. P., Graham, R. C., and Kellermeyer, R. W. (1975). Hemochromatosis. Pathophysiologic and genetic considerations, *Am. J. Clin. Pathol.*, **63**, 179-91.

Saab, G., Green, R., Jurjus, A., and Sarrou, E. (1986). Monocyte ferritin in idiopathic haemochromatosis, thalassemia and liver disease, *Scand. J. Haematol.*, **36**, 65-70.

Sheldon, J. H. (1935). *Haemochromatosis*, Oxford University Press.

Simon, M., Bourel, M., Fauchet, R., and Genetet, B. (1976). Association of HLA A3 and HLA B-14 antigens with idiopathic haemochromatosis, *Gut*, **17**, 332-4.

Simon, M., Le Mignon, L., Fauchet, R., Yauanq, J., David, V., Edan, G., and Bourel, M. (1987). A study of 609 haplotypes marking for the hemochromatotic gene, *Am. J. Hum. Genet.*, **41**, 89-105.

Sizemore, D. J., and Bassett, M. L. (1984). Monocyte transferrin iron uptake in hereditary hemochromatosis, *Aust. J. Haematol.*, **16**, 347-54.

Valberg, L. S., Simon, J. B., Manley, P. N., Corbett, W. E., and Ludwig, J. (1975). Distribution of storage iron as body iron stores expand in patients with haemochromatosis, *J. Lab. Clin. Med.*, **86**, 479-89.

van Asbeck, B. S., Verbrugh, H. A., van Oost, B. A., Marx, J. J. M., Imhof, H., and Verhoef, J. (1982). Listeria monocytogenes meningitis and decreased phagocytosis associated with iron overload, *Br. Med. J.*, **284**, 542-4.

van Asbeck, B. S., Marx, J. J. M., Struyvenberg, A., van Kats, J. H., and Verhoef, J. (1984a). Effect of iron (III) in the presence of various ligands on the phagocytic and metabolic activity of human polymorphonuclear leukocytes, *J. Immunol.*, **132**, 851-6.

van Asbeck, B. S., Marx, J. J. M., Struyvenberg, A., and Verhoef, J. (1984b). Functional defects in phagocytic cells from patients with iron overload, *J. Infect.*, **85**, 232-40.

Waterlot, Y., Cantinieaux, B., Hariga-Mulier, C., de Maertelaere-Laurent, E., Vanherweghem, J. L., and Fondu, P. (1985). Impairment of neutrophil phagocytosis in haemodialysed patients—the critical role of iron overload, *Br. Med. J.*, **291**, 501-4.

Part V

Iron and Malignancy

Iron in Immunity, Cancer and Inflammation
Edited by M. de Sousa and J. H. Brock
© 1989 John Wiley & Sons Ltd.

12
Iron and Tumor Cell Growth

Howard H. Sussman

Stanford University School of Medicine, Stanford, California 94305, USA

INTRODUCTION

This chapter is directed to a presentation of iron metabolism in lymphomyeloid cells in malignancy. It will address the importance of iron as an obligate requirement for cell proliferation and its role in other cell functions. Lymphomyeloid cells evolve from a pluripotent stem cell which differentiates into myeloid and lymphoid progenitor cells. The myeloid progenitor stem cell can be further differentiated to form cells of the erythroid series, granulocytes and monocyte–macrophages, megakaryocytes, and eosinophils. The lymphoid progenitor cell can be further differentiated into the T and B lymphocyte series of cells. The commitment of the pluripotential stem cell into the myeloid and lymphoid progenitor cells and the subsequent differentiation into the functionally active cell lines is a process which is controlled by growth factors and which responds to signals related to the requirement for the functional roles of the cells. A characteristic property of these cells is to undergo clonal expansion to ensure that adequate numbers of fully differentiated, competent cells are present to meet the body's needs. The clonal expansion that occurs in response to activation of the normal myeloid and lymphoid progenitor cells represents controlled proliferation that precedes differentiation to the functionally active cell. Malignant counterparts of lymphomyeloid cells exist. These can possess the phenotype characteristic of the stage of commitment of the cell at which time neoplastic transformation occurred. As is characteristic of malignant cells, these have the property of unremitting proliferation; however, some of these malignant lymphomyeloid cells can show response to the same growth factors which regulate controlled proliferation of non-malignant lymphomyeloid cells undergoing clonal expansion.

Iron is a necessary factor for cell proliferation. The control of proliferation in lymphomyeloid cells is governed by growth factors which are specific to cells of each line of differentiation. Examples would be IL-2 and IL-3 to stimulate production of lymphoid and myeloid cells respectively, or granulocyte–macrophage colony-stimulating factor (GM-CSF), which enhances production of the myeloid cell derivatives, macrophages, neutrophils, eosinophils and possibly erythroid cells, erythropoietin, which stimulates hematopoietic cells to erythrocyte production, and colony-stimulating factors which are specific to the production of macrophages (M-CSF) and granulocytes (G-CSF). Species of the principal iron-binding proteins, transferrin, lactoferrin and ferritin, have been implicated as having a role in the modulation of clonal expansion and the subsequent differentiation of cells of the lymphomyeloid cell system (see Chapters 9 and 10). The specific mechanisms by which these proteins act to regulate cell growth have not been elucidated and have not been defined in relationship to the iron-binding properties of these proteins.

The similarity in the steps involved in the clonal expansion of stem cells and activated progenitor cells to develop adequate numbers of competent differentiated cells has been a major accomplishment of research conducted during the past decade. The ability to manipulate these events in cell lines which are well characterized has provided models for evaluating the role of iron in both proliferation and differentiation. The identification of malignant cell lines which can be made to undergo terminal differentiation has been of critical importance for these studies.

PHYSICAL PROPERTIES OF IRON AND THE PRINCIPAL IRON COMPOUNDS OF CELLULAR IRON METABOLISM

These aspects are discussed in detail elsewhere in this volume, and will therefore be only mentioned briefly here. The obligate requirement for iron in cell and microbial proliferation reflects the fact that it is an essential element for all forms of life. It participates in key biochemical reactions which govern cellular metabolism, and is a component of the enzyme systems that conduct the principal respiration and electron-transfer reactions which are essential for cell viability (Neilands, 1972; Lehninger, 1982) (see also Chapter 3) Iron is also a component of enzymes involved in oxidation–reduction reactions and DNA synthesis.

The extracellular transport of iron in vertebrates is mediated by transferrin proteins which are evolutionarily old (Feeney and Komatsu, 1966); cellular iron is stored chiefly by ferritin (Aisen and Listowsky, 1980). A membrane receptor for transferrin provides a mechanism for incorporation of iron as is needed by the cell for essential metabolic functions, including proliferation (Seligman, Schleicher and Allen, 1979; Wada, Hass and Sussman, 1979). The structure and function of these proteins are described in detail elsewhere (Chapters 3 and 4) and are therefore mentioned here in brief.

Transferrins

Human serum transferrin synthesized in the liver is the principal extracellular iron-transport protein which delivers iron to the cell. It is a glycoprotein with a molecular mass of approximately 80 kDa. It contains 678 amino acids in a single chain and two carbohydrate chains (MacGillivray, Mendez and Sihna, 1982). There are two iron-binding sites, each of which is on one of the globular domains that correspond to the N- or C-terminal halves of the protein, and Fe^{3+} binding is always accompanied by concomitant anion binding, usually bicarbonate, and the release of protons (Aisen and Listowsky, 1980; Schlabach and Bates, 1975). The affinity constants for the two sites at pH 7.4 are approximately 10^{22}, although the N-terminal site has one-fifth the affinity of the C-terminal site. Below pH 5 both sites lose their ability to bind iron. Another factor which may play a role in the binding and release of iron from transferrin is the oxidation to Fe^{3+}, since transferrin has a much lower affinity for Fe^{2+} (Gaber and Aisen, 1970), but this requires displacement of the co-anion bicarbonate from the protein–iron complex for it to be rapid (Ankel and Petering, 1980). The rate of iron binding to transferrin depends on the chelation state of the ferric ion; ferric nitrilotriacetate and ferric bis-citrate bind to transferrin in a few seconds whereas ferric citrate takes many hours to reach equilibrium with diferric transferrin (Spiro and Saltman, 1969).

Lactoferrin is an iron-binding protein of similar molecular mass, 80 kDa, and structure, to serum transferrin. It is synthesized by granulocytes and is also found in tears and milk (Aisen and Listowsky, 1980). The function of this protein is to protect against microbial infection by limiting the availability of iron to the micro-organisms, thus inhibiting microbial proliferation. Lactoferrin also has a function in regulating myelopoiesis (see Chapters 9 and 10).

Transferrin receptor

The transferrin receptor is a membrane-bound glycoprotein which regulates the incorporation of iron by cells through the process of receptor-mediated endocytosis. Extensive studies have characterized the physical and binding properties of the transferrin receptor and these have been reviewed (Seligman, 1983; Newman *et al.*, 1983; May and Cuatrecasas, 1985) (see also Chapter 4). The transferrin receptor is a dimer with a subunit molecular mass of 94 kDa (Enns and Sussman, 1981; Schneider *et al.*, 1982). Transferrin receptors have been isolated from normal and transformed human cells, including human placenta and leukaemic T cells; no subtypes have been observed from peptide maps (Stein and Sussman, 1983), and the cDNA sequences obtained by different investigators have been the same (Schneider *et al.*, 1984; McClelland, Kuhn and Ruddle,

1984). The greater part of the molecule, including its C-terminal end, is in the extracellular environment; the N-terminal end is exposed to the intracellular environment (Schneider et al., 1984; McClelland, Kuhn and Ruddle, 1984). The cytoplasmic domain is essential for endocytosis, possibly enabling the receptor to be selectively concentrated in the coated pit (Rothenberger, Iacopetta and Kuhn, 1987). The affinity of the transferrin receptor for transferrin is approximately 10^9 M^{-1} and it forms a complex containing two subunits each of transferrin and receptor (Enns and Sussman, 1981; Schneider et al., 1982). Given the micromolar concentration of transferrin in human serum, most receptors will be occupied. The transferrin receptor does not show specific binding for lactoferrin.

Ferritin

Ferritin is the major storage form of iron in all tissues; highest concentrations are present in the liver and spleen. Natural human ferritin is composed of two types of peptide subunits, L and H, of molecular masses 19–21 kDa (Otsuka, Maruyama and Listowsky, 1981). These are synthesized from different mRNAs, suggesting that these are coded by separate genes (Watanabe and Drysdale, 1981) (see Chapter 4). The ferritin protein consists of 24 cylindrical subunits arranged about an iron-containing core which has the potential for storing up to 4500 iron atoms in the core as a hydrated ferric oxide polymer (Aisen and Listowsky, 1980; Ward, Kusher and Kaplan, 1984) (see also Chapter 3).

The ferritins which consist of larger numbers of the L subunit have a relatively basic p*I* and are called basic ferritins. They are present in iron-storage organs such as spleen and liver, and are in the plasma. Acidic ferritins consist principally of the H subunit, have a more acidic p*I*, and are present in tissues of low non-heme iron concentration. These tissues include heart, erythroid, and lymphomyeloid (monocytes, lymphocytes) series cells (Dezza et al., 1986). Malignant tissues tend to be rich in acidic ferritin (Matzner et al., 1985) (see also Chapters 13 and 14). Small amounts of extracellular ferritins are found in body fluids and on the surface of lymphocytes. In the serum these are predominantly basic ferritins and normally do not contain significant amounts of iron (Ward, Kushner and Kaplan, 1984).

Ferritin receptors

Specific binding of serum ferritin to cell surface membranes has been demonstrated on a variety of cells, including erythroblasts, macrophages, fibroblasts and placental brush border membranes (Takami et al., 1986), and K562, HL-60 and other cell lines (Fargion et al., 1988). The trophoblast membrane receptor binds ferritin at 37°C and pH 7.4 with a $K_a = 2.3 \times 10^7$ M^{-1}; the K562 receptor binds ferritin at 37°C with $K_a = 3 \times 10^8 M^{-1}$. The placental receptor has greater binding affinity for apoferritin than for ferric ferritin. The K562 ferritin receptor binds the H subunit preferentially, and Western blotting demonstrated the K562 receptor to be a 100 kDa protein (Fargion et al., 1988).

CELLULAR METABOLISM OF IRON

Iron incorporation—malignant and non-malignant cells

The ferric transferrin in the serum is the major source of iron for all cells in the body. Transferrin is synthesized in hepatic parenchymal cells. These cells incorporate iron by endocytosis of heme–hemopexin and hemoglobin–haptoglobin complexes circulating in the blood. The heme and hemoglobin in these complexes is derived from breakdown of erythrocytes and from dietary sources (Kino et al., 1987). The principal mechanism for cellular iron incorporation occurs by receptor-mediated endocytosis through the transferrin cycle (Karin and Mintz, 1981; Dautry-Varsat, Ciechanover and Lodish, 1983; Klausner et al., 1983; Yamashiro et al., 1984). The transferrin cycle consists of the binding of ferric transferrin to the transferrin receptor in the cell membrane, internalization of the receptor–ligand complex in acidified endosomes, release of the iron across the membrane to the intracellular compartment, and recycling of transferrin receptor and apotransferrin to the cell surface, where the apotransferrin is released and the transferrin receptor is available for another endocytotic cycle.

In the transferrin cycle, following receptor-mediated endocytosis, the iron released from transferrin in the acid vesicle passes into the cell compartment by a mechanism which is not clearly known. Upon entry into the cell compartment the iron is partitioned between that bound to ferritin and that bound to non-ferritin compounds. The non-ferritin pool includes organic compounds such as heme iron-containing proteins, and an active, low molecular weight soluble iron fraction which may exist as iron bound to small molecules or chelates (Borova, Ponka and Neuwirt, 1973; White, Bailey-Wood and Jacobs, 1976; Egyed, 1983).

The incorporation of ^{59}Fe into the different intracellular iron compartments has been studied in a variety of cells, including those of the lymphomyeloid series (Bomford, Young and Williams, 1986; Mattia et al., 1986). In all of these studies the results demonstrated that the uptake of iron by the cell is initially to the non-ferritin compartment, and this is followed by a time-dependent fractional accumulation of iron into ferritin which occurs gradually over a 2–5-hour period. The initial binding of iron to ferritin occurs within 10 minutes, and gradually the amount bound increases over a 5-hour period, after which there is a loss of ^{59}Fe from ferritin. These findings suggest that the non-ferritin component is initially the most active for maintenance of cell iron.

The principal mechanism for modulating cellular iron uptake is by the regulation of expression of the transferrin receptor (Rudolph et al., 1985; see also Chapter 4). Intracellular iron has been reported to regulate the transcription rate of the gene for the transferrin receptor in experiments which showed that transferrin receptor mRNA decreases when iron is delivered to the cells and increases when cells are deprived of iron (Mattia et al., 1984; Rao et al., 1986). However, there may be several levels of regulatory control (Pelosi et al., 1986; Taetle et al., 1987). The observation of different patterns of DNA protein binding in the promoter region of the receptor gene in a variety of cell types has suggested that different regulatory mechanisms exist (Miskimins et al., 1985). The increase in these DNA-binding proteins precedes the increase in transferrin receptor mRNA, which precedes entry of the cell into the S-phase of the cell cycle (Miskimins et al., 1986). Owen and Kuhn (1987) identified sequences in the 3' non-coding region of the receptor gene that are necessary for iron-dependent feedback regulation of receptor expression. They also reported data consistent with post-transcriptional regulation of the receptor.

A non-transferrin-mediated pathway of iron incorporation has been demonstrated in malignant cell-derived lines in culture (Taetle et al., 1985; Basset, Quesneau and Zwiller, 1986). This pathway may not be functional under normal conditions, because free iron is not present in serum or other biological fluid. However, it is possible that iron exchange at the cell surface from non-transferrin iron is important in certain circumstances such as cell–cell interaction and could utilize this pathway. Iron-binding proteins have been identified in the membranes of neoplastic and neoplasm-derived cell culture lines. The p97 glycoprotein found in melanoma cells has a high degree of homology with transferrin and is an example of a membrane-located iron-binding protein that could participate in such a mechanism (Brown et al., 1982). The non-transferrin mechanism of cellular iron incorporation has been useful in showing experimentally the relationship of cellular iron concentration and regulation of the transferrin receptor, transferrin, and ferritin.

The rate of iron uptake by mitogen-stimulated human lymphocytes and other non-erythroid cells is low in comparison to uptake in erythroid cells, in spite of comparable receptor numbers, indicating an independence of the number of transferrin receptors on the cell surface and cellular iron incorporation (Bomford et al., 1983). This may also reflect the needs for iron by the differentiating erythroid cell. Mitogen-stimulated lymphocytes from different individuals have been shown to take up iron at different rates, even though the receptor number and the characteristics of binding were the same (Bomford, Young and Williams, 1986). In these studies, lymphocytes from different subjects were submitted to mitogen stimulation and the iron uptake was shown to vary between groups. However, even though the rate of uptake varied, the proportion of iron in each intracellular iron compartment was similar. These iron-incorporation studies showed that after 3 hours a majority of the iron was present in ferritin, that incorporation into heme was fairly constant over a 3-hour period, and that the amount in the non-heme, non-ferritin fraction initially increased rapidly, and then reached a steady state. This observation appeared to match the same steady-state partitioning as was seen in similar studies using K562 cells, an erythroleukemia cell line which makes heme and which has a greater uptake of iron (Mattia *et al.*, 1986). Similar results showing that the distribution of iron in the intracellular pools was not influenced by the rate of iron uptake have been reported by other investigators. The finding that ^{59}Fe was incorporated into the intracellular components in a proportionally similar manner independent of the rate of iron uptake indicates that there is an obligatory relationship for the distribution of iron in each of these compartments. The amount of iron going into ferritin may be defined for a given ferritin level (Mattia *et al.*, 1986).

Calculation has indicated that at steady state there may be as much as 15% iron that is not identified as being associated with ferritin, heme or transferrin bound to transferrin receptor. Although this fraction has not been identified, this observation lends further support for a small molecular, or chelated, component in the intracellular iron pool. The iron in this component may act as a precursor for subsequent incorporation into functional components (Bomford, Young and Williams, 1986; Bottomley, Wolfe and Bridges, 1985).

CELL CYCLE AND CELLULAR IRON

As shown earlier, iron is a component of many proteins and enzymes which participate in reactions essential for cell viability. Normal and malignant cell growth is arrested when growing cells are cultured without transferrin (Barnes and Sato, 1980), if transferrin receptor function of cells in culture is blocked by anti-receptor antibodies which inhibit transferrin binding resulting in decreased cellular iron uptake (Taetle *et al.*, 1985; Trowbridge and Lopez, 1982), or if gallium transferrin is used to compete with ferric transferrin (Chitambar and Seligman, 1986; see also Chapter 15). All of these studies suggest that iron is an absolute requirement for cell growth. The events in the cell cycle at which iron deprivation exerts its inhibitory effect on proliferation have been studied.

Cell cycle

The cell cycle includes the events involved in cell proliferation (Alberts et al., 1983; Darnell, Lodish and Baltimore, 1986). These events have been divided into two periods. The first, cell division, is concerned with the separation into progeny cells and is designated the M or mitotic period. In the process of mitosis, each of the progeny cells receives identical copies of DNA in a complex process that assigns equal chromosomes to each progeny cell. The M period is divided into four phases, prophase, metaphase, anaphase, and telophase. Cytokinesis is co-ordinated closely with the four phases during mitosis. The second period, interphase, begins following completion of cytokinesis. Interphase has been divided into three phases, G_1, S and G_2. The replication of DNA and the synthesis of histone proteins occurs during the synthetic (S) phase. During S phase, each double-helical DNA molecule is replicated into two identical progeny DNA molecules. Histones and other chromosomal proteins which are synthesized during interphase rapidly bind to the newly synthesized progeny DNA molecules. The S phase of interphase is bounded by two gap periods, G_1 and G_2. During these gap periods there is no net synthesis of DNA, although DNA repair can occur. In the G_2 period, which follows S phase, the cell contains two copies of each of the DNA molecules present in the G_1 period. The times for the S, G_2, and M periods are relatively constant, being 7, 3 and 1 hour in different mammalian cells. The G_1 period can vary widely. A G_0 stage is defined as a period in which cells have ceased to grow and are not preparing for DNA replication. Cells that are lacking nutrients or essential growth factors can be reversibly stopped in G_0, but can progress to G_1 when the essential compound is resupplied. Cells that are terminally differentiated are also in G_0.

Lymphomyeloid stem and progenitor cells exist in a resting state, G_0, and can be induced to proliferate following exposure to an antigen or a mitogen for a finite number of cell divisions, followed by terminal differentiation resulting in an expanded set of cells of functional importance. During interphase there is also the synthesis of other macromolecules, such as RNA and proteins, and the assembly of organelles, such as the plasma membrane and mitochondria, which are necessary for each progeny cell to conduct those essential metabolic processes necessary for cell viability.

Mitochondria are the organelles in which enzymes of the respiratory and oxidative phosphorylation reactions are located. The growth and division of mitochondria are not co-ordinated with the events of the cell cycle, but occur throughout interphase (Posakony, England and Attardi, 1977). However, the synthesis of the macromolecules for the mitochondria and the assembly of this organelle must be complete prior to cell division (M), so that during cytokinesis each daughter cell will have the capability of performing the oxidative and energy-generating reactions essential for cell viability.

It is important to review the properties of this organelle, because the enzymes and electron-transport proteins in the mitochondria which perform these reactions contain iron, and because heme is essential for incorporation of nuclear-coded protein into mitochondria (Lehninger, 1982; Darnell, Lodish and Baltimore, 1986). Mitochondria contain DNA which encodes proteins that are mainly integral proteins of the inner mitochondrial membrane, or are subunits of multimeric complexes concerned with oxidative phosphorylation. Mitochondrial DNA also encodes the RNAs that form mitochondrial ribosomes and the tRNAs that are used to translate the mRNAs on mitochondrial ribosomes. There is no export of RNA or protein from the mitochrondria. All transcripts of mitochondrial DNAs and their translation products remain within the organelle.

Most mitochondrial proteins are encoded by nuclear DNA, are synthesized in the cytosol as precursors, and are then incorporated in the mitochondria. These include most of the proteins required for oxidative phosphorylation, and they are destined for localization into the matrix, the intramembrane space, or the inner mitochondrial membrane. The cytosol-synthesized precursor proteins have an N-terminal signal piece which is cleaved by a metalloenzyme as part of the process of incorporation of the protein into the mitochondrion. The cleavage is believed to result in a necessary conformational change of the protein, which ensures that it remains in the mitochondrion. These steps have been elucidated in yeast, but are proposed to be universal to mitochondria in all species. The process by which b_2 and c_1 cytochromes are localized to the intramembrane space and the outer face of the inner membrane consists of two steps: (a) part of the N-terminal signal sequence is removed by the metalloenzyme after partial insertion of the signal sequence into the mitochondrion; (b) the resulting intermediate is converted to the final or mature form by the removal of the rest of the signal sequence and the addition of heme. The final step occurs concomitantly with final localization of the protein. The addition of heme occurs concomitantly with uptake of the protein. As an example, the cytoplasmic cytochrome c lacks heme and is called the apo form. Only the apo form is incorporated into the mitochondrion. It is believed that the heme causes conformational change in the protein so that it fits into the membrane; it may also enable the metalloenzyme to recognize the correct cleavage site to remove the rest of the signal sequence. Energy is required for mitochondria to add precursor protein. ATP is the energy source; hydrolysis of ATP provides a protonmotive force. In the presence of poisons that uncouple oxidative phosphorylation, the precursor proteins can bind to the receptors' outer mitochondrial membrane but are not translocated. If the poisons are removed so that energy generation proceeds, the precursors are incorporated.

The assembly of the mitochondrion requires close co-ordination of the nuclear and mitochondrial genomes. This is especially the case for the multienzyme complexes such as the F_0F_1-ATPases and cytochrome c oxidase which are assembled from both mitochondrial and nuclear-coded multimeric proteins. Studies in yeast have demonstrated that heme is a requirement for the nuclear gene coding for cytochrome c, and possibly for the mitochondrial gene. Thus heme may serve to co-ordinate the transcription of nuclear and mitochondrial genes in mammalian cells as well. Such a role may be involved in the effects of iron deprivation in erythroid cells during differentiation when hemoglobinization results in large demands for heme. Ponka and Schulman (1985a) have proposed that 'free' intracellular heme regulates the utilization of iron from transferrin for heme synthesis but does not regulate ferrochelatase activity, or the enzyme of protoporphyrin synthesis. These investigators also showed that heme synthesis in reticulocytes is regulated by the acquisition of transferrin iron (Ponka and Schulman, 1985b). In an experimental system to study erythroid differentiation, as heme becomes a limiting factor, its lack results in death of cells committed to differentiation, and cell death could not be prevented by treatment with iron. It could result from competition for heme between hemoglobin-synthesizing pathways and pathways necessary for viability which require heme, or reflect the fact that heme was needed at a critical, temporal point in the differentiation program (Schmidt et al., 1986).

Iron in cell proliferation

The importance of iron in proliferating cells has been studied relative to the cell cycle in malignant epithelial, malignant lymphomyeloid, and mitogen- and antigen-activated proliferating normal lymphomyeloid cells. Studies in which transferrin endocytosis was impaired showed that iron is required in cells for completion of S phase of the cell cycle in mitogen-activated lymphocytes (Neckers and Cossman, 1983) and leukemia cell lines (Trowbridge and Lopez, 1982).

The effects of iron depletion on the cell cycle in studies using human mammary epithelial cancer cells (Reddel, Hedley and Sutherland, 1985) showed that at low concentration of fetal calf serum, cells proliferated very slowly and that there was an increase in the number of cells of the G_2 phase of the cell cycle and an increase in the number of polyploid cells. Inhibition of cell growth, with an increase in the number of cells in G_2, was also induced by adding an iron chelator (desferrioxamine) to the culture medium. The effects of growth inhibition could be overcome by the addition of diferric transferrin or ammonium ferric citrate. The conclusion from these data is that the limitation of cellular iron was the factor responsible for decreased proliferation and the G_2 arrest. From the study, one can conclude that iron is not limiting for DNA synthesis since the cells were in G_2 and there was an increased number of hyperdiploid cells. Similar experiments using graded doses of desferrioxamine were conducted with the K562 human leukemia cell line (Bomford et al., 1986). The results were the same, showing inhibition of cell proliferation, arrest of cells in the S and $G_2 + M$ phases of the cell cycle, and the continuation of DNA synthesis.

The best interpretation of the G_2 arrest observed in iron deprivation is that there is not enough iron for the enzymes and proteins of the respiratory and oxidation cycles in the progeny cells. The assembly of these organelles with the requisite complement of proteins necessary to conduct electron transport and oxidative phosphorylation must have taken place by the time of cytokinesis because each daughter cell must have a full complement of the iron-containing enzymes that conduct respiratory-chain phosphorylation. Functional incompetence of these organelles and enzyme systems must provide some as yet undetermined signal which results in inhibition of cytokinesis associated with cell division, as has been observed by G_2 arrest. An example of the importance of these enzyme systems is the observation in yeast that the availability of heme is necessary for synthesis of the cytochromes; yeast grown in the absence of heme will not perform aerobic glycolysis (Darnell, Lodish and Baltimore, 1986).

Iron in differentiation

The separate effects of iron on important processes in proliferation and differentiation of lymphomyeloid cells have been evaluated. The events following mitogenesis have been studied in detail in normal and malignant lymphomyeloid cells. Studies with lymphocytes have shown that mitogenesis is followed by the expression of growth factors and receptors for these growth factors as the initial step in expansion to a set of progeny cells with a common function. However, if proliferation is to ensue following mitogen or antigen activation, the transferrin receptor must be induced (Neckers and Cossman, 1983; Lum et al., 1986). The obligate expression of the transferrin receptor indicates the essential need for iron for cell growth in the normal lymphocytes, which have been activated to expand that set of cells. Similarly, expression of the transferrin receptor is recognized as a feature of malignant cells which have the property of continuous proliferation. Thus, there does not seem to be a difference in the need for iron between the malignant state and the normal state, but there is a need for iron for cell proliferation.

Studies have been performed with neoplasm-derived lymphomyeloid cell lines which could be induced to terminally differentiate, thus losing their ability to proliferate (Collins et al., 1978, 1980; Breitman, Selonick and Collins, 1980). This property has allowed the effect of iron on proliferation to be studied distinct from those of differentiation (Hunt, Ruffin and Yang, 1984; Taetle et al., 1985). Studies using the HL-60 cell line, a promyelocytic leukemia which can be induced to terminally differentiate to either granulocytes or to monocytes using selective agents, have shown a loss of transferrin receptor as the cells underwent terminal differentiation. This indicated that when differentiation occurs, these cells do not have the high requirements for iron, and iron incorporation is then reduced (Rhyner et al., 1985). The requirement of iron for cell proliferation but not for cell differentiation was shown in experiments in which deprivation of iron by inhibition of transferrin binding with antibodies resulted in growth inhibition, but did not affect dimethyl sulfoxide-induced terminal differentiation of HL-60 cells (Taetle et al., 1985).

Investigation of the requirement for iron by cells of the differentiated erythroid phenotype has been studied with leukemia cell lines which can be induced to erythroid differentiation as assessed by hemoglobin synthesis. In these cells the need for iron for hemoglobin, a product of differentiation, is distinct from the need for proliferation (Tsiftsoglou et al., 1983). One of the best studies used an avian erythroleukemia line in which viral transformation was used to develop temperature-sensitive mutants which synthesize hemoglobin at the viral non-permissive temperature (42°C) but not at the permissive temperature (33°C) at which proliferation is favored (Schmidt et al., 1986). The synthesis of hemoglobin at the 42°C temperature places a great demand on these cells for iron to be used in heme synthesis. These studies showed that the limiting factors regulating iron metabolism during proliferation are different from those operating during differentiation. Under normal proliferation heme synthesis appears to be rate limiting, as is evidenced by the fact that δ-aminolevulinic acid, which is one of the precursors of heme synthesis, is the limiting compound, and the enzyme responsible for its synthesis, aminolevulinic acid synthetase, is the rate-limiting enzyme. In contrast, at 42°C with increased hemoglobin synthesis, the availability of iron for the heme is the limiting factor. These studies may have additional value for interpreting the effect of iron deprivation on proliferating cells. Iron deprivation results in cessation of proliferation of tumor cell lines. An explanation consistent with the above studies is that under extreme conditions of iron deprivation in erythroid cells, the availability of iron for heme synthesis may be the limiting factor regulating cell proliferation, rather than the synthesis of heme precursors which should not be affected by the iron restriction (Ponka and Schulman, 1985b).

The central role of iron in cell growth and the regulatory role of transferrin receptors has been shown in experiments performed to determine whether receptor expression and cell proliferation could be independently regulated by perturbing available iron in growing cells in serum-free, transferrin-free medium containing supplemental iron (Rhyner et al., 1985), by blocking transferrin receptor function with anti-receptor antibodies (Trowbridge and Lopez, 1982), or by providing iron to the cell outside of the transferrin cycle by using heme or hemin (Ward, Kushner and Kaplan, 1984), soluble iron salts in the absence of ferric transferrin (Rudolph et al., 1985) or chelators (Taetle et al., 1985). The experiments which provided iron incorporation outside of the transferrin cycle resulted in decreased numbers of transferrin receptor displayed, but increased ferritin concentration. There is an increase in the fraction of iron delivered to ferritin under conditions that lead to an increase in iron delivery to the cells, such as incubating cells with diferric transferrin or hemin. Agents that lower the availability of iron to the cells, such as binding the OKT9 anti-transferrin receptor antibody to the surface transferrin receptor, decrease the fractional delivery of iron to ferritin. Chelation of iron from an intracellular iron pool was found to result in biosynthesis of transferrin receptors (Bridges and Cudkowicz, 1984). These data demonstrated the role of iron in regulating transferrin receptor and intracellular ferritin levels. The regulation of these proteins is closely linked but inversely related. Conditions which augment receptor expression downregulate the expression of ferritin and vice versa.

The relationship between regulation of the transferrin receptor and intracellular ferritin has also been studied in relation to proliferation and differentiation in the HL-60 cell line (Rhyner et al., 1985; Taetle et al., 1985). Induction of terminal differentiation of HL-60 cells into granulocytes and/ or monocyte–macrophages resulted in a decrease in the transferrin receptor display and an increase in ferritin content. The result of a series of these experiments was to establish that an *inverse* or *reciprocal* relationship exists between the presence of surface numbers of transferrin receptor and intracellular ferritin concentration in both the proliferating and terminally differentiating myeloid leukemia cells. The regulation of the proteins which are responsible for iron incorporation and for cell storage of iron is closely linked. These data are in support of the experiments with K562 cells which demonstrated that the presence of available iron within cells is the key regulator of transcription of the transferrin receptor (Rao et al., 1986). The reciprocal relation between the regulation of ferritin synthesis and that of the transferrin receptor may be important in the mechanisms which regulate growth and metabolism in myeloid cells. When there is a decrease in the incorporation of iron, the increase in ferritin provides a mechanism for ensuring storage of an adequate amount of cellular iron. Thus the conclusion from all of these studies is that during differentiation, intracellular ferritin concentration increases, as receptor concentration decreases.

The effect is to provide a stable pool of iron sequestered within the cells. These results also demonstrate that the iron incorporated into the cell by means other than endocytosis of ferric transferrin, i.e. cells grown in $FeCl_2$ or other iron salts, is partitioned into the intracellular iron compartments the same as is iron from transferrin and so is similarly prevented from being toxic to the cell.

IRON-BINDING PROTEINS AS MODULATORS OF GROWTH

The demonstration that the iron-binding proteins, transferrin, lactoferrin and ferritin, are synthesized by lymphocytes, granulocytes and macrophages, and are present on the surface of these cells in disease states, raised the question of the role of these proteins synthesized by lymphomyeloid cells in cell function (de Sousa, Smithyman and Tan, 1978). Subsequent studies have shown that these proteins act as modulators of clonal expansion and subsequent differentiation of cells of the lymphomyeloid cell system. The mechanism(s) by which these proteins act in this role are complex and have not been elucidated.

Lum et al. (1986) used hybridization with a cDNA probe to transferrin and demonstrated that transferrin is synthesized by the T4+ inducer subset of T lymphocytes and proposed that it participates in an autocrine mechanism for regulating growth. T lymphocyte proliferation is dependent on the presence of interleukin-2 (IL-2) and transferrin, and the receptors for each. Induction of IL-2 mRNA transcription and IL-2 receptor expression precedes transferrin mRNA transcription and transferrin receptor expression respectively. All of these events precede the initiation of DNA synthesis, suggesting that they are all functionally linked in an autocrine loop.

Proteoglycans are involved in growth regulation. The transferrin receptor has been shown to be the core protein of proteoheparan sulfate, and to be capable of binding diferric and apotransferrin species in human fibroblasts (Fransson et al., 1984). The importance of the transferrin receptor in the core protein to a regulatory role of heparan sulfate is not defined, and the ability of the proteoglycan to bind transferrin *in situ* may not be great but may be important in the micro-environment of the bone marrow or lymph node. Shedding of heparan sulfate into the medium of rapidly dividing cells has been observed in the G_2 phase of the cell cycle, and rapidly dividing cells have lower amounts of heparan sulfate than do non-dividing ones. It is possible that enzymatic cleavage of the sulfate from the proteoglycan core protein may be a mechanism for regulating exposure of the transferrin receptor in dividing cells (Fransson et al., 1984).

A role of inhibitory regulators of lymphomyeloid cell expansion has been described for transferrin, lactoferrin and acidic isoferritins, based upon *in vitro* experiments using neoplasm-derived lymphomyeloid cell lines and upon observations *in vivo* of anemia, neutropenia, decreased granulocyte–macrophage colony-forming units (CFU-GM) and depressed cellular immunity in patients with infections, malignancies, and proliferative disorders (Leiderman *et al.*, 1987).

Lactoferrin has independent action as a regulator of lymphomyeloid cells (Pelus, Broxmeyer and Moore, 1981) and as a suppressor of myelopoiesis (Gentile and Broxmeyer, 1983) (see Chapters 9 and 10). Iron-free transferrin has been shown to act as an inhibitor of lymphocyte proliferation. Initially this inhibitory activity was thought to be by a mechanism that was independent of its properties as an iron donor, but further studies have suggested otherwise. Experiments in which measured amounts of iron-free human or mouse transferrin were added to mouse lymphocytes grown *in vitro* in 5% fetal calf serum resulted in better than 80% inhibition of cell proliferation (Brock, Mainou-Fowler and Webster, 1986). However, addition of iron to achieve 30% saturation of the transferrin resulted in a 40–70% increase in proliferation, suggesting that the action of transferrin was not independent of its function as an iron donor. Other investigators (Broxmeyer *et al.*, 1986) used iron-saturated transferrin to inhibit release of granulocyte–macrophage colony-stimulating factor (GM-CSF) from MHC class II antigen-positive subsets of OKT4 T lymphocytes and showed that this effect could be blocked by antibody to to transferrin receptor. Shau, Shen and Golub (1986) showed that NK+ and NK-like activity was induced in the active large granular lymphocyte Percoll fraction of lymphocytes following stimulation by IL-2 and that transferrin was necessary for this induction. These experiments can be interpreted to indicate that transferrin is necessary as an iron donor to allow expansion of the subpopulation of NK+ and NK-like cells following stimulation, and is consistent with the conclusion drawn from the experiments described above.

High serum ferritin levels are present in conditions of iron overload, inflammation, solid tissue tumors, and malignancies of the lymphomyeloid system (Matzner *et al.*, 1985). Broxmeyer *et al.* (1981) identified a leukocyte-associated inhibition factor directed against lymphomyeloid progenitor cells as being an acidic isoferritin. Subsequent studies (see Chapter 9) have shown that acidic isoferritins are potent inhibitors of hematopoietic progenitors at concentrations of 10^{-10}–10^{-16} mol litre^{-1} and can suppress phytohemagglutinin (PHA) and concanavalin A (Con-A) induced blastogenesis at concentrations as low as 0.25 μg ml^{-1} (Matzner *et al.*, 1985).

The identification of receptors with high specific binding on the cell membranes of lymphocytes and other cells indicates that ferritin binding to cell membranes is not fortuitous. Studies of the binding of acidic ferritins using both the natural ligand and recombinant human ferritin have characterized the binding properties and the expression of binding sites on lymphomyeloid and other human cell lines. Studies using the H subunit of purified recombinant human ferritin with the erythroleukemic K562 cell line have demonstrated the H subunit specificity for binding (Fargion et al., 1988). Specificity was demonstrated by the fact that only ferritin containing a large proportion of the H subunit could displace the recombinant H subunit as ligand. Saturable binding gave an affinity coefficient of 10^8 M^{-1} at 37°C and showed 17 000–23 000 binding sites per cell in culture. Western blotting showed the binding protein was of $M_r = 100\,000$. The specific binding of the H subunit was also demonstrated on HL-60 cells as well as on other cells in culture. The number of ferritin-binding sites was shown to be highest during exponential growth and to progressively decrease and disappear when cells reached a plateau phase. Evidence that expression of the membrane ferritin receptor is not independent of iron metabolism is the finding that ferritin H subunit binding is increased when cells are treated with desferrioxamine and that K562 cells induced to differentiate with hemin failed to bind H subunit.

The ferritin H subunit has been shown to inhibit colony formation in normal human granulocyte-macrophage (CFU-GM) and erythroid (BFU-E) progenitor cells (Broxmeyer et al., 1982). These studies suggest that acidic isoferritins act as a normal feedback mechanism for the granulocyte-macrophage progenitor cell, and are described in Chapter 9. It should be noted that inconsistencies in the data reported by different investigators exist and have been addressed (Dezza, 1986; Chapter 10). The mechanism by which the acid ferritins act is not known and may be as part of complex interactions with other proteins and cells that have been implicated in regulating lymphomyelopoiesis. Both lactoferrin and C3 complement bind to acid ferritins, and interferons modulate the receptivity of lymphomyeloid progenitor cells to respond to these iron-binding proteins

Endogenously produced interferon-β has been demonstrated to participate in an autocrine system of growth inhibition in several cell lineages of the myeloid cell system, including macrophages, granulocytes and erythroid cells. The induction of interferon-β is independent of the nature of the agent initiating differentiation but includes natural inducers such as CSF-1 (Resnitzky et al., 1986). Interferon-γ was shown to modulate transferrin receptor downward as one of the biochemical changes accompanying macrophage activation (Hamilton, Gray and Adams, 1984). Exogenous interferon-γ was reported to induce responsiveness of colony-forming cells of a human monoblast cell line to the inhibitory actions of transferrin, lactoferrin and acidic isoferritins (Broxmeyer et al., 1986). That this was a direct effect of interferon was indicated from experiments showing that its activity was abolished by antiserum to interferon. The interpretation of the experiments was that interferon acts by perturbing transferrin–transferrin receptor interaction from the observation that the suppressive effect of transferrin could be blocked by treatment with anti-receptor antibody. Similar experiments with interferon-α showed that it was less effective (a higher dose was required) in inhibiting proliferation of cells with high transferrin receptor levels (Besancon, Bourgeade and Testa, 1985). In these studies interferon-α was shown to have an antiproliferative action on human lymphoblastoid cells and on mitogen-induced lymphocytes. The effect of interferon was to lower the transferrin receptor number in cells, and this correlated with the decrease in cell growth. These experiments showed that after PHA stimulation, interferon inhibited the increase in transferrin receptor and the increase in [^{3}H]thymidine incorporation. These data were consistent with this being the mechanism for the antiproliferative effect of interferon. These data are also in agreement with the requirement for iron from transferrin to enable completion of the S phase and transition into the mitotic phase of the cell cycle.

All of these studies suggest that the regulation of expansion of progenitor cells in myelopoiesis and the clonal expansion of activated lymphocytes in the immune response are governed by a complex set of interactions involving growth factors and other biological compounds which act as stimulators or inhibitors, and by cell–cell interactions. To better understand these interactions is an active area of research, and new glycoproteins which can inhibit activity of stem cells and more mature precursors to suppress granulopoiesis, hematopoiesis and lymphocyte proliferation in disease states are being identified (Leiderman et al., 1987). The demonstration that the major iron-binding proteins may have a critical role in the processes is in accord with the fact that iron is essential for the cell proliferation required for myelopoiesis or clonal expansion of activated lymphocytes.

ACKNOWLEDGEMENTS

This work was supported by the National Institutes of Health, Grant CA13533.

REFERENCES

Aisen, P., Leibman, A., and Zweier, J. (1978). Stoichiometric and site characteristics of the binding of iron to human transferrin, *J. Biol. Chem.*, **253**, 1930–7.
Aisen, P., and Listowsky, I. (1980). Iron transport and storage proteins, *Annu. Rev. Biochem.*, **49**, 357–93.

Alberts, B., Bray, D., Lewis, J., Raff, M., Roberts, K., and Watson, J. D. (1983). In *Molecular Biology of the Cell*, Garland Publishing Inc., New York.

Ankel, E., and Petering, D. H. (1980). Iron-chelating agents and the reductive removal of iron from transferrin, *Biochem. Pharmacol.*, **29**, 1833–7.

Barnes, D., and Sato, G. (1980). Serum free cell culture: a unifying approach, *Cell*, **22**, 649–55.

Basset, P., Quesneau, Y., and Zwiller, J. (1986). Iron-induced L1210 cell growth—evidence of a transferrin-independent iron transport, *Cancer Res.*, **46**, 1644–7.

Besancon, F., Bourgeade, M.-F., and Testa, U. (1985). Inhibition of transferrin receptor expression by interferon-alpha in human lymphoblastoid cells and mitogen induced lymphocytes, *J. Biol. Chem.*, **260**, 13074–80.

Bomford, A., Young, S. P., and Williams, R. (1986). Intracellular forms of iron during transferrin iron uptake by mitogen-stimulated human lymphocytes, *Br. J. Haematol.*, **62**, 487–94.

Bomford, A., Young, S. P., Nouri-Aria, K., and Williams, R. (1983). Uptake and release of transferrin and iron by mitogen stimulated human lymphocytes, *Br. J. Haematol.*, **55**, 93–101.

Bomford, A., Isaac, J., Roberts, S., Edwards, A., Young, S., and Williams, R. (1986). The effect of desferrioxamine on transferrin receptors, the cell cycle and growth rates of human leukaemic cells, *Biochem. J.*, **236**, 243–9.

Borova, J., Ponka, P., and Neuwirt, J. (1973). Study of intracellular iron distribution in rabbit reticulocytes with normal and inhibited heme synthesis, *Biochem. Biophys. Acta*, **320**, 143–56.

Bottomley, S. S., Wolfe, L. C., and Bridges, K. R. (1985). Iron metabolism in K562 erythroleukemic cells, *J. Biol. Chem.*, **260**, 6811–15.

Breitman, T. R., Selonick, S., and Collins, S. J. (1980). Induction of differentiation of the human promyelocytic leukemia cell lines (HL-60) by retinoic acid, *Proc. Natl Acad. Sci. USA*, **77**, 2936–40.

Bridges, K. R., and Cudkowicz, A. (1984). Effect of iron chelators on the transferrin receptor in K562 cells, *J. Biol. Chem.*, **259**, 12970–7.

Brock, J. H., Mainou-Fowler, T., and Webster, L. M. (1986). Evidence that transferrin may function exclusively as an iron donor in promoting lymphocyte proliferation, *Immunology*, **57**, 105–10.

Brown, J. P., Hewick, R. D., Hellstrom, I., Hellstrom, K. E., Doolittle, R. F., and Dreyer, W. J. (1982). Human melanoma-associated antigen p97 is structurally and functionally related to transferrin, *Nature*, **296**, 171–3.

Broxmeyer, H. E., Bognacki, J., Dorner, M. H., and de Sousa, M. (1981). The identification of leukemia-associated inhibitory activity (LIA) as acidic isoferritins: a regulatory role for acidic isoferritins in the production of granulocytes and macrophages, *J. Exp. Med.*, **153**, 1426–44.

Broxmeyer, H. E., Bognacki, J., Ralph, P., Dorner, M. H., Lu, L., and Castro-Malaspina, H. (1982). Monocyte–macrophage derived acidic isoferritins: normal feedback regulators of granulocyte–macrophage progenitor cells, *Blood*, **60**, 595–607.

Broxmeyer, H. E., Piacibello, W., Juliano, L., Platzer, E., Berman, E., and Rubin, Y. B. (1986). Gamma interferon induces colony-forming cells of the human macroblast line U937 to respond to inhibition by lactoferrin, transferrin, and acidic isoferritins, *Exp. Hematol.*, **14**, 35–43.

Chitambar, C. R., and Seligman, P. A. (1986). Effects of different transferrin forms on transferrin receptor expression, iron uptake, and cellular proliferation of human leukemic HL60 cells, *J. Clin. Invest.*, **78**, 1538–46.

Collins, S. J., Ruscetti, F. W., Gallagher, R. E., and Gallo, R. C. (1978). Terminal differentiation of promyelocytic leukemia cells induced by dimethyl sulfoxide and other polar compounds, *Proc. Natl Acad. Sci. USA*, **75**, 2458–62.

Collins, S. J., Bodner, A., Ting, R., and Gallo, R. C. (1980). Induction of morphological and functional differentiation of human promyelocytic leukemia cells (HL-60) by compounds which induce differentiation of murine leukemic cells, *Int. J. Cancer*, **25**, 312–18.

Darnell, J., Lodish, H., and Baltimore, D. (1986). In *Molecular Cell Biology*, Scientific American Books Inc., W. H. Freeman and Co., New York.

Dautry-Varsat, A., Ciechanover, A., and Lodish, H. F. (1983). pH and the recycling of transferrin during receptor-mediated endocytosis, *Proc. Natl Acad. Sci. USA*, **80**, 2258–62.

de Sousa, M., Smithyman, A., and Tan, C. (1978). Suggested models of ecotaxopathy in lymphoreticular malignancy. *Am. J. Pathol.*, **90**, 497–520.

Dezza, L., Cazzola, M., Piacibello, W., Arosio, P., Levi, S., and Aglietta, M. (1986). Effect of acidic and basic isoferritins on *in vitro* growth of human granulocyte–monocyte progenitors, *Blood*, **67**, 789–95.

Egyed, A. (1983). Studies on the partition of transferrin-donated iron in rabbit reticulocytes, *J. Haematol.*, **53**, 217–25.

Enns, C. A., and Sussman, H. H. (1981). Physical characterization of the transferrin receptor in human placentae, *J. Biol. Chem.*, **256**, 9820–3.

Fargion, S., Arosio, P., Fracanzoni, A. L., Cislaghi, V., Levi, S., Cozzi, A., Piperno, A., and Fiorelli, G. (1988). Characteristics and expression of binding sites specific for ferritin H chain on human cell lines, *Blood*, **71**, 753–7.

Feeney, R. E., and Komatsu, S. K. (1966). The transferrins, *Structure and Bonding*, **1**, 149–206.

Fransson, L.-A., Carlstedt, L. C., Coster, L., and Malmström, A. (1984). Binding of transferrin to the core protein of fibroblast proteoheparan sulfate, *Proc. Natl Acad. Sci. USA*, **81**, 5657–61.

Gaber, B. P., and Aisen, P. (1970). Is divalent iron bound to transferrin? *Biochim. Biophys. Acta*, **221**, 228–33.

Gentile, P., and Broxmeyer, H. E. (1983). Suppression of mouse myelopoiesis by administration of human lactoferrin *in vitro* and comparative action of human transferrin, *Blood*, **61**, 982–93.

Hamilton, T. A., Gray, P. W., and Adams, D. O. (1984). Expression of the transferrin receptor in murine peritoneal macrophages is modulated by *in vitro* treatment with interferon-γ, *Cell. Immunol.*, **89**, 478–88.

Hunt, R. C., Ruffin, R., and Yang, Y.-S. (1984). Alterations in the transferrin receptor of human erythroleukemic cells after induction of hemoglobin synthesis, *J. Biol. Chem.*, **259**, 9944–52.

Karin, M., and Mintz, B. (1981). Receptor-mediated endocytosis of transferrin in developmentally totipotent mouse teratocarcinoma stem cells, *J. Biol. Chem.*, **256**, 3245–52.

Kino, H., Mizumoto, K., Watanabe, J., and Tsunoo, H. (1987). Immunohistochemical studies on hemoglobin–haptoglobin and hemoglobin catabolism sites, *J. Histochem. Cytochem.*, **35**, 381–6.

Klausner, R. D., Ashwell, G., van Renswoude, J., Harford, J. B., and Bridges, K. R. (1983). Binding of apotransferrin to K562 cells: explanation of the transferrin cycle, *Proc. Natl Acad. Sci. USA*, **80**, 2263–6.

Lehninger, A. L. (1982). *Principles of Biochemistry*, pp. 486–542, Worth Publishers Inc., New York.

Leiderman, I. A., Greenberg, M. L., Adelsberg, B. R., and Siegel, F. P. (1987). A glycoprotein inhibitor of *in vitro* granulopoiesis associated with AIDS, *Blood*, **70**, 1267–72.

Lum, J. B., Infante, A. J., Makker, D. M., Yang, F., and Bowman, B. H. (1986). Transferrin synthesis by inducer T lymphocytes, *J. Clin. Invest.*, **77**, 841–9.

MacGillivray, R. T. A., Mendez, E., and Sihna, S. K. (1982). The complete amino acid sequence of human serum transferrin, *Proc. Natl Acad. Sci. USA*, **79**, 2504–8.

Mattia, E., Rao, K., Shapiro, D. S., Sussman, H. H., and Klausner, R. D. (1984). Biosynthetic regulation of the human transferrin receptor by desferrioxamine in K562 cells, *J. Biol. Chem.*, **259**, 2689–92.

Mattia, E., Josic, D., Ashwell, G., Klausner, R., and van Renswoude, J. (1986). Regulation of intracellular iron distribution in K562 human erythroleukemia cells, *J. Biol. Chem.*, **261**, 4587–93.

Matzner, Y., Konijn, A. M., Shlomai, Z., and Ben-Basset, H. (1985). Differential effect of isolated placental isoferritin on *in vitro* T lymphocyte function, *Br. J. Haematol.*, **59**, 443–8.

May, W. S., and Cuatrecasas, P. (1985). Transferrin receptor: its biological significance, *J. Membr. Biol.*, **88**, 205–15.

McClelland, A., Kuhn, L. C., and Ruddle, R. H. (1984). The human transferrin receptor gene: genomic organization, and the complete primary structure of the receptor deduced from a cDNA sequence, *Cell*, **39**, 267–74.

Miskimins, W. K., McClelland, A., Roberts, M. P., and Ruddle, F. H. (1986). Cell proliferation and expression of the transferrin receptor gene: promoter sequence homologies and protein interactions, *J. Cell Biol.*, **103**, 1781–8.

Neckers, L. M., and Cossman, J. (1983). Transferrin receptor induction in mitogen stimulated T lymphocytes is required for DNA synthesis and cell division and is regulated by IL-2, *Proc. Natl Acad. Sci. USA*, **80**, 3494–8.

Neilands, J. B. (1972). Evolution of biological iron binding center, *Structure and Bonding*, **11**, 145–70.

Newman, R., Schneider, C., Sutherland, R., Vodinelich, L., and Greaves, M. (1983). The transferrin receptor, *Trends Biochem. Sci.*, **7**, 397–400.

Otsuka, S., Maruyama, H., and Listowsky, I. (1981). Structure, assembly, conformation, and immunological properties of the two subunit classes of ferritin, *Biochemistry*, **20**, 5226–32.

Owen, D., and Kuhn, L. C. (1987). Noncoding 3' sequences of the transferrin receptor gene are required for mRNA regulation by iron, *EMBO J.*, **6**, 1287–93.

Pelosi, E., Testa, U., Louache, F., Thomopoulos, P., Salvo, G., Samoggia, P., and Peschle, C. (1986). Expression of transferrin receptors in phytohemagglutinin-stimulated human T-lymphocytes, *J. Biol. Chem.*, **261**, 3036–42.

Pelus, L. M., Broxmeyer, H. E., and Moore, M. A. S. (1981). Regulation of human myelopoieses by prostaglandin and lactoferrin, *Cell Tissue Kinet.*, **14**, 515–26.

Ponka, P., and Schulman, H. M. (1985a). Regulation of heme synthesis in erythroid cells: hemin inhibits transferrin iron utilization but not protoporphyrin synthesis, *Blood*, **65**, 850–7.

Ponka, P., and Schulman, H. M. (1985b). Acquisition of iron from transferrin regulates heme synthesis, *J. Biol. Chem.*, **260**, 14717–21.

Posakony, J. W., England, J. W., and Attardi, G. (1977). Mitochondrial growth and division during the cell cycle, *J. Cell Biol.*, **74**, 468–91.

Rao, K., Harford, J. B., Rouault, T., McClelland, A., Ruddle, F. H., and Klausner, R. D. (1986). Transcriptional regulation by iron of the gene for the transferrin receptor, *Mol. Cell. Biol.*, **6**, 236–40.

Reddel, R. P., Hedley, D. W., and Sutherland, R. L. (1985). Cell cycle effects of iron depletion on T-470 human breast cancer cells, *Exp. Cell Res.*, **161**, 277-84.

Resnitzky, D., Yarden, A., Zipori, D., and Kimchi, A. (1986). Autocrine β-interferon controls c-myc suppression and growth arrest during hematopoietic cell differentiation, *Cell*, **46**, 31-40.

Rhyner, K., Taetle, R., Bering, H., and To, D. (1985). Transferrin receptors coupled to intracellular ferritin in proliferating and differentiating HL60 leukemia cells, *J. Cell. Physiol.*, **125**, 608-12.

Rothenberger, S., Iacopetta, B. J., and Kuhn, L. C. (1987). Endocytosis of the transferrin receptor requires the cytoplasmic domain but not its phosphorylation site, *Cell*, **49**, 423-31.

Rudolph, N. S., Ohlsson-Wilhelm, B. M., Leary, J. F., and Rowley, P. T. (1985). Regulation of K562 cell transferrin receptors by exogenous iron, *J. Cell Physiol.*, **122**, 441-50.

Schlabach, M. R., and Bates, G. W. (1975). The synergistic binding of anion and Fe^{3+} by transferrin, *J. Biol. Chem.*, **250**, 2182-8.

Schmidt, J. A., Marshall, J., Hayman, M. J., Ponka, P., and Beug, H. (1986). Control of erythroid differentiation: possible role of the transferrin cycle, *Cell*, **46**, 41-51.

Schneider, C., Sutherland, R., Newman, R. A., and Greaves, M. F. (1982). Structural features of the cell surface receptor for transferrin that is recognized by the monoclonal antibody OKT9, *J. Biol. Chem.*, **257**, 8516-22.

Schneider, C., Owen, M. J., Banville, D., and Williams, J. G. (1984). Primary structure of human transferrin receptor deduced from the mRNA sequence, *Nature*, **311**, 675-8.

Seligman, P. A. (1983). Structure and function of the transferrin receptor, *Prog. Hematol.*, **13**, 131-47.

Seligman, P. A., Schleicher, R. B., and Allen, R. H. (1979). Isolation and characterization of the transferrin receptor from human placenta, *J. Biol. Chem.*, **254**, 9943-6.

Shau, H., Shen, D., and Golub, S. H. (1986). The role of transferrin in natural killer cell and IL-2 induced cytotoxic cell function, *Cell. Immunol.*, **97**, 121-30.

Spiro, T., and Saltman, P. (1969). Polynuclear complexes of iron and their biological implications, *Structure and Bonding.*, **6**, 117-56.

Stein, B. S., and Sussman, H. H. (1983). Peptide mapping of the human transferrin receptor in normal and transformed cells, *J. Biol. Chem.*, **258**, 2668-73.

Taetle, R., Rhyner, K., Castagnola, J., To, D., and Mendelsohn, J. (1985). Role of transferrin, Fe, and transferrin receptors in myeloid leukemia cell growth, *J. Clin. Invest.*, **75**, 1061-7.

Taetle, R., Ralph, S., Smedsrud, S., and Trowbridge, I. (1987). Regulation of transferrin receptor expression in myeloid leukemic cells, *Blood*, **70**, 852-4.

Takami, M., Mizumoto, K., Kasuya, I., Kino, K., Sussman, H. H., and Tsunoo, H. (1986). Human placental ferritin receptor, *Biochim. Biophys. Acta*, **884**, 31-8.

Trowbridge, I. S., and Lopez, F. (1982). Monoclonal antibody to transferrin receptor blocks transferrin binding and inhibits tumor cell growth *in vitro*, *Proc. Natl Acad. Sci. USA*, **79**, 1175-9.

Tsiftsoglou, A. S., Nunez, M. T., Wang, W., and Robinson, S. H. (1983). Dissociation of iron transport and heme biosynthesis from commitment to terminal maturation of murine erythroleukemia cells, *Proc. Natl Acad. Sci. USA*, **80**, 7528-32.

Wada, H. D., Hass, P. E., and Sussman, H. H. (1979). Transferrin receptor in human placental brush border membranes, *J. Biol. Chem.*, **254**, 12629–35.

Ward, J. H., Kushner, J. P., and Kaplan, J. (1984). Iron: metabolism and clinical disorders, *Curr. Hematol. Oncol.*, **3**, 1–50.

Watanabe, N., and Drysdale, J. (1981). Evidence for distinct mRNAs for ferritin subunits, *Biochem. Biophys. Res. Commun.*, **98**, 507–11.

White, G. P., Bailey-Wood, R., and Jacobs, A. (1976). The effect of chelating agents on cellular iron metabolism, *Clin. Sci. Mol. Med.*, **50**, 145–52.

Yamashiro, D. J., Tycko, B., Fluss, S. R., and Maxfield, F. R. (1984). Segregation of transferrin to a mildly acidic pathway, *Cell*, **37**, 789–800.

13
Ferritin as a Marker of Malignancy

Chaya Moroz and Hanna Bessler

Rogoff Medical Research Institute, Beilinson Medical Center and Sackler School of Medicine, Tel-Aviv University, Petah-Tikva, Israel

THE MOLECULAR STRUCTURE OF ISOFERRITINS ISOLATED BY MONOCLONAL ANTIBODIES FROM HUMAN PLACENTA AND BREAST CANCER CELLS

Ferritin is an iron-storage protein designed to maintain iron in an available non-toxic form. However, in recent years there has been considerable interest in ferritin as a protein related to malignancies.

As reviewed in detail in Chapter 4, analysis of cDNA clones revealed that the H and L subunits are encoded by rather complex families of genes (Brown, Leibold and Munro, 1983; Costanzo *et al.*, 1984; Boyd *et al.*, 1985), suggesting that the heterogeneity of ferritin molecules may be even greater than presently determined.

Adult human heart, kidney, pancreas and placental ferritins, as well as ferritins derived from several neoplasms, show more acidic isoferritins on isoelectric focusing than liver and spleen ferritin (Drysdale, 1970, 1971). Therefore, the term carcinofetal isoferritins has been used by Drysdale and Singer (1974) to describe the acidic isoferritins isolated from human placenta and HeLa cells.

In an attempt to investigate whether carcinofetal ferritin is of a unique molecular and/or antigenic structure, hybridomas producing monoclonal antibodies (McAbs) to human placental ferritin were developed. The production and characterization of two McAbs against human placental ferritin have been reported (Moroz *et al.*, 1985). One of the McAbs (CM-H-9) was found to bind exclusively to placental ferritin (Figure 13.1), and the second McAb (CM-G-8) bound to placental ferritin and cross-reacted with ferritins isolated from human spleen and liver (Figure 13.2). The two ferritin antigenic determinants recognized by CM-H-9 and CM-G-8 McAbs were molecularly associated, since placental ferritin first bound to CM-G-8

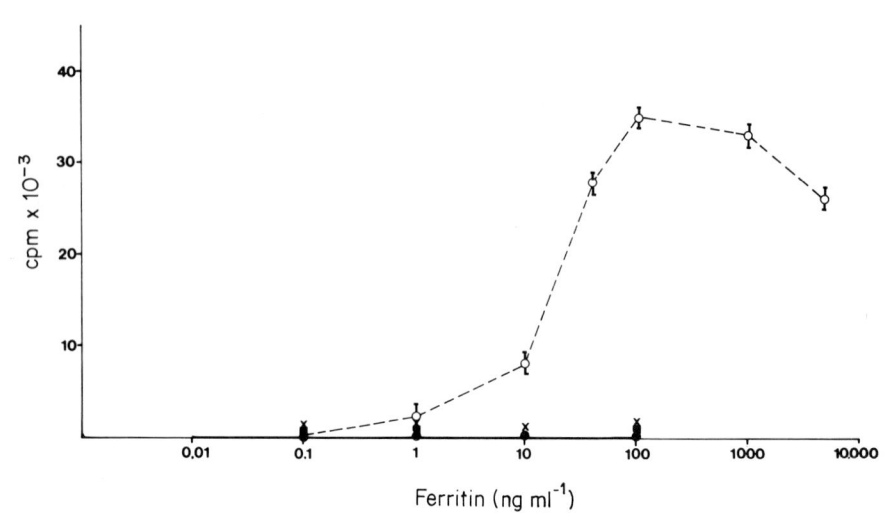

Figure 13.1 Characterization of the specificity of CM-H-9 McAb. The binding activity and specificity of CM-H-9 McAb was determined by the solid-phase radioimmunoassay in which plastic microtiter plates were coated with 20 μg purified CM-H9 McAb. Binding of different concentrations of human placenta, liver and spleen ferritin to CM-H-9 McAb was determined using [^{125}I]CM-H-9 McAb (10^5 cpm well^{-1}, ~ 1 μCi μg^{-1}). The bars represent SEM of triplicate assays. O----O, placental ferritin; ●———●, spleen ferritin; ■———■, liver ferritin; ×——×, human albumin. Data from Moroz et al. (1985). Reproduced by permission of Elsevier Science Publishers B.V. (Biomedical Division) Amsterdam

McAb was further capable of reacting with either [^{125}I]CM-G-8 or [^{125}I]CM-H-9 McAbs (Moroz et al., 1985). These results indicate that placental ferritin has a specific antigenic epitope reactive with CM-H-9 McAb.

Controversial results were reported by several investigators on the subunit composition of placental ferritin studied using gradients of differing gel pore size and/or discontinuous buffer systems. Some studies revealed two and sometimes three subunits of similar but distinctive mobility (Stefanini, 1982; Linder, 1981). In contrast, using similar techniques, placental ferritin was reported to be composed of a single subunit type which comigrated with liver-type ferritin on SDS-acrylamide under reducing conditions (Brown et al., 1979). Konijn et al. (1985) isolated five placental isoferritins with different isoelectric points and subunit compositions. The most basic isoferritin was identical to splenic ferritin, whereas in acidic ferritin fractions the H subunit content was similar to that found in heart ferritin.

A different subunit composition of placental ferritin has been described by Parhami-Seren and Moroz (1986). The placental ferritins were obtained using affinity purification by CM-G-8 and CM-H-9 McAbs. These studies

Ferritin as a Marker of Malignancy 285

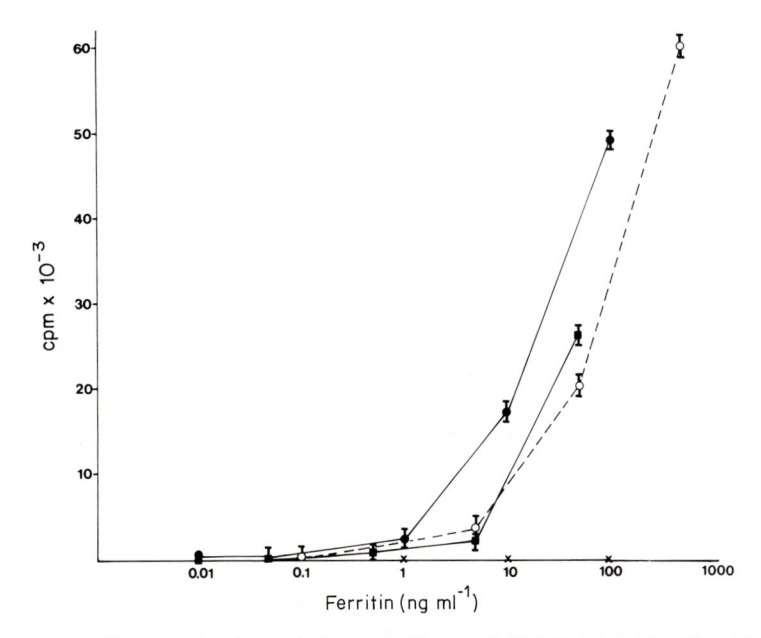

Figure 13.2 Characterization of the specificity of CM-G-8 McAb. The binding activity and specificity of CM-G-8 McAb was determined by solid-phase radio-immunoassay in which plastic microtiter plates were coated with 20 µg purified CM-G-8 McAb. Binding of different concentrations of ferritins isolated from human placenta, spleen and liver to CM-G-8 McAb was determined using [^{125}I]CM-G-8 McAb (10^5 cpm well^{-1}, ~ 1 µCi µg^{-1}). The bars represent SEM of triplicate assays. ○---○, placental ferritin; ●——●, spleen ferritin; ■——■, liver ferritin; ×——×, human albumin. Data from Moroz et al. (1985). Reproduced by permission of Elsevier Science Publishers B.V. (Biomedical Division) Amsterdam

revealed that placental ferritin immunoprecipitated with CM-G-8 McAb when dissociated under exhaustive reducing conditions exhibited three subunits (Figure 13.3). These included 18 kDa light (L) and 20 kDa heavy (H) subunits which have been shown previously to make up spleen and liver ferritins (Cragg, Wagstaff and Worwood, 1981; Adelman, Arosio and Drysdale, 1975; Otsuka, Maruyama and Listowsky, 1981), and in addition a high molecular mass subunit (43 kDa) was evident. Furthermore, ferritin immunoprecipitated with the specific antiplacental ferritin CM-H-9 McAb when dissociated was composed of the 43 kDa subunit (P43) only, indicating the presence of a homopolymer of this subunit type. This unique subunit could not be further dissociated into smaller peptides under exhaustive reducing conditions, indicating that it is not a polymerized H or L subunit dimer.

The presence of the 43 kDa subunit associated with human placental ferritin was not observed by other investigators who isolated ferritin from

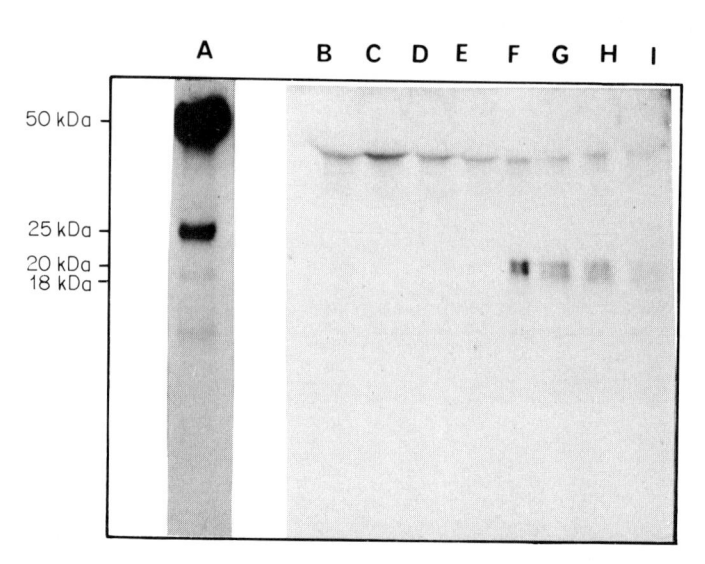

Figure 13.3 Subunit composition of [^{125}I]CM-H-9/Fer and [^{125}I]CM-G8/Fer. Placenta ferritin affinity purified on McAbs CM-H-9 (CM-H-9/Fer) or CM-G-8 (CM-G-8/Fer) coupled to Sepharose was radioiodinated. [^{125}I]CM-H-9/Fer and [^{125}I]CM-G-8/Fer were immunoprecipitated with CM-H-9 and CM-G-8 respectively. The precipitates were subjected to SDS-PAGE (15%) under reducing conditions and were then blotted on to a nitrocellulose paper for 16 h at 100 V, 0.36 A, dried and exposed for autoradiography. A: Marker for molecular weight determination; B–E: [^{125}I]CM-H-9/Fer immunoprecipitated with 100, 10, 1, 0.1 µg CM-H-9 McAb respectively; F–I: [^{125}I]CM-G-8/Fer immunoprecipitated with 100, 10, 1, 0.1 µg CM-G-8 McAb respectively. Data from Parhami-Seren and Moroz (1986)

human placenta (Drysdale and Singer, 1974; Brown et al., 1979; Konijn et al., 1985). This discrepancy might be due to the difference in the isolation procedures for placental ferritin used by the different investigators. A high molecular mass subunit (45 kDa) specific for rat placenta and fetal liver ferritins was reported by Shinjo et al. (1984).

The physicochemical and antigenic heterogeneity of placental isoferritins was further revealed using western blots of the isoelectric focused ferritins with CM-G-8 and CM-H-9 McAbs. As seen in Figure 13.4, CM-H-9 McAb reacted with placental ferritin at pH ranging from 4.7 to 5.2 (Figure 13.4A), whereas G-8 McAb reacted with placental ferritin at pH 5.1–5.4 (Figure 13.4C). In comparison, spleen ferritin did not react with CM-H-9 McAb (Figure 13.4B) whereas it reacted with CM-G-8 McAb at pH 5.4–5.5 (Figure 13.4D). These results exhibit the physicochemical and antigenic heterogeneity of placental ferritin and indicate that the most acidic ferritin (p*I* 4.7–5.0) is reactive with CM-H-9 McAb, whereas the less acidic molecules (p*I* 5.1–5.2) are reactive with both CM-H-9 and CM-G-8 McAbs.

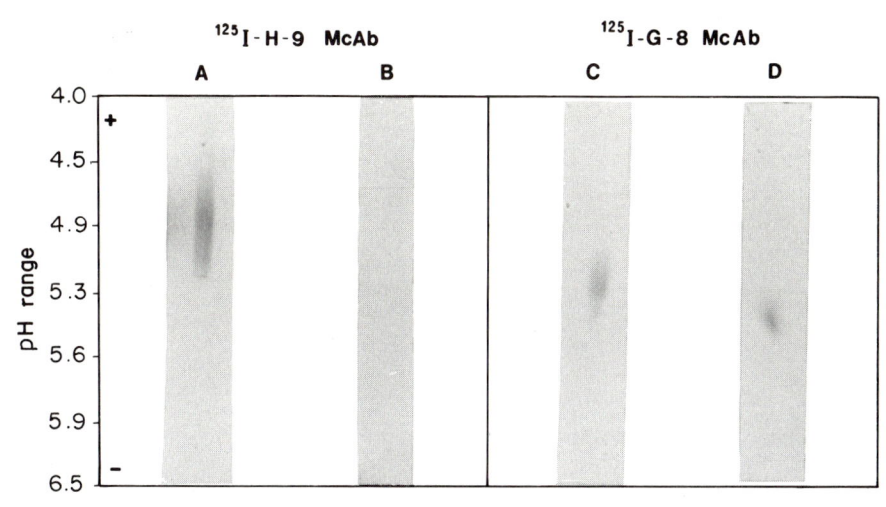

Figure 13.4 Analysis of the heterogeneity of human placenta and spleen ferritins by isoelectric focusing (IEF) following reactivity with CM-H-9 and CM-G-8 McAbs. IEF was performed in agarose containing Pharmalyte, pH 4.0–6.5. Focused placenta (A and C) and spleen (B and D) ferritins were detected following incubation with either [^{125}I]CM-H-9 (A,B) or [^{125}I]CM-G-8 McAbs (C,D) (100 μCi). Data from Parhami-Seren and Moroz (1986)

In many tissues affected by cancer the level of ferritin is elevated; these ferritins often have a relatively low iron content and are mostly more acidic than normal tissue ferritin as judged by isoelectric focusing. The finding of acidic isoferritin not present in normal adult tissues has been reported for a variety of tumor tissues such as breast cancer (Marcus and Zinberg, 1974), neuroblastoma (Hann, Stahlhut and Evans, 1985), leukemia and Hodgkin's disease (Cavaña et al., 1983; White et al., 1976). There has been much controversy about whether cancer ferritins are different from those of normal tissues (Drysdale et al., 1975). It was suggested that they contain specific carcinofetal sequences or that they are acidic because of the presence of higher proportions of the normal H subunit compared to the L subunit.

The use of the antiplacental ferritin McAbs for purification of ferritins synthesized *de novo* by cancer cell lines enabled Parhami-Seren and Moroz (1986) to characterize the subunit structure of carcinofetal ferritins. These studies revealed that ferritin synthesized *de novo* by breast cancer cells (HT-24 and T-47D) (Figure 13.5), when immunoprecipitated with CM-G-8 monoclonal anti-ferritin antibody, constituted three subunits, L (18 kDa), H (20 kDa) and a high molecular mass subunit of 43 kDa (designated P43) (Figure 13.5). In addition, a homopolymer of *de novo* synthesized P43 was precipitated with CM-H-9 McAb.

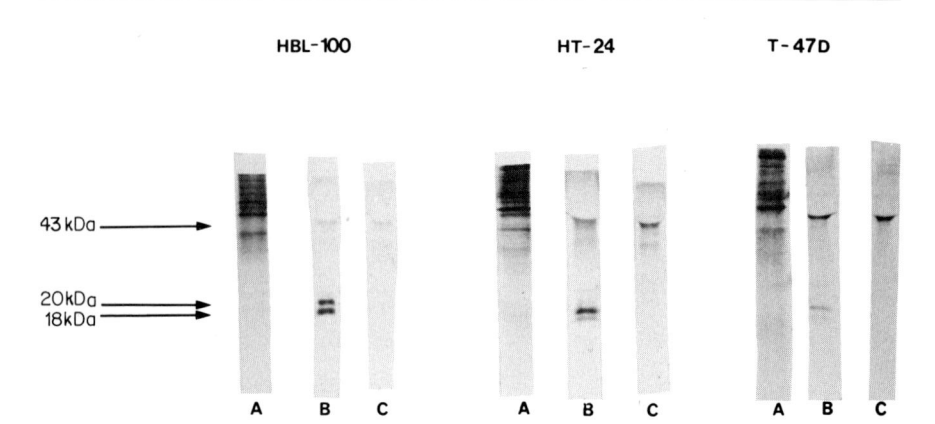

Figure 13.5 Autoradiograph of SDS-PAGE profile of lysates from breast cell lines labeled with [^{35}S]methionine and of the nascent isoferritins immunoprecipitated by McAbs. Total radiolabeled proteins in lysate (A) (1/200 of the amount used for immunoprecipitation), ferritin immunoprecipitated by CM-G-8 McAb (B), and ferritin immunoprecipitated by CM-H-9 McAb (C)

The above results exhibit similarity between the structure of ferritin in the placenta and that of ferritins isolated from breast cancer cells.

In contrast, ferritin synthesized *de novo* by cells which originated from normal breast epithelium (HBL-100) (Figure 13.5) or, for example, ferritin synthesized by monocyte–macrophages isolated from healthy donors (Figure 13.6), contained mostly L and H subunits with only trace amounts of P43.

Since P43 was isolated by CM-H-9 McAb both from the placenta (Parhami-Seren and Moroz, 1986) and from cancer cells, but none or very minute amounts were isolated from normal cells, it may be considered as a tumor-associated fetal antigen.

The acidic nature of isoferritins isolated from the heart, monocytes, placenta and tumors was considered previously to be due to the high proportion of H subunits in the molecule (Drysdale *et al.*, 1975). The high proportion of H subunits is indeed characteristic of acidic ferritins; however, within the family of acidic ferritins, the carcinofetal ferritins isolated either from breast cancer cells or from placenta (Parhami-Seren and Moroz, 1986) are unique in the high content of P43 as opposed to acidic ferritin isolated from normal non-malignant cells (HBL-100, monocytes), which lack P43. Since P43 identified by its binding to CM-H-9 McAb on western blots was found to be of the most acidic nature (Parhami-Seren and Moroz, 1986) (p*I* 4.7), its presence in high proportions further contributes to the acidic nature of oncofetal ferritin.

It may be appropriate to note that Dörner *et al.* (1980) reported the *de novo* synthesis of H-rich ferritin molecules by T cells of Hodgkin's disease

Ferritin as a Marker of Malignancy 289

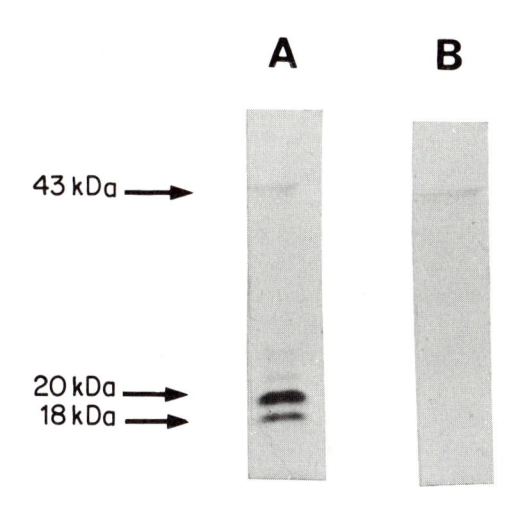

Figure 13.6 Autoradiograph of SDS-PAGE profile of [^{35}S]methionine-labeled ferritins immunoprecipitated from lysates of monocyte–macrophages with anti-placental ferritin McAbs. Ferritin immunoprecipitated by CM-G-8 McAb (A) and by CM-H-9 McAb (B)

patients. In their study, the *de novo* synthesized ferritin was immunoprecipitated by anti-spleen ferritin and electrophoresed under reducing conditions on SDS-polyacrylamide gel. The autoradiographs exhibited a peptide corresponding to a molecular mass of 43kDa, in addition to the L and H chains (Dörner *et al.*, 1980). Although the authors did not comment on this finding, the 43 kDa peptide which was sometimes exhibited (M. de Sousa, personal communication) may correspond to the 43 kDa peptide of placenta and breast cancer ferritins.

THE IMMUNOLOGICAL FUNCTION OF ONCOFETAL FERRITIN; ITS EFFECT ON T LYMPHOCYTES

Ferritin acts in the cell as an iron-storage protein, yet it may have other roles such as inducing regulation of myelopoiesis (Broxmeyer *et al.*, 1984; see also Chapter 9) and immunoregulation of the T cell function (Moroz and Kupfer, 1981; Matzner *et al.*, 1985). Different isoferritins may exert different functional activities.

Initial observations made by Moroz and coworkers revealed that lymphocytes isolated from patients with Hodgkin's disease and breast cancer possess surface-bound ferritin (Moroz *et al.* 1977a, 1977b, 1977c; Giler *et al.*, 1979). Evidence was presented that the binding of ferritin caused the inhibition of the formation of sheep red blood cell E-rosettes by a T cell subset (Moroz et al., 1977a). This was supported by experiments in which removal of the surface-bound ferritin following incubation with Levamisole or fetal calf serum resulted in the restoration of E-rosette formation. It was further established that the ferritin bound to the surface of the patients' T cells was of acidic nature and interacted with the McAb CM-H-9, which is specific for isoferritins found in placenta and breast cancer cells (Moroz et al., 1984). The specific inhibition of E-rosette formation by acidic ferritin derived from tumor cells and not by basic liver isoferritin was also observed by Hann, Stahlhut and Chung (1984). Other investigators have shown that Hodgkin's spleen ferritin may be acting as a tumor-associated sensitizing substance and as an immune response blocking agent (Hancock et al., 1979).

The interaction of the tumor-derived or placental acidic ferritin with T cells appears to have an immunosuppressive effect. This is supported by the following observations. In breast cancer patients the removal of the surface acidic ferritin from the T cells resulted in restoration of the T cells' reactivity in mixed lymphocyte culture (Moroz and Kupfer, 1981). *In vitro* experiments revealed that tumor ferritin suppresses the blastogenic response of lymphocytes to mitogens (Buffe et al., 1978; Niitsu et al., 1976). Other studies have shown that different isoferritins may have varying degrees of immunosuppressive activity. Matzner et al. (1985) demonstrated that acidic and basic isoferritins isolated from human placenta differ in their suppressive potential on T lymphocyte function *in vitro*. Acidic isoferritins suppressed T lymphocyte transformation by both phytohemagglutinin (PHA) and concanavalin-A (Con-A) mitogens, whereas the basic isoferritins did not affect the PHA transformation and had a lower suppressive effect on the blastogenic response to Con-A (Matzner et al., 1985).

The above described function of ferritin may be attributed to the unique molecular structure of acidic ferritins derived from placenta or tumor cells. Some T cells may express specific surface receptors for oncofetal ferritin, and its interaction with the ferritin ligand may result in immunosuppression. In a recent study, Moroz et al. (1987b) demonstrated that high levels of placental ferritin (PLF) isoform were measured in the sera of pregnant women at 17 weeks of gestation up to term delivery as compared with adult non-pregnant women, who are mostly lacking PLF. The level of PLF was independent of the total ferritin level. It was further found that in the blood of women who delivered at early gestational age (29–36 weeks), PLF was undetected or very low (Moroz et al., 1987b). Although direct association between the preterm delivery and absence of PLF in the serum has not been proven, it was suggested that PLF may play a regulatory role in pregnancy. Thus the high blood levels of PLF during pregnancy may be one of the factors responsible for the suppression of the immune system of the mother, enabling the development of a full-term pregnancy. Oncofetal ferritin may thus play an important role in modulation of the host immune response, enabling both cancer and embryonic development.

ONCOFETAL FERRITIN AS A MARKER FOR MALIGNANCY

Ferritin-bearing lymphocytes as a marker for early breast cancer

During the past several years, tumor marker testing has progressed from research into clinical practice. The low clinical sensitivity and specificity of tumor markers for neoplastic disease limits their usefulness in screening for cancer in an asymptomatic population. However, tumor markers are useful in establishing a diagnosis of cancer when they are used along with other diagnostic procedures.

Immunologic markers for breast cancer include ferritin (Marcus and Zinberg, 1974, 1975a, 1975b). Elevation in the serum ferritin level may simply reflect increased iron stores and block of reticuloendothelial uptake of iron or even release of ferritin from inflammatory or necrotic tissue. Serum ferritin levels in cancer patients are influenced by these factors, and in addition ferritin may be secreted directly by proliferating tumor cells (Marcus and Zinberg, 1974, 1975a). Elevation of serum ferritin in breast cancer patients has been reported (Marcus and Zinberg, 1975; Jacobs et al., 1976; Tappin, 1979). Serum levels greater than 200 μg l^{-1} in early breast cancer are predictive of clinical recurrence; however, only 10% of breast cancer patients have these high concentrations (Jacobs et al., 1976). A drop in the elevated serum ferritin occurred after surgical removal of the tumors (Tappin, 1979). Generally, the high serum concentrations of ferritin at presentation correlated with widespread disease and poor prognosis (Jacobs et al., 1976).

Moroz et al. studied the use of oncofetal ferritin bound to peripheral blood lymphocytes as a potential biomarker for the diagnosis of breast cancer. A blood test was developed in which ferritin-bearing lymphocytes (FBLs) were enumerated by an antibody-mediated cytotoxic assay using the specific anti-placental ferritin McAb CM-H-9 and rabbit complement (Moroz et al., 1984). Women who had above 5% FBLs in the circulation were considered as FBL-positive. This assay was further developed into a radioimmunossay in which the binding of [^{125}I]CM-H-9 McAb to peripheral blood lymphocytes was determined. These assays were applied to 496 women who underwent a breast biopsy. The FBL test results were compared to histopathological diagnosis of the breast tumor.

The results of the FBL test obtained in these studies revealed that among the patients with stages I and II breast cancer 81.7% were FBL-positive, whereas in patients with benign breast disease only 27.5% were FBL-positive. All three patients with *in situ* carcinoma were FBL-positive (Table 13.1).

A poor correlation between the FBL test and locally advanced breast cancer (stage III) was noted. Chernovskaia, Polevaia and Tuzhikova (1986) also reported that the maximum amount of FBLs was present in the blood of breast cancer patients with stage I–IIA disease and that a low or negative score was associated with advanced breast cancer. This is an unexplained observation. One hypothesis assumes that with the advancement of the disease there is an increased quantity of ferritin secreted by the tumor which saturates the receptors on the membrane of the lymphocytes, which are consequently removed from the circulation by the spleen. This could be supported by the reported observation of a significant enlargement of the spleen in locally advanced breast cancer (Roberts *et al.*, 1979). Another explanation could be the development of yet unidentified masking factors (antibodies, immune complexes) which inhibited the interaction of the ferritin with the CM-H-9 McAbs. It is interesting to note that among 25 patients who had breast cancer at stages I or II and 16 patients with stage III for whom 4 years follow-up data were available, those with negative FBL scores had a shorter disease-free survival than those with positive FBL (Moroz *et al.*, 1988). This would suggest that an FBL-negative test in histopathologically diagnosed breast cancer patients is an indicator for advanced disease and poor prognosis.

Because the large majority (81.9%) of patients with stage III breast cancer were negative in FBL testing it is clear that this test is only suitable for early disease. However, in the majority of patients with disseminated disease (stage IV), the FBL test was positive (Moroz *et al.*, 1984; Fereberger, 1984), indicating that the test could be used for the follow-up of metastatic disease. Similar results were obtained by Fereberger (1984) using the CM-H-9 FBL cytotoxic assay in patients with all stages of breast cancer and in patients with benign breast tumors. Other investigators confirmed the presence of FBLs in the circulation of breast cancer patients (Papenhausen *et al.*, 1984; Steinhoff *et al.*, 1984).

Multivariate analysis was used to evaluate a positive FBL score as a potential risk factor for early breast cancer (Moroz *et al.*, 1988). The analysis revealed that in addition to the known risk factors, age >50 years at examination and a positive family history of breast cancer, the next strongest risk factor was a positive FBL test, which had a significantly increased odds ratio estimate of 2.9 with a 95% confidence interval of 1.4–5.8.

Being a measure of systemic immune reaction, the positive FBL test appears to be an early manifestation of breast cancer (Moroz *et al.*, 1984). In contrast, elevated levels of ferritin in the serum may indicate a progression

TABLE 13.1 Sensitivity of the FBL test for breast cancer diagnosis: data from two studies utilizing different assay systems. By permission of the American Cancer Society

Histopathological diagnosis of breast disease	Ferritin-bearing lymphocytes					Study I + II	
	Study I (Cytotoxic assay)[a] || Study II (RIA)[b,d]				
	No. of patients tested ($n = 176$)	% with positive FBL[c]	No. of patients tested ($n = 320$)	% with positive FBL[d]	No. of patients tested ($n = 496$)	% with positive FBL
Benign	96	30.2	148	25.7	244	27.5
Premalignant	12	100.0	21	42.9	33	63.6
In situ	—		3	100.0	3	100.0
Stage I, II	47	89.0	57	75.4	104	81.7
Stage III	18	22.0	87	17.2	105	18.1
Stage IV	3	100.0	4	50.0	7	71.4

[a] Ferritin-bearing lymphocytes were enumerated by an antibody-mediated cytotoxic assay using CM-H-9 McAb and rabbit complement (data from Moroz et al. (1984)).
[b] Ferritin-bearing lymphocytes were measured by a competitive binding assay with [^{125}I]CM-H-9 McAb.
[c] FBL 0–5% = negative, FBL ≥ 6% = positive (data from Moroz et al. (1988)).
[d] $\text{FBL} = \dfrac{\text{Total [}^{125}\text{I]CM-H-9 McAb bound (cpm) to PBL}}{\text{Nonspecific [}^{125}\text{I]CM-H-9 McAb bound (cpm) to PBL}}$.   FBL < 1.59 = negative, FBL ≥ 1.60 = positive

of the disease (Jacobs et al., 1976). A direct relation between a rise of the serum ferritin concentration, a drop in the amount of FBLs and breast cancer spreading was established by Chernovskaia, Polevaia and Tuzhikova (1986). Therefore, in order for the ferritin marker to have the potential of being a population-screening test, it may be necessary to measure both the FBL level and the serum ferritin concentration to identify the patients with early as well as advanced breast cancer.

Ferritin-bearing lymphocytes as a marker in other malignancies

The presence of a subpopulation of lymphocytes bearing surface ferritin in the circulation has also been demonstrated in patients with Hodgkin's disease (Moroz et al., 1977; Steinhoff et al., 1984; Koprivova et al., 1986) as well as in patients with carcinomas of the head and neck, colon and lung (Papenhausen et al., 1984; Steinhoff et al., 1984). As in breast cancer, no correlation was demonstrated between the presence of FBLs and serum ferritin levels (liver isotype) in the above-described malignancies (Steinhoff et al., 1984; Fereberger, 1984). It was suggested that in the above malignancies the determination of the FBLs may be a biomarker of an early manifestation, and may be better than the serum ferritin concentration.

Placental ferritin isoform detected in the serum by CM-H-9 monoclonal antibody as a biomarker in lymphoproliferative disease

Elevated concentrations of serum ferritin were found in patients suffering from a variety of malignant diseases other than breast cancer (Jacobs et al., 1976), such as acute lymphatic leukemia (ALL) (Matzner, Konijn and Hershko, 1980), hepatoma (Giannoulis, 1984; see also Chapter 14) and Hodgkin's disease (Dörner et al., 1983).

The structural and immunological heterogeneity of different isoferritins gives rise to a variation in their reactivity to various antibody preparations (Worwood, Jones and Jacobs, 1976; Hazard and Drysdale, 1977; Jones, 1980).

It has been suggested that a specific assay for acidic ferritin in the serum may be of value in the diagnosis of cancer. Assays which utilized antibodies to HeLa cell ferritin and spleen ferritin revealed that HeLa-type ferritin concentrations were greater in patients with advanced breast cancer than in patients with early cancer. However, the same was true for spleen-type ferritin, which was present in considerable excess (Jones, Worwood and Jacobs, 1980).

Some investigators reported high liver-type ferritin levels in patients with lymphoproliferative disorders (Matzner, Konijn and Hershko, 1980). In Hodgkin's disease the high serum ferritin levels correlated with the disease activity without being related to the amount of iron storage (Ramot et al., 1976; Hancock et al., 1979; Cazzola et al., 1983; Dorner et al., 1983). In assays based on antibodies against HeLa cell ferritin (acidic type), Hazard and Drysdale (1977) found higher concentrations of ferritin in sera from patients with various tumors than when assayed by antibodies directed against normal liver ferritin. Others have failed to demonstrate a consistent pattern of isoferritins in tumor tissues (Halliday, McKeeting and Powell, 1976; Jones and Worwood, 1978) or in sera obtained from patients with tumors (Jones and Worwood, 1978; Jones, Worwood and Jacobs, 1980).

Moroz et al. developed a new enzyme-linked immunosorbent assay (ELISA) specific for placental ferritin isoform (PLF). Using this assay, the level of PLF was measured in the sera of patients with lymphoproliferative diseases and multiple myeloma (the amount of PLF which bound 25 pg of conjugated CM-H-9 McAB was considered as 1u) (Moroz et al., 1987a). In 40 healthy individuals the mean serum concentration of PLF was 8.1 ± 0.8 u ml^{-1}, with 70% of the sera containing no detectable PLF. The PLF concentrations were significantly elevated in the sera of patients with Hodgkin's disease (47 ± 43 u ml^{-1}) and in non-Hodgkin's lymphoma of low and intermediate grade (97.1 ± 39.0 u ml^{-1}; 41.9 ± 35.8 u ml^{-1} respectively). During remission the PLF levels in patients with Hodgkin's lymphoma decreased to levels similar to those of healthy individuals. No PLF or very low PLF concentrations were found in the sera of patients with multiple myeloma and chronic lymphatic leukemia (CLL) (6.3 ± 13.5 u ml^{-1}). All the sera exhibiting high PLF levels had elevated liver-type ferritin as well.

Malignant cells such as leukemic blast cells or reactive lymphocytes may have increased rates of ferritin synthesis and may be responsible for an abnormally high serum concentration (White et al., 1976; Cavana et al., 1983). Sarcione and coworkers (Sarcione, Stutzman and Mittelman, 1975; Sarcione et al., 1977) presented evidence of elevated synthesis of ferritin by peripheral lymphocytes and involved spleen cells in Hodgkin's disease patients.

The serum ferritin may represent a specific tumor product and/or may result from inflammation, iron overload, hepatic damage, drug toxicity or blood transfusions. Since PLF was not detected in the serum of the majority of normal individuals, but in patients with Hodgkin's and non-Hodgkin's lymphoma high levels were measured, it may be considered a tumor-associated antigen and thereby serve as a more specific marker for the diagnosis and follow-up of these diseases.

REFERENCES

Adelman, T. G., Arosio, P., and Drysdale, J. W. (1975). Multiple subunits in human ferritins: evidence for hybrid molecules, *Biochem. Biophys. Res. Commun.*, **63**, 1056–62.
Arosio, P., Adelman, T. G., and Drysdale, J. W. (1978). On ferritin heterogeneity— further evidence for heteropolymers, *J. Biol. Chem.*, **253**, 4451–8.
Bezwoda, W. R., Derman, D. P., Bothwell, T. H., Baynes, R., Hesdorffer, C., and MacPhail, A. P. (1985). Serum ferritin and Hodgkin's disease, *Scand. J. Haematol.*, **35**, 505–10.
Boyd, D., Vecoli, C., Belchert, D. M., Jain, S. K., and Drysdale, J. W. (1985). Structural and functional relationships of human ferritin H and L chains deduced from cDNA clones, *J. Biol. Chem.*, **260**, 11755–61.
Brown, A. J., Leibold, E. A., and Munro, H. H. (1983). Isolation of cDNA clones for the light subunit of rat liver ferritin: evidence that the light subunit is encoded by a multigene family, *Proc. Natl Acad. Sci. USA*, **80**, 1265–9.
Brown, J. P., Johnson, P. M., Ogbimi, A. O., and Tappin, I. A. (1979). Characterization and localization of human placental ferritin, *Biochem. J.*, **182**, 763–9.
Broxmeyer, H. E., Gentile, D., Listowsky, E., Cavanna, F., Feickert, H. J., Dorner, M. H., Ruggeri, G., Cazzola, M., and Cooper, S. (1984). Acidic isoferritins in the regulation of hematopoiesis in vitro and in vivo. In A. Albertini (ed.) *Ferritins and Isoferritins as Biochemical Markers*, pp. 97–111, Elsevier Science, Amsterdam.
Buffe, D., Rimbaut, C., and Erard, D. (1978). Immunosuppressive activity of alpha 2 H-'isoferritin' as compared to normal crystallized ferritin, *Scand. J. Immunol.*, **8** (supplement), 633–40.
Cavanna, F., Rugeri, G., Iacobello, C., Chieregatti, G., Murada, F., Albertini, A., and Arosio, P. (1983). Development of monoclonal antibody against heart ferritin and its application in an immunoradiometric assay, *Clin. Chim. Acta*, **134**, 347–56.
Cazzola, M., Arosio, P., Gobbi, P. G., Barosi, G., Bergamaschi, G., Dezza, L., Iacobello, C., and Ascari, E. (1983). Basic and acidic isoferritins in the serum of patients with Hodgkin's disease, *Eur. J. Cancer Clin. Oncol.*, **19**, 339–45.
Chernovskaia, E. M., Polevaia, E. B., and Tuzhikova, N. K. (1986). Relationship of blood serum ferritin and ferritin bearing lymphocytes in breast cancer, *Med. Radiol. (Mosk).*, **31**, 7–15.
Cragg, S. J., Wagstaff, M., and Worwood, M. (1981). Detection of glycosylated subunit in human serum ferritin, *Biochem. J.*, **199**, 565.
Costanzo, F., Santoro, C., Colantuoni, V., Bensi, G., Raugei, G., Romano, V., and Cortese, R. (1984). Cloning and sequencing of a full length cDNA coding for a human apoferritin H chain: evidence for multigenic family, *EMBO J.*, **3**, 23–27.
Dörner, M. H., Silverstone, A., Nishiya, K., De Sostoa, A., Munn, G., and De Sousa, M. (1980). Ferritin synthesis by human T lymphocytes, *Science*, **209**, 1019–21.
Dörner, M. H., Abel, U., Fritze, D., Manke, H. G., and Drings, P. (1983). Serum ferritin in relation to the course of Hodgkin's disease, *Cancer*, **52**, 2308–12.
Drysdale, J. W. (1970). Microheterogeneity of ferritin molecules, *Biochim. Biophys. Acta*, **207**, 256–8.
Drysdale, J. W. (1977). Human isoferritins in normal and disease states, *Ciba Found. Symp.*, **51**, 41–7.
Drysdale, J. W., and Singer, R. M. (1974). Carcinofetal human isoferritins in placenta and HeLa cells, *Cancer Res.*, **34**, 3352–4.

Drysdale, J. W., Adelman, T. G., Arosio, P., Casareale, D., Fitzpatrick, P., Hazard, J. T. and Yokota, M. (1971). Human isoferritins in normal and disease states, *Semin Hematol.*, **14**, 71–88.
Drysdale, J. W., Arosio, P., Adelman, T., Hazard, J. T., and Brooke, D. (1975). Isoferritins in normal and diseased states. In R. R. Crichton (ed.) *Proteins of Iron Storage and Transport in Biochemistry and Medicine*, pp. 359–66, North Holland, Amsterdam.
Fereberger, W. (1984). Iron and iron binding proteins in inflammation and cancer, *Wien. Med. Wochensch.*, **134** (supplement 79).
Giannoulis, E. (1984). Diagnostic value of serum ferritin in primary hepatocellular carcinoma, *Digestion*, **30**, 236–41.
Giler, S., Kupfer, B., Urca, I., and Moroz, C. (1979). Immunodiagnostic test for the early detection of carcinoma of the breast, *Surg. Gynaecol. Obstet.*, **149**, 655–7.
Halliday, J. W., McKeeting, L. V., and Powell, L. W. (1976). Isoferritin composition of tissues and serum in human cancers, *Cancer Res.*, **36**, 4486–90.
Hancock, B. W., Bruce, L., May, K., and Richmond, J. (1979). Ferritin, a sensitizing substance in the leukocyte migration inhibition test in patients with malignant lymphoma, *Br. J. Haematol.*, **43**, 223–33.
Hann, H.-W. L., Stahlhut, M. W., and Chung, L. C. (1984). Inhibitory effects of isoferritins from tumour and non-tumour tissues on E-rosette formation, *Lancet*, **1**, 43–4.
Hann, H.-W. L., Stahlhut, M. W., and Evans, A. E. (1985). Serum ferritin as a prognostic indicator in neuroblastoma, biological effects of isoferritins, *Adv. Neuroblast. Res.*, 331–45.
Hazard, J. T., and Drysdale, J. W. (1977). Ferritinemia in cancer, *Nature*, **265**, 755–6.
Hazard, J. T., Yokota, M., Arosio, P., and Drysdale, J. W. (1977). Immunologic differences in human isoferritins: implication for immunologic quantitation of serum ferritin, *Blood*, **49**, 139–46.
Jacobs, A., Jones, B., Ricketts, C., Boolbrook, R. D., and Wang, D. Y. (1976). Serum ferritin concentration in early breast cancer, *Br. J. Cancer*, **34**, 286–90.
Jain, S. K., Barrett, K. J., Boyd, D., Favreau, M. F., Crampton, J., and Drysdale, J. W. (1985). Ferritin H and L chains are derived from different multigene families, *J. Biol. Chem.*, **260**, 11762–8.
Jones, B. M., and Worwood, M. (1978). An immunoradiometric assay for the acidic ferritin of human heart: Application to human tissues, cells and serum, *Clin. Chim. Acta*, **85**, 81–8.
Jones, B. M., Worwood, M., and Jacobs, A. (1980). Serum ferritin in patients with cancer: Determination with antibodies to HeLa and spleen ferritin, *Clin. Chim. Acta*, **106**, 203–14.
Konijn, A. M., Tal, R., Levy, R., and Matzner, Y. (1985). Isolation and fractionation of ferritin from human term placenta—a source for human isoferritins, *Anal. Biochem.*, **144**, 423–8.
Koprivova, H., Hermanska, Z., Novak, F., Blehova, Z., and Dienstbier, Z. (1986). Ferritin-bearing lymphocytes in Hodgkin's disease, *Neoplasma*, **33**, 63–9.
Linder, M. C., Nagel, G. M., Roboz, M., and Hungerford, D. M. (1981). The size and shape of heart and muscle ferritins analyzed by sedimentation, gel-filtration and electrophoresis, *J. Biol. Chem.*, **256**, 9104–10.
Marcus, D. M., and Zinberg, N. (1974). Isolation of ferritin from human mammary and pancreatic carcinomas by means of antibody immunoadsorbents, *Arch. Biochem. Biophys.*, **162**, 493–501.

Marcus, D. M., and Zinberg, N. (1975a). Serum ferritin levels in patients with breast cancer, *Clin. Res.*, **23**, 447–50.

Marcus, D. M., and Zinberg, N. (1975b). Measurement of serum ferritin by radioimmunoassay: Results in normal individuals and patients with breast cancer, *J. Natl Cancer Inst.*, **55**, 791–5.

Matzner, Y., Konijn, A.M., and Hershko, C. (1980). Serum ferritin in hematologic malignancies, *Am. J. Hematol.*, **9**, 13–22.

Matzner, Y., Konijn, A. M., Shlomai, Z., and Ben-Bassat, H. (1985). Differential effect of isolated placental isoferritins on in vitro T-lymphocyte function, *Br. J. Haematol.*, **59**, 443–8.

Moroz, C., and Kupfer, B. (1981). Suppressor-cell activity of ferritin-bearing lymphocytes in patients with breast cancer, *Isr. J. Med. Sci.*, **17**, 879–81.

Moroz, C., Lahat, N., Biniaminov, M., and Ramot, B. (1977a). Ferritin on the surface of lymphocytes in Hodgkin's disease patients. A possible blocking substance removed by levamisole, *Clin. Exp. Immunol.*, **29**, 30–5.

Moroz, C., Giler, S. H., Kupfer, B., and Urca, I. (1977b). Lymphocytes bearing surface ferritin in patients with Hodgkin's disease and breast cancer, *N. Engl. J. Med.*, **296**, 1173.

Moroz, C., Giler, S. H., Kupfer, B., and Urca, I. (1977c). Ferritin-bearing lymphocytes and T cell levels in peripheral blood of patients with breast cancer, *Cancer Immunol. Immunother.*, **3**, 101–5.

Moroz, C., Kan, M., Chaimof, C., Marcus, H., Kupfer, B., and Cuckle, H. S. (1984). Ferritin-bearing lymphocytes in the diagnosis of breast cancer, *Cancer*, **54**, 84–9.

Moroz, C., Kupfer, B., Twig, S., and Parhami-Seren, B. (1985). Preparation and characterization of monoclonal antibodies specific to placenta ferritin, *Clin. Chim. Acta*, **148**, 111–18.

Moroz, C., Bessler, H., Lurie, Y., and Shaklai, M. (1987a). A new monoclonal antibody enzymoassay for the specific measurement of placental ferritin isotype in hematologic malignancies, *Exp. Hematol.*, **15**, 258–62.

Moroz, C., Bessler, H., Sirota, L., Dulitzky, F., and Djaldetti, M. (1988b). Difference in the placental ferritin levels measured by a specific monoclonal antibody enzymoassay in preterm and term delivery, *Clin. Exp. Immunol.*, **69**, 702–6.

Moroz, C., Kahn, M., Ron, E., and Chaimoff, C. (1988c). Oncofetal ferritin bearing lymphocytes as a marker for early breast malignancy (submitted for publication).

Niitsu, Y., Kohgo, Y., Ohtsuka, S. et al. (1976). Ferritin in serum and tissues and their implications in malignancy. In W. H. Fishman and S. Sell (eds) *Onco-developmental Gene Expression*, pp. 757–62, Academic Press.

Otsuka, S., Maruyama, H., and Listowsky, I. (1981). Structure assembly conformation and immunological properties of the two subunit classes of ferritin, *Biochemistry*, **20**, 5226–32, Academic Press, New York.

Papenhausen, P. R., Emeson, E. E., Croft, C. B., and Borowiecki, B. (1984). Ferritin-bearing lymphocytes in patients with cancer, *Cancer*, **53**, 267–71.

Parhami-Seren, B., and Moroz, C. (1986). A unique subunit structure of human placental ferritin identified by the use of monoclonal antibodies, *Ital. J. Clin. Pathol.*, **1**, 17–23.

Ramot, B., Biniaminov, M., Shohan, C., and Rosenthal, E. (1976). Effect of levamisole on E-rosettes forming cells in vivo and in vitro in Hodgkin's disease, *N. Engl. J. Med.*, **294**, 809–11.

Roberts, J. G., Chare, M. J. B., Leach, K. G., and Baum, M. (1979). Spleen size in women with breast cancer, *Clin. Oncol.*, **5**, 317–23.

Sarcione, E. J., Stutzman, L., and Mittelman, A. (1975). Ferritin synthesis by splenic tumor tissues of Hodgkin's disease, *Experientia*, **31**, 1334–5.

Sarcione, E. J., Smalley, J. R., Lenia, M. J., and Stutzman, L. (1977). Increased ferritin synthesis and release by Hodgkin's disease peripheral blood lymphocytes, *Int. J. Cancer*, **20**, 339–46.

Shinjo, S., Kitajima, Y., Hirai, Y., and Yoshino, Y. (1984). The role of ferritin isomers on the maternofetal iron transfer in rats, *Acta Haematol. (Japan)*, **47**, 829–37.

Stefanini, S., Chiancone, E., Arosio, P., Finazzi-Argo, A., and Antonini, E. (1982). Structural heterogeneity and subunit composition of horse ferritins, *Biochemistry*, **21**, 2293–9.

Steinhoff, G., Van der Heul, C., Van Eijk, H., Rice, L., and Alfrey, C. (1984). Elevated lymphocyte surface ferritin in malignant diseases and mononucleosis infection, a lymphocyte ferritin antibody binding test. In A. Albertini *et al.* (eds) *Ferritins and Isoferritins as Biochemical Markers*, pp. 181–4, Elsevier, Amsterdam.

Toppin, J. A., George, W. D., and Bellingham, A. S. (1979). Effect of surgery on serum ferritin concentrations in patients with breast cancer, *Br. J. Cancer*, **40**, 658–67.

Watanabe, N., and Drysdale, J. W. (1981). Natural enrichment of ferritin in mRNA in mRNP particles, *Biochem. Biophys. Res. Commun.*, **103**, 207–12.

White, G. P., Worwood, M., Parry, D., and Jacobs, A. (1976). Ferritin synthesis in normal and leukaemic leukocytes, *Nature*, **250**, 584–6.

Worwood, M., Jones, B. M., and Jacobs, A. (1976). The reactivity of isoferritins in a labelled antibody assay, *Immunochemistry*, **13**, 447–8.

Iron in Immunity, Cancer and Inflammation
Edited by M. de Sousa and J. H. Brock
© 1989 John Wiley & Sons Ltd.

14
Iron-related Markers in Liver Cancer

Jonathan L. Israel, Katherine A. McGlynn, Hie-Won L. Hann and
Baruch S. Blumberg
*Division of Population Oncology, Fox Chase Cancer Center, Philadelphia,
Pennsylvania 19111, USA*

INTRODUCTION

There are approximately 210 million chronic carriers of the hepatitis B virus worldwide. Chronic hepatitis B infection can progress through chronic active hepatitis to postnecrotic cirrhosis and eventually to primary hepatocellular carcinoma (PHC). The disease progression may stop at any stage or, alternatively, may bypass stages, although that sequence is rare. Based on a large prospective study of male government workers in Taiwan, it is estimated that 40% of viral carriers develop liver cancer (Beasely, 1982). While hepatitis B virus is known to be the single greatest risk factor for PHC, it is not known why some carriers develop liver cancer and others do not. It is the purpose of this chapter to review the role of iron as a possible co-factor in the pathogenesis of hepatitis B infection.

IRON, HEPATITIS B VIRUS AND LIVER CANCER

Over the past 15 years a variety of epidemiologic studies have implicated iron and iron-related proteins in the pathogenesis of hepatitis B virus (HBV) infection and PHC. More recently, a number of laboratory studies have supported and expanded the epidemiologic observations and suggested possible mechanisms whereby iron may be involved in the development of liver cancer in chronic carriers of the hepatitis B virus.

Interest in the role of iron in host response to infection and cancer has been stimulated by Weinberg's comprehensive analysis of this subject (Weinberg, 1981). Based on an extensive body of evidence that suggests iron is important in host response to infection, particularly bacterial infection, Weinberg has proposed that analogous mechanisms are involved in host defense against neoplasia. The underlying hypothesis is that the mammalian host responds to infection and growth of tumor cells by denying iron to the invading agent or replicating cells. Various mechanisms are proposed for withholding of iron, including: (1) the binding of iron at the site of infection or tumor to prevent its utilization by the pathogen or cancer, (2) diminished absorption of iron by the gastrointestinal tract, and (3) increased synthesis of the iron-binding protein ferritin, resulting in increased storage of iron.

As withholding iron appears to be a defense mechanism, the converse, excess total body iron, has been associated with higher rates of carcinogenesis (Weinberg, 1984). Evidence suggests that iron may interfere with the tumoricidal action of macrophages as well as with the circulation of lymphocytes and thus may impair antitumor cell defense (de Sousa, 1978; de Sousa, Smithyman and Tan, 1978; de Sousa and Potaznik, 1984).

Studies have demonstrated that the parenteral administration of iron dextran induces sarcomas at the site of injection in rats, rabbits, and humans (Richmond, 1959; Greenberg, 1976; Magnusson, Flodh and Malmfors, 1977). Additionally, a number of cases of primary liver cancer, as well as other neoplasms, have been observed in persons who had developed siderosis because of excessive ingested iron and/or inordinate absorption of the metal (Berman, 1958; Robertson, Harington and Bradshaw, 1971; Weinberg, 1981). Furthermore, hemochromatosis, a disease of idiopathic iron overload, is associated with an increased incidence of primary liver cancer. In idiopathic hemochromatosis, iron deposits in numerous tissues in addition to the liver, prompting expectations of an increased incidence of many tumors as well as hepatocellular carcinoma. In fact, this expectation has been borne out in a study by Bomford and Williams who observed that of 46 patients with idiopathic hemochromatosis, followed for at least 15 years, 13 died of hepatoma while 12 succumbed to a variety of other neoplasms (Bomford and Williams, 1976). In yet another example, miners who smoke and are exposed to iron oxides appear to have a higher incidence of lower respiratory cancers than non-miners who smoke, although epidemiologists have since questioned these results (Axelson, and Sjoberg, 1979; Antoine et al., 1979).

Soon after the identification of the HBV and its association with clinical hepatitis, it became clear that patients' responses to HBV infection were not uniform (Blumberg et al., 1967). The spectrum of clinical response ranged from no symptoms to fulminant hepatitis and death. Serologically, patients could develop antibody to the hepatitis B surface antigen (anti-HBs) and clear the virus, or alternatively, remain persistently positive for HBsAg (HBsAg(+)), thereby becoming chronic viral carriers.

By the 1970s evidence had accumulated that persistent infection with

HBV was associated with an increased risk of PHC. However, while some HBV carriers develop PHC, it was not a universal sequela and, conversely, there have been cases of primary liver cancer not apparently associated with HBV. It became apparent that other factors were also involved. In order to better understand the pathogenesis of this process, investigations into a possible role for iron and iron-related proteins were begun.

In 1971, Kolk-Vegter et al. reported on 11 patients with end stage kidney disease undergoing renal dialysis (Kolk-Vegter, 1971). Ten of these patients had developed anicteric hepatitis associated with HBsAg positivity. These patients, on average, experienced a spontaneous rise in hemoglobin level and required fewer transfusions than a group of similar patients who were HBsAg(−). Subsequently, Sutnick et al. reported a study comparing 20 HBsAg(+) asymptomatic carriers with Down's syndrome with 20 HBsAg(−) Down's syndrome patients (Sutnick, Blumberg and Lustbader, 1974). Consistent with the work of Kolk-Vegter et al., serum iron, hemoglobin, and hematocrit were significantly higher in the HBsAg(+) patients than in the HBsAg(−) patients. The total serum iron-binding capacity was also higher in the HBsAg(+) group. Elevation of serum iron did not correlate with elevation of serum glutamic pyruvic transaminase (SGPT), suggesting that hepatic cell necrosis did not account for the observed increase in serum iron.

In 1979, Felton et al. studied 201 patients undergoing renal dialysis (Felton et al., 1979). Among these patients with end-stage renal disease were 39 HBsAg(+) persons, 76 anti-HBs(+) persons and 86 persons without evidence of previous hepatitis B exposure. As previously demonstrated in Down's syndrome patients, the HBsAg(+) patients had higher serum iron levels, greater percentage iron saturation and higher SGPT levels than anti-HBs(+) persons. No difference was seen in hemoglobin concentration, hematocrit or red blood cell count. A logistic regression analysis determined that there were two-way interactions between serum iron and SGPT and between serum iron and HBV status, suggesting several possible explanations for the elevation of iron levels. Elevated iron could be a consequence of liver cell breakdown as indicated by the elevated SGPT levels. An additional explanation is that HBV infection could be more prevalent in persons with high iron levels.

Felton's observations were made in patients with end-stage renal disease on dialysis. Many of the study group were on iron therapy, had anemia of chronic disease and/or were taking aluminum hydroxide which affects iron absorption. Feret et al. sought to extend Felton's findings to other populations, including non-hospitalized populations in regions of the world with high frequencies of hepatitis B infection (Blumberg, 1986). Feret studied the population of the small village of Tip, Senegal in west Africa. Sera were obtained from 193 persons: 40 HBsAg(+) persons, 59 anti-HBs(+) persons and 94 with no HBV markers. Although the SGPT level was higher in the HBsAg(+) group, serum iron level was independently associated with HBV status, confirming the finding of the Felton and Sutnick studies (Blumberg, 1986).

The question left unanswered by Feret's work was the temporal relationship of iron level to HBV infection. Were the raised iron levels a consequence of HBV infection or did elevated iron levels make persons more prone to chronic infection with HBV? To study the transmission of HBV, Blumberg and colleagues had monitored for 10 years a group of renal dialysis patients with a high incidence HBV infection (Blumberg, Lustbader and Whitford, 1981). Patients were divided into two groups: those that became HBV carriers and those that developed transient infections. Serum iron levels were determined for both groups one month before, at the time of, and 6–12 months after infection. In the patients destined to become carriers, serum iron levels were not elevated before infection but rose immediately after infection and remained elevated. In patients only transiently infected, the serum iron levels were not elevated before infection, rose at the time of infection, but decreased in the follow-up period. The results, therefore, were consistent with the interpretation that elevated serum iron was caused by HBV infection.

During the 1970s a sensitive assay for serum ferritin, an iron-binding protein, became available. Serum ferritin is more highly correlated with total body iron stores than serum iron. The introduction of the assay enabled further investigation of the relationship of iron to HBV. Lustbader *et al.* hypothesized that individuals fated to become carriers would have higher ferritin levels before infection than those who were to become transiently infected (Lustbader, Hann and Blumberg, 1983). A study similar to the serum iron study of Blumberg *et al.* was carried out among the same renal dialysis patients. Data obtained on the serum sample collected prior to the positive sample were to be used to predict the outcomes (persistent or transient HBV infection). The analysis showed that persistently infected individuals had significantly higher ferritin values prior to infection than persons transiently infected. Based on their results, the authors postulated that liver cells with an increased propensity to ferritin production were also more likely to become infected with HBV and to provide a suitable environment for replication. Infection with HBV, in turn, stimulated the production of even more ferritin in a positive feedback mechanism. This accounted for the increased levels of ferritin seen prior to infection and the even higher levels after infection had become persistent.

The model postulated by the authors can be extended to include PHC, a common sequela of chronic HBV infection. If an iron-rich environment predisposes to the development of PHC, as suggested by Weinberg (1984), ferritin levels would be expected to start higher and increase to an even larger extent in chronic carriers of HBV who develop hepatocellular carcinoma.

Stevens *et al.* studied the relationship of iron-binding proteins (ferritin and transferrin) to mortality in an historical–prospective study of Solomon Islanders (Stevens *et al.*, 1983). The authors found that high ferritin levels and low transferrin levels were associated with increased mortality. The causes of death could not be determined in this study. To test the model more directly, Stevens *et al.* conducted a synthetic case-control study using Beasley's cohort of male Taiwanese government workers (Stevens, Beasely and Blumberg, 1986). The authors confirmed the hypothesis; men who subsequently developed cancer had higher ferritin levels and lower transferrin levels, at the beginning of the study, than did those men who did not develop cancer.

Synthesizing the accumulated data, Blumberg has proposed a model to explain the pathogenesis of HBV infection and its progression to chronic liver disease and hepatocellular carcinoma (Blumberg, 1986). According to the model, some individuals infected with HBV have liver cells that contain large amounts of ferritin, or an augmented ability, possibly under genetic control, to synthesize the protein. Within a single liver, the cells will be heterogeneous with respect to their ferritin content and potential to generate it. Cells with higher amounts of ferritin or the capacity to synthesize it would be more likely to be infected with HBV. HBV infection, in turn, would enhance ferritin production and increase the iron content of the cell. When the iron content exceeded the binding capacity of the ferritin, iron levels would increase in the cell. Iron would stimulate the production of oxygen radicals with consequent damage to the liver cell. Cell death would be followed by regeneration and scarring, leading to the pathological picture of advanced liver disease and cirrhosis.

London and Blumberg extended the model to include hepatocellular carcinoma (Blumberg and London, 1982). An important feature of the pathology of hepatocellular carcinoma is the absence of stainable iron in the neoplastic cells of the tumor. High levels of iron, however, are often seen in the non-malignant cells surrounding the tumor (Edmundson, 1954). In addition, malignantly transformed cells contain few or no viral particles. The surrounding non-malignant cells, those with large amounts of storage iron, may contain whole hepatitis B virions, viral surface antigen and core antigen particles. All cells including malignant cells require iron to grow and divide. Fernandez-Pol has shown experimentally that removal of iron with a chelating agent decreases the growth of live tumors in tissue culture (Fernandez-Pol, 1977). The Blumberg–London model suggests that the iron-containing cells, infected with replicating HBV, can supply the iron to malignant cells and thereby stimulate their growth and division. The model suggested the possibility that diminishing the availability of iron to tumor cells would inhibit neoplastic growth.

Hann et al. tested this hypothesis in laboratory animals. They showed that a variety of murine tumors grew faster and larger in mice fed an iron-rich diet than in animals fed an iron-deficient diet (Hann, Stahlhut and Blumberg, 1988). This observation was confirmed in a subsequent study of spontaneous mammary tumors in C3H/HeN-MTV$^+$ mice. These are mice that are congenitally infected with mammary tumor virus and develop spontaneous mammary tumors between age 7.2 and 9.2 months. A group of 15 of these mice were fed an iron-rich diet while a control group of 15 mice consumed a low-iron diet. As hypothesized, spontaneous mammary tumors grew faster and larger in the mice fed an iron-rich diet (Hann et al., in preparation).

Several recent *in vitro* experiments have also evaluated the relationship of iron supply and tumor growth. Hann et al. have shown: (1) PHC cells (PLC/PRF/5) grow proportionally with increasing amounts of iron contained in the tissue medium (Hann, Hann and Stahlhut, 1988); and (2) an iron chelating agent, desferoxamine, caused cell death in three PHC cell lines (PLC/PRF/5, Hep G2 and Hep 3B) in tissue culture (Hann, Stahlhut and London, 1988).

A number of intriguing questions have been raised by these studies of iron and HBV in the pathogenesis of PHC. Among the most clinically significant of these is speculation that ferritin could be used as a marker in liver cancer.

FERRITIN AS A MARKER IN LIVER CANCER

Since Reissman and Dietrich first reported ferritin fluctuations in the sera of 9 patients with hepatocellular disease, investigators have been interested in the use of ferritin as a tumor marker (Reissman and Dietrich, 1956; see Chapter 13). Studies have addressed at least five basic questions: Why is ferritin raised in PHC? Is ferritin useful as a diagnostic marker in PHC in comparison with AFP? Is ferritin useful in distinguishing PHC from other liver diseases? Can ferritin be used to monitor therapy of PHC patients? Is the ferritin from patients with liver disease different from normal serum ferritin?

Why is ferritin raised in PHC?

In 1972 a sensitive radioimmunoassay for detecting ferritin in serum became available (Addison et al., 1972) and was shortly thereafter used to establish that ferritin was raised in many liver disease patients (Prieto, Barry and Sherlock, 1975). In a landmark study published in 1978, Kew *et al.* explored why serum ferritin levels were elevated in some patients with PHC (Kew *et al.*, 1978). They posed four hypotheses: (1) growth of the tumor could cause death of hepatocytes with subsequent ferritin leakage into the serum; (2) ferritin could be raised due to cirrhosis which was frequently found in PHC patients; (3) hepatic uptake of serum ferritin could be adversely affected in the presence of PHC; and (4) the tumor itself could secrete ferritin into the serum. To test their hypotheses, they correlated serum ferritin in 76 PHC patients with four variables: extent of cell damage, cirrhosis, hepatic storage iron content, and size of the tumor. They also correlated ferritin with alpha-fetoprotein (AFP), an accepted tumor marker for PHC. The patients were black South Africans and, with a single exception, were male.

The serum ferritin concentrations ranged from 30 $\mu g\, l^{-1}$ to 25 600 $\mu g\, l^{-1}$ with 58 of the 76 patients having values in the abnormal range ($\geq 300 \mu g\, l^{-1}$). There was no correlation between (1) serum ferritin and tumor size, (2) ferritin and the presence of cirrhosis or (3) ferritin and two indices of liver cell damage (SGOT, SGPT). Interestingly, there was a negative correlation between ferritin and AFP. There was a weak correlation between ferritin and a histological assessment of liver iron stores derived from liver biopsies, although there was no correlation between ferritin and a more sensitive chemical quantitation of liver iron concentration. In examining the livers of three PHC patients to assess whether the ferritin in the tumor tissue was distinguishable from that in normal tissue, the authors found that the tumor tissue ferritin was more acidic.

These findings indicated that (1) the elevated serum ferritin levels were not simply a reflection of high body iron stores, (2) cryptogenic cirrhosis was not the explanation of elevated ferritin levels because patients without cirrhosis were as likely to have elevated ferritin as patients with cirrhosis, (3) leakage of stored ferritin from necrotic hepatocytes at the edge of the tumor was an unlikely answer because there was no correlation with either liver enzyme levels or tumor size, and (4) decreased hepatic uptake of ferritin was probably not a factor because the study patients maintained liver function until the terminal stages of their disease. The most likely explanation for the raised serum ferritin in patients with PHC seems to be ferritin production by the tumor itself. The authors note that the negative correlation between AFP and ferritin suggests that ferritin, particularly an acidic isoferritin, might be useful as a valuable second marker for PHC. The reason for the variability in elevations of AFP and serum ferritin among different patients that develop PHC is unknown.

Tumor as a source of serum ferritin has been established for another cancer, namely neuroblastoma (Hann, Levy and Evans, 1980). The authors had shown that ferritin levels correlated with clinical status, elevated ferritin at diagnosis, normal level in remission and reappearance of increased ferritin in relapse. Furthermore, six neuroblastoma cell lines in culture showed ferritin in the culture supernatant, whereas the normal cell line in the same culture did not secrete ferritin into the medium. Direct demonstration of tumor secretion of ferritin has come from two *in vivo* experiments. Watanabe *et al.* transplanted various primary carcinomas into nude mice and showed ferritinemia in some of these tumor-bearing mice (Watanabe *et al.*, 1979). Hann *et al.* have expanded this observation by transplanting human PHC and neuroblastoma cells grown in culture into nude mice and shown increased amounts of human ferritin in murine serum of many of the animals (Hann, Stahlhut and Millman, 1984).

Cohen *et al.* (1984) sought to investigate the cause of elevated ferritin by examining the liver tissue of PHC patients. The authors found that ferritin was present in the tumor tissue of 43% of black South African patients and 63% of American patients. In both groups of patients, the ferritin was present in a higher percentage of normal tissue, 82% and 100% respectively. These authors concluded that the elevated ferritin levels seen in PHC could be due to secretion from the tumor itself or related to co-existing iron overload.

Zhou *et al.* (1987) examined the tumor and normal tissue of 40 PHC patients from China. Stainable iron was present in 65% of the normal tissues and 10% of the tumors. Ferritin was demonstrated in 75% of the normal tissues and 40% of the tumors. The authors' interpretation of these data was that immunohistochemical ferritin is not due to increased stainable iron and more likely is due to another source, such as synthesis by the tumor.

Therefore, it appears most likely that at least part of the marked elevation of serum ferritin is a result of production by the tumor.

Is ferritin useful as a diagnostic marker compared with AFP?

In a 1982 report by Chapman *et al.*, the authors examine three issues. (1) Was ferritin useful in distinguishing between PHC and other liver disease? (2) Was the serum ferritin in PHC patients different from the serum ferritin in other liver disease patients or in normal controls? (3) Was serum ferritin a useful marker in monitoring PHC patients? In contrasting 30 Caucasian PHC patients with 33 liver disease patients, the authors noted that the mean ferritin level was significantly higher in the PHC patients, although there was appreciable overlap in the two groups. Seventy per cent of the PHC group had elevated AFP levels, while none of the liver disease group did. There was no correlation between AFP and ferritin in the PHC group. Both the sensitivity (70% vs. 63%) and the specificity (100% vs. 67%) of

AFP were superior to those of ferritin. Among AFP(−) PHC patients, the sensitivity of ferritin improved to 78%.

To answer the second question, the concentration of ferritin binding to concanavalin A was measured in the sera of PHC patients and liver disease patients and a control group. Although the proportion of bound ferritin was decreased in the majority of PHC patients compared with the controls, there was no difference between the PHC patients and the liver disease patients, suggesting similar ferritin was present in both groups of patients. To answer the final question, the authors monitored 3 patients with AFP and ferritin during chemotherapy. There was parallel production of AFP and ferritin in 2 of the 3 patients, both of whom had elevated levels of both markers. The authors suggested that ferritin might have a role in monitoring AFP(−) patients, although it is not clear how the data influenced this recommendation.

Giannoulis et al. (1984) studied a similar problem among a Greek population. They identified two patient groups (PHC patients and chronic liver disease patients (CLD)) and one normal control group. Although the authors note that the ages of the three groups were not statistically different, the control group was 50% male, while the study groups were 80% male. All three groups were tested for: (1) liver enzymes, (2) serum ferritin, (3) serum AFP, and (4) hepatitis B virus markers. The authors found that PHC patients had significantly higher ferritin levels than either the CLD patients or the controls. While the CLD patients' mean level was significantly higher than the controls' mean level, the PHC patients' mean level was significantly higher than the CLD groups' mean level. Only one PHC patient had a value in the control range, while there was considerable overlap between the CLD group and the controls.

In comparing the AFP levels of the PHC and CLD groups, the authors noted that the mean level of the PHC group was significantly higher than the CLD group. However, the overlap between the two groups was great. Ten of the 17 PHC patients had AFP values within the CLD range, and of these 10, 7 were in the normal range. In total 59% of the PHC patients had abnormal AFP values (>25 ng ml^{-1}), while 88% had abnormal ferritin values (>450 ng ml^{-1}). No significant correlation was noted between AFP and ferritin. The sensitivity of ferritin was greater than that of AFP (88% vs. 59%), as was the specificity (85% vs. 68%).

In 1984, Nakano et al. reported on a comparison of AFP and ferritin in the diagnosis of PHC. Their previous work (Nakano, 1979; Kumada, 1981) had determined that ferritin tended to be high in low-AFP-producing PHC. They contrasted the abilities of ferritin and AFP to distinguish between PHC and cirrhosis. They found that ferritin was elevated in all liver diseases, but was more elevated in PHC than cirrhosis. Furthermore, use of a ferritin/iron, ferritin/SGOT, or ferritin/SGPT ratio was an even better distinguisher between PHC and cirrhosis. Compared with AFP, however, ferritin was neither as sensitive nor as specific in diagnosing PHC. When the PHCs were stratified by size, AFP showed a higher positive rate for tumors greater than 3 cm in diameter and ferritin a better positive rate in tumors of diameter 3 cm or less. When examined by HBV status, the authors reported that, in those cases where only AFP was elevated, 46.8% of the cases were HBsAg(+). Conversely, among those cases where only ferritin was abnormal, none of the cases were HBsAg(+) and all were long-term alcohol drinkers. By comparing the sensitivities and specificities of AFP and ferritin, separately and together, the authors concluded that the use of both tests improved the sensitivity of diagnosis, but decreased the specificity over that of AFP alone.

Tatsuta et al. (1986) determined whether ferritin was more sensitive than AFP in diagnosing small PHC (<3 cm). For their research, they tested 224 healthy persons, 55 persons with liver disease and 44 PHC patients for both AFP and ferritin. Overall, they found that both markers were highly specific (98.6%), but that AFP outperformed ferritin in sensitivity (65.9% vs. 56.8%, respectively). The two tests combined had a sensitivity of 88.6% and a specificity of 97.8%. While their specificity rates of ferritin were higher than some of the other studies, it was most likely due to the higher limit of normal employed (350 ng ml^{-1} rather than 300 ng ml^{-1}). When stratified by size, ferritin did not improve upon the sensitivity of AFP in either small or large tumors. The combined results, however, greatly improved upon the use of AFP alone.

In sum, while serum ferritin levels appear to be a useful adjunct to AFP in the monitoring of HBV carriers, they are too insensitive to be used alone. Ongoing work aimed at the development of a monoclonal antibody to PHC ferritin might improve sensitivity.

Is ferritin useful in monitoring therapy in PHC?

Melia et al., in a complicated study, explored the use of ferritin as a marker in monitoring response to therapy (Melia et al., 1983). They followed 35 PHC patients with both AFP and serum ferritin to see whether ferritin would accurately reflect response status based on a clinical assessment. Serum ferritin was raised, prior to treatment, in 97% of the PHC patients, but also in 87% of 23 cirrhotic patients. Among the 35 PHC patients, 4 achieved remission post-therapy. The authors did not report initial AFP levels. They did indicate that, in all the PHC patients with raised levels prior to treatment (tumor devascularization and subsequent chemotherapy), AFP levels fell post-treatment. In contrast, serum ferritin levels rose in the PHC patients post-treatment. All 4 patients who achieved remission subsequent to treatment had decreases in both their AFP level and their ferritin level. Among the 27 patients not achieving remission, 2 had decreases in their AFP level and 4 had decreases in their ferritin level. The authors concluded that ferritin was a poor diagnostic tool to distinguish PHC from cirrhosis, but that it was a useful monitoring tool. Their data, however, argue that ferritin is less valuable as a diagnostic tool than AFP. While they indicate that some other marker is needed in AFP(−) patients, their data shed no light on the usefulness of ferritin in such a situation.

In research conducted at the University of Palermo, Simonetti concluded that serum ferritin was not useful to distinguish PHC from cirrhosis; nor was it useful for monitoring therapy (Simonetti et al., 1985). The authors age- and sex-matched 85 PHC patients with 62 cirrhosis patients and tested both groups for AFP and ferritin. Fifty-four per cent of the PHC patients and 35% of the cirrhotics had abnormal ferritin values (>300 ng ml^{-1}). Among the PHC patients, 70% had elevated AFP levels (>50 ng ml^{-1}) and there was no correlation between AFP and ferritin levels. Ferritin performed equally poorly as a marker in therapy monitoring. While not presenting their data, the authors noted that ferritin levels did not decrease in the 7 of 61 patients who had an objective response to treatment.

Nagasue et al. (1986) also found that ferritin was not a useful marker for monitoring PHC patients post-therapy. They followed 24 PHC patients who had undergone tumor resection with both AFP and total serum ferritin. Stratifying by tumor size, they found that ferritin did not decrease in patients post-operatively, as AFP did. There was no indication that ferritin was a valuable predictor in patients whose AFP level was normal.

As a monitor of therapy, there is no indication that serum ferritin level is of clinical use.

Is there a tumor specific ferritin?

Much research has attempted to determine whether the elevated serum ferritin seen in PHC patients is different from serum ferritin seen in normal persons.

Ferritin is composed of two parts: an outer protein shell and an inner iron core. The outer protein shell is made of a total of 24 subunits of two major types: H (heavy, molecular weight (MW) 21 000) and L (light, MW 19 000) subunits (see Chapter 4). Different combinations of these subunits produce various forms of ferritins (isoferritins) which differ immunologically (Drysdale, 1977). These isoferritins can be characterized by different isoelectric points. The more basic ferritins (pI 5.3–5.8), rich in L subunits, are predominant in liver and spleen. The liver ferritin contains 80% to 90% L and 10% to 20% H subunits. On the other hand the more acidic isoferritins (pI 4.7–5.2), rich in H subunits, are predominant in heart, erythroid cells, monocytes, and HeLa cells (Drysdale, 1977; Worwood,

1982). HeLa ferritins contain 90% H and 10% L subunits and are some of the most acidic ferritins among human isoferritins.

In malignancy, ferritins in cancer tissues become different from ferritins in the corresponding normal tissues; isoferritins from hepatoma tissue have more acidic isoelectric points than those from the neighboring normal tissue (Alpert, Coston and Drysdale, 1973; Niitsu et al., 1975; Kew et al., 1978) and a similar shift of tumor ferritins toward the acidic side was seen in breast cancer and Hodgkin's disease (Marcus and Zinburg, 1974; Coombes et al., 1977; Hancock et al., 1979; see also Chapter 13).

Noting, in 1975, that it was clinically important to identify tumor-associated substances, Niitsu et al. sought to characterize ferritins from hepatoma and normal tissues on isoelectric focusing. They confirmed their previous finding that hepatoma ferritin was more acidic than normal liver ferritin, but not more acidic than heart and kidney ferritins. In contrasting PHC patients with liver disease patients and controls by noting the number of patients outside the normal range, they found that both PHC and acute hepatitis patients had abnormal values, while chronic hepatitis patients and cirrhotics did not.

As mentioned previously, a number of other investigators have demonstrated that hepatoma ferritin has a more acidic isoelectric focusing pattern than normal liver. Alpert et al. (1978) have suggested that the isoelectric focusing pattern of the hepatoma ferritin indicates that the tumor synthesizes not only normal ferritin subunits, but also a distinct carcinofoetal subunit.

Massover (1985), characterizing the tumor and normal liver ferritins derived from mice, reported that although there were differences in the two ferritins, both were composed of the same subunit types and the difference was explained by the different proportions of the subunits.

In 1984, Niitsu et al. demonstrated that the isoelectric point of ferritin was related to the iron content of the tissue. In an experiment which involved iron-depleting and iron-overloading tumor-bearing mice, the authors demonstrated that the ferritins of all tissues varied with the iron. In the anemic animals there was a shift to acidic ferritin in tumor, heart and liver tissues and, conversely, a shift to basic ferritin in the tissues of iron-supplemented mice. For both the normal tissues and the tumor tissues, they demonstrated a direct correlation between the iron content of the tissue and the ferritin subunit composition. In comparison with the normal liver, where the L (light) type subunit predominated, they noted an increase in the proportion of H (heavy) subunits in the liver of the anemic mice. Conversely, the tumors of the iron-overloaded mice showed a shift toward a greater proportion of L type subunits, in comparison with tumors of normal mice.

In total, while current evidence suggests that a tumor-specific ferritin subunit may exist, further research is necessary.

CONCLUSIONS

In conclusion, a sizeable body of evidence from epidemiologic, animal and laboratory studies supports the positive association of increased body iron stores and the risk of primary liver cancer. While the biological underpinning of the relationship has not yet been conclusively determined, the epidemiologic association is well substantiated. The evidence indicates that high body iron stores predispose persons to persistent hepatitis B infection. Among these chronic HBV carriers, increased iron appears to place individuals at even greater risk of primary liver cancer. High iron levels may also promote the growth of liver tumors once malignant change has occurred.

Once a liver cancer has developed, serum ferritin appears to be a useful adjunct to AFP in detecting the tumor. Though ferritin levels are less specific than AFP, they are clearly raised in some cases where AFP is not. An exciting area of research is aimed at the development of an antibody to PHC-specific ferritin. While PHC-specific ferritin may result from an alteration in the different known subunits, a provocative possibility is that a distinct molecule is synthesized by the tumor. Work aimed at identifying this molecule is ongoing. Currently, total serum ferritin levels have not proved useful in monitoring therapy of PHC.

ACKNOWLEDGEMENTS

This work was supported by USPHS grants CA-40737, RR-05895 and CA-06927 from the National Institutes of Health and by an appropriation from the Commonwealth of Pennsylvania.

REFERENCES

Addison, G. M., Beamish, M. R., Hales, C. N., Hodgkins, M., Jacobs, A., and Llewellin, P. (1972). An immunoradiometric assay for ferritin in the serum of normal subjects and patients with iron deficiency and iron overload, *J. Clin. Pathol.*, **25**, 326–9.

Alpert, E., Coston, R. L., and Drysdale, J. W. (1973). Carcino-fetal human liver ferritins, *Nature*, **242**, 194–5.

Antoine, D., Braun, P., Cervoni, P., Schwartz, P., and Lamy, P. (1979). Le cancer bronchique des mineurs de fer de Lorraine peut-il être consideré comme une maladie professionelle? *Rev. Fr. Mal. Resp.*, **7**, 63–5.

Axelson, O., and Sjoberg, A. (1979). Cancer incidence and exposure to iron oxide dust, *Occup. Med.*, **21**, 419–42.

Beasley, P. (1982). Hepatitis B virus as the etiologic agent in hepatocellular carcinoma/epidemiologic considerations, *Hepatology*, **2** 21S–26S.

Berman, C. (1958). Primary carcinoma of the liver, *Adv. Cancer Res.*, **5**, 55–96.

Blumberg, B. S. (1986). Hepatitis B virus, iron and iron-binding proteins, In A. Szentivanyi and H. Freidman (eds) *Viruses, Immunity and Immunodeficiency*, pp. 81–99. Plenum Press, New York.

Blumberg, B. S., and London, W. T. (1982). Hepatitis B virus: pathogenesis and prevention of primary cancer of the liver, *Cancer*, **50**, 2657–65.

Blumberg, B. S., Lustbader, E. D., and Whitford, P. L. (1981). Changes in serum iron levels due to infection with hepatitis B virus, *Proc. Natl. Acad. Sci. (USA)*, **78**, 3222–4.

Blumberg, B. S., Gerstley, B. J. S., Hungerford, D. A., London, W. T., and Sutnick, A. I. (1967). A serum antigen (Australian antigen) in Down's syndrome, leukemia and hepatitis, *Ann. Intern. Med.*, **66**, 924–31.

Bomford, A., and Williams, R. (1976). Long term results of venesection therapy in idiopathic haemochromatosis, *Q. J. Med.*, **45**, 611–23.

Chapman, R. W., Bassendine, M. F., Laulicht, M., Gorman, A., Thomas, H. C., Sherlock, S., and Hoffbrand, A. V. (1982). Serum ferritin and binding of serum ferritin to concanavalin A as a tumor marker in patients with primary liver cell cancer and chronic liver disease, *Digest. Dis. Sci.*, **27**, 111–16.

Cohen, C., Berson, S. D., Shulman, G., and Budgeon, L. R. (1984). Immunohistochemical ferritin in hepatocellular carcinoma, *Cancer*, **53**, 1931–5.

Coombes, R. C., Powles, T. J., Gazet, J. C., Ford, H. T., Nash, A. G., Sloane, J. P., Hillyard, C. J., Thomas, P., Keyser, J. W., Marcus, D., Zinberg, N., Stimson, W. H., and Munro, N. A. (1977). A biochemical approach to the staging of human breast cancer, *Cancer*, **40**, 937–44.

De Sousa, M. (1978). Lymphoid cell positioning: a new proposal for the mechanism of control of lymphoid cell migration, *Soc. Exp. Biol. Symp.*, **32**, 393–409.

De Sousa, M., and Potaznik, D. (1984). Proteins of the metabolism of iron, cells of the immune system and malignancy. In J. S. Prasad (ed.) *Vitamins, Nutrition and Cancer*, pp. 231–9. Karger, Basel.

De Sousa, M., Smithyman, A., and Tan, C. T. C. (1978). Suggested models of ecotaxopathy in lymphoreticular malignancy. A role for iron-binding proteins in the control of lymphoid cell migration, *Am. J. Pathol.*, **90**, 497–520.

Drysdale, J. W. (1977). Ferritin phenotypes: structure and metabolism, *Ciba Found. Symp.*, **51**, 41–57.

Edmundson, H. A., and Steiner, P. C. (1954). Primary carcinoma of the liver, *Cancer*, **7**, 462–503.

Felton, C., Lustbader, E. D., Merten, C., and Blumberg, B. S. (1979). Serum iron levels and response to hepatitis B virus, *Proc. Natl. Acad. Sci. (USA)*, **76**, 2438–41.

Fernandez-Pol, J. A. (1977). Iron: possible cause of the G_1 arrest induced in NRK cells by picolinic acid, *Biochem. Biophys. Res. Commun.*, **78**, 136–43.

Giannoulis, E., Arvanitakis, C., Nikopoulos, A., Doutsos, I., and Tourkantonis, A. (1984). Diagnostic value of serum ferritin in primary hepatocellular carcinoma, *Digestion*, **30**, 236–41.

Greenberg, G. (1976). Sarcoma after intramuscular iron injection, *Br. Med. J.*, **1**, 1508–9.

Hancock, B. W., Bruce, L., May, K., and Richmond, J. (1979). Ferritin: a sensitizing substance in the leukocyte migration inhibition test in patients with malignant lymphoma, *Br. J. Haematol.*, **43**, 223–33.

Hann, H. L., Hann, C. L., and Stahlhut, M. W. (1988). Increased *in vitro* ferritin synthesis and cell growth of a human hepatoma cell line induced by iron. *Proc. Am. Assoc. Cancer Res.*, **29**, 79 (abstract 314).

Hann, H. L., Levy, H. M., and Evans, A. E. (1980). Ferritin and cancer: study of isoferritins in patients with neuroblastoma, In A. E. Evans (ed.) *Advances in Neuroblastoma Research*, Raven Press, New York, pp. 43–8.

Hann, H. L., Stahlhut, M. W., and Blumberg, B. S. (1988). Iron nutrition and tumor growth: decreased tumor growth in iron deficient mice, *Cancer Res.*, **48**, 2168–4170.

Hann, H. L., Stahlhut, M. W., and London, W. T. (1988). Anti-tumor activity of an iron chelating agent (desferoxamine) on human hepatoma cell lines, *Clin. Res.*, **36**, 495A.

Hann, H. L., Stahlhut, M. W., and Millman, I. (1984). Human ferritins present in the sera of nude mice transplanted with human neuroblastoma or hepatocellular carcinoma, *Cancer Res.*, **44**, 3898–901.

Kew, M. C., Torrance, J. D., Dermna, D., Simon, M., MacNab, G. M., Charlton, R. W., and Bothwell, T. H. (1978). Serum and tumour ferritins in primary liver cancer, *Gut*, **19**, 294–9.

Kolk-Vegter, A. J., Bosch, E., and Leeuwen, A. M. (1971). Influence of serum hepatitis on haemoglobin level in patients on regular haemodialysis, *Lancet*, **i**, 526–8.

Kumada, T., Nakano, S., Ohta, H., Kitamura, K., Wataniki, H., Takeda, I., and Sasaki, T. (1981). Clinical evaluation on the diagnosis for hepatocellular carcinoma, *Nippon Shokakibyo Gakkai Zasshi*, **78**, 2367–75 (English abstract).

Lustbader, E. D., Hann, H. L., and Blumberg, B. S. (1983). Serum ferritin as a predictor of host response to hepatitis B virus infection, *Science*, **220**, 423–5.

Magnusson, G., Flodh, H., and Malmfors, T. (1977). Oncological study in rats of Ferastral, an iron-poly-(sorbitol–gluconic acid) complex, after intramuscular administration, *Scand. J. Hemat. Suppl.* **32**, 87–98.

Marcus, D. M., and Zinberg, N. (1974). Isolation of ferritin from human mammary and pancreatic carcinomas by means of antibody immunoabsorbance, *Arch. Biochem. Biophys.*, **162**, 493–501.

Massover, W. M. (1985). Molecular size heterogeneity of ferritin in mouse liver, *Biochim. Biophys. Acta*, **829**, 377–86.

Melia, W. M., Bullock, S., Johnson, P. J., and Williams, R. (1983). Serum ferritin in hepatocellular carcinoma: a comparison with alphafetoprotein, *Cancer*, **51**, 2112–5.

Nagasue, N., Yukaya, H., Chang, Y.-C., and Ogawa, Y. (1986). Serum ferritin level after resection of hepatocellular carcinoma: correlation with alpha-fetoprotein level, *Cancer*, **57**, 1820–3.

Nakano, S., Kumada, T., Kitamura, K., Wataniki, H., Takeda, I., Imoto, M., and Kazawa, H. (1979). Clinical evaluation of serum ferritin on the diagnosis for hepatocellular carcinoma, *Nippon Shokakibyo Gakkai Zasshi*, **78**, 2367–75 (English abstract).

Nakano, S., Kumada, T., Sugiyama, K., Watahiki, H., and Takeda, I. (1984). Clinical significance of serum ferritin determination for hepatocellular carcinoma, *Am. J. Gastroenterol.*, **79**, 623–7.

Niitsu, Y., Ohtsuka, S., Kohgo, Y., Watanabe, N., Koseki, J., and Urushizaki, I. (1975). Hepatoma ferritin in the tissue and serum, *Tumor Res.*, **10**, 31–42.

Niitsu, Y., Watanabe, N., Onodera, Y., Goto, Y., Kohgo, Y., and Urushizaki, I. (1984). Correlations between iron content and isoferritin profiles of normal and malignant tissues, *Gann*, **75**, 699–702.

Prieto, J., Barry, M., and Sherlock, S. (1975). Serum ferritin in patients with iron overload and with acute and chronic liver diseases, *Gastroenterology*, **68**, 525–33.

Reissman, K. R., and Dietrich, M. R. (1956). On the presence of ferritin in the peripheral blood of patients with hepatocellular disease, *J. Clin. Invest.*, **35**, 588–95.

Richmond, H. G. (1959). Induction of sarcoma in the rat by iron-dextran complex, *Br. Med. J.*, **1**, 947–9.

Robertson, M. A., Harington, J. S., and Bradshaw, E. (1971). The cancer pattern in African gold miners, *Br. J. Cancer*, **25**, 395–402.

Simonetti, R. G., Craxi, A., Dardanoni, G., Lanzarone, F., Barbaria, F., Cottone, M., and Pagliaro, L. (1985). The clinical value of serum ferritin in hepatocellular carcinoma, *Hepatogastroenterology.*, **32**, 276–8.

Stevens, R. G., Beasley, R. P., and Blumberg, B. S. (1986). Iron-binding proteins and risk of cancer in Taiwan, *J. Natl. Cancer Inst.*, **76**, 605–10.

Stevens, R. G., Kuvibidila, S., Kapps, M., Friedlaender, J., and Blumberg, B. S. (1983). Iron-binding proteins, hepatitis B virus, and mortality in the Solomon Islands, *Am. J. Epidemiol.*, **118**, 550–61.

Sutnick, A. I., Blumberg, B. S., and Lustbader, E. D. (1974). Elevated serum iron levels and persistent Australia antigen (HBsAg), *Ann. Intern. Med.*, **81**, 855–6.

Tatsuta, M., Yamamura, H., Iishi, H., Kasugai, H., and Okuda, S. (1986). Value of serum alpha-fetoprotein and ferritin in the diagnosis of hepatocellular carcinoma, *Oncology*, **43**, 306–10.

Watanabe, N., Niitsu, Y., Koseki, J., Okikawa, J., Yukata, K., Ishii, T., Goto, Y., Oncodera, Y., and Urushizaki, I. (1979). Ferritinemia in nude mice bearing various human carcinomas, In F. G. Lehman (ed.) *Carcinoembryonic Proteins*, vol. 1. Elsevier/North-Holland Biomedical Press, Amsterdam, pp. 273–8.

Weinberg, E. D. (1981). Iron and neoplasia, *Biol. Trace Element Res.*, **3**, 55–80.

Weinberg, E. D. (1984). Iron withholding: a defense against infection and neoplasia, *Physiol. Rev.*, **64**, 65–102.

Worwood, M. (1982). Ferritin in human tissues and serum, *Clin. Haematol.*, **11**, 275–307.

Zhou, X.-D., DeTolla, L., Custer, P., and London, W. T. (1987). Iron, ferritin, hepatitis B surface antigens in the livers of Chinese patients with hepatocellular carcinoma, *Cancer*, **59**, 1430–7.

Part VI

Implications for Diagnosis and Therapy

Iron in Immunity, Cancer and Inflammation
Edited by M. De Sousa and J. H. Brock
© 1989 John Wiley & Sons Ltd

15

The Iron-binding Proteins in Nuclear Medicine: Uses in Diagnosis and Therapy

Michael R. Zalutsky
Duke University Medical Center, Box 3808, Durham, North Carolina 27710, USA

INTRODUCTION

The development of radiopharmaceuticals for diagnostic and therapeutic applications has largely been an empirical process. Until about ten years ago, successful radiotracers generally resulted from serendipitous observation rather than rational design. It should not be surprising, therefore, that the role of iron-binding proteins in nuclear medicine has not always been explicit. Until recently, transferrin, ferritin and lactoferrin had rarely been exploited directly in strategies for radiopharmaceutical design. However, these proteins have been shown to play critical roles in mediating the transport of tracers to their tissue targets, and in determining the selectivity of tracer uptake and retention in tissues of interest.

By far the most commonly used radiopharmaceutical whose utility is related to the action of metal-binding proteins is gallium-67 citrate. This compound is used routinely both in the diagnosis of cancer and for the identification of inflammatory processes (Hoffer, Beckerman and Henkin, 1978; Beckerman, Hoffer and Bitran, 1984). It is worth noting that ^{67}Ga was being evaluated as a potential bone-scanning agent when its selective uptake in tumors was first recognized (Edwards and Hayes, 1969).

In addition to ^{67}Ga, other nuclides of the group IIIB elements have been utilized in nuclear medicine. Properties pertinent to the use of these isotopes for imaging applications are summarized in Table 15.1. [67]Ga and ^{111}In are produced routinely using a cyclotron and have half-lives of approximately three days. These nuclides are available for use at almost

TABLE 15.1 Nuclides of iron, gallium and indium of potential utility for imaging

Nuclide	Half-life	Gamma energies (keV)	Gamma abundance (%)
^{52}Fe	8.27 h	169	99
		511 (positron annihilation)	57
^{67}Ga	78.3 h	93	38
		185	24
		300	16
		394	4
^{68}Ga	68.3 min	511 (positron annihilation)	100
^{111}In	67.9 h	171	87
		245	94

every medical center in the United States and western Europe. These nuclides decay by the emission of gamma rays with energies suitable for use with either planar gamma cameras or single photon emission tomographs. ^{68}Ga, despite its short half-life, is available for widespread use because it can be supplied on a regular basis from a ^{68}Ge (275 days half-life) radionuclide generator. Since ^{68}Ge decays by positron emission, this nuclide permits the utilization of positron emission tomography, a technology which offers increased spatial resolution and the potential for superior quantitation (Reivich and Alavi, 1985). Unfortunately, use of ^{68}Ga is limited to the study of those biological phenomena which occur in a time-frame compatible with its 68-minute half-life.

At least two isotopes of iron itself have been used in clinical studies. ^{59}Fe has been employed by Chauduri and coworkers as a marrow-scanning agent (Chauduri *et al.*, 1974; DeGowin *et al.*, 1974). However, ^{59}Fe was not included in Table 15.1 because its long half-life (46 days) and high-energy gamma emissions (1095 and 1292 keV) result in high radiation dose to the patient and poor image quality, rendering this isotope of little value for clinical applications. Iron 52 citrate has been used for investigating the distribution of erythropoietically active marrow (Anger and Van Dyke, 1964; Van Dyke, Anger and Pollycove, 1964). The short half-life of ^{52}Fe limits the use of this nuclide to medical centers in close proximity to a relatively large cyclotron.

This chapter will be confined to the discussion of nuclear medical applications of ^{67}Ga and ^{111}In for which reasonable evidence of iron-binding protein involvement can be documented. In addition, the utilization of ferritin, transferrin, and/or specific receptors for these proteins as targets for the selective uptake of radiopharmaceuticals will be discussed.

TRANSFERRIN-MEDIATED ^{67}Ga AND ^{111}In TRANSPORT

In the clinical applications described in the following sections, ^{67}Ga and ^{111}In are administered intravenously as the citrate and chloride, respectively. However, almost immediately after injection, most of the radioactivity is bound to serum proteins (Gunasekera, King and Lavender, 1972). Using affinity chromatography, Vallabhajosula et al. (1980) have shown that ^{67}Ga in the plasma is present almost exclusively as a ^{67}Ga–transferrin complex. This is presumably related to the fact that the formation constant for gallium–transferrin is high, almost 10^{24} (Kulprathipanja et al., 1979). As shown in Table 15.2, the formation constant for indium–transferrin is even higher, approximating that of iron–transferrin (Kulprathipanja et al., 1979; Moerlein and Welch, 1981). Also listed in Table 15.2 are the log K for the conversion of the metal–transferrin complexes to the highly insoluble hydroxides. Both iron–transferrin and gallium–transferrin are thermodynamically unstable to hydrolysis, while indium–transferrin is not. This difference may play some role in explaining the eventual disposition of ^{67}Ga and ^{111}In in the body.

It is worth noting that the affinity of lactoferrin for ^{67}Ga at physiological pH is greater than that of transferrin (Hoffer, Huberty and Khayam-Bashi, 1977). Weiner, Schreiber and Hoffer (1983) have shown that incubation of ^{67}Ga–transferrin with ferritin in vitro resulted in the formation of a significant amount of ^{67}Ga–ferritin. However, the concentrations of lactoferrin and ferritin in plasma are about 1000-fold less than that of transferrin (Tsan, 1985). Thus, it is not unexpected that, despite these observations, the majority of ^{67}Ga is present in the plasma as a ^{67}Ga–transferrin complex.

TABLE 15.2 Formation constants for iron–transferrin, gallium–transferrin and indium–transferrin and hydrolysis of metal–transferrin complex. Adapted from Moerlein and Welch (1981)

Metal	Metal–transferrin formation (log K)	Metal–transferrin hydrolysis (log K)
Iron	30.3	3.9
Gallium	23.7	7.2
Indium	30.5	−1.2

MARROW IMAGING

Several groups have investigated the potential utility of iron-52 citrate (Van Dyke, Anger and Pollycove, 1964; Anger and Van Dyke, 1964) and indium-111 chloride (Lilien et al., 1973; Farrer, Saha and Katz, 1973; Merrick et al., 1975; Parmentier et al., 1977) as erythropoietic bone marrow-imaging agents. Both nuclides are taken up by red marrow-containing bones and exhibit similar distributions in focal marrow lesions. However, the distribution of ^{111}In did not follow that of ^{52}Fe in patients with red cell aplasia (Merrick et al., 1975) or with polycythemia or anemia (Parmentier et al., 1977), suggesting that indium nuclides are less than ideal analogs of iron for the purpose of the assessment of the hematopoietic marrow system.

The metabolism of indium–transferrin appears to differ significantly from that of iron–transferrin. In the rat, ^{59}Fe–transferrin is taken up rapidly by the placenta and the ^{59}Fe activity is transferred almost immediately through the placenta (Graber et al. 1970). With ^{113m}In–transferrin, placental uptake is not followed by fetal uptake of ^{113m}In. The plasma clearance of ^{111}In activity following injection of ^{111}In–transferrin in the dog and the human is considerably slower than that of ^{59}Fe–transferrin (McIntyre et al., 1974; McIntyre, 1975). In addition, McIntyre and coworkers have reported that ^{111}In is incorporated into circulating erythrocytes after ^{111}In–transferrin administration; however, the magnitude of uptake was only about one-tenth of that seen with ^{59}Fe–transferrin.

CANCER-RELATED APPLICATIONS

Transferrin receptor

The transferrin receptor is a potential cell surface target that could be exploited for the preferential delivery of both diagnostic and therapeutic isotopes to specific cell populations. Specific receptors for transferrin have been found on rapidly proliferating malignant and normal tissues (see Chapter 12). Transferrin receptors have been identified in human breast cancer tissue (Faulk, Hsi and Stevens, 1980; Shindelman, Ortmeyer and Sussman, 1981), non-Hodgkin's lymphoma (Habershaw et al., 1983) and leukemic cells (Goding and Burns, 1981). However, transferrin receptors are also found on normal tissue substructures such as hemopoietic precursors in bone marrow, gastrointestinal epithelium, basal epidermis, hepatocytes and Kupffer cells (Gatter et al., 1983; Lebman et al., 1982).

If strategies can be developed for minimizing receptor-mediated binding in normal tissues, radiolabeled monoclonal antibodies directed against the

TABLE 15.3 Some mouse monoclonal antibodies to the human transferrin receptor

Antibody	Class	Reference
B3/25	IgG$_1$	Omary, Trowbridge and Minowada (1980)
5E9	IgG$_1$	Haynes et al. (1981)
L5.1	IgG$_{2a}$	Lebman et al. (1982)
OKT9	IgG$_1$	Sutherland et al. (1981)
BK19.9	IgG	Brown et al. (1981)
24-17.1	IgG$_{2a}$	Thompson et al. (1983)
454A12	IgG$_1$	Frankel et al. (1985)
D$_{51}$	IgG$_1$	Gross (1985)

transferrin receptor might be valuable tools for radioimmunoscintigraphy and therapy (see Chapter 16). Mouse monoclonal antibodies which recognize the human transferrin receptor have been developed in a number of laboratories (Table 15.3). The fact that these antibodies exhibit different patterns of binding to normal tissues is a property which suggests that these antibodies may differ with regard to epitope recognition and/or binding affinity.

To date, radiolabeled anti-transferrin antibodies have yet to be exploited for imaging or therapeutic applications. A conceptually similar approach to the latter is the use of peptide toxins linked to a monoclonal antibody to the transferrin receptor. These conjugates have been synthesized and shown to be extremely potent cytotoxic agents which are selective for transferrin receptor-positive cells (Trowbridge and Domingo, 1981; Lesley et al., 1984; see also Chapter 16).

In order to minimize the problem of normal tissue binding, administration of a labeled anti-transferrin receptor antibody by a non-intravenous route would be recommended. For example, we are currently considering the use of intraperitoneal administration for treating ovarian carcinoma and the intrathecal route for leptomeningeal tumors. The nuclide of choice for therapeutic applications will depend on the nature of the tumor target. Because of the rapid internalization of the receptor–transferrin complex, nuclides which decay by the emission of radiation of subcellular range might be of particular utility. Factors pertinent to the selection of beta-, alpha- and low-energy electron-emitting nuclides for antibody-mediated radiotherapy have been reviewed recently (Zalutsky, 1988).

^{67}Ga and ^{111}In complexes

Gallium-67 citrate, indium-111 chloride and the transferrin complexes of these nuclides have been shown to accumulate preferentially in a variety of rodent tumors (Hunter and de Kock, 1969; Wagner et al., 1971; Serafini et al., 1971; Anghileri, Ottaviani and Raynaud, 1983; Saha and Boyd, 1983). Despite the fact that ^{67}Ga and ^{111}In exhibit similar tumor selectivity in these models, ^{111}In has rarely been used for tumor imaging clinically (Goodwin et al., 1971) while gallium-67 citrate is one of the most frequently utilized radiopharmaceuticals for imaging cancer patients (Hoffer, Beckerman and Henkin, 1978; Beckerman, Hoffer and Bitran, 1984).

For this reason, the mechanism of gallium-67 citrate accumulation in tumors has been investigated more extensively (Tsan and Scheffel, 1986). As one might expect, iron-binding proteins play an important role in most hypotheses for the mechanism of ^{67}Ga uptake in tumors. After injection of gallium-67 citrate, essentially all the ^{67}Ga activity is present as a transferrin complex; therefore, it is not surprising that the addition of transferrin to tumor cells in culture enhances the binding of ^{67}Ga to the cells (Sephton and Harris, 1975, 1981; Larson et al., 1979).

Larson and coworkers (Larson et al., 1979; Larson, 1981) have suggested that tumor uptake of ^{67}Ga is mediated by the binding of ^{67}Ga–transferrin to transferrin receptors on the tumor cell surface. The ^{67}Ga-labeled receptor complex is then internalized into the cell, where the ^{67}Ga activity is transcomplexed to an intracellular acceptor macromolecule which is retained within the tumor cell. There is evidence to suggest that ^{67}Ga is bound intracellularly by ferritin (Clausen, Edeling and Fogh, 1974; Hegge, Mahler and Larson, 1977) and/or lactoferrin (Tsan and Scheffel, 1986). The transcomplexation of ^{67}Ga from transferrin to both ferritin (Weiner, Schreiber and Hoffer, 1983) and lactoferrin (Hoffer, Huberty and Khayam-Bashi, 1977) has been shown to occur *in vitro*.

Although the transferrin receptor hypothesis is supported by the majority of *in vitro* data, conflicting results have been obtained in animal models. Decreased tumor uptake of ^{67}Ga has been observed in rat tumors in animals with both elevated (Hayes et al., 1981) and reduced (Bradley et al., 1978) unsaturated iron-binding capacities. Using the H-4-II-E hepatoma cell line, Scheffel et al. (1985) have shown that, *in vitro*, addition of transferrin enhances ^{67}Ga uptake at low doses and inhibits uptake at higher doses. However, uptake of ^{67}Ga by hepatic tumors in perfused livers or intact animals is not enhanced by low concentrations of transferrin. These results suggest that multiple mechanisms may be involved in the accumulation of ^{67}Ga in tumors *in vivo*. Since some tumors have been shown to contain ferritin and/or lactoferrin, it seems plausible that these proteins may also be involved in the tumor uptake and retention of ^{67}Ga.

Whatever the mechanism of ^{67}Ga accumulation in tumors, this radiopharmaceutical is used extensively as a tumor-imaging agent. The current status of gallium-67 citrate in the clinical evaluation of cancer has been documented by Beckerman, Hoffer and Bitran (1984) and Neumann and

Hoffer (1984). As described in these reviews and the references cited therein, ^{67}Ga imaging is particularly useful for the evaluation of Hodgkin's lymphoma, metastatic melanoma, certain types of non-Hodgkin's lymphomas and possibly carcinomas of the lung. Because of the accumulation of ^{67}Ga by some normal tissues, in particular the bowel, the reliability of tumor detection is somewhat dependent upon the location of a lesion.

The formation constant and thermodynamic stability towards hydrolysis of indium–transferrin are significantly higher than those of gallium–transferrin (Table 15.2). In addition, the gamma rays emitted in the decay of ^{111}In are more favorable than those of ^{67}Ga for gamma camera imaging (Table 15.1). For these reasons, we have investigated the distribution and mechanism of uptake of ^{111}In activity following the injection of indium-111 chloride in a tumor model for lymph node metastases (de Sousa et al., 1985). These experiments were performed in ACI rats inoculated in the foot with H-4-II-E hepatoma cells. This model is of particular value for the study of metastatic lymph node imaging, because in males, tumors metastasize to regional popliteal lymph nodes, while in females, regional lymph node involvement rarely occurs.

Groups of animals were injected with both indium-111 chloride and [^{3}H]thymidine in order to determine whether ^{111}In localization was related to cellular proliferation. Uptake of ^{111}In in primary tumors in both males and females and in the regional lymph nodes of females was not correlated with ^{3}H accumulation. However, as shown in Figure 15.1, the uptake of ^{111}In in the metastatic regional lymph nodes of the males exhibited a significant correlation with [^{3}H]thymidine levels, suggesting that ^{111}In uptake in metastatic nodes is related to cellular proliferation.

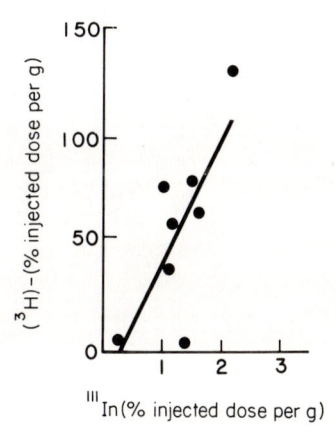

Figure 15.1 Correlation between uptake of ^{3}H and ^{111}In in draining lymph nodes of males following injection of [^{3}H]thymidine and indium-111 chloride. From de Sousa et al. (1985). Reproduced by permission of Pergamon Press

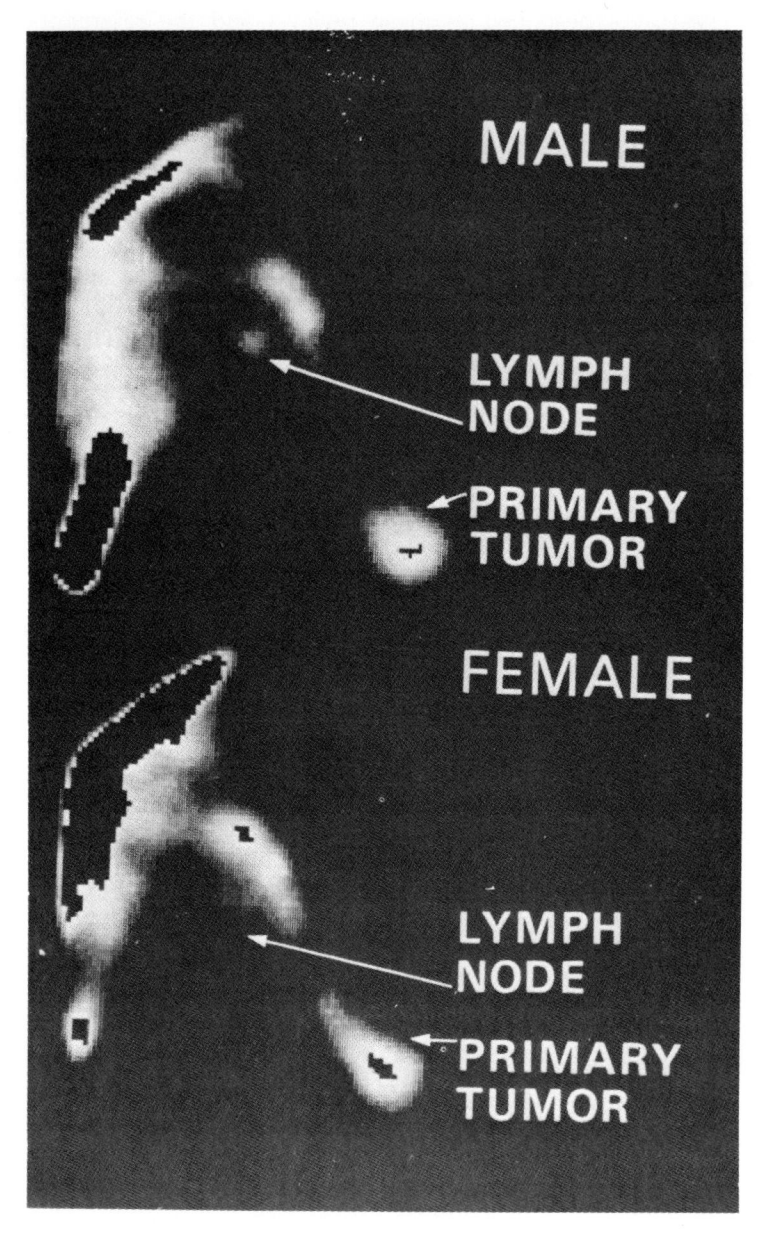

Figure 15.2 Gamma camera images of a male and a female rat 48 hours after injection of indium-111 chloride. Both animals have H-4-II-E tumors in foot; male has 31 mg metastatic lymph node, female has 37 mg normal node ($r = 0.74$) From de Sousa *et al.* (1985). Reproduced by permission of Pergamon Press

External gamma camera imaging was performed in both male and female rats 24 hours after injection of indium-111 chloride. Figure 15.2 compares the images obtained in a female and a male rat. At necropsy, the two animals were shown to have similar lymph node weights. The metastatic node (confirmed by histology) of the male could be visualized, whereas the draining node in the female could not. This difference could be related in part to the fact, demonstrated by autoradiographic studies, that dividing cells in the male nodes were packed in metastatic foci, in contrast to female nodes, where they were distributed more uniformly.

Antibodies directed against ferritin

Ferritin is currently under investigation as a potential tumor-associated target for use in radioimmunotherapy. Ferritin has been found in a wide range of tumors, including breast and pancreatic cancers (Marcus and Zinberg, 1974), Hodgkin's disease (Eshar, Order and Katz, 1974) and hepatomas (Beck and Bollack, 1977). Synthesis and secretion of ferritin by tumors have both been reported (Eshar, Order and Katz, 1974; Kew *et al.*, 1978; see Chapter 14).

With regard to the potential utility of ferritin as a tumor-specific target, it is important to realize that many normal tissues contain ferritin, including the liver, bone marrow, spleen, kidney, heart and lung (Munro and Linder, 1978). However, in these tissues, ferritin is present intracellularly, whereas in tumor, ferritin is also located extracellularly. Because of the greater availability of ferritin for antigen-mediated binding, it would be expected that tumor uptake of an anti-ferritin antibody would be higher than in normal tissues.

The efficacy of selectively localizing ^{131}I-labeled rabbit anti-ferritin polyclonal antibodies in a ferritin-containing tumor has been investigated in the H-4-II-E syngeneic rat hepatoma model (Rostock *et al.*, 1983). Two groups of animals were injected with 200 μg of either ^{131}I-labeled anti-ferritin or normal IgG and the integrated radiation doses to both tumor and normal tissues were compared. Tumors of animals receiving anti-ferritin received a 2.9 times higher dose than those injected with normal IgG, while normal tissues received the same dose from both labeled proteins. Tumor uptake after injection of ^{131}I-labeled anti-ferritin was about 2.4% of the injected dose per gram at 24 hours and 1.7% per gram at 72 hours.

Interpretation of these results is hindered by the fact that different sets of animals were used for measurement of anti-ferritin and control IgG biodistribution. Since tumor size, flow, permeability and other variables known to influence tumor uptake of antibody may have differed in the two groups, it might have been more relevant to have performed a paired-label experiment (^{131}I-labeled anti-ferritin and ^{125}I-labeled control IgG).

Since the most promising application of ^{131}I-labeled anti-ferritin antibodies is as a radiotherapeutic agent, it is important to determine the effects of increasing the specific activity and total protein dose on the specificity of tumor uptake. Rostock et al. (1984a) have shown that the uptake of ^{131}I activity in the H-4-II-E hepatoma does not vary when antibody is radioiodinated at specific activities ranging from 0.1 to 15 μCi μg^{-1}. The ratio of anti-ferritin to control IgG radiation dose was determined at protein doses ranging between 0.7 μg and 5 mg per rat. For normal tissues, the anti-ferritin to normal IgG uptake ratio was approximately 1 and dose-invariant. With tumors, the maximum dose advantage was observed at a dose level of 200 μg per animal. The authors suggested that subtle differences in normal tissue uptake may have been obscured by the fact that the immunospecificity of the anti-ferritin was only 20%.

The effects of tumor size, vascularity and ferritin concentration on tumor uptake have also been investigated in the rat hepatoma model. The anti-ferritin to control IgG dose ratio decreased with increasing tumor size, with no specific uptake being observed in large necrotic areas (Rostock et al., 1984b). Autoradiography using ^{125}I-labeled anti-ferritin revealed that antibody deposition at 24 hours is perivascular, with ^{125}I activity decreasing at increasing distances from vessels. Although diffusion of activity throughout the tumor was observed with time, avascular regions always exhibited less ^{125}I activity. A recent study by Klein, Kopher and Rostock (1986) has shown that greater targeting of smaller tumors with anti-ferritin antibodies might also be related to the fact that the ferritin content of H-4-II-E tumors decreases with increasing size.

In parallel with these studies, Order and coworkers have been investigating the therapeutic efficacy of ^{131}I-labeled anti-ferritin antibodies in several patient populations. Phase I–II studies involved the administration of single doses of up to 150 mCi to hepatoma patients who had previously received chemotherapy and external-beam radiotherapy (Order et al., 1980; Order, Klein and Leichner, 1981). No major organ toxicity was reported; however, one patient had 3 weeks of marrow aplasia. The half-life for clearance of ^{131}I activity from the tumor, determined by external probe counting, was 7.7 days.

Radiation dosimetric evaluation of ^{131}I-labeled anti-ferritin therapy has been performed by Leichner et al. (1983). The ratio of uptake of ^{131}I by tumor and normal liver tissue was found to be dependent on the volume of the tumor; for tumors less than 1700 cm^3, the tumor to liver ratio was 4.8 : 1, while for tumors larger than 2300 cm^3, the tumor to liver ratio fell to 1.6 : 1. The doses received by the tumor, normal liver and total body were calculated to be about 1850, 700 and 165 rad, respectively.

More recently, Order et al. (1985) have reported the results of ^{131}I-labeled anti-ferritin antibody therapy in 105 patients with hepatoma. Patients received various combinations of external beam irradiation and chemotherapy prior to injection of 1–4 cycles of labeled antibody. One cycle of antibody consisted of a 30 mCi dose of anti-ferritin of one species of origin, followed 5 days later by 20 mCi of anti-ferritin derived from a different species. An initial dose of 30 mCi was selected because it was thought that at a specific activity of 8–10 mCi mg^{-1}, this dose was sufficient to saturate the tumor.

In this study, computed tomographic tumor volume measurement was the criterion used to document complete response in 7% of patients and partial response in 43% of patients. Thrombocytopenia was the major toxicity observed. The half-life of tumor activity was found to be dependent on the species of origin of the antibody, varying from between 3 and 5 days for rabbit, pig, monkey and cow, to 2 days or less for sheep, goat, chicken or turkey-derived antibodies. The need for multiple species antibodies for retreatment protocols was confirmed in a later study which demonstrated the production of species-specific antibodies in 50% of hepatoma patients treated with anti-ferritin (Klein *et al.*, 1986).

Lenhard *et al.* (1985) have studied the therapeutic efficacy of ^{131}I-labeled anti-ferritin for treating patients with Hodgkin's disease who had not responded to combination chemotherapy. Because of the relative radiosensitivity of this tumor and the documented presence of ferritin in Hodgkin's disease (Eshar, Order and Katz, 1974), treatment with labeled anti-ferritin is a particularly favorable approach. Partial remission and symptomatic response were observed in 40% and 77% of patients, respectively.

More recently, Order *et al.* (1986) have initiated a phase I–II trial of anti-ferritin antibodies labeled with yttrium-90 in hepatoma patients. The advantage of ^{90}Y is that its beta particles have a significantly higher range in tissue and deposit more energy. Together with its shorter half-life, this means that ^{90}Y-labeled antibodies offer the potential of increasing the dose rate compared to that obtained with ^{131}I-labeled antibodies.

Partial remissions were seen in two of six patients treated with ^{90}Y-labeled anti-ferritin. Some hematologic toxicity was reported. The authors observed that pretreatment of patients with 3 × 300 rad of external beam radiation increased tumor to liver ratios from 1.8 : 1 to 4.6 : 1 and increased integrated tumor dose from 424 rad to 1072 rad. These changes were attributed to increased tumor permeability resulting from the external beam irradiation.

INFLAMMATION

Gallium-67 citrate and, to a lesser extent, indium-111 chloride, have been used for the detection of various inflammatory diseases. In a recent review, Neumann and Hoffer (1984) have evaluated the clinical utility of ^{67}Ga scintigraphy for identification of inflammatory lesions. They observed that this radiopharmaceutical is of greatest value for detecting chronic inflammatory lesions, detecting sites of inflammation which are not focal anatomically such as cellulitis and peritonitis, and documenting osteomyelitis and other acute lesions which sometimes escape detection by other imaging modalities.

Indium-111 chloride has also been used as a radiopharmaceutical for the evaluation of abscesses and other inflammatory lesions. The potential utility of this tracer for these applications was first described by Hussein, Breen and Leslie (1978). More recently, Sayle, Balachandran and Rogers (1983) reported that the specificity and accuracy of lesion detection in 258 patients with suspected inflammatory disease by indium-111 chloride imaging were 95% and 94%, respectively. They observed that these values are greater than those found in the literature for gallium-67 citrate and ^{111}In-labeled white blood cell imaging of inflammatory processes. Potential advantages of indium-111 chloride over gallium-67 citrate include the lack of uptake in the gastrointestinal tract and in normally healing wounds. In addition, use of indium-111 chloride does not involve the lengthy radiopharmaceutical preparation step required for ^{111}In-labeled white cell imaging.

The exact mechanism of ^{67}Ga and ^{111}In uptake in inflammatory lesions remains unknown; however, iron-binding proteins are implicated in most hypotheses (Tsan, 1985). It is generally believed that ^{67}Ga is transported to the site of inflammation as a ^{67}Ga–transferrin complex. Lactoferrin has been shown to be present in inflammatory exudates, presumably due to secretion by and/or death of stimulated neutrophils (Leffel and Spitznagel, 1975). Alternatively, bacterial siderophores capable of binding iron and its analogs could be involved in the retention of ^{67}Ga in inflammatory lesions (Emery and Hoffer, 1980).

ARTHRITIS

Iron and proteins which bind iron have been implicated in the pathogenesis of rheumatoid arthritis (Blake et al., 1981, 1985; see also Chapter 7). Synovial cells and subsynovial macrophages have been shown to contain iron; indeed, there is an association between the presence of iron in a joint and the grade of disease assessed radiographically (Muirden, 1970; Blake et al., 1984). In addition, the degree of inflammatory activity in rheumatoid knees has been correlated with the amount of lactoferrin in the synovial fluid (Malmquist, Thorell and Wolheim, 1977).

Both gallium-67 citrate and indium-111 chloride have been evaluated as potential radiopharmaceuticals for the evaluation of rheumatoid arthritis. Tannenbaum et al. (1984) have investigated the tissue distribution of ^{67}Ga following the injection of gallium-67 citrate in rabbits with zymosan-induced arthritis. The ratio of ^{67}Ga in the affected to control knee reached a maximum value of 8.2 ± 0.8 : 1 five days after intra-articular zymosan administration. Tissue distribution measurements performed 48 hours after injection of gallium-67 citrate demonstrated preferential uptake of radioactivity in the synovia from arthritic knees. Accumulation of ^{67}Ga in the inflamed synovium was about eight times higher than in synovial tissue from normal knees.

Since indium has a higher affinity than gallium for iron-binding proteins, we have been investigating the utility of indium-111 chloride as an agent for the quantitative assessment of rheumatoid arthritis. Gamma camera images were used to calculate joint to soft tissue ratios, which were used as an objective index of arthritic disease. This parameter has two potential advantages over those used previously. First, unlike the right to left joint ratio used by Tannenbaum et al. (1984), the knee to soft tissue ratio facilitates the evaluation of bilateral disease. Second, the uptake of ^{67}Ga and ^{111}In in muscle is lower than in bone, making the joint to soft tissue ratio a more useful index than the femur to joint ratio utilized by others (McCall et al., 1983).

Initial studies were performed in the collagen model of proliferative arthritis in the rat (de Sousa et al., 1986). The ratio of ^{111}In uptake in ankles and feet to adjacent soft tissue in animals immunized with collagen was 1.18 ± 0.04, a value which was significantly higher than that observed in control rats (0.39 ± 0.02).

More recently, we have studied the use of indium-111 chloride as a quantitative indicator of inflammatory activity in the knees of rabbits with antigen-induced arthritis (Zalutsky et al., 1988). As shown in Figure 15.3, the knee to soft tissue ^{111}In uptake ratio in control knees was constant with time, varying between 1.5 : 1 and 1.85 : 1. In contrast, the knee to soft tissue ratio in involved knees increased from 2.0 : 1 at 30 minutes to 4.6 : 1 at 96 hours after indium-111 chloride administration.

In arthritic knees, ^{111}In accumulates preferentially in intra-articular structures covered by the synovium (Table 15.4). While no significant difference in uptake in extra-articular structures was observed between involved and control knees, the synovium and tissues in contact with the synovium from arthritic knees generally exhibited at least a ten-fold higher uptake than control knees, particularly at 96 hours.

Synovial tissues from control and involved knees from six animals were evaluated histologically for the presence of hyperplasia, inflammatory cell infiltration and villus formation. The ^{111}In knee to soft tissue ratio determined from the gamma camera and the synovium to muscle ratio meas-

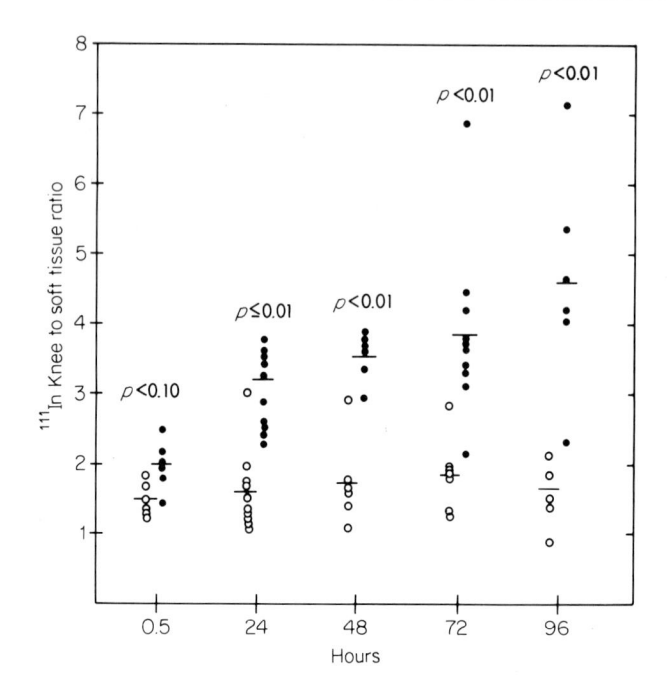

Figure 15.3 Knee to soft tissue ^{111}In uptake ratios for arthritic (closed circles) and control (open circles) knees. P value for the significance of the difference between uptake ratios for control and arthritic joints at each time point. From Zalutsky et al. (1988). Reproduced by permission of Lippincott/Harper & Row

ured at necropsy correlated well with the histological evaluation of joint status (Figure 15.4).

Several groups have attempted to use gallium-67 citrate and indium-111 chloride for the evaluation of septic and rheumatoid arthritis in patients. Coleman et al. (1982) did not find any correlation between the ^{67}Ga joint to bone uptake ratio and clinical symptoms of disease. In addition, no differences were observed in the joint to bone ratios of patients with septic versus rheumatoid arthritis. McCall et al. (1983) have reported that the ^{67}Ga femur to knee joint ratio in arthritic knees, 1.40 ± 0.22, was significantly different from that observed in clinically inactive knees (1.11 ± 0.12).

De Sousa et al. (1986) have begun to investigate the clinical utility of ^{111}In joint to soft tissue ratios as a quantitative index of rheumatoid arthritis. In two patients, joint to soft tissue ratios of about 1 were observed in clinically normal joints 72 hours after injection of 2 mCi of indium-111 chloride; in contrast, swollen joints yielded uptake ratios of between 2.5 : 1 and 4.7 : 1. Similar ratios have been obtained in subsequent studies evaluating the use of indium-111 chloride in patients with rheumatoid arthritis (A. Lima

TABLE 15.4 Distribution in the knee region of ^{111}In in AIA rabbits following injection of indium-111 chloride

	% Injected dose per gram tissue × 10^2				Arthritic/control	
	72 hour		96 hour			
	Control	Arthritic	Control	Arthritic	72 hour	96 hour
Extra-articular structure						
Muscle	0.9 ± 0.2	1.1 ± 0.4	1.9 ± 1.7	1.1 ± 0.7	1.2	0.6
Femur (midshaft)	1.9 ± 0.4	2.0 ± 0.4	1.5 ± 0.7	2.1 ± 0.8	1.0	1.4
Marrow	10.7 ± 2.8	11.6 ± 4.0	14.1 ± 7.5	14.3 ± 6.6	1.1	1.0
Intra-articular structures without synovial covering						
Femoral condyle	2.2 ± 0.5	8.2 ± 2.5	3.0 ± 1.7	11.9 ± 6.2	3.7	3.9
Tibia-fibular condyle, intra-articular tensor	5.7 ± 4.5	12.2 ± 3.6	3.9 ± 1.0	9.6 ± 4.7	2.1	2.5
Patella	1.3 ± 0.3	5.7 ± 1.0	1.7 ± 0.9	7.1 ± 2.1	4.6	4.1
Intra-articular structures covered by synovium						
Synovium	6.6 ± 4.5	34.1 ± 8.8	4.4 ± 1.4	44.3 ± 9.8	5.2	10.2
Fat pad	2.3 ± 0.8	9.3 ± 4.5	1.9 ± 1.0	10.7 ± 3.1	4.1	5.8
Quadriceps tendon	1.7 ± 0.6	13.2 ± 9.6	1.6 ± 0.4	14.7 ± 9.6	7.8	9.5
Collateral ligament	6.5 ± 2.1	53.0 ± 16.7	4.1 ± 1.3	44.3 ± 15.3	8.2	10.7
Menisci	4.4 ± 1.3	30.7 ± 9.8	2.6 ± 1.6	39.8 ± 11.8	7.0	15.6
Intra-articular tendon	3.0 ± 1.0	36.4 ± 10.7	2.7 ± 0.9	37.8 ± 9.0	12.0	13.9

$n = 6 \pm$ SD

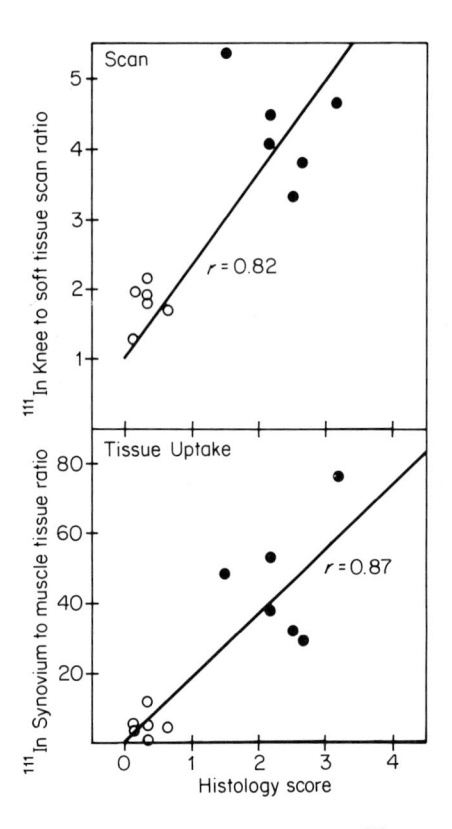

Figure 15.4 Correlation between histology score and ^{111}In knee to soft tissue ratio from gamma camera images (upper) and synovium to muscle tissue ratio determined at necropsy (lower). Open and closed circles represent control and arthritic joints, respectively. From Zalutsky et al. (1988). Reproduced by permission of Lippincott/Harper & Row

Bastos, Gomes Duarte and M. de Sousa, personal communication). Figure 15.5 illustrates a typical gamma image of the knees of a patient obtained 72 hours after injection of 2mCi of indium-111 chloride. Increased uptake of ^{111}In is evident both in subjective evaluation of the image and by comparison of the knee to proximal bone ratios (clinically normal knee, 0.94; swollen knee, 2.2).

SUMMARY

Iron-binding proteins play an important role in the mechanism of localization of radiopharmaceuticals used for imaging bone marrow, cancer and

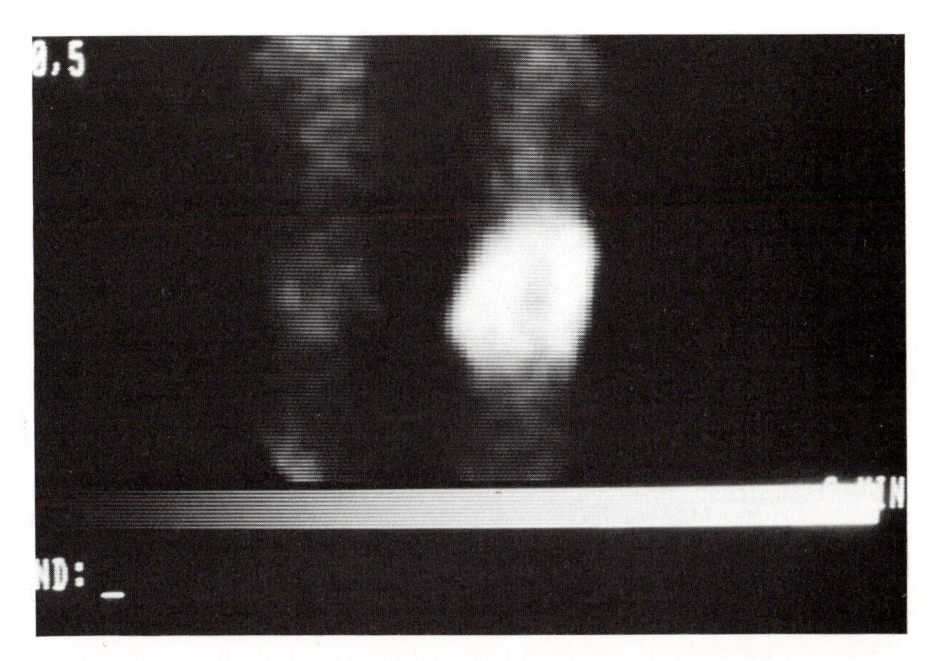

Figure 15.5 Gamma camera image of knees of a rheumatoid arthritis patient obtained at 72 hours after the intravenous injection of ^{111}In chloride (2 mCi). Increased uptake of ^{111}In in affected knee (right) is evident both in subjective evaluation and by comparison of the knee/proximal bone ratios (2.2 in swollen knee; 0.94 in clinically normal knee)

various inflammatory processes, including rheumatoid arthritis. Radio-labeled antibodies may also be useful in the treatment of tumors which contain elevated levels of ferritin. As our knowledge of the involvement of iron and iron-binding proteins in the pathogenesis of these and other diseases increases, we will be able to exploit more fully the diagnostic and therapeutic potential of these tracers. In addition, ^{111}In and ^{67}Ga, as well as antibodies to iron-binding proteins (and their receptors), may also be useful as probes for studying the etiology of these diseases *in vivo*.

ACKNOWLEDGEMENTS

Research support from the National Institutes of Health (NIADDKD AM-23063 and NCI CA-42324) and the American–Portuguese Biomedical Research Fund is gratefully acknowledged. The author wishes to thank Dr Arthur Frankel for helpful discussions and Mr John Hess for manuscript preparation.

REFERENCES

Anger, H. O., and Van Dyke, D. (1964). Human bone marrow distribution shown in vivo by ^{52}Fe and the positron scintillation camera, *Science*, **144**, 1587–9.

Anghileri, L. J., Ottaviani, M., and Raynaud, C. (1983). In vivo distribution of ^{67}gallium and ^{111}indium complexes with transferrin: Uptake by DS sarcoma tumors, *J. Nucl. Med. Allied Sci.*, **27**, 17–20.

Beck, G., and Bollack, C. (1977). Synthesis of ferritin in cultured hepatoma cells, *Fed. Exp. Biol. Soc.*, **47**, 14–17.

Beckerman, C., Hoffer, P. B., and Bitran, J. D. (1984). The role of gallium-67 in the clinical evaluation of cancer, *Semin. Nucl. Med.*, **14**, 296–323.

Blake, D. R., Hall, N. D., Bacon, P. A., Dieppe, P. A., Halliwell, B., and Gutteridge, J. M. C. (1981). The importance of iron in rheumatoid disease, *Lancet*, **ii**, 1142–3.

Blake, D. R., Gallagher, P. J., Potter, A. R., Bell, M. J., and Bacon, P. A. (1984). The effect of synovial iron on the progression of rheumatoid disease, *Arthritis Rheum.*, **27**, 495–501.

Blake, D. R. Lunec, J., Ahern, M., Ring, E. F. J., Bradfield, J., and Gutteridge, J. M. C. (1985). Effect of intravenous iron dextran on rheumatoid arthritis, *Ann. Rheum. Dis.*, **44**, 183–8.

Bradley, W. P., Alderson, P. O., Eckelman, W. C., Hamilton, R. G., and Weiss, J. F. (1978). Decreased tumor uptake of gallium-67 in animals after whole body irradiation, *J. Nucl. Med.*, **19**, 204–9.

Brown, G., Kourilsky, F., Fisher, A., Bastin, J., and MacLennan, I. C. M. (1981). Strategy for screening for monoclonal antibodies against cellular antigens expressed on minor cell populations or in low amounts, *Hum. Lymph Differentiation*, **1**, 167–82.

Chauduri, T. K., Ehrhart, J. C., DeGowin, R. L., and Christie, J. H. (1974). ^{59}Fe whole body scanning, *J. Nucl. Med.*, **15**, 667–73.

Clausen, J., Edeling, C. J., and Fogh, J. (1974). Ga binding to human serum protein and tumor components, *Cancer Res.*, **43**, 1931–7.

Coleman, R. E., Samuelson, C. O. Jr, Baim, S., Christian, P. E., and Ward, J. R. (1982). Imaging with Tc-99m MDP and Ga-67 citrate in patients with rheumatoid arthritis and suspected septic arthritis, *J. Nucl. Med.*, **23**, 479–82.

DeGowin, R. L., Chaudhuri, T. K., Christie, J. H., Callis, M. N., and Mueller, A. L. (1974). Marrow scanning in the evaluation of hemopoiesis after radiotherapy, *Arch. Intern. Med.*, **134**, 297–303.

de Sousa, M., Carroll, A. M., Herman, P. G., Kerr, S., Boulton, J., and Zalutsky, M. R. (1985). Distribution and mechanism of uptake of ^{111}InCl$_3$ in a tumor model for lymph node metastases, *Int. J. Nucl. Med. Biol.*, **12**, 89–96.

de Sousa, M., Bastos, A. L., Dynesius-Trentham, R., Kerr, S., Bernardo, A., Duarte, J. G., and Trentham, D. E. (1986). Potential of indium-111 to measure inflammatory arthritis, *J. Rheum.*, **13 : 6**, 1108–16.

Edwards, C. L., and Hayes, R. L. (1969). Tumor scanning with ^{67}Ga-citrate, *J. Nucl. Med.*, **10**, 103–5.

Emery, T., and Hoffer, P. B. (1980). Siderophore-mediated mechanism of gallium-uptake demonstrated in the microorganism *Ustilago sphaerogena*, *J. Nucl. Med.*, **21**, 935–9.

Eshar, Z., Order, S. E., and Katz, D. H. (1974). Ferritin-A Hodgkin's disease associated antigen, *Proc. Natl Acad. Sci. USA*, **75**, 3956–60.

Farrer, P. A., Saha, G. B., and Katz, M. (1973). Further observations on the use of

[111]In–transferrin for the visualization of bone marrow in man, *J. Nucl. Med.*, **14**, 394–5.

Faulk, W. P., Hsi, B.-L., and Stevens, P. J. (1980). Transferrin and transferrin receptors in carcinoma of the breast, *Lancet*, **ii**, 390–2.

Frankel, A., Ring, D., Tringale, F., and Hsieh-Ma, S. (1985). Tissue distribution of breast cancer associated antigens defined by monoclonal antibodies, *J. Biol. Response Mod.*, **4**, 273–86.

Gatter, K., Brown, G., Trowbridge, I., Woolston, R.-E., and Mason, D. Y. (1983). Transferrin receptors in human tissues: Their distribution and possible clinical relevance, *J. Clin. Pathol.*, **36**, 539–45.

Goding, J. W., and Burns, G. F. (1981). Monoclonal antibody OKT-9 recognizes the receptor for transferrin on human acute lymphocytic leukaemia cells, *J. Immunol.*, **127**, 1256–8.

Goodwin, D. A., Goode, R., Brown, L., and Imborne, C. (1971). ^{111}In-labeled transferrin for the detection of tumors, *Radiology*, **100**, 175–9.

Graber, S. E., Hurley, P. J., Heyssel, R. M., and McIntyre, P. A. (1970). Behavior of iron-, indium-, and iodine-labeled transferrin in the pregnant rat, *Proc. Soc. Exp. Biol. Med.*, **133**, 1093–6.

Gross, H.-J. (1985). A monoclonal antibody D_{51} recognizes the transferrin-receptor structure, *Blut*, **51**, 117–22.

Gunasekera, S. W., King, L. J., and Lavender, P. J. (1972). The behavior of tracer gallium-67 towards serum proteins, *Clin. Chim. Acta*, **39**, 401–6.

Habershaw, J. A., Lister, T. A., Stansield, A. G., and Greaves, M. F. (1983). Correlation of transferrin receptor expression with histological class and outcome in non-Hodgkin's lymphomas, *Lancet*, **i**, 498–501.

Hayes, R. L., Rafter, J. J., Byrd, B. L., and Carlton, J. E. (1981). Studies of the in vivo entry of Ga-67 into normal and malignant tissue, *J. Nucl. Med.*, **22**, 325–32.

Haynes, B., Hemler, M., Cotner, T., Mann, D., Eisenbarth, G., Strominger, J., and Fauci, A. (1981). Characterization of a monoclonal antibody (5E9) that defines a human cell surface antigen of cell activation, *J. Immunol.*, **127**, 347–51.

Hegge, F. N., Mahler, D. J., and Larson, S. M. (1977). The incorporation of Ga-67 into the ferritin fraction of rabbit hepatocytes in vivo, *J. Nucl. Med.*, **18**, 937–9.

Hoffer, P. B., Beckerman, C., and Henkin, R. E. (eds) (1978). *Gallium-67 Imaging*, Wiley Medical, New York.

Hoffer, P. B., Huberty, J., and Khayam-Bashi, H. (1977). The association of Ga-67 and lactoferrin, *J. Nucl. Med.*, **10**, 713–17.

Hunter, W. W., and de Kock, H. W. (1969). [111]In for tumor localization, *J. Nucl. Med.*, **10**, 343.

Hussein, M. A. D., Breen, J., and Leslie, E. V. (1978). Clinical experience with [^{111}In]indium chloride scanning in inflammatory diseases, *Clin. Nucl. Med.*, **3**, 196–201.

Kew, M. C., Torrance, J. D., Derman, D., Dimon, M., McNab, G. N., Charlton, R. W., and Bothwell, T. H. (1978). Serum tumor ferritins in primary liver cancer, *Gut*, **19**, 294–9.

Klein, J. L., Kopher, K. A., and Rostock, R. A. (1986). Ferritin concentration and ^{131}I-antiferritin tumor localization in an experimental hepatoma, *Int. J. Radiat. Oncol. Biol. Phys.*, **12**, 137–40.

Klein, J. L., Sandoz, J. W., Kopher, K. A., Leichner, P. K., and Order, S. E. (1986). Detection of specific anti-antibodies in patients treated with radiolabeled antibody, *Int. J. Radiat. Oncol. Biol. Phys.*, **12**, 939–43.

Kulprathipanja, S., Hnatowich, D. J., Beh, R., and Elmaleh, D. (1979). Formation constants of gallium and indium transferrin, *Int. J. Nucl. Med. Biol.*, **6**, 138–41.

Larson, S. M. (1981). Factors determining tumor affinity for gallium-67 citrate. In R. P. Spencer (ed.) *Radiopharmaceuticals: Structure Activity Relationships*, pp. 167–81, Grune Stratton, New York.

Larson, S. M., Rasey, J. S., Allen, D. R., and Nelson, N. J. (1979). A transferrin mediated uptake of gallium-67 by EMT-6 sarcoma. I. Studies in tissue culture, *J. Nucl. Med.*, **20**, 837–42.

Lebman, D., Trucco, M., Bottero, L., Lange, B., Pessano, S., and Rovera, G. (1982). A monoclonal antibody that detects expression of transferrin receptor in human erythroid precursor cells, *Blood*, **59**, 671–8.

Leffel, M. S., and Spitznagel, J. K. (1975). Fate of human lactoferrin and myeloperoxidase in phagocytizing human neutrophils: Effect of immunoglobulin G subclasses and immune complexes coated on latex beads, *Infect. Immun.*, **12**, 813–20.

Leichner, P. K., Klein, J. L., Siegelman, S. S., Ettinger, D. S., and Order, S. E. (1983). Dosimetry of ^{131}I-labeled antiferritin in hepatoma: Specific activities in the tumor and liver, *Cancer Treat. Rep.*, **67**, 647–58.

Lenhard, R. E. Jr, Order, S. E., Spunberg, J. J., Asbell, S. O., and Leibel, S. A. (1985). Isotopic immunoglobulin: A new systemic therapy for advanced Hodgkin's disease, *J. Clin. Oncol.*, **3**, 1296–300.

Lesley, J., Domingo, D., Schulte, R., and Trowbridge, I. (1984). Effect of an antimurine transferrin receptor-ricin A conjugate on bone marrow stem and progenitor cells treated in vitro, *Exp. Cell Res.*, **150**, 400–7.

Lilien, D. L., Berger, H. G., Anderson, D. P., and Bennett, L. R. (1973). ^{111}In-chloride: A new agent for bone marrow imaging, *J. Nucl. Med.*, **14**, 184–6.

Malmquist, J., Thorell, J. I., and Wolheim, F. A. (1977). Lactoferrin and lysozyme in arthritic exudates, *Acta Med. Scand.*, **202**, 313–18.

Marcus, D. M., and Zinberg, N. (1974). Isolation of ferritin from human mammary and pancreatic carcinomas by means of antibody immunoadsorbents, *Arch. Biochem. Biophys.*, **162**, 495–501.

McCall, I. W., Sheppard, H., Haddaway, M., Park, W. M., and Ward, D. J. (1983). Gallium 67 scanning in rheumatoid arthritis, *Br. J. Radiol.*, **56**, 241–3.

McIntyre, P. A. (1975). Agents for bone marrow imaging: An evaluation. In G. Subramaniun, B. A. Rhodes, J. F. Cooper, and V. J. Sodd (eds) *Radiopharmaceuticals*, pp. 343–8, The Society of Nuclear Medicine, New York.

McIntyre, P. A., Larson, S. M., Eikman, E. A., Colman, M., Scheffel, U., and Hodkinson, B. A. (1974). Comparison of the metabolism of iron-labeled transferrin (Fe TF) and indium-labeled transferrin (In TF) by the erythropoietic marrow, *J. Nucl. Med.*, **15**, 856–62.

Merrick, M. V., Gordon-Smith, E. C., Lavender, J. P., and Szur, L. (1975). A comparison of ^{111}In with ^{52}Fe and ^{99m}Tc-sulfur colloid for bone marrow scanning, *J. Nucl. Med.*, **16**, 66–8.

Moerlein, S. M., and Welch, M. J. (1981). The chemistry of gallium and indium as related to radiopharmaceutical production, *Int. J. Nucl. Med. Biol.*, **8**, 277–87.

Muirden, K. D. (1970). The significance of iron deposits in the synovial membrane, *Austr. Ann. Med.*, **19**, 97–104.

Munro, H. N., and Linder, M. C. (1978). Ferritin: Structure, biosynthesis, and role in iron metabolism, *Physiol. Rev.*, **58**, 317–96.

Neumann, R. D., and Hoffer, P. B. (1984). Gallium-67 scintigraphy for detection of inflammation and tumors. In L. M. Freeman (ed.) *Freeman and Johnson's Clinical Radionuclide Imaging*, pp. 1319–64. Grune and Stratton, Orlando.

Omary, M., Trowbridge, I., and Minowada, J. (1980). Human cell-surface glycoprotein with unusual properties, *Nature*, **286**, 888–91.

Order, S. E., Klein, J. L., and Leichner, P. K. (1981) Antiferritin IgG antibody for isotopic cancer therapy, *Oncology*, **38**, 154–60.

Order, S. E., Klein, J. L., Ettinger, D., Alderson, P., Siegelman, S., and Leichner, P. (1980). Phase I–II study of radiolabeled antibody integrated in the treatment of primary hepatic malignancies, *Int. J. Radiat. Oncol. Biol. Phys.*, **6**, 703–10.

Order, S. E., Stillwagon, G. B., Klein, J. L., Leichner, P. K., Siegelman, S. S., Fishman, E. K., Ettinger, D. S., Haulk, T., Kopher, K., Finney, K., Surdyke, M., Self, S., and Leibel, S. (1985). Iodine 131 antiferritin, a new treatment modality in hepatoma: A radiation therapy oncology group study, *J. Clin. Oncol.*, **3**, 1573–82.

Order, S. E., Klein, J. L., Leichner, P. K., Frincke, J., Lollo, C., and Carlo, D. J. (1986). Yttrium antiferritin—A new therapeutic radiolabeled antibody, *Int. J. Radiat. Oncol. Biol. Phys.*, **12**, 277–81.

Parmentier, C., Therain, F., Charbord, P., Aubert, B., and Morardet, N. (1977). Comparative study of ^{111}In and ^{59}Fe bone marrow scanning, *Eur. J. Nucl. Med.*, **2**, 89–92.

Reivich, M., and Alavi, A. (eds) (1985). *Positron Emission Tomography*, Alan R. Liss, New York.

Rostock, R. A., Klein, J. L., Leichner, P., Kopher, K. A., and Order, S. E. (1983). Selective tumor localization in experimental hepatoma by radiolabeled antiferritin antibody, *Int. J. Radiat. Oncol. Biol. Phys.*, **9**, 1345–50.

Rostock, R. A., Klein, J. L., Leichner, P. K., and Order, S. E. (1984a). Distribution of and physiologic factors that affect ^{131}I-antiferritin tumor localization in experimental hepatoma, *Int. J. Radiat. Oncol. Biol. Phys.*, **10**, 1135–41.

Rostock, R. A., Klein, J. L., Kopher, K. A., and Order, S. E. (1984b). Variables affecting the tumor localization of ^{131}I-antiferritin in experimental hepatoma, *Am. J. Clin. Oncol.*, **6**, 9–18.

Saha, G. B., and Boyd, C. M. (1983). Tissue distribution of [^{67}Ga]citrate and ^{111}InCl$_3$ in mouse with adenocarcinoma, *Int. J. Nucl. Med. Biol.*, **10**, 223–5.

Sayle, B. A., Balachandran, S., and Rogers, C. A. (1983). Indium-111 chloride imaging in patients with suspected abscesses, *J. Nucl. Med.*, **24**, 1114–18.

Scheffel, U., Wagner, H. N. Jr, Klein, J. L., and Tsan, M.-F. (1985). Gallium-67 uptake by hepatoma: Studies in cell cultures, perfused livers, and intact rats, *J. Nucl. Med.*, **26**, 1438–44.

Sephton, R. G., and Harris, A. W. (1975). Gallium-67 citrate uptake by cultured tumor cells stimulated by serum transferrin, *J. Natl Cancer Inst.*, **54**, 1263–6.

Sephton, R. G., and Harris, A. W. (1981). Studies on the uptake of ^{67}Ga and ^{59}Fe and the binding of transferrin by cultured mouse tumour cells, *Int. J. Nucl. Med. Biol.*, **8**, 333–9.

Serafini, A. N., Dunning, W., Charyulu, K., and Weinstein, M. B. (1971). Concentration of ^{111}In-chloride and ^{67}Ga-chloride in the irradiated rat lymphosarcoma, *J. Nucl. Med.*, **12**, 464.

Shindelman, J. E., Ortmeyer, A. E., and Sussman, H. H. (1981). Demonstration of the transferrin receptor in human breast cancer tissue. Potential marker for identifying dividing cells, *Int. J. Cancer*, **27**, 329–34.

Sutherland, R., Delia, D., Schneider, C., Newman, R., Kemshead, J., and Greaves, M. (1981). Ubiquitous cell surface glycoprotein on tumor cells is proliferation associated receptor for transferrin, *Proc. Natl Acad. Sci. USA*, **78**, 4515–19.

Tannenbaum, H., Rosenthall, L., Greenspoon, M., and Ramelson, H. (1984). Quantitative joint imaging using ^{67}gallium citrate in a rabbit model of zymosan induced arthritis, *J. Rheum.*, **11**, 687–91.

Thompson, C., Jones, S., Whitehead, R., and McKenzie, I. (1983). A human breast tissue-associated antigen detected by a monoclonal antibody, *J. Natl Cancer Inst.*, **70**, 409–19.

Trowbridge, I., and Domingo, D. (1981). Anti-transferrin receptor monoclonal antibody and toxin–antibody conjugates affect growth of human tumour cells, *Nature*, **294**, 171–3.

Tsan, M.-F. (1985). Mechanism of gallium-67 accumulation in inflammatory lesions, *J. Nucl. Med.*, **26**, 88–92.

Tsan, M.-F., and Scheffel, U. (1986). Mechanism of gallium-67 accumulation in tumors, *J. Nucl. Med.*, **27**, 1215–19.

Vallabhajosula, S. R., Harwig, J. F., Siemsen, J. K., and Wolf, W. (1980). Radiogallium localization in tumors: Blood binding and transport and the role of transferrin, *J. Nucl. Med.*, **21**, 650–6.

Van Dyke, D., Anger, H. O., and Pollycove, M. (1964). The effect of erythropoietic stimulation on marrow distribution in man, rabbit and rat as shown by ^{59}Fe and ^{52}Fe, *Blood*, **24**, 356–71.

Wagner, M. S., Huemer, R. P., Spolter, L., and Bickert, C. (1971). Radioindium localization in mouse tumors, *J. Nucl. Med.*, **12**, 470.

Weiner, R. E., Schreiber, G. J., and Hoffer, P. B. (1983). In vitro transfer of Ga-67 from transferrin to ferritin, *J. Nucl. Med.*, **24**, 608–14.

Zalutsky, M. R. (1988). Antibody-mediated radiotherapy: Future prospects. In M. R. Zalutsky (ed.) *Antibodies in Radiodiagnosis and Therapy*, pp. 213–36. CRC Press, Boca Raton.

Zalutsky, M. R., de Sousa, M., Venkatesan, P., Shortkroff, S., Zuckerman, J., and Sledge, C. (1987). Evaluation of indium-111 chloride as a radiopharmaceutical for joint imaging in a rabbit model of arthritis, *Invest. Radiol.*, **22**, 733–40.

Iron in Immunity, Cancer and Inflammation
Edited by M. de Sousa and J. H. Brock
© 1989 John Wiley & Sons Ltd

16
Potential Clinical Uses of Anti-transferrin Receptor Monoclonal Antibodies

Ian S. Trowbridge

Department of Cancer Biology, The Salk Institute, Post Office Box 85800, San Diego, California 92138, USA

INTRODUCTION

Since 1980, there have been major advances in our understanding of iron uptake by mammalian cells and its relationship to cell growth (Trowbridge and Shackelford, 1985). As described elsewhere in this volume (see Chapter 3), vertebrates have evolved an iron-transport system consisting of the iron-binding protein transferrin and a specific cell surface receptor that binds transferrin and facilitates its uptake into the cell. The human transferrin receptor has been extensively characterized biochemically and its primary structure deduced from the nucleotide sequence of cDNA clones. It has been established that iron bound to transferrin is transported into the cell via receptor-mediated endocytosis, and the major features of this process have been determined. Further, it is now known that transferrin receptors are expressed on essentially all cultured cells and that their expression is co-ordinately regulated with cell growth. Studies to establish the structure–function relationship of the transferrin receptor and to determine the molecular basis of the regulation of its expression have begun (Jing and Trowbridge, 1987; Rothenberger, Iacopetta and Kuhn, 1987; Miskimins *et al.*, 1986; Owen and Kuhn, 1987; see also Chapter 4). Monoclonal antibodies against the human transferrin receptor were identified in 1981 and have proved to be invaluable in the study of various aspects of the basic biology of the transferrin receptor. At that time, there was considerable interest in the use of monoclonal antibodies against tumor cell surface antigens as therapeutic agents in the treatment of malignant disease. It seemed to us that monoclonal antibodies against the transferrin receptor might have practical applications in cancer immunotherapy from two different perspectives: first, because the transferrin receptor was a well-characterized cell surface molecule involved in receptor-mediated endocytosis and abundantly expressed on tumor cell lines, it offered several advantages as a model to study the targeting of antibody–toxin conjugates to tumor cells; and second, as a cell surface receptor found on proliferating cells, it offered an opportunity to explore a novel approach to immunotherapy based on the ability for monoclonal antibodies to directly interfere with the function of a receptor essential to cell growth. In this chapter I review the studies that have been performed to investigate both of these approaches to the use of anti-transferrin receptor monoclonal antibodies as anti-tumor agents.

MONOCLONAL ANTIBODIES THAT BLOCK TRANSFERRIN RECEPTOR FUNCTION

Monoclonal antibodies against the transferrin receptor were initially identified during a search for antibodies specific for human hematopoietic differentiation antigens. The monoclonal antibody B3/25, defining a major cell surface glycoprotein associated with cell proliferation (Omary, Trowbridge and Minowada, 1980), and the monoclonal antibody OKT9, which originally was thought to define an early thymocyte differentiation antigen (Reinherz et al., 1980), were both independently shown to be directed against the human transferrin receptor by virtue of their ability to co-precipitate labeled transferrin as a receptor–ligand complex (Trowbridge and Omary, 1981; Sutherland et al., 1981). Binding of these antibodies to the transferrin receptor did not interfere with receptor function. It was, therefore, of considerable interest to determine whether it was possible to obtain antibodies that blocked receptor function and, if so, what the effects of such antibodies would be on cell growth. To derive additional monoclonal antibodies against the human transferrin receptor, mice were immunized with purified receptor glycoprotein isolated from deoxycholate-solubilized membranes of the leukemic cell line CCRF-CEM, by affinity chromatography on a column of B3/25 monoclonal antibody covalently coupled to Sepharose. Anti-receptor antibodies produced by hybridomas derived from the spleen cells of the immunized mice were identified by immunoprecipitation studies and then tested for their ability to block transferrin binding to the human leukemic cells. This approach led to the identification of one monoclonal antibody, 42/6, which inhibited transferrin binding (Figure 16.1). Moreover, this monoclonal antibody was shown to specifically inhibit the growth of CCRF-CEM cells and provided

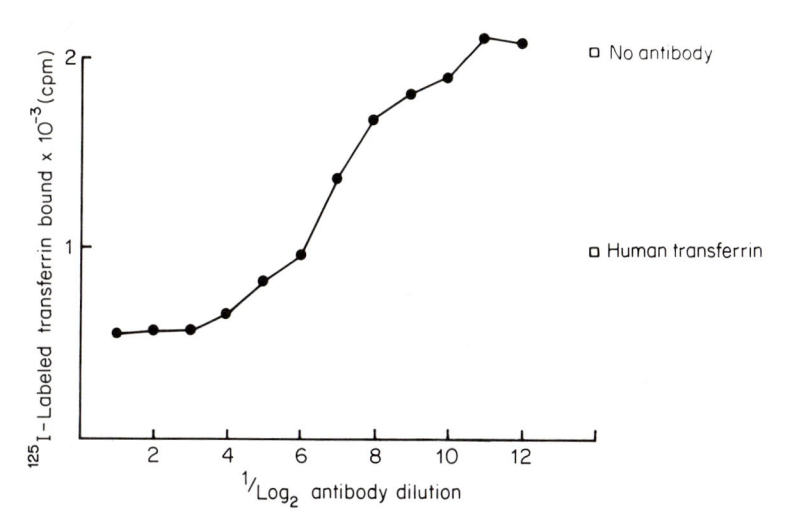

Potential Clinical Uses of Monoclonal Antibodies 343

Figure 16.1 Blocking of transferrin binding by 42/6 monoclonal antibody. CCRF-CEM cells were incubated with various dilutions of an antibody-containing culture supernatant, washed, and then reincubated with ^{125}I-labeled human transferrin (solid circles). Tissue culture medium was used as a negative control, and non-radioactive transferrin was used as a positive control for blocking (□, controls). Data from Trowbridge and Omary (1981)

the first direct evidence that the transferrin receptor performed a function essential for cell proliferation (Trowbridge and Lopez, 1982). In subsequent studies, two monoclonal antibodies that inhibit the function of the murine transferrin receptor have also been identified by directly testing anti-receptor antibodies for their ability to inhibit the growth of murine lymphoma cell lines (Trowbridge, Lesley and Schulte, 1982; Lesley and Schulte, 1985). Another monoclonal antibody that blocks the function of the human transferrin receptor was obtained by screening antibodies against a human B cell lymphoma for the ability to inhibit cell growth (Vaickus and Levy, 1985).

The biological effects of the antibodies against the human and murine transferrin receptors that block function are similar in most respects. The results of a typical experiment are shown in Figure 16.2. Transferrin-mediated iron uptake and cell growth are inhibited at antibody concentrations of 10–20 μg ml^{-1}. Inhibition of iron uptake occurs rapidly and is detectable within 1–2 hours. Inhibition of cell growth occurs within 1–2 days. Initially, the inhibition of cell growth by the antibodies is reversible, but substantial cell death occurs in cultures of the most sensitive murine cell lines within a day. Although the initial effects of anti-transferrin receptor monoclonal antibodies on cell growth are cytostatic rather than

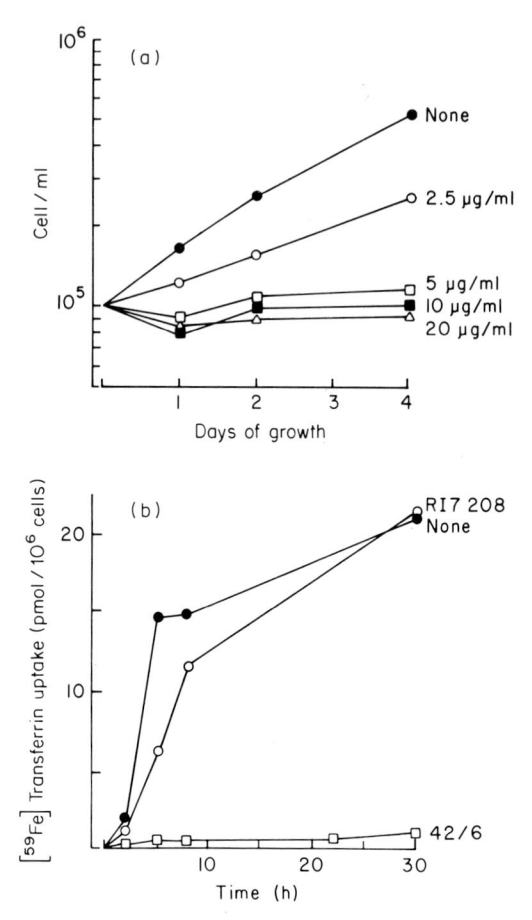

Figure 16.2 Effects of 42/6 monoclonal antibody on iron uptake and growth of CCRF-CEM cells. (a) shows the inhibition of growth of CCRF-CEM cells by purified 42/6 monoclonal antibody. Experimental details are given in Trowbridge and Lopez (1982). (b) shows the specific inhibition by 42/6 monoclonal antibody of transferrin-mediated iron uptake by CCRF-CEM cells. Experimental details of the assay are described in Trowbridge, Lesley and Schulte (1982)

cytotoxic, clonal assays show that prolonged exposure to the antibodies kills virtually all cells. The treatment of murine lymphoma cells with either of the two anti-receptor antibodies that inhibit iron uptake reduces their cloning efficiency by a factor of more than 1×10^4 (Lesley and Schulte, 1985). It has been shown that treatment of the human T leukemic cell line CCRF-CEM with 42/6 monoclonal antibody causes the cells to accumulate in S-phase of the cell cycle (Trowbridge and Omary, 1981). It is noteworthy that iron chelators which inhibit cell growth by iron deprivation also lead to the accumulation of cells in S-phase (Gurley and Jett, 1981; Lederman et al., 1984; Cavanaugh et al., 1985; Bergeron et al., 19886). This suggests that, at least for some cells, the major effect of iron deprivation involves a metabolic process associated with DNA synthesis. One candidate for this is the enzyme ribonucleotide reductase, which plays a key regulatory role in DNA synthesis and requires iron for the formation of an organic free radical required for the catalytic reduction of ribonucleotides (Reichard, 1978). However, some cell types do not accumulate in S-phase after treatment with either anti-transferrin receptor antibodies or iron chelators, suggesting that the metabolic consequences of iron deprivation are complex and may be cell-specific (Trowbridge, Lesley and Schulte, 1982; Fernandez-Pol, Bono and Johnson, 1977; see Chapter 12).

The effects of monoclonal antibodies against the mouse and human transferrin receptors on the growth of a variety of normal and malignant cells in tissue culture have been evaluated. Several general conclusions can be reached; as might be expected from the fact that transferrin is an essential factor for the growth of most cultured cells (Barnes and Sato, 1980), both normal and malignant cells are susceptible to the growth-inhibitory effects of the antibodies. For example, the growth of normal human peripheral blood T lymphocytes is inhibited by monoclonal antibody 42/6 to the same degree as leukemic cell lines derived from T cells (Mendelsohn, Trowbridge and Castagnola, 1983). However, there is a wide variation in the sensitivity of different cell types to the anti-transferrin receptor monoclonal antibodies grown in tissue culture. Whereas anti-receptor antibodies completely inhibit *in vitro* growth of normal lymphocytes, hematopoietic progenitor cells, and many leukemic and lymphoma cell lines (Mendelsohn, Trowbridge and Castagnola, 1983; Taetle, Honeysett and Trowbridge, 1983; Lesley and Schulte, 1984; Rammensee et al., 1985), the antibodies have little or no effect on the growth of a variety of carcinoma, melanoma and fibroblast cell lines (Taetle and Honeysett, 1987; Trowbridge et al., 1988). The reason for the large differences in the sensitivity of individual cell types to the growth-inhibitory effects of anti-transferrin receptor antibodies is unclear. However, it cannot be explained by differences in the number of transferrin receptors expressed on sensitive and resistant cell lines. One variable may be how different cells respond to iron deprivation. Intracellular iron metabolism is still poorly understood, and how iron is made accessible to essential iron-requiring enzymes such as ribonucleotide reductase is obscure. It has generally been thought that ferritin serves as an intracellular iron store that can be mobilized for use within the cell. However, an alternative suggestion has recently been made that ferritin serves as a detoxification mechanism to sequester excess iron, and that once associated with ferritin, iron is not available for use within the cell (Mattia et al., 1986). If so, it is possible that the utilizable intracellular iron pool could be small and turn over rapidly. Differences in the size and kinetics of turnover of this mobilizable iron pool in specific cell types could then account for their variable sensitivity to monoclonal antibodies that block iron uptake.

If anti-receptor antibodies inhibit the growth of cells by depriving them of iron, then it might be expected that soluble iron complexes such as Fe^{3+}-nitrilotriacetic acid or Fe^{3+}-fructose might prevent the effects of the antibodies on cell growth. In the case of some cells, this is true. Inhibition of the growth of the human myeloid leukemic cell line KG-1 by the anti-transferrin receptor antibody 42/6 is completely prevented by 20 μM Fe^{3+}-nitrilotriacetic acid (Taetle, Honeysett and Trowbridge, 1983). However, the capacity of iron chelates to reverse growth inhibition by anti-receptor antibodies depends upon cell type. Antibody inhibition of the growth of peripheral blood lymphocytes is only partially reversed by Fe^{3+}-nitrilotriacetic acid and the growth of CCRF-CEM cells is completely inhibited by 42/6 monoclonal antibody even in the presence of soluble iron (Mendelsohn, Trowbridge and Castagnola, 1983; Trowbridge and Lopez, 1982). This variability may reflect differences in the capacity of different cells to utilize the iron complexes. Alternatively, in the instances where cell growth cannot be restored by iron chelates, anti-receptor antibodies may not only block iron uptake but may also inhibit other processes required for cell growth. It could be envisaged, for example, that anti-transferrin receptor antibodies may indirectly interfere with receptor-mediated uptake of other nutrients or growth factors by sterically blocking access to coated pits.

MECHANISM BY WHICH MONOCLONAL ANTIBODIES INHIBIT TRANSFERRIN-MEDIATED IRON UPTAKE

It is now known that transferrin-mediated iron uptake involves a series of discrete steps, including binding of transferrin to its receptor, endocytosis of the receptor–ligand complex, dissociation of iron from transferrin in an acidic endosomal compartment, and recycling of apotransferrin and its receptor back to the cell surface, whereupon apotransferrin is then released (see Chapters 3 and 12). It is evident, therefore, that monoclonal antibodies against the transferrin receptor could act at a number of different points during receptor-mediated endocytosis to inhibit iron uptake. The ability of monoclonal antibodies against the transferrin receptor to block iron uptake is correlated with their antibody class (Trowbridge and Shackelford, 1985). Both monoclonal antibodies against the mouse transferrin receptor, R17 208 and REM 17, that block function are IgMs (Lesley and Schulte, 1985). One of the monoclonal antibodies against the human receptor that blocks receptor function, 42/6, is an IgA, whereas the other is also an IgM (Trowbridge and Lopez, 1982; Vaickus and Levy, 1985). In contrast, IgG antibodies against the mouse or human transferrin receptors that have been studied generally have little or no effect on cell growth (Lesley and Schulte, 1985; Mendelsohn, Trowbridge and Castagnola, 1985; Trowbridge, unpublished results). This suggests that the polymeric nature of the IgM and IgA antibodies is an important prerequisite for their biological activity. Direct evidence consistent with this mechanism was obtained in experiments in which cells were incubated with rat IgG monoclonal antibodies against the mouse transferrin receptor in the presence of various concentrations of anti-rat immunoglobulin antibody (Lesley and Schulte, 1985). It was found that cross-linking of the IgG monoclonal antibodies by the second layer of anti-immunoglobulin antibody mimicked the effects of the polymeric antibodies and inhibited cell growth. Further, it was shown that neither of the IgM antibodies against the murine transferrin receptor block transferrin binding to the receptor, but instead they inhibit internalization of receptors (Lesley and Schulte, 1985). Thus, these antibodies appear to block iron uptake by extensive cross-linking of transferrin receptors. In similar studies, Taetle *et al.* (1986) have shown that 42/6 monoclonal antibody also inhibits the internalization of transferrin by transferrin receptors on human cells. Thus, it is possible that, although this antibody was originally selected for its ability to block transferrin binding, this may not be the major mechanism by which it blocks iron uptake and inhibits cell growth.

Although IgG monoclonal antibodies have little effect on the rate of internalization of the transferrin receptor, it has been shown that they induce increased degradation of receptors and a reduction in the steady-state expression of receptors on the cell surface (Lesley and Schulte, 1985; Weissman *et al.*, 1986). Because of the rapid recycling of transferrin receptors relative to their half-life, only a small change in recycling efficiency can lead to a large increase in the rate of receptor turnover. Thus, it has been calculated that a reduction in recycling efficiency of receptors from 99.1% to 98.2% would reduce the half-life on receptors in K562 cells from 16 to 8 hours, assuming that receptors which are not recycled are degraded (Weissman *et al.*, 1986). The downregulation of receptors induced by the anti-receptor IgG antibodies may be sufficient to account for the inhibitory effects of some IgG antibodies on the growth of primary hematopoietic cells that have been reported (Shannon *et al.*, 1986; Kemp *et al.*, 1987).

IMMUNOTHERAPY WITH MONOCLONAL ANTIBODIES THAT BLOCK TRANSFERRIN RECEPTOR FUNCTION

The availability of anti-murine transferrin receptor monoclonal antibodies that block iron uptake has provided the opportunity to investigate the effectiveness of such antibodies as anti-tumor agents and at the same time assess their toxicity in a murine syngeneic tumor model system (Sauvage *et al.*, 1987). The model that was chosen to investigate the therapeutic potential of anti-transferrin receptor monoclonal antibodies was the AKR transplantable leukemia, SL-2. This tumor system had been extensively used previously by Bernstein and coworkers to study the parameters which influence the effectiveness of serotherapy with anti-Thy-1 monoclonal antibodies (Bernstein, Tam and Nowinski, 1980; Badger and Bernstein, 1983; Denkero *et al.*, 1985). Preliminary studies established that the SL-2 cells were sensitive to the effects of anti-receptor monoclonal antibodies *in vitro*. As shown in Figure 16.3, both R17 208 and REM 17.2 monoclonal antibodies completely inhibited the growth of cultured SL-2 cells at a concentration of 10–20 μg ml^{-1}. Thus, the sensitivity of SL-2 cells to each of the antibodies was similar to that previously observed for a

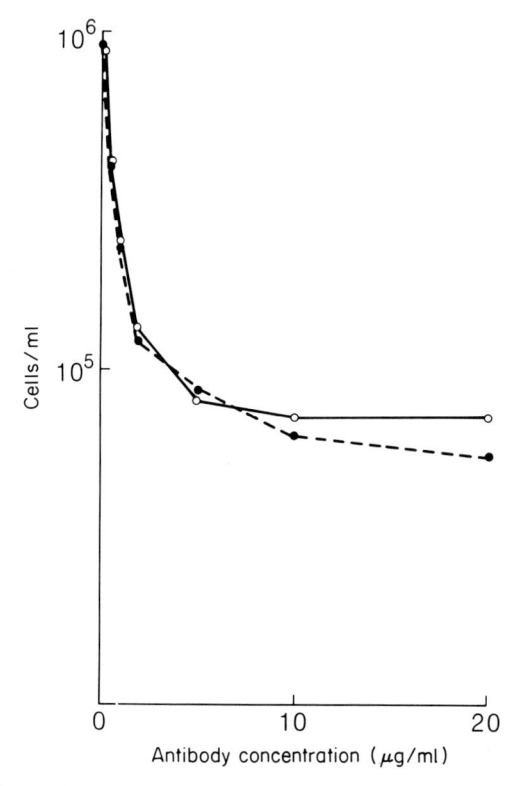

Figure 16.3 Effects of anti-murine transferrin receptor monoclonal antibodies on the growth of mouse SL-2 leukemic cells *in vitro*. Cells were cultured at an initial cell density of 5 × 10^4 ml^{-1} in the presence of various concentrations of R17 208 (●) and REM 17.2 (○) monoclonal antibodies. The cells were harvested 3 days later and counted. Reproduced from Sauvage *et al.* (1987)

variety of other murine hematopoietic cell lines. To determine the effects of R17 208 and REM 17.2 monoclonal antibodies on the growth of SL-2 leukemic cells *in vivo*, groups of mice were inoculated with various doses of leukemic cells at a subcutaneous site on the back and then immediately given graded amounts of monoclonal antibody administered as a single intraperitoneal injection. As shown in Figure 16.4, administration of R17 208 monoclonal antibody prolonged survival of the mice in a dose-dependent manner. The anti-tumor activity of R17 208 monoclonal antibody was also manifested by a delay in the appearance of palpable primary tumors at the site of inoculation. However, not all tumor cells were eliminated, even at the highest dose of monoclonal antibody, and the single-dose treatment did not result in long-term survivors, even among the group challenged with the smallest inoculum of leukemic cells.

Fluorescence-activated cell surface analysis showed that the leukemic cells from the monoclonal antibody-treated mice that survived antibody treatment still bound antibody, and when they were cultured *in vitro* their growth was inhibited by R17 208 monoclonal antibody. These data indicate that the eventual development of tumors in the antibody-treated mice was not the result of the selective growth of antibody-resistant mutant cells but instead reflects the failure of a single dose of monoclonal antibody to kill all the potentially sensitive leukemic cells. Although REM 17.2 monoclonal antibody was as effective as R17 208 in inhibiting the growth of SL-2 leukemic cells *in vitro*, its effect on the survival of tumor-bearing mice was much less marked. The reason for this difference in the *in vivo* anti-tumor activity of the two monoclonal antibodies is unclear, as their tissue localization and *in vivo* pharmacokinetics were similar (Sauvage et al., 1987).

On the basis of the *in vitro* studies indicating that the growth inhibitory effects of anti-receptor antibodies are initially reversible, it seemed probable that maintaining therapeutic serum levels of antibody for several days would be important in producing a maximum kill of tumor cells. Serum clearance studies of monoclonal antibodies metabolically labeled with [^{75}Se]methionine showed that a single dose of 2 mg of antibody was sufficient to maintain antibody serum levels of greater than 5 μg ml^{-1} for 2–3 days. Based upon these results, two different schedules of antibody administration were used: either 3 mg of antibody at 3–4 day intervals or 1 mg of antibody daily. As shown in Figure 16.5, these multiple dose schedules were much more effective than a single injection of antibody. Administration of anti-transferrin receptor antibody over several weeks using either schedule resulted in the long-term survival of the majority of mice challenged with leukemic cells, with no evidence of tumor (Sauvage et al., 1987).

One of the reasons for selecting the SL-2 leukemia model for immunotherapy studies was the previously demonstrated anti-tumor activity of

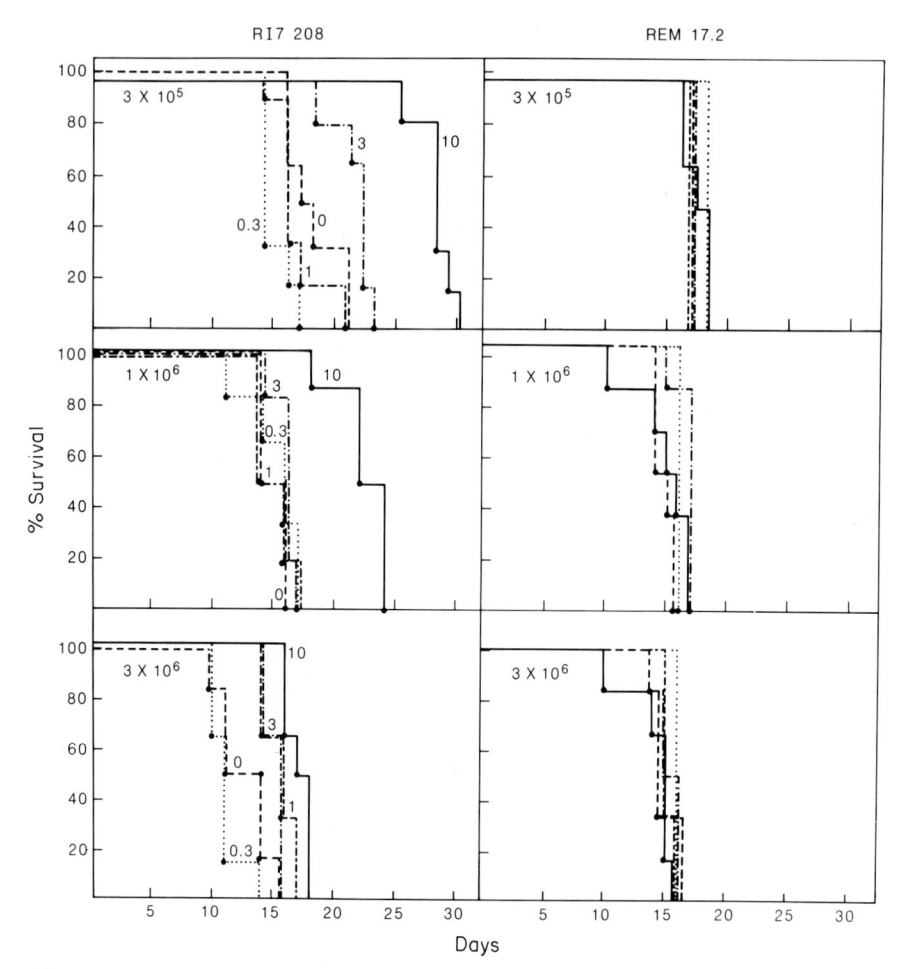

Figure 16.4 Determination of the anti-tumor effects of single doses of anti-murine transferrin receptor monoclonal antibodies. Groups of five to six AKR/J mice were challenged subcutaneously with either 3×10^5 (top panels), 1×10^6 (middle panels) or 3×10^6 (lower panels) SL-2 leukemic cells. Within 1–2 hours, groups of mice were treated with a single i.p. dose of either R17 208 or REM 17.2 monoclonal antibodies in the milligram amounts indicated. Shown are the survival times of individual mice. Reproduced from Sauvage et al. (1987)

anti-Thy-1 antibodies in this system. This provided a standard with which to compare the effectiveness of therapy using anti-transferrin receptor monoclonal antibodies that block receptor function and conventional serotherapy. It was also possible to ask the question whether a combination of an anti-transferrin receptor antibody that blocks growth directly and an antibody which produces anti-tumor effects by activation of the host

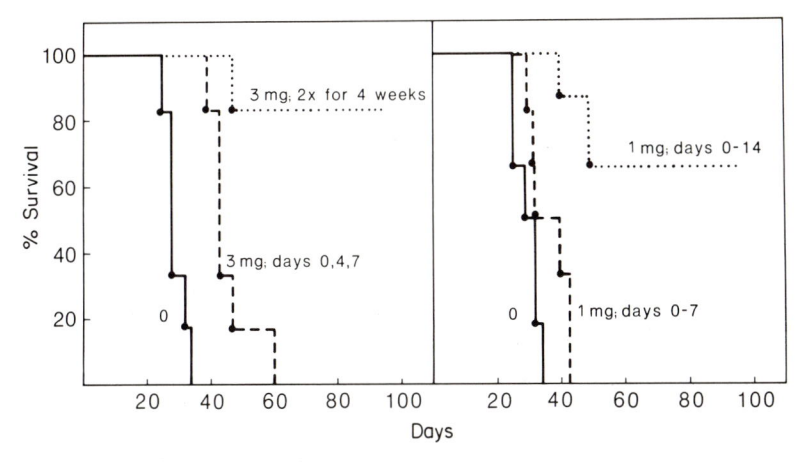

Figure 16.5 Effect of multiple doses of R17 208 monoclonal antibodies on AKR/J mice challenged with SL-2 leukemic cells. Groups of six mice were challenged with 1×10^6 SL-2 leukemic cells and then multiple doses of R17 208 monoclonal antibody were given i.p. on the schedules indicated. Reproduced from Sauvage et al. (1987)

immunological effector mechanisms would result in greater therapeutic effects. As shown in Figure 16.6, the anti-tumor activity of R17 208 anti-transferrin receptor antibody was similar to that of the anti-Thy-1 monoclonal antibody 19E12. The most striking result, however, was that combination therapy with both antibodies resulted in significantly greater anti-tumor effects than either antibody alone. This raises the possibility that anti-transferrin receptor antibodies that block function may generally complement other monoclonal antibodies that mediate their anti-tumor activity by activation of immunological effector mechanisms.

Although multiple-dose therapy with R17 208 monoclonal antibody or combination therapy with anti-Thy-1 and anti-receptor antibodies together led to long-term survival of the majority of mice inoculated with SL-2 leukemic cells if treatment was initiated immediately, neither protocol was as effective against the established tumors. If therapy was delayed for 7 days, treatment prolonged the life of tumor-bearing mice but did not lead to long-term survival. This indicates that, as with conventional serotherapy, tumor load is an important factor limiting the effectiveness of treatment. For this reason, the treatment of mice bearing established tumors with either cyclophosphamide or cytosine arabinoside in combination with anti-transferrin receptor monoclonal antibody is presently being investigated to determine whether the antibody can eliminate residual tumor cells following conventional chemotherapy.

As transferrin receptors are expressed on some cells of normal tissues (Gatter et al., 1983), an important question concerning the *in vivo* adminis-

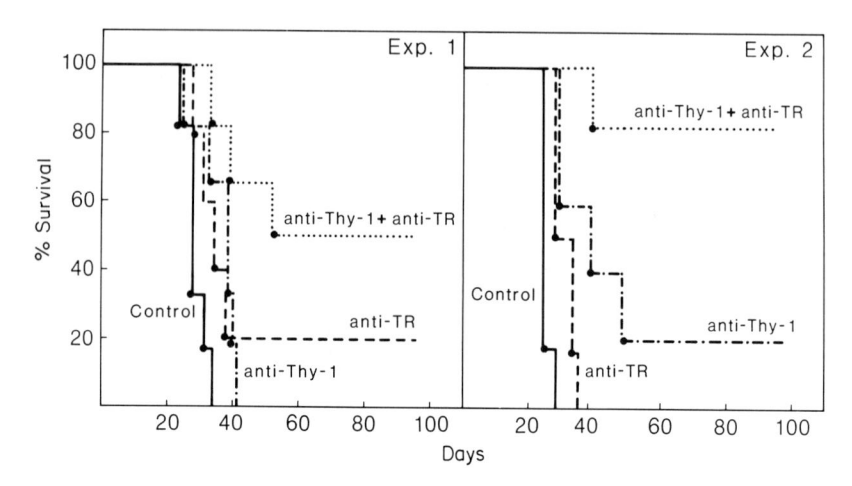

Figure 16.6 Combination therapy with anti-Thy-1 and anti-transferrin receptor (anti-TR) monoclonal antibodies. Groups of 5–6 mice were challenged with 1×10^6 SL-2 leukemic cells and then given 3 mg of RI7 208 or 19E12 monoclonal antibodies on day 0, 4 and 7 in the combinations indicated. Survival of the mice was followed for 90 days. Reproduced from Sauvage et al. (1987)

tration of anti-receptor monoclonal antibodies is that of toxicity. Analysis of the biodistribution of R17 208 monoclonal antibody showed that the major sites of localization one day after administration were the liver, kidney and spleen (Sauvage et al., 1987). However, histological examination of these and other tissues showed no evidence of cellular damage after administration of anti-receptor antibody according to the same multiple-dose schedules used in immunotherapy. Further, no decreases in circulating erythrocytes or leukocytes were detected in the antibody-treated mice. However, in mice given 1 mg of R17 208 monoclonal antibody daily for 7 days, there was clear evidence of splenomegaly. Assay of myeloid (CFU-c) and erythroid (CFU-e) progenitor cells in the bone marrow and spleens of these mice revealed significant changes in both populations. The cellularity of the bone marrow in antibody-treated mice was not significantly different from that of the controls but there was a two-fold decrease in the number of CFU-e per 10^6 cells (Figure 16.7). Concomitantly, an almost three-fold increase in CFU-e per 10^6 spleen cells was also observed. Further, there was an approximately four-fold increase in the number of cells in the spleens of the antibody-treated mice. Similar but less dramatic changes were observed in the CFU-c in bone marrow and spleen. Thus, although there is no evidence of acute toxicity, administration of the anti-transferrin receptor antibody R17 208 depresses erythropoiesis and myelopoiesis in the bone marrow. The increases in CFU-e and

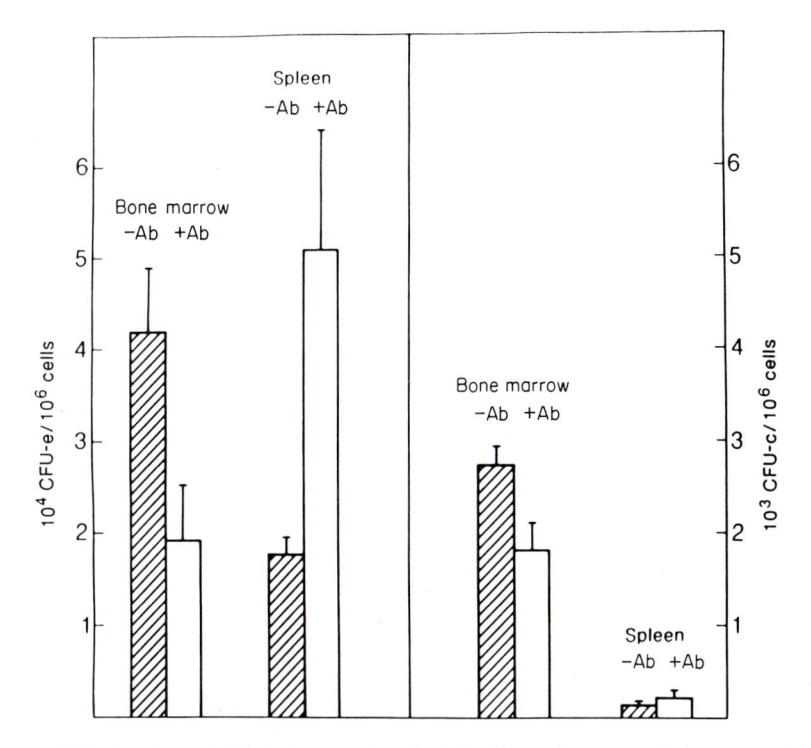

Figure 16.7 Effect of R17 208 monoclonal antibody on hematopoietic stem cells in the bone marrow and spleens of treated mice. Groups of four AKR/J mice were either untreated or treated with 1 mg of R17 208 monoclonal antibody i.p. daily for 7 days. CFU-c and CFU-e in the bone marrow and spleens of individual mice were then assayed. Reproduced from Sauvage et al. (1987)

CFU-c in the spleen, which in the mouse is a secondary site of hematopoiesis, is presumably another reflection of the stress antibody administration imposes on the hematopoietic system. These effects on the hematopoietic system are consistent with the *in vitro* studies documenting the expression of transferrin receptors on most CFU-e and a significant fraction of CFU-c (Sieff et al., 1982; Lesley et al., 1984a).

ANTI-TRANSFERRIN RECEPTOR IMMUNOTOXINS

As discussed earlier, monoclonal antibodies against the transferrin receptor have been used to prepare antibody–toxin conjugates or immunotoxins. Immunotoxins consist of antibodies covalently bound to a plant or bacterial toxin. Most toxins consist of two components, usually single polypeptides, which mediate different functions: an A chain which has enzymatic properties and inactivates its intracellular target to produce toxic effects, and a B chain which binds to the cell surface and facilitates the entry of the A chain into the cell. Immunotoxins have been constructed by covalently coupling monoclonal antibodies to the toxic A chains of plant or bacterial toxins. Thus, the specificity of this type of immunotoxin is determined exclusively by the antibody, whereas the cytotoxic activity is provided by the toxin A chain. For general reviews of the structure and mechanism of action of toxins, the reader is referred to Olsnes and Pihl (1976) and Olsnes and Sandvig (1985), and for reviews on immunotoxins to Vitetta *et al.* (1983) and Pastan, Willingham and Fitzgerald (1986). Potential advantages of such immunotoxins are their high specificity and potency. Because the toxin A chains kill cells by catalytic inactivation of protein synthesis or some other essential function, delivery of only a few molecules of immunotoxin to the site of action within the cell is sufficient to kill the cell. The cytotoxic activity of the immunotoxin requires binding of the antibody–toxin conjugate to the cell surface, followed by internalization and finally translocation of a biologically active A chain across a cell membrane. These processes are normally facilitated by the B chain in the native toxin, and it was found that ricin A chain conjugated to monoclonal antibodies directed against a variety of cell surface antigens was much less toxic than the intact ricin toxin (Trowbridge and Domingo, 1982). It seemed possible that this was because immunotoxins against most cell surface target antigens were only poorly internalized. If so, we hypothesized that antibodies against the transferrin receptor would make effective immunotoxins, since the normal role of the receptor was to transport its ligand into the cell via receptor-mediated endocytosis. Further, because of the abundant expression of transferrin receptors on some tumor cells, it was possible that such immunotoxins may have sufficient selectivity as an antitumor agent to be of practical clinical importance in certain circumstances.

In our initial studies, immunotoxins were prepared by covalently coupling the ricin A toxic subunit to the monoclonal antibody B3/25 using the bifunctional cross-linking reagent N-succinimidyl-3-(2-pyridyldithio)-propionate (Trowbridge and Domingo, 1981). This immunotoxin was extremely potent and in *in vitro* studies specifically killed human cells with an IC_{50} of 10^{-10} M (Figure 16.8). Clonal assays showed that the frequency with which cells escape killing by the immunotoxin was less than 2×10^{-5}. However, although the anti-transferrin receptor immunotoxin had activity against a human melanoma cell line, M2I, grown as a subcutaneous tumor in nude mice, the immunotoxin was not more effective than unconjugated antibody. One obstacle to *in vivo* use of currently available immunotoxins is their rapid clearance from the circulation (Bourrie *et al.*, 1986).

From a clinical viewpoint, an important question was the effect that an immunotoxin directed against the transferrin receptor might have on bone

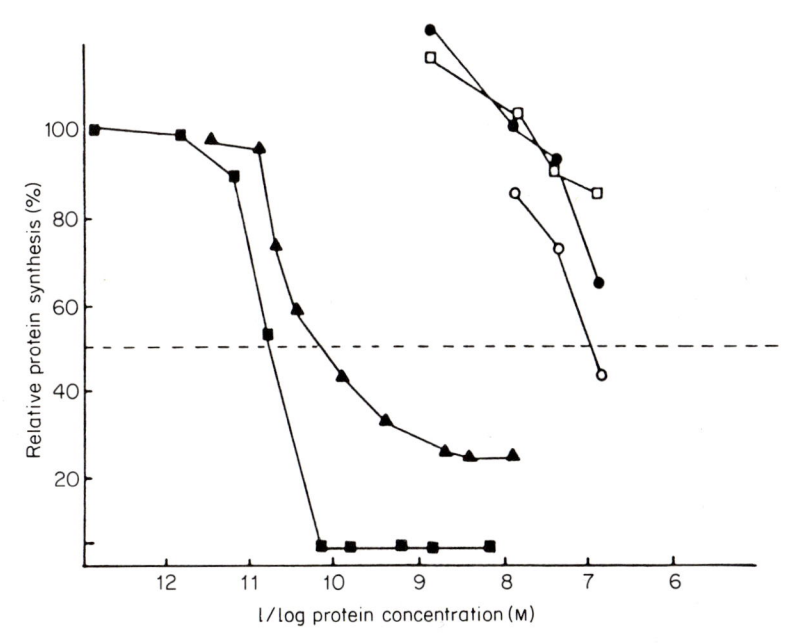

Figure 16.8 Inhibition of protein synthesis in the human leukemic cell line CCRF-CEM by an anti-transferrin receptor–ricin A conjugate. Ricin A was covalently coupled to the B3/25 anti-human transferrin receptor monoclonal antibody using the bifunctional reagent N-succinimidyl-3-(2-pyridyldithio)-propionate. Cells were cultured for 20 hours with various concentrations of ricin toxin (■), anti-transferrin receptor–ricin A conjugate (▲), ricin A subunit (●), anti-transferrin receptor antibody (□), anti-transferrin receptor antibody plus ricin A subunit (○). Protein synthesis in cultures was then assayed by measuring incorporation of [^{3}H]leucine into protein. Further experimental details can be found in Trowbridge and Domingo (1981), from which these data are reproduced

marrow hematopoietic progenitor cells. It was shown that even brief exposure of murine bone marrow cells to the immunotoxin constructed with the anti-murine transferrin receptor monoclonal antibody R17 217 and ricin A chain resulted in the killing of virtually all late CFU-e and a fraction of CFU-c. However, the pluripotent stem cells (CFU-s) capable of repopulating the hematopoietic system of lethally irradiated animals were not killed by exposure to the immunotoxin *in vitro* (Lesley *et al.*, 1984b). These results correlate well with the proportion of each progenitor cell population in cycle in normal bone marrow and their expression of transferrin receptors determined by fluorescence-activated cell sorting.

Several other groups have prepared immunotoxins consisting of antibodies against the transferrin receptor covalently coupled to various toxins to explore their potential clinical value. FitzGerald *et al.* (1983) prepared an immunotoxin in which B3/25 monoclonal antibody against the human transferrin receptor was covalently coupled to *Pseudomonas* exotoxin and showed that this conjugate gave specific and potent killing *in vitro*. Furthermore, it was shown by electronmicroscopy and immunofluorescence studies that the conjugates entered the cells from coated pits into endocytotic vesicles, recapitulating the early stages of the normal pathway of transferrin-mediated iron uptake. In these studies it was shown that adenovirus enhanced toxicity of the immunotoxin and it was postulated that this was the result of virus-mediated disruption of the endocytotic vesicles allowing more toxin molecules to be delivered to the cytoplasm. This type of immunotoxin also proved to be extremely effective at killing human ovarian carcinoma cell lines *in vitro* (Pirker et al., 1985). Death from ovarian cancer usually occurs at a time when the cancer cells are mainly confined to the peritoneal cavity and surrounding tissues. Thus, therapeutic agents can be effective against ovarian cancer when delivered directly to the peritoneal cavity. Because of their potential toxicity if given systemically, the delivery of anti-transferrin receptor immunotoxins locally is an attractive idea and thus ovarian tumors may represent a practical clinical target for such immunotoxins. FitzGerald et al. (1987) have studied the anti-tumor activity of an immunotoxin composed of an antibody to the human transferrin receptor (454A12) and ricin A chain in a nude mouse model of human ovarian cancer. It was shown that the immunotoxin inhibited the growth of the ovarian tumor cells (NIH:OVCAR-3) growing in the peritoneal cavity of a nude mouse in a dose-dependent manner. Significant prolongation of life of the tumor-bearing mice was obtained at doses of $10\,\mu g$ or greater of immunotoxin given 4, 7 and 10 days after inoculation of 6×10^7 cells into the peritoneal cavity. Similar studies were performed using *Pseudomonas* exotoxin coupled to a different monoclonal antibody against the human transferrin receptor (FitzGerald, Willingham and Pastan, 1986). This immunotoxin was even more potent and doses of $1-2\,\mu g$ given on days 5–8 after inoculation of tumor cells produced marked increases in the survival of the treated mice. Although these results are encouraging, this model does not directly address the question of the potential toxicity of anti-transferrin receptor immunotoxins, as the immunotoxins used are specific for the human transferrin receptor and do not react with normal mouse tissues. Information on this point could be obtained by a study in mice of the toxicity of immunoconjugates constructed with monoclonal antibodies against the murine transferrin receptor.

CONCLUDING REMARKS

In the past seven years, the transferrin receptor has been characterized and its primary structure determined. The major features of the role the receptor plays in mediating cellular iron uptake via receptor-mediated endocytosis have been defined and its importance in relationship to cell growth has been shown. It has also been clearly established that monoclonal antibodies against the transferrin receptor can block iron uptake and inhibit cell growth. Thus, the transferrin receptor is one of only a few molecules accessible on the cell surface that offer the potential as a target for antibodies or other agents to directly modulate cell growth. Because of its role as a transport molecule, the receptor is also of considerable interest from the perspective of specific drug targeting. As the structure–function relationship of the transferrin receptor is elucidated, this should provide further opportunities to explore the practical applications of anti-receptor monoclonal antibodies in cancer therapy and other areas.

REFERENCES

Badger, C. C., and Bernstein, I. D. (1983). Therapy of murine leukemia with a monoclonal antibody against a normal differentiation antigen, *J. Exp. Med.*, **157**, 828–41.

Barnes, D., and Sato, G. (1980). Serum-free cell culture: A unifying approach, *Cell*, **22**, 649–55.

Bergeron, R. J., Braylan, R., Goldey, S., and Ingeno, M. (1986) Effects of the *Vibrio cholerae* siderophore vibriobactin on the growth characteristics of L1210 cells, *Biochem. Biophys. Res. Commun.*, **136**, 273–80.

Bernstein, I. D., Tam, M. R., and Nowinski, R. C. (1980). Mouse leukemia: therapy with monoclonal antibodies against a thymus differentiation antigen, *Science*, **207**, 68–73.

Bourrie, B. J. P., Casellas, P., Blythman, H. E., and Jansen, F. K. (1986). Study of the plasma clearance of antibody-ricin-A-chain immunotoxins. Evidence for specific recognition sites on the A chain that mediate rapid clearance of the immunotoxin, *Eur. J. Biochem.*, **155**, 1–10.

Cavanaugh, P. F. Jr, Porter, C. W., Tukalo, C., Frankfurt, O. S., Pavelic, Z. P., and Bergeron, R. J. (1985). Characterization of L1210 cell growth inhibition by bacterial iron chelators parabactin and compound II, *Cancer Res.*, **45**, 4754–9.

Denkero, E. Y., Badger, C. C., Ledbetter, J. A., and Bernstein, I. D. (1985) Influence of antibody isotype on passive serotherapy of lymphoma, *J. Immunol.*, **135**, 2182–6.

Fernandez-Pol, J. A., Bono, V. H., and Johnson, G. S. (1977). Control of growth by picolinic acid: Differential response of normal and transformed cells, *Proc. Natl Acad. Sci. USA*, **74**, 2889–93.

FitzGerald, D., Willingham, M. C., and Pastan, I. (1986). Anti-tumor effects of an immunotoxin made with Pseudomonas exotoxin in a nude mouse model of human ovarian cancer, *Proc. Natl Acad. Sci. USA*, **83**, 6627–30.

FitzGerald, D. J. P., Trowbridge, I. S., Pastan, I., and Willingham, M. C. (1983). Enhancement of toxicity of antitransferrin receptor antibody–Pseudomonas exotoxin conjugates by adenovirus, *Proc. Natl Acad. Sci. USA*, **80**, 4134–8.

FitzGerald, D., Bjorn, M. J., Ferris, R. J., Winkelhake, J. L., Frankel, A. E., Hamilton, T. C., Ozols, R. F., Willingham, M. C., and Pastan, I. (1987). Anti-tumor activity of an immunotoxin in a nude mouse model of human ovarian cancer, *Cancer Res.*, **47**, 1407–10.

Gatter, K. C., Brown, G., Trowbridge, I. S., Woolston, R., and Mason, D. Y. (1983). Transferrin receptors in human tissues: their distribution and possible clinical relevance, *J. Clin. Pathol.*, **36**, 539–45.

Gurley, L. R., and Jett, J. H. (1981). Cell cycle kinetics of Chinese hamster (CHO) cells treated with the iron-chelating agent picolinic acid, *Cell Tissue Kinet.*, **14**, 269–83.

Jing, S., and Trowbridge, I. S. (1987). Identification of the intermolecular disulphide bonds of the human transferrin receptor and its lipid-attachment site, *EMBO J.*, **6**, 327–31.

Kemp, J. D., Thorson, J. A., McAlmont, T. H., Horowitz, M., Cowdery, J. S., and Ballas, Z. K. (1987). Role of the transferrin receptor in lymphocyte growth: a rat IgG monoclonal antibody against the murine transferrin receptor produces highly selective inhibition of T and B cell activation protocols. *J. Immunol.*, **138**, 2422–6.

Lederman, H. M., Cohen, A., Lee, J. W. W., Freedman, M. H., and Gelfand, E. W. (1984). Deferoxamine: a reversible S-phase inhibitor of human lymphocyte proliferation, *Blood*, **64**, 748–53.

Lesley, J. F., and Schulte, R. J. (1984). Selection of cell lines resistant to antitransferrin receptor antibody: Evidence for a mutation in transferrin receptor, *Mol. Cell. Biol.*, **4**, 1675–81.

Lesley, J. F., and Schulte, R. J. (1985). Inhibition of cell growth by monoclonal antitransferrin receptor antibodies, *Mol. Cell. Biol.*, **5**, 1814–21.

Lesley, J., Hyman, R., Schulte, R., and Trotter, J. (1984a). Expression of transferrin receptor on murine hematopoietic progenitors, *Cell. Immunol.*, **83**, 14–25.

Lesley, J., Domingo, D. L., Schulte, R., and Trowbridge, I. S. (1984b). Effect of an anti-murine transferrin receptor-ricin A conjugate on bone marrow stem and progenitor cells treated *in vitro*, *Exp. Cell Res.*, **150**, 400–7.

Mattia, E., Josic, D., Ashwell, G., Klausner, R., and van Renswoude, J. (1986). Regulation of intracellular iron distribution in K562 human erythroleukemic cells, *J. Biol. Chem.*, **261**, 4587–93.

Mendelsohn, J. M., Trowbridge, I. S., and Castagnola, J. (1983). Inhibition of human lymphocyte proliferation by monoclonal antibody to transferrin receptor, *Blood*, **62**, 821–6.

Miskimins, W. K., McClelland, A., Roberts, M. P., and Ruddle, F. H. (1986). Cell proliferation and expression of the transferrin receptor gene: promoter sequence homologies and protein interactions, *J. Cell Biol.*, **103**, 1781–8.

Olsnes, S., and Pihl, A. (1976). Abrin, ricin and their associated agglutinins. In P. Cuatrecasas (ed.) *The Specificity and Action of Animal, Bacterial and Plant Toxins (Receptors and Recognition)*, Series B, Vol. 1, pp. 131–71, Chapman and Hall, London.

Olsnes, S., and Sandvig, K. (1985). Entry of polypeptide toxins into animal cells. In I. Pastan and M. C. Willingham (eds) *Endocytosis*, pp. 195–234, Plenum Publishing Corp., New York.

Omary, M. B., Trowbridge, I. S., and Minowada, J. (1980). Human cell-surface glycoprotein with unusual properties, *Nature*, **286**, 888–91.

Owen, D., and Kuhn, L. C. (1987). Noncoding 3' sequences of the transferrin receptor gene are required for mRNA regulation by iron, *EMBO J.*, **6**, 1287–93.

Pastan, I., Willingham, M. C., and Fitzgerald, D. J. P. (1986). Immunotoxins, *Cell*, **47**, 641–8.

Pirker, R., Fitzgerald, D. J. P., Hamilton, T. C., Ozols, R. F., Willingham, M. C., and Pastan, I. (1985). Anti-transferrin-receptor antibody linked to pseudomonas exotoxin as a model immunotoxin in human ovarian carcinoma cell lines, *Cancer Res.*, **45**, 751–7.

Rammensee, H. G., Lesley, J., Trowbridge, I. S., and Bevan, M. J. (1985). Antibodies against the transferrin receptor block the induction of cytotoxic T lymphocytes. A new method for antigen-specific negative selection *in vitro*, *Eur. J. Immunol.*, **15**, 687–92.

Reichard, P. (1978). From deoxynucleotides to DNA synthesis, *Fed. Proc.*, **37**, 9–14.

Reinherz, E. L., Kung, P. C., Goldstein, G., Levey, R. H., and Schlossman, S. F. (1980). Discrete stages of human intrathymic differentiation: analysis of normal thymocytes and leukemic lymphoblasts of T-cell lineage, *Proc. Natl Acad. Sci. USA*, **77**, 1588–92.

Rothenberger, S., Iacopetta, B. J., and Kuhn, L. C. (1987). Endocytosis of the transferrin receptor requires the cytoplasmic domain but not its phosphorylation site, *Cell*, **49**, 423–31.

Sauvage, C. A., Mendelsohn, J. C., Lesley, J. F., and Trowbridge, I. S. (1987). Effects of monoclonal antibodies that block transferrin receptor function on the *in vivo* growth of a syngeneic murine leukemia, *Cancer Res.*, **47**, 747–53.

Shannon, K. M., Larrick, J. W., Fulcher, S. A., Burck, K. B., Pacely, J., Davis, J. C., and Ring, D. B. (1986). Selective inhibition of the growth of human erythroid bursts by monoclonal antibodies against transferrin or the transferrin receptor, *Blood*, **67**, 1631–8.

Sieff, C., Bicknell, D., Caine, G., Robinson, J., Lam, G., and Greaves, M. F. (1982). Changes in cell surface antigen expression during erythropoietic differentiation, *Blood*, **60**, 703–13.

Sutherland, R., Delia, D., Schneider, C., Newman, R., Kemshead, J., and Greaves, M. (1981). Ubiquitous cell surface glycoprotein on tumor cells is proliferation associated receptor for transferrin, *Proc. Natl Acad. Sci. USA*, **78**, 4515–19.

Taetle, R., and Honeysett, J. M. (1987). Effects of monoclonal anti-transferrin receptor antibodies on the *in vitro* growth of human solid tumor cells, *Cancer Res.*, **47**, 2040–4.

Taetle, R., Castagnola, J., and Mendelsohn, J. (1986). Mechanisms of growth inhibition by anti-transferrin receptor monoclonal antibodies, *Cancer Res.*, **46**, 1759–63.

Taetle, R., Honeysett, J. M., and Trowbridge, I. (1983). Effects of anti-transferrin receptor antibodies on growth of normal and malignant myeloid cells, *Int. J. Cancer*, **32**, 343–9.

Trowbridge, I. S., and Domingo, D. (1981). Anti-transferrin receptor monoclonal antibody and toxin–antibody conjugates affect growth of human tumor cells, *Nature*, **294**, 171–3.

Trowbridge, I. S., and Domingo, D. L. (1982). Prospects for the clinical use of cytotoxic monoclonal antibody conjugates in the treatment of cancer, *Cancer Surveys*, **1**, 543–56.

Trowbridge, I. S., Lesley, J., and Schulte, R. (1982). Murine cell surface transferrin receptor: Studies with an anti-receptor monoclonal antibody, *J. Cell. Physiol.*, **112**, 403–10.

Trowbridge, I. S., and Lopez, F. (1982). Monoclonal antibody to transferrin receptor blocks transferrin binding and inhibits human tumor cell growth *in vitro*, *Proc. Natl Acad. Sci. USA*, **79**, 1175–9.

Trowbridge, I. S., and Omary, M. B. (1981). Human cell surface glycoprotein related to cell proliferation is the receptor for transferrin, *Proc. Natl Acad. Sci. USA*, **78**, 3039–43.

Trowbridge, I. S., and Shackelford, D. A. (1985). Structure and function of transferrin receptors and their relationship to cell growth, *Biochem. Soc. Symp.*, **51**, 117–29.

Trowbridge, I. S., Lesley, J. F., Domingo, D., Schulte, R., Sauvage, C., and Rammensee, H.-G. (1988). Monoclonal antibodies to transferrin receptor and assay of their biological effects, *Methods Enzymol.*, **147**, 265–79.

Vaickus, L., and Levy, R. (1985). Antiproliferative monoclonal antibodies: detection and initial characterization, *J. Immunol.*, **135**, 1987–97.

Vitetta, E. S., Krolick, K. A., Miyama-Inaba, M., Cushley, W., and Uhr, J. W. (1983). Immunotoxins: a new approach to cancer therapy, *Science*, **219**, 644–50.

Weissman, A. M., Klausner, R. D., Rao, K., and Harford, J. B. (1986). Exposure of K562 cells to anti-receptor monoclonal antibody OKT9 results in rapid redistribution and enhanced degradation of the transferrin receptor, *J. Cell. Biol.*, **102**, 951–8.

Iron in Immunity, Cancer and Inflammation
Edited by M. de Sousa and J. H. Brock
© 1989 John Wiley & Sons Ltd

17

Clinical Use of Iron Chelation

Martin J. Pippard
*Department of Haematology, Ninewells Hospital and Medical School, Dundee
DD1 9SY, Scotland*

INTRODUCTION

Previous chapters have discussed the role of iron in essential physiological processes, as well as its potential involvement in a variety of diseases associated with cellular and tissue damage. This chapter will be concerned with attempts to divert iron from existing metabolic pathways by using iron-chelating agents, with the hope of modifying the course of disorders in which iron is thought to play either a primary or secondary role.

Iron overload in man is an obvious target for iron-chelation therapy, particularly when it complicates dyserythropoietic anaemias such as the thalassaemia disorders, where there is excessive iron absorption from the diet or the need for regular blood transfusions (Weatherall and Clegg, 1981). Here the disordered marrow function prevents the removal of iron by the regular phlebotomy which is used so effectively to reduce morbidity and mortality in the inherited iron-loading disorder idiopathic haemochromatosis (Bomford and Williams, 1976). More speculative is the potential use of iron-chelating agents in modifying tissue damage resulting from a wide range of different insults (including inflammation, ischaemia and certain drugs). Here the possible involvement of iron through its ability to catalyse the formation of highly toxic, oxygen-derived free radicals (Halliwell and Gutteridge, 1984) has led to the investigation of this novel approach to therapy (Editorial, 1985). The requirement for ribonucleotide reductase in proliferating cells (Hoffbrand *et al.*, 1976) has stimulated further studies of iron-chelating agents as inhibitors of the growth of malignant cells or of the replication of infecting organisms. Most work in these areas has been with experimental models, though there have been limited studies in the clinic. In many cases the interpretation of the data is difficult because of the extreme complexity of the pathophysiological processes involved in tissue injury or the multitude of potential sites of action of the iron-chelating agents. As yet, only in disorders associated with iron overload has a clinical role for iron chelation been unequivocally established.

In addition to agents designed specifically as iron-chelating compounds, the effects of a number of drugs already in clinical use may, at least in part, be dependent upon chelation of iron. These include the therapeutic effects of some cytotoxic agents used in cancer chemotherapy as well as unwanted reactions to a variety of agents.

Before considering these aspects further, the nature of iron chelation and the factors which may influence this *in vivo*, as well as the agents which are available for experimental and clinical use, will be reviewed.

IRON CHELATION

An iron chelator is an organic molecule containing two or more functional ligand groups which are capable of forming co-ordinate bonds with iron to form a heterocyclic iron-containing ring (a chelate). The shared electrons of the co-ordinate bonds are usually donated by atoms of nitrogen, oxygen or sulphur in the ligand groups. Fe^{2+} is readily oxidized to virtually insoluble Fe^{3+} under physiological conditions, and many naturally occurring iron-chelating molecules have evolved with the function of maintaining iron in solution as it is transported within the body and made available for essential metabolic processes. These molecules include the plasma transport protein, transferrin (Williams, 1985), and many low molecular weight chelators (ATP, amino acids, sugars, ascorbate, etc.) have been suggested as potential intracellular iron-binding agents (Jacobs, 1977).

Micro-organisms have also evolved specific iron-chelating compounds, usually catechols or hydroxamates, with which they obtain essential iron from their surrounding medium (Neilands, 1972). These microbial siderophores have been a fertile area for the investigation of iron-chelating agents of potential pharmacological use. Indeed, the only chelator in widespread clinical use at present, desferrioxamine (DF), is a hydroxamate siderophore produced by *Streptomyces pilosus* (Keberle, 1964). Unfortunately this agent has to be given by injection since the ligand is not stable to gastric acid, and the drug is also expensive to produce. Other agents of potential use are summarized in Table 17.1. Of particular interest are a number of synthetic agents which, unlike DF, have been shown in various animal models to have substantial iron-chelating activity when given by mouth. However, there have been long delays between the identification of promising ligands and the undertaking of the extensive toxicity studies necessary before clinical trials (Hershko, 1988). This relates in part to the perception

TABLE 17.1 Iron-chelating agents

Groups and examples	Comments	References
Hydroxamates (fungal origin)		
Desferrioxamine (DF)	See text	See text
Rhodotorulic acid	Pain on injection. No oral effect.	Grady et al. (1979)
Catechols (bacterial origin)		
2,3-Dihydroxybenzoic acid (DHB)	Active ligand of enterobactin. Oral activity in rats, but not in thalassaemia.	Graziano, Grady and Cerami (1974) Peterson et al (1976)
Desferrithiocin (Streptomycetes origin)		
	Unique structure. High oral activity. Neurotoxic in rats?	Peter (1983)
Polycarboxylic amines (synthetic origin)		
Ethylene diamine tetra-acetic acid (EDTA)	Low selectivity for Fe^{3+}.	Waxman and Brown (1969)
Diethylene triamine pentaacetic acid (DTPA)	Inactive by mouth. Confined to extracellular space. Zinc depletion in chronic use.	Fahey et al. (1961) Herskho (1975) Pippard et al. (1987)
N,N'-Ethylene bis-(2-hydroxyphenyl-glycine) (EHPG)	EHPG and HBED have added phenolic groups. EHPG active in man	Martell et al. (1987) Cleton, Turnbull and Finch (1963)
N,N'-bis-(2-hydroxy-benzoyl)-ethylene-diamine N,N'-diacetic acid (HBED)	Dimethyl esters are orally active pro-drugs. Extremely powerful iron chelators in rodents. Some phenolic chelators toxic, but ? HBED non-toxic in rodents.	Pitt et al. (1986) Hershko, Grady and Link (1984) Kim, Huebers and Finch (1987) Rosenkrantz, Metterville and Fleischman (1986)
Aroyl hydrazones (synthetic origin)		
Pyridoxal isonicotinoyl hydrazone (PIH)	Active by mouth in animals, but ? in man.	Cikrt et al. (1980) Hoy et al. (1979)
Pyridoxal benzoyl hydrazone (PBH)	? liable to hydrolysis in gut.	Hershko et al. (1981) Williams et al. (1982) Johnson et al. (1982)
Hydroxypyridones (synthetic origin)		
3-Hydroxypyrid-4-ones (e.g. 1,2-dimethyl-3-hydroxypyrid-4-one)	Combines hydroxamate and catechol features. Oral activity in man. Oral and parenteral activity comparable.	Porter et al. (1986) Kontoghiorghes et al. (1987) Gyparaki et al. (1987)

This is a highly selective list of compounds and references. Further information may be obtained from the following reviews and comprehensive reports of screening for iron-chelating activity: Waxman and Brown (1969), Pitt et al. (1979), Grady and Jacobs (1981), Martell et al. (1987), Hershko and Weatherall (1988).

TABLE 17.2 Factors influencing iron chelation

Chemistry of chelator
Affinity of chelator for iron relative to other metals (under physiological conditions of pH and metal concentrations).
Competition with other ligands *in vivo*.
Size, charge and lipophilicity (governing ability to cross cell membranes).

Pharmacology of chelator
Stability (e.g. to acid or enzymes in the gut or after uptake by tissues).
Rate and route of clearance from the plasma and the body.
Pattern of distribution in the body, determining site(s) of action:
    gut lumen
    plasma and extracellular fluids
    intracellular—which tissue?
        —which iron?
Metabolism *in vivo* to active or inactive compounds (e.g. some metabolites of DF retain chelating properties).

Properties of chelate
Retention or exit from cells after intracellular chelation of iron (e.g. highly charged molecules of enterobactin iron chelates may be trapped in the cell).
Pattern of excretion in bile, urine or other body fluids.
Resorption by gut or kidney tubules?
Possible transport to other tissues and/or utilization for metabolic processes.
Reactivity of the complex—possible toxicity resulting from redox reactions.

---

that the use of iron-chelating agents, and thus the potential market, may be restricted to the relatively uncommon disorders of iron overload. It gives added impetus to the need to understand any potential role for iron chelation in the much more common disorders of inflammation and infection to be discussed in this chapter. Despite the difficulties, in short-term studies in iron-loaded patients with thalassaemia, one of the hydroxypyridones (1,2-dimethyl-3-hydroxypyrid-4-one) has already been shown to chelate iron effectively when given by mouth (Kontoghiorghes *et al.*, 1987), and oral pyridoxal nicotinoyl hydrazone (PIH) is also under investigation in man (Hershko, 1988).

The factors which may influence iron chelation *in vivo* are summarized in Table 17.2. They range from the basic chemistry of the chelator to how it is handled *in vivo* (particularly to which compartments of body iron it has access) and the metabolism and reactivity of any resulting iron chelate. These aspects are best worked out for DF, though even with this agent, in clinical use for over 20 years, understanding is incomplete. Experience with DF in treating iron overload provides a background for considering the more experimental uses for iron chelators (Table 17.3).

TABLE 17.3 Clinical situations or experimental models in which iron chelators have been used in an attempt to modify iron-dependent pathological processes

Tissue damage (probable free radical involvement)	
Iron overload	Iron-loading anaemias[a]
	Acute iron poisoning[a]
Post-ischaemic reperfusion injury	Myocardial ischaemia
	Intestinal ischaemia
	Cerebral ischaemia
	Organ transplants
Inflammatory/immune-mediated disease	Rheumatoid arthritis[a]
	Pulmonary vasculitis
	Immune-complex induced vasculitis
	Allergic encephalomyelitis
	Pancreatic islet cell rejection
	Graft versus host disease[a]
Chemical toxicity—Lung	e.g. Bleomycin, paraquat
—Liver	e.g. Aspirin
Effects on haem synthesis	
Increased activity of uroporphyrinogen decarboxylase	Porphyria cutanea tarda[a]
Improved erythropoiesis with reduction in red cell protoporphyrin	Anaemia of renal failure[a]
Inhibition of cell division	
Inhibition of lymphocyte proliferation	Immune modulation in inflammatory diseases
Cancer chemotherapy	Leukaemia[a]
	Other tumours
Infection	Inhibition of malaria and *Trypanosoma* growth

[a]Studies carried out using desferrioxamine in man.

IRON OVERLOAD

Although DF given by mouth is not absorbed, it chelates inorganic food iron in the gut lumen (Balcerzak, Jenson and Pollak, 1966), and would thus be an expensive and inefficient way to reduce the rate of iron loading in patients with excessive food iron absorption, e.g. patients with thalassaemia intermedia syndromes (Pippard and Weatherall, 1987). Development of a less expensive, perhaps non-absorbable, iron chelator might be valuable in this context. Chelation of iron within the gut lumen is also the basis for instilling DF into the stomach to prevent further iron absorption in acute iron poisoning, the first clinical indication for the use of DF (Ciba Pharmaceutical Company, 1969).

The progressive accumulation of iron from regular blood transfusions in the major thalassaemia syndromes leads to cardiac, endocrine and liver damage, with death usually by the end of the second decade of life from heart failure or arrhythmias (Modell, 1979). Initial attempts to mobilize excess storage iron using intramuscular injections of DF were disappointing because urine iron excretion was minimal until a very substantial excess of tissue iron had accumulated (Modell and Beck, 1974). Nevertheless, even this apparently inadequate therapy prevented the progression of liver fibrosis (Barry et al., 1974) in thalassaemic children, and stabilized liver iron concentrations, albeit at very high levels. This suggests that the benefits of DF therapy may result from the removal of a particularly toxic fraction of total body iron, or that interference with an iron-dependent process such as fibroblast proliferation (Hunt et al., 1979) may be important.

Prolonged infusions of DF were known to be more effective in promoting iron excretion than single bolus doses (Model and Beck, 1974) and, stimulated by the encouraging results of Barry et al. (1974), Propper, Shurin and Nathan (1976) undertook a reappraisal of this approach. As a result, overnight subcutaneous infusions of around 50 mg kg^{-1} DF became the norm for treatment of iron-loading anaemias, offering the hope of preventing the development of iron overload even from a very early age (Pippard et al., 1978). Despite the greater iron-chelating efficiency, the rapid improvement in liver function seen in thalassaemic patients after starting subcutaneous DF therapy preceded any marked fall in total liver iron (Hoffbrand et al., 1979). This again suggested that continual removal of a particularly toxic, chelatable fraction of iron might be especially important in preventing tissue damage from iron overload. Over the subsequent ten years the ability of regular subcutaneous infusions of DF to prevent liver iron loading (Cohen, Martin and Schwartz, 1984), and to reduce (Wolfe et al., 1985) and perhaps treat (Marcus et al., 1984) cardiac complications, has become clearer. However, the arduous nature of the treatment means that non-compliance is a major problem, and the expense of the DF has limited its availability. In addition, though DF has proved generally remarkably non-toxic over prolonged periods of heavy use, a number of adverse effects of continued high doses have gradually emerged—these will be considered later in this chapter.

In pharmacological studies with DF in man, the drug was rapidly cleared from the plasma (Summers et al., 1979). Animal studies have suggested that this is due to a combination of urinary excretion, avid uptake by hepatocytes, and enzymatic destruction within the plasma, the last of these being less important in man (Peters *et al.*, 1966; Meyer-Brunot and Keberle, 1967). The short half-life of the drug in the blood (5–10 minutes) probably accounts for the greater iron removal seen with DF infusions. It should be noted for comparison with later experimental studies that the peak concentrations of DF in plasma after bolus intravenous injection of 10 mg kg^{-1} in man were around 100 μmol l^{-1}, and that even with high doses given as an intravenous infusion (100 mg kg^{-1} over 24 hours) the maximum plasma concentration that was reached was only around 20 μmol l^{-1}.

It became clear that biliary excretion of the iron chelate, ferrioxamine, was a substantial fraction of the total (Harker, Funk and Finch, 1968; Cumming *et al.*, 1969). This could exceed 50% with infusions of large doses of DF (Pippard, Callender and Finch, 1982), and became the predominant route of excretion when iron stores had been reduced to near normal (Pippard and Weatherall, 1987). Since ferrioxamine is not reabsorbed to any significant extent from the gut, and unlike DF is not taken up from the plasma by liver cells, measurement of faecal iron excretion gives an estimate of chelation of iron by DF specifically within hepatocytes. Here the iron available for chelation is thought to be iron in transit between the main iron-containing proteins, particularly iron released by the degradation of ferritin within lysosomes (Pippard, Johnson and Finch, 1981; Laub *et al.*, 1985; Pippard, Tikerpae and Peters, 1986). The source of urinary iron excretion is less clear, but probably includes chelation of any non-transferrin-bound iron in the plasma (Hershko and Peto, 1987). This is a fraction of iron which is increased in iron-loaded patients with fully saturated plasma transferrin (Hershko *et al.*, 1978), and which is likely to be particularly toxic by reason of its ready availability to take part in the generation of oxygen-derived free radicals (see below). Iron which is capable of exchanging with plasma transferrin at cell membranes as part of the normal cycle of internal iron exchange is also thought to be an important source of iron chelated by DF: both hepatocytes (Pippard, Callender and Finch, 1982; Pippard, Johnson and Finch, 1982) and macrophages (Hershko, 1978; Hershko and Rachmilewitz, 1979) may contribute to the urinary iron in this way. Direct chelation by DF of iron from transferrin (Hallberg and Hedenberg, 1965), or from intracellular ferritin (Pippard, Johnson and Finch, 1982), is probably insignificant *in vivo*, though it occurs slowly *in vitro* (Crichton, Roman and Roland, 1980), and may be more important for some of the newer iron-chelating agents (Kontoghiorghes, 1986). Iron locked up in the porphyrin ring of haem is not thought to be available for chelation (Keberle, 1964).

In occasional patients with adverse reactions to DF, subcutaneous infusions of the synthetic agent, diethylene triamine pentaacetic acid (DTPA) have been used to prevent further accumulation of iron (B. Wonke, personal communication). Unlike DF, this drug is confined to the extracellular compartment and produces no faecal iron excretion (Hershko,

1975; Pippard et al., 1986). A major drawback is its relative non-selectivity for iron, and oral zinc supplements are required since symptomatic zinc depletion can occur with prolonged use, perhaps accounting for the life-threatening toxicity seen in one early study (Fairbanks, Warson and Beutler, 1963). There is no information on whether this agent may prevent iron-related tissue damage.

These studies illustrate the varying penetration of chelators to different body sites, with DF having a preferential clearance to hepatocytes. They show how interaction with particular fractions of total body iron may be important in moderating iron toxicity. They also demonstrate how the precise method of drug administration may greatly influence its effect as an iron-chelating agent. These pharmacological considerations should be borne in mind when assessing the effects, or lack of effects, of DF and other newer chelating agents (whose behaviour *in vivo* may be less well understood) in disorders other than iron overload.

TISSUE DAMAGE AND IRON CHELATION

Increased lipid peroxidation is an important effect of both acute and chronic iron toxicity. The resulting damage to cell membranes and increased lysosomal fragility (Seymour and Peters, 1978) is likely to account for much of the cell and tissue damage in iron overload, though degradation of DNA or hyaluronic acid may also be important. The pathogenesis of these lesions is thought to involve iron in catalysing the production of highly toxic hydroxyl radicals (OH·) from superoxide (O_2^-) and peroxide via the Haber–Weiss reaction:

$$Fe^{3+} + O_2^- \rightarrow Fe^{2+} + O_2 \tag{17.1}$$

$$Fe^{2+} + H_2O_2 \rightarrow Fe^{3+} + OH\cdot + OH^- \tag{17.2}$$

In this classical formulation, catalytic Fe^{2+} for the second (Fenton) reaction is made available by the reduction of Fe^{3+} by superoxide. Other cellular reducing substances (e.g. ascorbate and glutathione) also recycle Fe^{3+}, as do a number of extremely reactive organic radicals, including paraquat and the adriamycin semiquinone (Vile, Winterbourn and Sutton, 1987). The ability of ascorbate both to mobilize iron from ferritin and to increase the availability of Fe^{2+} (Sirivech, Frieden and Osaki, 1974) has given rise to concern about its clinical use to enhance urinary iron excretion in response to DF in patients with iron overload (Wapnick et al., 1969), particularly in relation to possible exacerbation of cardiac toxicity (Nienhuis, 1981): as a result, doses of supplemental ascorbate have been kept to a minimum and there has been little evidence of clinical toxicity.

Superoxide is produced *in vivo* (e.g. as part of the respiratory burst of phagocytic cells) and is normally removed (at the expense of forming hydrogen peroxide) by superoxide dismutase (Halliwell and Gutteridge, 1986). The precise source of the iron which is available to take part in the Haber–Weiss reaction is unknown, but it seems likely that metabolically active transit iron, such as that chelated by DF within hepatocytes, plays a major role. Such chelatable labile iron is increased in iron overload, but 'decompartmentalization' of protein-bound iron associated with other causes of tissue injury—e.g. as the result of liberation of lysosomal hydrolases—might be expected to promote further oxidative tissue damage. Haemosiderin iron is relatively inert in this respect (O'Connell *et al.*, 1986), but ferritin iron can be mobilized by superoxide (Biemond *et al.*, 1986a; Bolann and Ulvik, 1987). Furthermore, though iron in transferrin, lactoferrin, and haemoglobin is normally too tightly bound to catalyse the Haber–Weiss reaction, oxidative protein damage could release the iron (Aruoma and Halliwell, 1987; Puppo and Halliwell, 1988), thus setting up a vicious cycle of cellular damage. It is these considerations that have prompted investigation of iron chelation as a possible means of interrupting propagation of free radical damage in a variety of forms of tissue injury.

It should be noted that while hydrogen peroxide is poorly reactive, it is able to cross biological membranes, while the hydroxyl radical is so highly reactive that its formation and any damage produced will be limited to the location of the iron catalyst (Halliwell and Gutteridge, 1986); a corollary of this 'site specificity' is that the effects of an iron chelator will be highly dependent on the precise tissue and cellular compartments to which the drug has access. Furthermore, once access is gained to the correct site, the effects of the drug could include direct scavenging of the superoxide or hydroxyl radicals as well as interference with iron-catalysed free radical formation. DF has such a dual action (Hoe, Rowley and Halliwell, 1982) and, indeed, in concentrations much greater than those normally achieved in the plasma *in vivo* (> 1 mM), it can itself be oxidized to a nitroxide free radical (Morehouse, Flitter and Mason, 1987). It is important that any iron chelate formed should be inert in terms of the propagation of free radical formation—this appears to be true for ferrioxamine (Gutteridge, Richmond and Halliwell, 1979), but iron chelates of drugs such as EDTA and the pyridoxal hydrazones, which have a high affinity for Fe^{2+} as well as Fe^{3+}, may undergo redox cycling and thus make Fe^{2+} available to catalyse hydroxyl radical formation. With the possible exception of potential cytotoxic agents, it would be most undesirable for a chelator to mobilize relatively safe protein-bound iron to a more reactive soluble chelate.

POST-ISCHAEMIC REPERFUSION INJURY

Interruption of the blood supply to vital organs is a major cause of death in Western societies, e.g. from ischaemic heart or cerebrovascular diseases. Although cell disruption due to anoxia will itself eventually lead to irreversible tissue damage, recovery of the flow of oxygen-rich blood may cause further injury, in which membrane lipid peroxidation induced by oxygen-derived free radicals may play an important part (McCord, 1985; see also Chapter 7). The main source of superoxide is thought to be the enzyme xanthine oxidase, which is formed from xanthine dehydrogenase under anoxic conditions, perhaps as a result of an influx of calcium ions into the cells; the latter may activate a number of enzymes, including phospholipases, which give rise to toxic lipid metabolites. Unlike the dehydrogenase, xanthine oxidase transfers electrons to molecular oxygen rather than NAD^+ during the conversion of xanthine to uric acid. As already described, the resulting superoxide may give rise to the hydroxyl radical in the presence of iron, and both superoxide and xanthine oxidase are able to mobilize ferritin iron (Biemond et al., 1986a).

There are thus a number of possible points at which the cycle of reperfusion injury might be interrupted; these include the use of calcium channel-blocking agents, the use of allopurinol to inhibit xanthine oxidase, the use of exogenous scavengers for oxygen metabolites (e.g. N-acetyl cysteine), or the use of iron-chelating agents to block formation of more reactive radicals from superoxide. The last will now be discussed in more detail, but it would be unrealistic to expect a single agent to provide a complete answer to these complex problems.

Myocardial ischaemia

Occlusion of a coronary artery produces myocardial ischaemia and infarction, and cardiac arrest during open-heart surgery a more generalized cardiac ischaemia. In experimental models of these clinical situations, both allopurinol and superoxide dismutase ameliorate the damage, suggesting a role for toxic oxygen metabolites in the injury (McCord, 1985). Furthermore, in isolated perfused hearts, recovery of myocardial function and energy metabolism was much greater if DF was given at the time of post-ischaemic reflow (Ambrosia et al., 1987). This was interpreted as indicating a role for iron in the generation of hydroxyl radical during reperfusion, and for the chelator in interrupting this process. It was not clear whether DF was acting extracellularly or was entering the heart muscle cells under these conditions: in vitro studies suggest that it may be able to enter iron-loaded fetal cardiac cells (Link, Pinson and Hershko, 1985). In other studies, DF, even in high doses, failed to protect the function of isolated hearts from the effect of oxygen radicals produced exogenously by addition of xanthine oxidase to the perfusion medium (Gupta and Singal, 1987). This was in contrast to the protection given by mannitol, a hydroxyl radical scavenger, and suggested that iron chelation may not always be successful in interrupting the production of hydroxyl radical *in vivo*.

Intestinal ischaemia

The intestinal mucosa is highly sensitive to reperfusion ischaemic injury: both superoxide dismutase and allopurinol block the resulting increased membrane permeability, suggesting that the high concentration of xanthine dehydrogenase in mucosal villi is involved via the production of superoxide and hydroxyl radicals. In cats, DF (50 mg kg^{-1}) infused intravenously from 5 minutes before reperfusion of an ischaemic ileal segment could also reduce the permeability change, consistent with a role for iron in catalysing this process (Hernandez, Grisham and Granger, 1987). In addition, gastric mucosal bleeding produced by haemorrhagic shock and retransfusion in rats could be reduced by a 30-minute intravenous infusion of 50 mg kg^{-1} DF, starting 10 minutes before retransfusion (Smith *et al.*, 1987).

Cerebral ischaemia following cardiac arrest

The brain is particularly vulnerable to short periods of anoxia, perhaps by reason of its high lipid content and vulnerability to lipid peroxidation (Babbs, 1985). In dogs subjected to 15 minutes cardiac arrest followed by resuscitation, brain tissue 2 hours later was found to have increased malondialdehyde and low molecular weight iron concentrations (Nayini *et al.*, 1985). Treatment with 50 mg kg^{-1} DF infused intravenously over 15 minutes at the time of reperfusion reduced both these biochemical changes, whereas treatment with a calcium channel-blocking agent (lidoflazine) reduced only the concentrations of low molecular weight iron. It is known that DF is able to penetrate the brain (Keberle, 1964), and it was suggested that the chelation of iron which had been liberated from protein-bound stores in the hypoxic brain prevented lipid peroxidation in the post-resuscitation period. However, these biochemical changes may not be directly related to the extent of brain damage, since other workers, using a similar protocol but including neurological assessment at 48 hours, found no evidence of protection of cerebral function by DF (Fleischer *et al.*, 1987). By contrast, rats subjected to 7 minutes cardiac arrest showed much improved survival if post-resuscitation treatment included ventilation with 7% carbon dioxide, intravenous lidoflazine, and DF 50 mg kg^{-1} intravenously over 15 minutes (Badylak and Babbs, 1986): because of the combined therapy, the effect of iron chelation alone cannot be assessed.

Organ transplantation

Organs removed for transplantation are inevitably subjected to a period of ischaemia followed by reperfusion in the recipient. In rabbit kidneys subjected to warm ischaemia by clamping the renal arteries for up to 2 hours, lipid peroxidation could be prevented by intravenous DF (15–50 mg kg^{-1}) given 15 minutes before reperfusion (Green *et al.*, 1986a). Similarly, lipid peroxidation products were much reduced in kidneys stored at 0°C for 24 hours if they were first treated with a single-passage arterial flush with cold medium containing a high concentration (60 mM) of DF or the hydroxyl radical scavenger, mannitol (Green *et al.*, 1986b). It is not known whether other possible damage (e.g. to proteins or nucleic acids) can be prevented by such therapy, or whether the viability of the organs following transplantation may be improved, though in general, measures of lipid peroxidation do mirror functional and histological changes (Green *et al.*, 1986c). It is thus too soon to make any recommendations for improved perfusion of organs in transit.

It is clear that the use of iron chelation in various types of reperfusion injury remains at the stage of pre-clinical assessment. There is a need for studies which pay particular attention to the relationships between metabolism of oxygen-derived free radicals, lipid peroxidation, and organ function, as well as to the effects of iron chelators.

INFLAMMATORY AND IMMUNE-MEDIATED DISEASES

Extracellular release of superoxide and peroxide from the respiratory burst of infiltrating phagocytic cells, and the subsequent formation of hydroxyl radical in the presence of iron, have been implicated in the pathogenesis of the tissue injury associated with various inflammatory conditions. (It may also be a factor adding to the post-ischaemic perfusion injury discussed in the previous section.) However, there are likely to be additional mechanisms for inflammatory tissue injury, including the local release of lysosomal proteases and cationic proteins from phagocytic cells (Henson and Johnston, 1987). These may sometimes confound any possible benefits of iron chelation.

Rheumatoid arthritis

The accumulation of iron in the synovial membrane of rheumatoid joints, and of reactive bleomycin-detectable iron (Gutteridge, 1987) and ferritin iron (Blake and Bacon, 1981; Biemond et al., 1986b) in synovial fluid, has lent support to the hypothesis that local iron-catalysed production of hydroxyl radicals may exacerbate the inflammatory joint disease (Blake et al., 1981; Winyard et al., 1987; see also Chapter 7). In experimental models, mild nutritional iron deficiency was found to reduce the severity of joint inflammation in rats with adjuvant disease (Andrews et al., 1987a), as did daily intraperitoneal injections of 100 or 200 mg kg^{-1} DF (Andrews et al., 1987b): in these latter experiments the DF did not affect systemic manifestations, suggesting a selective effect on iron-mediated joint inflammation. Other animal studies have suggested a more marked effect of the DF on reducing chronic rather than acute inflammation (Blake et al., 1983).

Unfortunately, limited studies in patients with rheumatoid arthritis have been unable to demonstrate any significant anti-inflammatory effect with DF. In one study, seven patients received 3 g DF as 8–12-hour subcutaneous infusions for 5 days, for a maximum of 3 weeks (Blake et al., 1985). Two patients showed improvement both clinically and in acute-phase reactants. However, the study was discontinued because of the development of coma in two patients (in association with additional prochlorperazine therapy) and of retinal changes in three patients. In another study (Polson et al., 1985), six patients received 2 g DF as subcutaneous infusion over 20 hours initially for 5 days a week, but after 4–12 days the onset of nausea and vomiting forced a reduction in dose to only 2 g once-weekly. In a further uncontrolled study, ten patients receiving 1 g DF intramuscularly each day for 2 weeks showed rather unconvincing improvements in rheumatoid symptoms and in associated anaemia, though no change in erythrocyte sedimentation rate (ESR) (Giordano et al., 1986).

The toxic effects seen in two of these studies will be considered later in this chapter. They meant the abandonment of therapy or reduction of DF dose to amounts that are unlikely to have had more than a very transient effect. It should also be noted that the ability of DF to penetrate into joints is not known. The effect of iron chelation in rheumatoid arthritis should thus be regarded as unproven.

Pulmonary vasculitis

After experimental thermal skin injury (Till et al., 1985), or infusion of cobra venom factor (Ward et al., 1983) in rats, there is systemic activation of complement, followed by sequestration of neutrophils in pulmonary capillaries, vascular endothelial damage, and the development of interstitial oedema, intra-alveolar haemorrhage, and fibrin deposition. In both models, pretreatment with DF (15 mg kg^{-1}), but not ferrioxamine, gave substantial protection against increased lung permeability, and reduced the appearance of products of lipid peroxidation. In similar studies using a rat model for immune complex vasculitis (an intradermal Arthus reaction that is also dependent on complement and neutrophil activation), both apolactoferrin and two intravenous injections of 5 mg DF were able to protect against injury, whereas iron infusion potentiated the damage. Whether these models, and the potential for treatment with iron chelators, have a parallel in human 'adult respiratory distress syndrome' is not known, though there is some evidence that toxic oxygen metabolites from neutrophils may be involved in the alveolar damage seen in this syndrome.

Allergic encephalomyelitis

Experimental allergic encephalomyelitis is a cell-mediated autoimmune demyelinating disease, induced in rats by injection of guinea-pig spinal cord homogenate with Freund's adjuvant. The inflammatory lesions in the white matter of the brain and spinal cord partly resemble the lesions of multiple sclerosis, with a cellular infiltrate of T helper cells and macrophages. Continuous DF infusion at a rate of 70 mg day^{-1} for 7 days, using an implanted subcutaneous osmotic pump, dramatically reduced the severity and duration of the disease (Bowern et al., 1984). This effect was accompanied by a diminished T cell, but not macrophage, responsiveness, and an absence of inflammatory cells in the lesions, suggesting that the drug might be acting as a mild immunosuppressive agent. However, in subsequent studies DF failed to prevent the development of the disease when purified myelin basic protein was used as the induction agent, nor could it block the development of passive disease after transfer of spleen cells from affected animals (Willenborg et al., 1988). This suggested that the action of DF might be relatively trivial, in preventing iron-dependent lipid breakdown in the crude spinal homogenate and thus interfering with antigen presentation. These careful studies reinforce the lesson that it is extremely difficult to be certain about the relative importance of the numerous different processes involved in tissue injury. They by no means rule out a potential therapeutic role for iron chelation in this kind of autoimmune disease.

Allograft surgery

Graft rejection involves an immune-mediated inflammatory response in which iron chelators might act either to alter lymphocyte function (see below) or to interrupt iron-catalysed free radical formation resulting from the respiratory burst of the inflammatory cell infiltrate. These possibilities were examined in studies using mouse pancreatic allografts (Bradley et al., 1986). DF (4 mg day^{-1} delivered for 28 days with an implanted subcutaneous osmotic pump) was started 3–8 days after the transplant, and after 100 days was found to have reduced chronic islet cell rejection, as compared with controls, from 62% to 13%. Since DF was started after the period when sensitization might have been expected to occur, the results suggested an affect of the iron chelation on the immune effector mechanism. Furthermore, although DF ($> 30\ \mu$M) inhibited *in vitro* activation of T lymphocytes, much lower concentrations of DF were achieved *in vivo*, where there was no evidence of any impairment of function of cytotoxic T cells. The results were thus felt to be consistent with DF interrupting the production of toxic hydroxyl radical by the local inflammatory cells, though no direct evidence for this was obtained. It is of great interest that after allogeneic bone marrow transplantation, two children showed prompt resolution of graft-versus-host disease with DF treatment (50 mg kg^{-1} day^{-1} continuously for two 5-day courses) (Weinberg *et al.*, 1986). Although this response was accompanied by a loss of circulating activated (interleukin-2 receptor-positive) T lymphocytes, the results from the mouse allograft model indicate how difficult it may be to be certain whether this is really the main mechanism for any therapeutic effect of the iron chelator. In any event, further experimental studies of this novel approach to management of the devastating problems of organ rejection and graft-versus-host disease seem warranted.

Chemical tissue injury

Paraquat is a widely used bipyridylium herbicide which is highly toxic to living cells in biological systems ranging from microbes to man (Korbashi *et al.*, 1986). In humans accidental or deliberate ingestion results in rapidly progressive lung damage and death from respiratory failure. The toxicity of this compound is believed to result from its ability to undergo redox cycling with production of hydroxyl radicals: paraquat is reduced enzymatically in mammalian tissue, probably by NADPH–cytochrome P450 reductase, and the paraquat radical thus formed reacts with molecular oxygen to produce superoxide, as well as making available Fe^{2+} by reducing Fe^{3+} (Vile, Winterbourn and Sutton, 1987).

In paraquat-treated mice, DF (5 mg intraperitoneally once before, and twice-daily for 2 days after, paraquat injection) increased survival, whereas iron enhanced the effect of paraquat (Kohen and Chevion, 1985). However, in rats given subcutaneous injections of 300 mg DF daily for 10 days, there appeared to be an accentuation of the paraquat-induced lung damage (Osheroff *et al.*, 1985). The authors raised the possibility that this unexpected result could reflect the enormous doses of DF used: they suggested that a direct attack of the paraquat radical on increased amounts of ferrioxamine might enhance the availability of iron to take part in hydroxyl radical formation. However, as in many of the other conditions discussed in this chapter, the ability of the chelator to penetrate to the critical sites of toxicity (in this case the lung) is not known. It is of interest that a continuous intravenous infusion of DF in rats produced a striking reduction in mortality after paraquat administration (Van Asbeck et al., 1986). This suggests that a constant inhibition of hydroxyl radical formation may be necessary for therapeutic effect (Hershko and Weatherall, 1988). Clinical studies of this approach to the therapy of paraquat poisoning now appear justified in view of the appalling outlook with severe poisoning and the absence of any other effective therapy.

Bleomycin is a glycopeptide antibiotic which is used in the treatment of selected human malignancies. Its action depends upon the formation of an Fe^{2+}-bleomycin complex and its ability to bind to DNA, where its oxidation leads to the production of superoxide and hydroxyl radicals and consequent damage both to DNA (Sausville, Peisach and Horwitz, 1978; Sausville et al., 1978; Gutteridge, Rowley and Halliwell, 1981) and to other cellular structures (Martin and Kachel, 1987). This damage is likely to account for both the anti-tumour cytotoxic effects and the unwanted adverse effects of bleomycin, including progressive lung fibrosis. Studies *in vitro* indicate that the DNA and cellular damage can be blocked by DF (Sausville, Peisach and Horwitz, 1978; Martin and Kachel, 1987). However, attempts to limit the pulmonary toxicity in animal models by the use of DF have given conflicting results. In hamsters, DF (5 mg intramuscularly twice-daily for 5 days before and 21 days after intratracheal injection of bleomycin) produced a significant reduction in lung collagen formation (Chandler and Fulmer, 1985). However, in rats no protective effect was seen with DF 100 mg kg^{-1} twice-daily beginning 2 days before bleomycin instillation (Cross et al., 1985). As with paraquat there are thus conflicting data, which may reflect species differences in the tissue and cellular distribution of DF. The potential role of iron chelation in the clinical management of bleomycin-induced fibrosis remains an open question.

Other agents may give rise to iron-mediated oxidative damage affecting organs other than the lung. For example, aspirin is known to be potentially hepatotoxic (Zimmerman, 1981), with a putative role in the development of Reye's syndrome in children. Recent studies with mouse liver microsomes and mitochondria suggest mediation of this toxicity by a reactive aspirin–iron chelate which enhances lipid peroxidation; this effect was blocked by DF *in vitro* (Schwarz et al., 1988), raising the question as to whether iron chelation might have a role in limiting hepatotoxicity in this condition.

EFFECTS ON HAEM SYNTHESIS

One potential site for toxic effects of iron chelation is at the level of haem synthesis, vital in cells throughout the body but particularly in red cell precursors and in the liver. Thus it is perhaps surprising to find clinical evidence of improvements with DF therapy in pathological conditions affecting haem synthesis in both these sites.

Porphyria cutanea tarda

This is a disorder characterized by cutaneous photosensitivity and liver dysfunction, and is due to deficiency of the haem synthetic enzyme, uroporphyrinogen decarboxylase. This deficiency results in the accumulation of abnormal photoreactive porphyrins and is usually an acquired (occasionally inherited) defect of the liver enzyme, finding expression only in association with moderately increased liver iron stores. Iron plays an important part in inhibiting the enzyme activity (Kushner, Steinmuller and Lee, 1979), and the disease responds to removal of the excess iron by regular phlebotomy (Ippen, 1977). More recently, a rapid reversal of symptoms of the disease has been seen in patients treated with 1.5 g DF as an 8–10-hour subcutaneous infusion five nights each week (Rocchi et al., 1986a). During therapy, iron stores (as judged by serum ferritin values) and urinary porphyrin excretions declined in parallel (Rocchi et al., 1986b), though the rapid effect of DF suggests a more direct interference with iron-dependent free radical formation in the skin. Patients selected for chelation therapy had severe liver or cardiovascular disease which made regular phlebotomy difficult. This was also true of a further responsive patient with haemodialysis-related porphyria cutanea tarda (Praga et al., 1987). In this patient with chronic renal failure an improvement in anaemia was seen during DF therapy, an aspect to be discussed below.

The anaemia of renal failure

This is multifactorial in origin, but is primarily due to lack of erythropoietin production (Cotes, 1988). However, when sixteen chronic haemodialysis patients with normal or high iron stores received DF 1 g intravenously at the end of each dialysis for 6 months, they showed a significant increase in haemoglobin and reticulocyte counts with respect to eight untreated controls (De La Serna et al., 1988). Serum ferritin and red cell protoporphyrin concentrations declined in the treated group, the latter suggesting an improvement in haem synthesis. Whether this effect was a result of chelation of iron or of aluminium will require further investigation. Aluminium excess is known to cause microcytic anaemia, as well as bone and encephalopathic problems, responsive to aluminium chelation with DF (Brown et al., 1982; Malluche et al., 1984), but there was no evidence of prior aluminium toxicity in these patients. One alternative suggestion is that iron-dependent free radical formation may have been limiting erythropoiesis by the induction of oxidative cellular damage. It is of interest that occasional patients with sideroblastic anaemia also show improved red cell production after phlebotomy treatment for accompanying iron overload (Bottomley, 1982), an effect attributed to improved mitochondrial function.

INHIBITION OF CELL DIVISION

Iron deficiency inhibits the replication of mammalian cells, iron being an essential cofactor for ribonucleotide reductase (Reichard and Ehrenberg, 1983), a rate-limiting enzyme in DNA synthesis. DF was also found to inhibit DNA synthesis in HeLa cells (Robbins and Pederson, 1970) and lymphocytes (Hoffbrand et al., 1976). In lymphocytes, micromolar concentrations which are easily achieved during DF therapy in man produced a reversible S-phase inhibition of proliferation after overnight incubation (Lederman et al., 1984). The pattern of the disturbance in DNA synthesis with DF and other hydroxamate chelators (e.g. rhodotorulic acid) was characteristic of inhibition of ribonucleotide reductase activity, but some other chelators, including benzoic acid derivatives, were able to inhibit DNA synthesis by a mechanism independent of this enzyme (Ganeshaguru et al., 1980; Barankiewicz and Cohen, 1987). An alternative mechanism for chelator effects on lymphocyte proliferation may involve inhibition of hydroxyl radical formation, since removal of hydroxyl radicals by scavengers (e.g. mannitol) inhibited the response to some mitogens and to interleukin-1 (Novogrodsky et al., 1982). These studies have suggested that some iron-chelating agents may have a potential role as immunoregulatory compounds or as cytotoxic drugs. Furthermore, the possibility that the growth of certain infections, notably intracellular protozoal parasites, might also be inhibited has been investigated.

Immunoregulatory actions

The difficulties in determining whether the actions of iron-chelating agents are primarily an interference with hydroxyl radical formation, or a modulation of immune response, have already been discussed, particularly in connection with the mechanisms of the effect of DF in experimental allergic encephalomyelitis and in human graft-versus-host disease. The prospect of an easily reversible immune suppression using a relatively non-toxic therapy should stimulate further work in this area, particularly as newer chelating agents become available.

Cytotoxic effects

In vitro studies with murine (Bergeron *et al.*, 1984) and human (Kontoghiorges, Piga and Hoffbrand, 1986) leukaemic cell lines have shown chelator cytotoxic effects which tend to be related to the lipophilicity (and thus the potential ease of cell penetration) of the compounds. In the murine studies, incubation (24–48 hours) with a range of spermidine catecholamide iron chelators inhibited growth of L1210 leukaemia cells (as well as replication of herpes simplex type 1 virus in monkey kidney cells): these effects were reversible by the addition of iron, consistent with an inhibition of ribonucleotide reductase. By contrast, although short-term incubations (4 hours) with the human myeloid leukaemia cell lines were unable to demonstrate any cytotoxicity with DF or the new orally active chelator, 1,2-dimethyl-3-hydroxypyrid-4-one, they did show a powerful cytotoxic effect of 1-hydroxypyridine-2-thione (omadine). This was augmented by the addition of iron, suggesting that it may be oxidative damage to DNA produced by redox reactions of the iron chelate of omadine which is important for cytotoxicity. Both these mechanisms, i.e. iron deprivation (potentially relatively safe and easily reversible) and chelate-induced cell damage (potentially highly damaging and irreversible), have their counterpart in the mode of action of established cytotoxic drugs used for the treatment of human malignancy.

Ribonucleotide reductase inhibition is well established as the mode of action of hydroxyurea, a drug widely used in the management of myeloproliferative disorders in man. The effects of this drug *in vitro* can be partially reversed by the addition of Fe^{2+}, while they are enhanced by simultaneous exposure to DF, raising the possibility that simultaneous treatment might alter the therapeutic index of hydroxyurea (Cory, Lasater and Sato, 1981), perhaps favourably. DF alone, infused intravenously at a dose of 10 mg kg^{-1} h^{-1}, produced a partial and temporary response in a single infant with a drug-resistant acute leukaemia (Estrov *et al.*, 1987), but its role as an anti-tumour agent remains highly speculative. The demonstration that parabactin (a polyamine catecholamide siderophore) has an enhanced ability to synchronize murine leukaemia cells compared with DF (Bergeron and Ingeno, 1987) may eventually bear fruit in the use of more efficient cell-synchronizing iron chelators to enhance the effect of other cytotoxic anti-tumour agents.

Oxidative damage to DNA is thought to be the mechanism of action of the important anthracycline anti-tumour antibiotics, including adriamycin. Adriamycin binds to DNA and also chelates Fe^{3+}, forming a ternary complex (Eliot, Gianni and Myers, 1984) in which redox cycling of both the iron and the quinone component of the drug lead to the site-specific production of hydroxyl free radicals: it is the latter which are thought to disrupt the DNA (Gutteridge and Quinlan, 1985; Myers et al., 1986). The use of these drugs is limited by dose-related cardiomyopathy, and the ability of adriamycin, through the production of superoxide, to mobilize iron from ferritin stores (Thomas and Aust, 1986), has been suggested as a possible mechanism contributing to cardiac damage. DF is able to inhibit the DNA damage caused by adriamycin *in vitro*, presumably by preventing iron-dependent hydroxyl radical formation (Gutteridge and Quinlan, 1985). Whether a site-selective action of an iron chelator *in vivo* could lead to cardiac protection while maintaining anti-tumour effect remains entirely speculative, but the increasing range of new iron chelators becoming available may enable this hypothesis to be tested.

Infections

There is a large and complex literature on the relationships between iron and infection, and the potential for iron-chelating agents to moderate infection (e.g. by *Salmonella* and *Neisseria* species) in a variety of *in vitro* and animal models (Weinberg, 1984; Brock, 1986). As well as depriving organisms of essential iron, it has also been suggested that iron chelators might enhance neutrophil phagocytic function by protecting them from self-induced toxic free radical damage (Van Asbeck et al., 1984). However, since many micro-organisms produce iron chelators to obtain iron from the environment, there is a risk that, far from inhibiting growth, the use of such chelators may sometimes help to provide iron for replication (Brock and Ng, 1983). Indeed, exacerbation of *Yersinia* infections may be a real hazard in iron-loaded thalassaemic patients receiving DF therapy (Chiu et al., 1986), though in renal dialysis patients the risk of septicaemia was related to iron overload rather than to DF therapy (Seifert, Von Herrath and Schaefer, 1987).

Plasmodium falciparum growth in human red cells *in vitro* was inhibited by DF, with minimum inhibitory concentrations as low as 10–15 μM (Raventos-Suarez, Pollack and Nagel, 1982; Peto and Thompson, 1986). These are values which are easily achieved *in vivo* with subcutaneous DF infusions. There is as yet no clinical information on this potential therapy for a form of malaria which shows a relentless ability to develop resistance to existing chemotherapy. However, in mice infected with *Plasmodium vinkei* (Fritsch et al., 1985), large doses of DF (300 mg kg^{-1} every 8 hours) suppressed parasite growth and prevented death, provided treatment was started from the time of infection: infection rapidly relapsed on early cessation of treatment. Similar suppressive effects were seen in Aotus monkeys infected with *Plasmodium falciparum*, and receiving continuous exposure to low doses of DF (2–4 mg h^{-1}) via an implanted subcutaneous pump (Pollack et al., 1987). Studies in rats infected with *Plasmodium berghei*

(Hershko and Peto, 1988) suggested that the severity of the infection and the effect of DF was independent of the overall iron status of the animals, and that DF inhibited the parasites by chelating a labile intracellular iron pool. DF has a rather poor penetration of red cells (though this may be better in parasitized cells), and it will be of great interest to assess the effect in these models of chelators with increased ability to traverse the red cell membranes.

Trypanosoma cruzi, another intracellular protozoan parasite and the cause of Chagas disease, also appears to be dependent on the availability of intracellular iron. In experimental Chagas disease in mice, where the parasite lodges in macrophages and muscle cells, depletion of host iron stores with DF therapy reduced the pathogenicity of the infection (Lalonde and Holbein, 1984). Studies of infected peritoneal macrophages exposed to DF *in vitro* suggested a relationship between reduced cellular iron stores and impaired parasite replication (Loo and Lalonde, 1984). However, it is not clear whether, as with malaria, removal of a labile intracellular iron pool could be more important than depletion of iron stores in their own right. There is a need in this disease for new treatments which are less toxic than existing chemotherapy, and several of a range of iron chelators proved active against trypanosomes when tested *in vitro* and in infected mice (Shapiro et al., 1982).

Antibiotic therapy illustrates a rather different aspect of the relationship between iron chelation and infection. Tetracycline is an iron-chelating agent, and deprivation of iron vital to micro-organism growth may be part of its mode of action. Conversely, the action of tetracycline against *Pseudomonas* species *in vitro* is neutralized by added iron (Weinberg, 1954), and *in vivo* the simultaneous oral administration of both iron and tetracycline may lead to impaired antibiotic action and malabsorption of the iron as a result of iron chelation within the gut lumen. By contrast, the activity of two aminoglycosides against *Klebsiella* was substantially reduced by the addition of the chelators DF and enterochelin (Miles and Maskell, 1986). This observation could reflect enhanced provision of iron from the growth medium in the presence of these siderophore chelators, and re-emphasizes the potential complexity of responses to iron chelation.

TOXICITY OF IRON CHELATORS

Adverse effects of iron chelators may be expected from the effects already discussed in this chapter. For example, depletion of essential trace metals other than iron may cause problems, particularly with less selective agents such as DTPA, and cytotoxicity may result when iron chelates are able to undergo redox cycling. Other adverse reactions with DF have been less predictable. Cataracts seen in dogs given high doses (Ciba Pharmaceutical Company, 1969) have not been a problem in clinical use. In man, there have been rare examples of anaphylactic reactions (Miller et al., 1981), but the major concern has been with neurological toxicity. This includes retinal and visual field abnormalities (Davies et al., 1983), as well as auditory impairment ranging from subclinical high tone loss to overt deafness (Olivieri et al., 1986). In addition, retardation of growth velocity has been seen in over 50% of chelated prepubertal thalassaemic children (Gabutti et al., 1987). These effects are largely confined to patients who continue to receive large doses of DF despite reduction of iron stores to low levels, suggesting that it is depletion of iron critical to the function of vital enzymes that is responsible, rather than any toxic effects of DF itself. The visual effects are usually reversible, though auditory damage may sometimes be permanent. In two patients with rheumatoid disease and normal iron stores, DF therapy led to the development of a transient coma when prochlorperazine was given simultaneously (Blake et al., 1985): increased amounts of 'loosely bound' copper, products of lipid peroxidation, and total iron were found in the CSF of one of these patients and in others with evidence of neuro-ophthalmic toxicity (Pall et al., 1986). In vitro and animal studies suggested that decompartmentalization of trace metals by DF may be enhanced by prochlorperazine, and that a combination of chelation of iron essential for neurotransmitter functions and copper-catalysed free radical damage might account for DF-induced neurotoxicity. The retina is also exposed to UV light which could enhance free radical reactions, including the formation of a toxic DF nitroxide radical (Morehouse, Flitter and Mason, 1987): this could provide an alternative mechanism for the transient abnormalities of the electroretinogram seen in response to single infusions of very high doses of DF (200–450 mg kg^{-1} over 24 hours) (De Virgiliis et al., 1988).

Investigation of adverse reactions encountered with DF has stimulated the development of animal models which should enable pre-clinical testing, at least for ocular toxicity, of potential new iron-chelating agents. However, the apparently greater liability of patients without iron overload to develop toxic effects with DF may limit the use of both this drug and newer agents in other disorders.

CONCLUSION

The field of iron chelation has reached an exciting stage with the coming together of increasing knowledge about the possible involvement of iron in a variety of causes of tissue damage, and the development of a range of new iron-chelating agents. The experience with DF has provided a legacy of animal models with which to assess the efficacy, site of action, and potential toxicity of these newer agents, from among which there is now real hope of one or more orally active chelators eventually emerging as suitable for general clinical use. As well as transforming the management of transfusional iron overload, the availability of agents that may have pharmacological behaviour and sites of action that differ from DF is likely to stimulate further investigation of iron chelation as potential therapy for the variety of inflammatory, infectious, and malignant conditions reviewed in this chapter.

REFERENCES

Ambrosio, G., Zweier, J. L., Jacobus, W. E., Weisfeldt, M. L., and Flaherty, J. T. (1987). Improvement of postischemic myocardial function and metabolism induced by administration of deferoxamine at the time of reflow: the role of iron in the pathogenesis of reperfusion injury, *Circulation*, **76**, 906–15.

Andrews, F. J., Morris, C. J., Lewis, E. J., and Blake, D. R. (1987a). Effect of nutritional iron deficiency on acute and chronic inflammation, *Ann. Rheum. Dis.*, **46**, 859–65.

Andrews, F. J., Morris, C. J., Kondratowicz, G., and Blake, D. R. (1987b). Effect of iron chelation on inflammatory joint disease, *Ann. Rheum. Dis.*, **46**, 327–33.

Aruoma, O. I., and Halliwell, B. (1987). Superoxide-dependent and ascorbate-dependent formation of hydroxyl radicals from hydrogen peroxide in the presence of iron. Are lactoferrin and transferrin promoters of hydroxyl radical generation? *Biochem. J.*, **241**, 273–8.

Babbs, C. F. (1985). Role of iron ions in the genesis of reperfusion injury following successful cardiopulmonary resuscitation: preliminary data and a biochemical hypothesis, *Ann. Emerg. Med.*, **14**, 777–83.

Badylak, S. F., and Babbs, C. F. (1986). The effect of carbon dioxide, lidoflazine and deferoxamine upon long term survival following cardiorespiratory arrest in rats, *Resuscitation*, **13**, 165–73.

Balcerzak, S. P., Jenson, W. N., and Pollak, S. (1966). Mechanism of action of deferoxaminum on iron absorption, *Scand. J. Haematol.*, **3**, 205–12.

Barankiewicz, J., and Cohen, A. (1987). Impairment of nucleotide metabolism by iron-chelating deferoxamine, *Biochem. Pharmacol.*, **36**, 2343–7.

Barry, M., Flynn, D. M., Letsky, E. A., and Risdon, R. A. (1974). Long-term chelation therapy in thalassaemia major: effect on liver iron concentration, liver histology, and clinical progress, *Br. Med. J.*, **2**, 16–20.

Bergeron, R. J., and Ingeno, M. J. (1987). Microbial iron chelator-induced cell cycle synchronization in L1210 cells: potential in combination chemotherapy, *Cancer Res.*, **47**, 6010–16.

Bergeron, R. J., Cavanaugh, P. F., Kline, S. J., Hughes, R. C., Elliott, G. T., and Porter, C. W. (1984). Antineoplastic and antiherpetic activity of spermidine catecholamide iron chelators, *Biochem. Biophys. Res. Commun.*, **121**, 848–54.

Biemond, P., Swaak, A. J. G., Beindorff, C. M., and Koster, J. F. (1986a). Superoxide-dependent and -independent mechanisms of iron mobilization from ferritin by xanthine oxidase, *Biochem. J.*, **239**, 169–73.

Biemond, P., Swaak, A. J. G., van Eijk, H. G., and Koster, J. F. (1986b). Intra-articular ferritin-bound iron in rheumatoid arthritis, *Arthritis Rheum.*, **29**, 1187–93.

Blake, D. R., and Bacon, P. A. (1981). Synovial fluid ferritin in rheumatoid arthritis: an index or cause of inflammation, *Br. Med. J.*, **282**, 189.

Blake, D. R., Hall, N. D., Bacon, P. A., Dieppe, P. A., Halliwell, B., and Gutteridge, J. M. C. (1981). The importance of iron in rheumatoid disease, *Lancet*, **ii**, 1142–4.

Blake, D. R., Hall, H. D., Bacon, P. A., Dieppe, P. A., Halliwell, B., and Gutteridge, J. M. C. (1983). Effect of a specific iron chelating agent on animal models of inflammation, *Ann. Rheum. Dis.*, **42**, 89–93.

Blake, D. R., Winyard, P., Lunec, J., Williams, A., Good, P. A., Crewes, S. J., Gutteridge, J. M. C., Rowley, D., Halliwell, B., Cornish, A., and Hider, R. C. (1985). Cerebral and ocular toxicity induced by desferrioxamine, *Q. J. Med.*, **56**, 345–55.

Bolann, B. J., and Ulvik, R. J. (1987). Release of iron from ferritin by xanthine oxidase, *Biochem. J.*, **243**, 55–9.

Bomford, A., and Williams, R. (1976). Long term results of venesection therapy in idiopathic haemochromatosis, *Q. J. Med.*, **45**, 611–23.

Bottomley, S. S. (1982). Sideroblastic anaemia, *Clin. Haematol.*, **11**, 389–409.

Bowern, N., Ramshaw, I. A., Clark, I. A., and Doherty, P. C. (1984). Inhibition of autoimmune neuropathological process by treatment with an iron-chelating agent, *J. Exp. Med.*, **160**, 1532–43.

Bradley, B., Prowse, S. J., Bauling, P., and Lafferty, K. J. (1986). Desferrioxamine treatment prevents chronic islet allograft damage, *Diabetes*, **35**, 550–5.

Brock, J. H. (1986). Iron and the outcome of infection, *Br. Med. J.*, **293**, 518–20.

Brock, J. H., and Ng, J. (1983). The effect of desferrioxamine on the growth of *Staphylococcus aureus*, *Yersinia enterocolitica* and *Streptococcus faecalis* in human serum: Uptake of desferrioxamine bound iron, *FEMS Microbiol. Lett.*, **20**, 439–42.

Brown, D. J., Ham, K. N., Dawborn, J. K., and Xipell, J. M. (1982). Treatment of dialysis osteomalacia with desferrioxamine, *Lancet*, **ii**, 343–5.

Chandler, D. B., and Fulmer, J. D. (1985). The effect of deferoxamine on bleomycin-induced lung fibrosis in the hamster, *Am. Rev. Respir. Dis.*, **131**, 596–8.

Chiu, H. Y., Flynn, D. M., Hoffbrand, A. V., and Politis, D. (1986). Infection with *Yersinia enterocolitica* in patients with iron overload, *Br. Med. J.*, **292**, 97.

Ciba Pharmaceutical Company (1969). Deferoxamine mesylate (Desferal mesylate). A specific iron-chelating agent for treating acute iron intoxication, *Clin. Pharmacol. Ther.*, **10**, 595–6.

Cikrt, M., Ponka, P., Necas, E., and Neuwirt, J. (1980). Biliary iron excretion in rats following pyridoxal isonicotinoyl hydrazone, *Br. J. Haematol.*, **45**, 275–83.

Cleton, F., Turnbull, A., and Finch, C. A. (1963). Synthetic chelating agents in iron metabolism, *J. Clin. Invest.*, **42**, 327–37.

Cohen, A., Martin, M., and Schwartz, E. (1984). Depletion of excessive liver iron stores with desferrioxamine, *Br. J. Haematol.*, **58**, 369–73.

Cory, J. G., Lasater, L., and Sato, A. (1981). Effect of iron-chelating agents on inhibitors of ribonucleotide reductase, *Biochem. Pharmacol.*, **30**, 979–84.

Cotes, P. M. (1988). Erythropoietin: the developing story, *Br. Med. J.*, **296**, 805–6.

Crichton, R. R., Roman, F., and Roland, F. (1980). Ferritin iron mobilisation by chelating agents, *FEBS Lett.*, **110**, 271–4.

Cross, C. E., Warren, D., Gerriets, J. E., Wilson, D. W., Halliwell, B., and Last, J. A. (1985). Deferoxamine injection does not affect bleomycin-induced lung fibrosis in rats, *J. Lab. Clin. Med.*, **160**, 433–8.

Cumming, R. L. C., Millar, J. A., Smith, J. A., and Goldberg, A. (1969). Clinical and laboratory studies on the action of desferrioxamine, *Br. J. Haematol.*, **17**, 257–63.

Davies, S. C., Marcus, R. E., Hungerford, J. L., Miller, M. H., Arden, G. B., and Huehns, E. R. (1983). Ocular toxicity of high-dose intravenous desferrioxamine, *Lancet*, **ii**, 181–4.

De La Serna, F.-J., Praga, M., Gilsanz, F., Rodicio, J.-L., Ruilope, L.-M., and Alcazar, J.-M. (1988). Improvement in the erythropoiesis of chronic haemodialysis patients with desferrioxamine, *Lancet*, **i**, 1009–11.

De Virgiliis, S., Congia, M., Turco, M. P., Frau, F., Dessi, C., Argiolu, F., Sorcinelli, R., Sitzia, A., and Cao, A. (1988). Depletion of trace elements and acute ocular toxicity induced by desferrioxamine in patients with thalassaemia, *Arch. Dis. Child.*, **63**, 250–5.

Editorial (1985). Metal chelation therapy, oxygen radicals, and human disease, *Lancet*, **i**, 143–5.

Eliot, H., Gianni, L., and Myers, C. (1984). Oxidative destruction of DNA by the adriamycin–iron complex, *Biochemistry*, **23**, 928–36.

Estrov, Z., Tawa, A., Wang, X.-H., Dubé, I. D., Sulh, H., Cohen, A., Gelfand, E. W., and Freedman, M. H. (1987). *In vitro* and *in vivo* effects of deferoxamine in neonatal acute leukemia, *Blood*, **69**, 757–61.

Fahey, J. L., Rath, C. E., Princiotto, J. V., Brick, I. B., and Rubin, M. (1961). Evaluation of trisodium calcium diethylenetriaminepentaacetate in iron storage disease, *J. Lab. Clin. Med.*, **57**, 436–48.

Fairbanks, V. F., Warson, M. D., and Beutler, E. (1963). Drugs for iron overload, *Br. Med. J.*, **1**, 1414–15.

Fleischer, J. E., Lanier, W. L., Milde, J. H., and Michenfelder, J. D. (1987). Failure of deferoxamine, an iron chelator, to improve neurologic outcome following complete cerebral ischemia in dogs, *Stroke*, **18**, 124–7.

Fligiel, S. E. G., Ward, P. A., Johnson, K. J., and Till, G. O. (1984). Evidence for a role of hydroxyl radical in immune-complex-induced vasculitis, *Am. J. Pathol.*, **115**, 375–82.

Fritsch, G., Treumer, J., Spira, D. T., and Jung, A. (1985). Plasmodium vinckei: suppression of mouse infections with desferrioxamine B, *Exp. Parasitol.*, **60**, 171–4.

Gabbutti, V., Luzzato, L., Sandri, A., Capalbo, P., D'Oria, A., Sacchetti, L., and Piga, A. (1987). Toxicity of desferrioxamine treatment, *Proceedings of the 2nd International Conference on Thalassemia and the Hemoglobinopathies*, p. 27, Heraklion, Crete.

Ganeshaguru, K., Hoffbrand, A. V., Grady, R. W., and Cerami, A. (1980). Effect of various iron chelating agents on DNA synthesis in human cells, *Biochem. Pharmacol.*, **29**, 1275–9.

Giordano, N., Sancasciani, S., Borghi, C., Fioravanti, A., and Marcolongo, R. (1986). Antianaemic and anti-inflammatory activity of desferrioxamine: possible usefulness in rheumatoid arthritis, *Clin. Exp. Rheumatol.*, **4**, 25–9.

Grady, R. W., and Jacobs, A. (1981). The screening of potential iron chelating drugs. In A. E. Martell, W. G. Anderson and D. G. Badman (eds) *Development of Iron Chelators for Clinical Use*, pp. 133–64, Elsevier, North Holland.

Grady, R. W., Peterson, C. M., Jones, R. L., Graziano, J. H., Bhargava, K. K., Berdoukas, V. A., Kokkini, G., Loukopoulos, D., and Cerami, A. (1979). Rhodotorulic acid—investigation of its potential as an iron-chelating drug, *J. Pharmacol. Exp. Ther.*, **209**, 342–8.

Graziano, J. H., Grady, R. W., and Cerami, A. (1974). The identification of 2,3-

dihydroxybenzoic acid as a potentially useful iron-chelating drug, *J. Pharmacol. Exp. Ther.*, **190**, 570–5.

Green, C. J., Healing, G., Simpkin, S., Lunec, J., and Fuller, B. J. (1986a). Desferrioxamine reduces susceptibility to lipid peroxidation in rabbit kidneys subjected to warm ischaemia and reperfusion, *J. Comp. Biochem. Physiol.*, **85B**, 113–17.

Green, C. J., Healing, G., Simpkin, S., Fuller, B. J., and Lunec, J. (1986b). Reduced susceptibility to lipid peroxidation in cold ischaemic rabbit kidneys after addition of desferrioxamine, mannitol or uric acid to the flush solution, *Cryobiology*, **23**, 358–65.

Green, C. J., Healing, G., Simpkin, S., Lunec, J., and Fuller, B. J. (1986c). Increased susceptibility to lipid peroxidation in rabbit kidneys: a consequence of warm ischaemia and subsequent reperfusion, *J. Comp. Biochem. Physiol.*, **83**, 603–8.

Gupta, M., and Singal, P. W. (1987). Oxygen radical injury in the presence of desferal, a specific iron-chelating agent, *Biochem. Pharmacol.*, **36**, 3774–7.

Gutteridge, J. M. C. (1987). Bleomycin-detectable iron in knee joint synovial fluid from arthritic patients and its relationship to the extracellular antioxidant activities of caeruloplasmin, transferrin and lactoferrin, *Biochem. J.*, **245**, 415–21.

Gutteridge, J. M. C., and Quinlan, G. J. (1985). Free radical damage to deoxyribose by anthrocycline, aureolic acid and aminoquinone antitumour antibiotics, *Biochem. Pharmacol.*, **34**, 4099–103.

Gutteridge, J. M. C., Richmond, R., and Halliwell, B. (1979). Inhibition of the iron-catalysed formation of hydroxyl radicals from superoxide and of lipid peroxidation by desferrioxamine, *Biochem. J.*, **184**, 469–72.

Gutteridge, J. M. C., Rowley, D. A., and Halliwell, B. (1981). Superoxide-dependent formation of hydroxyl radicals in the presence of iron salts, *Biochem. J.*, **199**, 263–5.

Gyparaki, M., Porter, J. B., Hirani, S., Streater, M., Hider, R. C., and Huehns, E. R. (1987). *In vivo* evaluation of hydroxypyridone iron chelators in a mouse model, *Acta Haematol.*, **78**, 217–21.

Hallberg, L., and Hedenberg, L. (1965). The effect of desferrioxamine on iron metabolism in man, *Scand. J. Haematol.*, **2**, 67–79.

Halliwell, B., and Gutteridge, J. M. C. (1984). Oxygen toxicity, oxygen radicals, transition metals and disease, *Biochem. J.*, **219**, 1–14.

Halliwell, B., and Gutteridge, J. M. C. (1986). Oxygen free radicals and iron in relation to biology and medicine: some problems and concepts, *Arch. Biochem. Biophys.*, **246**, 501–14.

Harker, L. A., Funk, D. D., and Finch, C. A. (1968). Evaluation of storage iron by chelates, *Am. J. Med.*, **45**, 105–15.

Henson, P. M., and Johnston, R. B. (1987). Tissue injury in inflammation, *J. Clin. Invest.*, **79**, 669–74.

Hernandez, L. A., Grisham, B. M., and Granger, D. N. (1987). A role for iron in oxidant-mediated ischemic injury to intestinal microvasculature, *Am. J. Physiol.*, **253**, G49–53.

Hershko, C. (1975). A study of the chelating agent diethylenetriaminepentaacetic acid using selective radioiron probes of reticuloendothelial and parenchymal iron stores, *J. Lab. Clin. Med.*, **85**, 913–21.

Hershko, C. (1978). Determinants of fecal and urinary iron excretion in desferrioxamine-treated rats, *Blood*, **51**, 415–23.

Hershko, C. (1988). Oral iron chelating drugs: coming but not yet ready for clinical use, *Br. Med. J.*, **296**, 1081–2.

Hershko, C., Grady, R. W., and Link, G. (1984). Phenolic ethylenediamine derivatives: a study of orally effective iron chelators, *J. Lab. Clin. Med.*, **103**, 337–46.
Hershko, C., and Peto, T. E. A. (1987). Non-transferrin plasma iron, *Br. J. Haematol.*, **66**, 149–51.
Hershko, C., and Peto, T. E. A. (1987). Deferoxamine-inhibition of malaria is independent of host iron status, *J. Exp. Med.*, **168**, 375–87.
Hershko, C., and Rachmilewitz, E. A. (1979). Mechanism of desferrioxamine-induced iron excretion in thalassaemia, *Br. J. Haematol.*, **42**, 125–32.
Hershko, C., and Weatherall, D. J. (1988). Iron chelating therapy, *CRC Crit. Rev.* (in press).
Hershko, C., Graham, G., Bates, G. W., and Rachmilewitz, E. A. (1978). Non-specific serum iron in thalassaemia: an abnormal serum iron fraction of potential toxicity, *Br. J. Haematol.*, **40**, 255–63.
Hershko, C., Avramovici-Grisaru, S., Link, G., Gelfand, L., and Sarel, S. (1981). Mechanism of *in vivo* iron chelation by pyridoxal isonicotinoyl hydrazone and other imino derivatives of pyridoxal, *J. Lab. Clin. Med.*, **98**, 99–108.
Hoe, S., Rowley, D. A., and Halliwell, B. (1982). Reactions of ferrioxamine and desferrioxamine with the hydroxyl radical, *Chem. Biol. Interact.*, **41**, 75–81.
Hoffbrand, A. V., Ganeshaguru, K., Hooton, J. W. L., and Tattersall, M. H. N. (1976). Effect of iron deficiency and desferrioxamine on DNA synthesis in human cells, *Br. J. Haematol.*, **33**, 517–26.
Hoffbrand, A. V., Gorman, A., Laulicht, M., Garidi, M., Economidou, J., Georgipoulou, P., Hussain, M. A. M., and Flynn, D. M. (1979). Improvement in iron status and liver function in patients with transfusional iron overload with long-term subcutaneous desferrioxamine, *Lancet*, **i**, 947–9.
Hoy, T., Humphrys, J., Jacobs, A., Williams, A., and Ponka, P. (1979). Effective iron chelation following oral administration of an isoniazid—pyridoxal hydrazone, *Br. J. Haematol.*, **43**, 443–9.
Hunt, J., Richards, R. J., Harwood, R., and Jacobs, A. (1979). The effect of desferrioxamine on fibroblasts and collagen formation in cell cultures, *Br. J. Haematol.*, **41**, 69–76.
Ippen, H. (1977). Treatment of porphyria cutanea tarda by phlebotomy, *Semin. Hematol.*, **14**, 253–9.
Jacobs, A. (1977). Low molecular weight intracellular iron transport compounds, *Blood*, **50**, 433–9.
Johnson, D. K., Pippard, M. J., Murphy, T. B., and Rose, N. J. (1982). An *in vivo* evaluation of iron-chelating drugs derived from pyridoxal and its analogs, *J. Pharmacol. Exp. Ther.*, **221**, 399–403.
Keberle, H. (1964). The biochemistry of desferrioxamine and its relation to iron metabolism, *Ann. N.Y. Acad. Sci.*, **119**, 758–68.
Kim, B.-K., Huebers, H. A., and Finch, C. A. (1987). Effectiveness of oral iron chelators assayed in the rat, *Am. J. Hematol.*, **24**, 277–84.
Kohen, R., and Chevion, M. (1985). Paraquat toxicity is enhanced by iron and reduced by desferrioxamine in laboratory mice, *Biochem. Pharmacol.*, **34**, 1841–3.
Kontoghiorghes, G. J. (1986). Iron mobilization from ferritin using α-oxohydroxy heteroaromatic chelators, *Biochem. J.*, **333**, 299–302.
Kontoghiorghes, G. J., Piga, A., and Hoffbrand, A. V. (1986). Cytotoxic effects of the lipophilic iron chelator omadine, *FEBS Lett.*, **204**, 208–12.
Kontoghiorghes, G. J., Aldouri, M. A., Hoffbrand, A. V., Barr, J., Wonke, B., Kourouclaris, T., and Sheppard, L. (1987). Effective chelation of iron in β

thalassaemia with the oral chelator 1,2-dimethyl-3-hydroxypyrid-4-one, *Br. Med. J.*, **295**, 1509–12.

Korbashi, P., Kohen, R., Katzhendler, J., and Chevion, M. (1986). Iron mediates paraquat toxicity in Escherichia coli, *J. Biol. Chem.*, **261**, 12472–6.

Kushner, J. P., Steinmuller, D. P., and Lee, G. R. (1979). The role of iron in the pathogenesis of porphyria cutanea tarda. II. Inhibition of uroporphyrinogen decarboxylase. *J. Clin. Invest.*, **56**, 661–7.

Lalonde, R. G., and Holbein, B. E. (1984). Role of iron in *Trypanosoma cruzi* infection of mice, *J. Clin. Invest.*, **73**, 470–6.

Laub, R., Schneider, Y.-J., Octave, J.-N., Trouet, A., and Crichton, R. (1985). Cellular pharmacology of deferrioxamine B and derivatives in cultured rat hepatocytes in relation to iron metabolism, *Biochem. Pharmacol.*, **34**, 1175–83.

Lederman, H. M., Cohen, A., Lee, J. W. W., Freedman, M. H., and Gelfand, E. W. (1984). Deferoxamine: a reversible S-phase inhibitor of human lymphocyte proliferation, *Blood*, **64**, 748–53.

Link, G., Pinson, A., and Hershko, C. (1985). Heart cells in culture: a model of myocardial iron overload and chelation, *J. Lab. Clin. Med.*, **106**, 147–53.

Loo, V. G., and Lalonde, R. G. (1984). Role of iron in intracellular growth of *Trypanosoma cruzi*, *Infect. Immun.*, **45**, 726–30.

Malluche, H. H., Smith, A. J., Abreo, K., and Faugere, M. C. (1984). The use of deferoxamine in the management of aluminium accumulation in bone in patients with renal failure, *N. Engl. J. Med.*, **311**, 140–4.

Marcus, R. E., Davies, S. C., Bantock, H. M., Underwood, S. R., Walton, S., and Huehns, E. R. (1984). Desferrioxamine to improve cardiac function in iron-overloaded patients with thalassaemia major, *Lancet*, **i**, 392–3.

Martell, A. E., Motekaitis, R. J., Murase, I., Sala, L. F., Stoldt, R., Ng, C. Y., Rosenkrantz, H., and Metterville, J. J. (1987). Development of iron chelators for Cooley's anemia, *Inorg. Chim. Acta*, **138**, 215–30.

Martin, W. J., and Kachel, D. L. (1987). Bleomycin-induced pulmonary endothelial cell injury: evidence for the role of iron-catalyzed toxic oxygen-derived species, *J. Lab. Clin. Med.*, **110**, 153–8.

McCord, J. M. (1985). Oxygen-derived free radicals in postischemic tissue injury. *N. Engl. J. Med.*, **312**, 159–63.

Meyer-Brunot, H. G., and Keberle, H. (1967). The metabolism of desferrioxamine B, *Biochem. Pharmacol.*, **16**, 527–37.

Miles, A. A., and Maskell, J. P. (1986). The neutralization of antibiotic action by metallic cations and iron chelators, *J. Antimicrob. Chemother.*, **17**, 481–7.

Miller, K. B., Rosenwasser, L. J., Bessette, J. M., Beer, D. J., and Rocklin, R. E. (1981). Rapid desensitisation for desferrioxamine anaphylactic reaction, *Lancet*, **i**, 1059.

Modell, B. (1979). Advances in the use of iron-chelating agents for the treatment of iron overload, *Prog. Hematol.*, **11**, 267–312.

Modell, C. B., and Beck, J. (1974). Long-term desferrioxamine therapy in thalassemia, *Ann. N.Y. Acad. Sci.*, **232**, 201–10.

Morehouse, K. M., Flitter, W. D., and Mason, R. P. (1987). The enzymatic oxidation of Desferal to a nitroxide free radical, *FEBS Lett.*, **222**, 246–50.

Myers, C., Gianni, L., Zweier, J., Muindi, J., Sinha, B. K., and Eliot, H. (1986). Role of iron in adriamycin biochemistry, *Fed. Proc.*, **45**, 2792–7.

Nayini, N. R., White, B. C., Aust, S. D., Huang, R. R., Indrieri, R. J., Evans, A. T., Bialek, H., Jacobs, W. A., and Komaro, J. (1985). Post resuscitation iron delocalisation and malondialdehyde production in the brain following prolonged cardiac arrest, *J. Free Radical Biol. Med.*, **1**, 111–16.

Neilands, J. B. (1972). Evolution of biological iron-binding centres, *Struct. Bonding*, **2**, 145–70.

Nienhuis, A. W. (1981). Vitamin C and iron, *N. Engl. J. Med.*, **304**, 170–1.

Novogrodsky, A., Ravid, A., Rubin, A. L., and Stenzel, K. H. (1982). Hydroxyl radical scavengers inhibit lymphocyte mitogenesis, *Proc. Natl Acad. Sci. USA*, **79**, 1171–4.

O'Connell, M., Halliwell, B., Moorehouse, C. P. Aruoma, O. I., Baum, H., and Peters, T. J. (1986). Formation of hydroxyl radicals in the presence of ferritin and haemosiderin, *Biochem. J.*, **234**, 727–31.

Olivieri, N. F., Buncic, J. R., Chew, E., Gallant, T., Harrison, R. V., Keenan, N., Logan, W., Mitchell, D., Ricci, G., Skarf, B., Taylor, M., and Freedman, M. H. (1986). Visual and auditory neurotoxicity in patients receiving subcutaneous deferoxamine infusions, *N. Engl. J. Med.*, **314**, 869–73.

Osheroff, M. R., Schaich, K. M., Drew, R. T., and Borg, D. C. (1985). Failure of desferrioxamine to modify the toxicity of paraquat in rats, *J. Free Radical Biol. Med.*, **1**, 71–82.

Pall, H., Blake, D. R., Good, P. A., Winyard, P., and Williams, A. C. (1986). Copper chelation and the neuro-ophthalmic toxicity of desferrioxamine, *Lancet*, **ii**, 1279.

Peter, H. H. (1983). Eisenchelierung. Biologische bedeutung und medizinische anwendungen', *Schweiz. Med. Wochenschr.*, **113**, 1428–33.

Peters, G., Keberle, H., Schmid, K., and Brunner, H. (1966). Distribution and renal excretion of desferrioxamine and ferrioxamine in the dog and in the rat, *Biochem. Pharmacol.*, **15**, 93–9.

Peterson, C. M., Graziano, J. H., Grady, R. W., Jones, R. L., Vlassara, H. V., Canale, V. C., Miller, D. R., and Cerami, A. (1976). Chelation studies with 2,3-dihydroxybenzoic acid in patients with β-thalassaemia major, *Br. J. Haematol.*, **33**, 477–85.

Peto, T. E. A., and Thompson, J. L. (1986). A reappraisal of the effects of iron and desferrioxamine on the growth of *Plasmodium falciparum in vitro*: the unimportance of serum iron, *Br. J. Haematol.*, **63**, 273–86.

Pippard, M. J., Callender, S. T., and Finch, C. A. (1982). Ferrioxamine excretion in iron-loaded man, *Blood*, **60**, 288–94.

Pippard, M. J., Johnson, D. K., and Finch, C. A. (1981). A rapid assay for evaluation of iron-chelating agents in rats, *Blood*, **58**, 685–92.

Pippard, M. J., Johnson, D. K., and Finch, C. A. (1982). Hepatocyte iron kinetics in the rat explored with an iron chelator, *Br. J. Haematol.*, **52**, 211–24.

Pippard, M. J., Tikerpae, J., and Peters, T. J. (1986). Ferritin iron metabolism in the rat liver, *Br. J. Haematol.*, **64**, 839.

Pippard, M. J., and Weatherall, D. J. (1987). Iron balance and the management of iron overload in β-thalassemia intermedia, *Birth Defects*, **23**(5B), 29–33.

Pippard, M. J., Letsky, E. A., Callender, S. T., and Weatherall, D. J. (1978). Prevention of iron loading in transfusion-dependent thalassaemia, *Lancet*, **i**, 1178–81.

Pippard, M. J., Jackson, M. J., Hoffmann, K., Petrou, M., and Modell, C. B. (1986). Iron chelation using subcutaneous infusions of diethylene triamine penta-acetic acid (DTPA), *Scand. J. Haematol.*, **36**, 466–72.

Pitt, C. G., Gupta, G., Estes, W. E., Rosenkrantz, H., Metterville, J. J., Crumbliss, A. L., Palmer, R. A., Nordquest, K. W., Sprinkle Hardy, K. A., Whitcomb, D. R., Byers, B. R., Arceneaux, J. E. L., Gaines, C. G., and Sciortino, C. V. (1979). The selection and evaluation of new chelating agents for the treatment of iron overload, *J. Pharmacol. Exp. Ther.*, **208**, 12–18.

Pitt, C. G., Bao, Y., Thompson, J., Wani, M. C., Rosenkrantz, H., and Metterville, J. (1986). Esters and lactones of phenolic amino carboxylic acids: prodrugs for iron chelation, *J. Med. Chem.*, **29**, 1231–7.

Pollack, S., Rossan, R. N., Davidson, D. E., and Escajadillo, A. (1987). Desferrioxamine suppresses Plasmodium falciparum in Aotus monkeys, *Proc. Soc. Exp. Biol. Med.*, **184**, 162–4.

Polson, R. J., Jawed, A., Bomford, A., Berry, H., and Williams, R. (1985). Treatment of rheumatoid arthritis with desferrioxamine: relation between stores of iron before treatment and side effects, *Br. Med. J.*, **291**, 448.

Porter, J. B., Gyparaki, M., Huehns, E. R., and Hider, R. C. (1986). The relationship between lipophilicity of hydroxypyrid-4-one iron chelators and cellular iron mobilisation, using an hepatocyte culture model, *Biochem. Soc. Trans.*, **14**, 1180.

Praga, M., Enriquez de Salamanca, R., Andres, A., Nieto, J., Oliet, A., Perpina, J., and Morales, J. M. (1987). Treatment of hemodialysis-related porphyria cutanea tarda with deferoxamine, *N. Engl. J. Med.*, **316**, 547–8.

Propper, R. D., Shurin, S. B., and Nathan, D. G. (1976). Reassessment of the use of desferrioxamine B in iron overload, *N. Engl. J. Med.*, **294**, 1421–3.

Puppo, A., and Halliwell, B. (1988). Formation of hydroxyl radicals from hydrogen peroxide in the presence of iron, *Biochem. J.*, **249**, 185–90.

Raventos-Suarez, C., Pollack, S., and Nagel, R. (1982). *Plasmodium falciparum*: inhibition of *in vitro* growth by desferrioxamine, *Am. J. Trop. Med. Hyg.*, **31**, 919–22.

Reichard, P., and Ehrenberg, A. (1983). Ribonucleotide reductase—a radical enzyme, *Science*, **221**, 514–20.

Robbins, E., and Pederson, T. (1970). Iron: its intracellular localization and possible role in cell division, *Proc. Natl Acad. Sci. USA*, **66**, 1244–51.

Rocchi, E., Gilbertini, P., Cassanelli, M., Pietrangelo, A., Borghi, A., Pantaleoni, M., Jensen, J., and Ventura, E. (1986a). Iron removal therapy in porphyria cutanea tarda: phlebotomy versus slow subcutaneous desferrioxamine infusion, *Br. J. Dermatol.*, **114**, 621–9.

Rocchi, E., Gibertini, P., Cassanelli, M., Pietrangelo, A., Borghi, A., and Ventura, E. (1986b). Serum ferritin in the assessment of liver iron overload and iron removal therapy in porphyria cutanea tarda, *J. Lab. Clin. Med.*, **107**, 36–42.

Rosenkrantz, H., Metterville, J. J., and Fleischman, W. (1986). Preliminary toxicity findings in dogs and rodents given the iron chelator ethylenediamine-N,N'-bis (2-hydroxyphenylacetic acid) (EDHPA), *Fundam. Appl. Toxicol.*, **6**, 292–8.

Sausville, E. A., Peisach, J., and Horwitz, S. B. (1978). Effect of chelating agents and metal ions on the degradation of DNA by bleomycin, *Biochemistry*, **17**, 2740–6.

Sausville, E. A., Stein, R. W., Peisach, J., and Horwitz, S. B. (1978). Properties and products of the degradation of DNA by bleomycin and iron(II), *Biochemistry*, **17**, 2746–54.

Schwarz, K. B., Arey, B. J., Tolman, K., and Mahanty, S. (1988). Iron chelation as a possible mechanism for aspirin-induced malondialdehyde production by mouse liver microsomes and mitochondria, *J. Clin. Invest.*, **81**, 165–70.

Seifert, A., Von Herrath, D., and Schaefer, K. (1987). Iron overload, but not treatment with desferrioxamine favours the development of septicaemia in patients on maintenance haemodialysis, *Q. J. Med.*, **65**, 1015–24.

Seymour, C. A., and Peters, T. J. (1978). Organelle pathology in primary and secondary haemochromatosis with special reference to lysosomal changes, *Br. J. Haematol.*, **40**, 239–53.

Shapiro, A., Nathan, H. C., Hutner, S. H., Garofalo, S. D., McLaughlin, S. D,. Rescigno, D., and Bacchi, C. J. (1982). In vivo and in vitro activity by diverse chelators against *Trypanosoma brucei*, *J. Protozool.*, **29**, 85–90.

Sirivech, S., Frieden, E., and Osaki, S. (1974). The release of iron from horse spleen ferritin by reduced flavins, *Biochem. J.*, **143**, 311–15.

Smith, S. M., Grisham, M. B., Manci, E. A., Granger, D. N., and Kvietys, P. R. (1987). Gastric mucosal injury in the rat. Role of iron and xanthine oxidase, *Gastroenterology*, **92**, 950–6.

Summers, M. R., Jacobs, A., Tudway, D., Perera, P., and Ricketts, C. (1979). Studies in desferrioxamine and ferrioxamine metabolism in normal and iron-loaded subjects, *Br. J. Haematol.*, **42**, 547–55.

Thomas, C. E., and Aust, S. D. (1986). Release of iron from ferritin by cardiotoxic anthracycline antibiotics, *Arch. Biochem. Biophys.*, **248**, 684–9.

Till, G. O., Hatherill, J. R., Tourtellotte, W. W., Lutz, M. J., and Ward, P. A. (1985). Lipid peroxidation and acute lung injury after thermal trauma to skin. Evidence of a role for hydroxyl radical, *Am. J. Pathol.*, **119**, 376–84.

Van Asbeck, B. S., Marx, J. J. M., Struyvenberg, A., Kats, J. H. V., and Verhoef, J. (1984). Deferoxamine enhances phagocytic function of human polymorphonuclear leukocytes, *Blood*, **63**, 714–20.

Van Asbeck, B. S., Hillen, S. C., Boonen, H. C. M., De Jong, Y., Doormans, J. A. M. A., Van der Wal, W. A. A., Marx, J. J. M., and Sangster, B. (1986). A new perspective of the putative role of iron chelation in oxygen toxicity: protection against paraquat poisoning by deferoxamine, *Abstracts of the European Iron Club Meeting*, Pavia, Italy, September.

Vile, G. F., Winterbourn, C. C., and Sutton, H. C. (1987). Radical-driven Fenton reactions: studies with paraquat, adriamycin, and anthraquinone 6-sulfonate and citrate, ATP, ADP, and pyrophosphate iron chelates, *Arch. Biochem. Biophys.*, **259**, 616–26.

Wapnick, A. A., Lynch, S. R., Charlton, R. W., Seftel, H. C., and Bothwell, T. H. (1969). The effect of ascorbic acid deficiency on desferrioxamine-induced urinary iron excretion, *Br. J. Haematol.*, **17**, 563–8.

Ward, P. A., Gill, G. O., Kunkel, R., and Beauchamp, C. (1983). Evidence for role of hydroxyl radical in complement and neutrophil dependent tissue injury, *J. Clin. Invest.*, **72**, 789–801.

Waxman, H. S., and Brown, E. B. (1969). Clinical usefulness of iron chelating agents, *Prog. Hematol.*, **6**, 338–73.

Weatherall, D. J., and Clegg, J. B. (1981). *The Thalassaemic Syndromes*, Blackwell Scientific, Oxford.

Weinberg, E. D. (1954). The influence of inorganic salts on the activity *in vitro* of oxytetracycline, *Antibiot. Chemother.*, **4**, 35–42.

Weinberg, E. D. (1984). Iron withholding: a defense against infection and neoplasia, *Physiol. Rev.*, **64**, 65–102.

Weinberg, K., Champagne, J., Lenarsky, C., Peterson, J., Nguyen, T., Felder, B., and Parkman, R. (1986). Desferrioxamine (DFO) inhibition of interleukin 2 receptor (IL2R) expression: potential therapy of graft versus host disease (GVHD), *Blood*, **68**, 286a.

Willenborg, D. O., Bowern, N. A., Danta, G., and Doherty, P. C. (1988). Inhibition of allergic encephalomyelitis by the iron chelating agent desferrioxamine: differential effect depending on type of sensitizing encephalitogen, *J. Neuroimmunol.*, **17**, 127–35.

Williams, A., Hoy, T., Pugh, A., and Jacobs, A. (1982). Pyridoxal complexes as potential chelating agents for oral therapy in transfusional iron overload, *J. Pharm. Pharmacol.*, **34**, 730–2.

Williams, J. (1985). The structure of transferrins. In G. Spik, J. Montreuil, R. R. Crichton and J. Mazurier (eds) *Proteins of Iron Storage and Transport*, pp. 13–23, Elsevier Science Publishers, Amsterdam.

Winyard, P. G., Blake, D. R., Chirico, S., Gutteridge, J. M. C., and Lunec, J. (1987). Mechanisms of exacerbation of rheumatoid synovitis by total-dose iron-dextran infusion: *in vivo* demonstration of iron-promoted oxidant stress, *Lancet*, **i**, 69–72.

Wolfe, L., Olivieri, N., Sallan, D., Colan, S., Rose, V., Propper, R., Freedman, M. H., and Nathan, D. G. (1985). Prevention of cardiac disease by subcutaneous deferoxamine in patients with thalassemia major, *N. Engl. J. Med.*, **312**, 1600–3.

Zimmerman, H. J. (1981). Effects of aspirin and acetaminophen on the liver, *Arch. Intern. Med.*, **141**, 333–42.

Iron in Immunity, Cancer and Inflammation
Edited by M. de Sousa and J. H. Brock
© 1989 John Wiley & Sons Ltd

18
Closing Overview

Allan Jacobs

Department of Haematology, University of Wales College of Medicine, Cardiff CF4 4XN, Wales

This final chapter is not, of course, a closing overview. Such a title supposes both that it is possible to have the last word—an unlikely event while scientific investigation continues—and that by an overview it is possible to see everything. I do not know of any study that has measured the half-life of accepted scientific facts, but there is no reason to believe that it is any longer in the fields of iron metabolism and immunity than in any other area of knowledge. Accumulated information and new techniques mean that we now see problems in a different light from ten or twenty years ago and the older knowledge needs to be re-evaluated rather than chiselled in tablets of stone. We have to ask new and relevant questions rather than try to fit our data to preconceived notions. The uncomfortable fact that doesn't fit, particularly if it is verifiable, is far more important than the twentieth fact that fits.

In this context the editors and contributors of this book have chosen not to retread the well-worn paths that have criss-crossed the field of iron metabolism for the last few decades, but have gone out into uncharted land on the periphery of the subject where exciting new phenomena can be observed. In many instances they appear to be on firm ground. Occasionally there is a risk of sinking into the mire. While much of the literature on iron metabolism relates to erythropoiesis, anaemia and the effects of iron overload, it has been known for many years that iron is essential to the normal function of all living cells and takes part in a large number of intracellular metabolic reactions (Wrigglesworth and Baum, 1980). Systemic iron deficiency leads to diverse functional defects which have been documented in many organs and many species (Jacobs, 1982). Brock (Chapter 5) draws particular attention to the importance of iron deficiency for the immune system, and de Sousa (Chapter 11) shows how immune function cannot escape the effects of systemic iron overload. So while it is clear that no system within the body can be uninfluenced by overall iron status, the time has come to explore non-erythroid iron metabolism and its relevance to function.

I do not understand the meaning of the term 'immune system' and may be it is best not to attempt a definition. It appears to include the lymphocytes, the myeloid-macrophage system, their protein products and the substances that interact with them. de Sousa points out the vital and substantial relationship that exists between the erythron and the macrophage system, the former being entirely degraded by the latter with recycling of the breakdown products. Thus all the progeny of the totipotential haemopoietic stem cell appear to interact in a complex but intimate manner. By considering iron and immunity we are actually considering iron and the totality of haemopoiesis. Current information does not allow us to omit from this system the rapidly growing number of cytokines (Morstyn and Burgess, 1988), maturation factors (Sachs, 1987) and leukaemia inhibitory substances (Gough *et al.*, 1988), or the stromal and endothelial cells and their extracellular matrix (Gordon, 1988). It is not surprising that a leap into this area of iron metabolism, where the permutations of cellular and humoral interactions are almost indefinable, does not yield easy answers but a number of hints and many questions. Often it is not clear whether we are looking at mechanisms of primary importance or at secondary epiphenomena that may lead to a dead end. Broxmeyer (Chapter 9) expresses the present state of knowledge when he points to the cell–cell biomolecular network that controls haemopoiesis—a concept that is developed by Torok-Storb (1988). The place of transferrin, ferritin or lactoferrin in this network and their influence *in vivo* are entirely unknown. Many of the *in vitro* experiments are far from physiological and, especially in the case of ferritin, difficult to interpret. Fletcher (Chapter 10) makes a case for a possible role of lactoferrin both in the local inflammatory lesion and in generating a signal to the myelopoietic cells in the bone marrow.

My own feeling is that we still need far more information about the basic biochemistry and physiology of iron before making too many speculative guesses about its role in disease. The investigation of pathological states can be used to that end. Discussion regarding possible cellular sites for the synthesis of transferrin and lactoferrin has been inconclusive for many years and we await the definitive studies using *in situ* hybridization to see where the genes are expressed and to determine the factors influencing expression. We need far more information about the nature of circulating non-transferrin iron and its interactions with transferrin and tissue cells. We have not begun to characterize the intracellular 'labile' iron pool. Can we really still talk about ferritin and transferrin rather than their families? How many of the genes are expressed in different cell types, what is the function of their products and how are these altered by post-translational modifications?

The leukaemic and preleukaemic syndromes with their common translocations and deletions involving chromosomes 3 and 11 could be a fruitful area for further study. It has been assumed that transferrin's importance is as an iron carrier, but we know little more of its role in trace metal metabolism since the review of Worwood (1974). No consideration of a possible physiological role for ferritin outside its function as an iron storage compound can ignore its ability to bind a variety of other molecules, such as α_2-macroglobulin (Santambrogio and Massover, 1989), which may themselves be active regulators. Should we consider ferritin as a carrier molecule?

Despite considerable speculation there is little evidence that iron proteins act as specific markers of malignant disease (Jacobs, 1984). Ferritin joins the list of acute-phase proteins that may be used to monitor the presence of disease but with no discernible advantages. Similarly, in the anaemia associated with chronic disease and malignancy the (still unexplained) fall in serum iron appears to be a secondary phenomenon. Nor have more recent studies supported defective erythropoietin production as a cause for this phenomenon (Cotes *et al.*, 1980; Birgegård *et al.*, 1987). There are no simple answers to be found in the control of the interactive haemopoietic network. Children with acute lymphoblastic leukaemia survive significantly longer when their transferrin saturation is less than 37% (Potaznik *et al.*, 1987). Is this due to a protective effect of unsaturated transferrin or to a stimulating effect of iron on the malignant cells? A far more likely explanation is that children with more advanced leukaemia have a greater degree of erythropoietic failure and hence a higher transferrin saturation. In all situations the effect of iron and erythropoietic status on all the usually measured parameters is overwhelming and cannot be ignored in considering other possibilities.

The possibility of utilizing our knowledge of iron metabolism for therapeutic intervention in the treatment of leukaemia is an enticing prospect. Trowbridge (Chapter 16) has shown how blocking the transferrin receptor can inhibit the progression of malignancy *in vivo* in mice. The experimental use of an antibody–toxin conjugate can also be effective *in vivo*, but we still seem a little way from the application of this methodology to human disease. The use of iron-chelating agents, however, offers a prospect of human studies at the present time. The inhibitory effect of desferrioxamine on DNA synthesis has been known for many years, but the recent demonstration of its transient effectiveness in a case of childhood acute leukaemia (Estrov *et al.*, 1987) encourages its further study as an adjuvant therapy.

Halliwell *et al.* (1988) have shown that therapy both with anthracycline and with other antileukaemia drugs may result in the rapid appearance of circulating iron that is not bound to transferrin. Much of the toxicity associated with anthracycline therapy has been attributed to the tissue effects of free radical damage that would undoubtedly be potentiated by the presence of unbound iron. Continued therapy with desferrioxamine might well eliminate the cardiotoxicity that currently limits the acceptable dosage of drugs such as daunorubicin and adriamycin. Whether desferrioxamine will be effective in the treatment of other conditions where tissue damage results from free radical formation, as suggested by Pippard (Chapter 17), will become clearer after the results of clinical trials are available. The balance between the beneficial therapeutic effect of a chelator, its potential toxicity to normal cells in terms of DNA or haem synthesis, and the possible availability of the iron chelate to increase the virulence of invading microorganisms, might be difficult to determine.

de Sousa and Brock have gathered together all their colleagues' contributions and forced us to look at iron metabolism in relation to the whole of haemopoiesis. This is a major step forward in our understanding of the pathophysiology of iron and we will no longer be able to ignore its problems beyond the bounds of nutritional requirements, erythropoiesis and iron overload. The problems outside the haemopoietic system remain uncharted.

REFERENCES

Birgegård, G., Hallgren, R., and Caro, J. (1987). Serum erythropoietin in rheumatoid arthritis and other inflammatory arthritides: relationship to anaemia and the effect of anti-inflammatory treatment, *Br. J. Haematol.*, **65**, 479–83.

Cotes, P. M., Brozovic, B., Mausel, M., and Samson, D. M. (1980). Radioimmunoassay of erythropoietin (EPO) in human serum: validation and application of an assay system, *Exp. Haematol.*, **8** (suppl.), 292–4.

Estrov, Z., Tawa, A., Wang, Z. H., Dube, I. D., Sulh, H., Cohen, A., Gelfland, E., and Freedman, M. H. (1987). In vitro and in vivo effects of deferoxamine in neonatal acute leukemia, *Blood*, **69**, 757–61.

Gordon, M. Y. (1988). Extracellular matrix of the marrow microenvironment, *Br. J. Haematol.*, **70**, 1–4.

Gough, N. M., Gearing, D. P., King, J. A., Willson, T. A., Hilton, D. J., Nicola, N. A., and Metcalf, D. (1988). Molecular cloning and expression of the human homologue of the murine gene encoding myeloid leukemia-inhibitory factor, *Cell Biol.*, **85**, 2623–7.

Halliwell, B., Aruoma, O. I., Mufti, G., and Bomford, A. (1988). Bleomycin-detectable iron in serum from leukaemic patients before and after chemotherapy. *Fed. Eur. Biochem. Soc. Lett.*, **241**, 202–4.

Jacobs, A. (1982). Non-haematological effects of iron-deficiency. *Clin. Haematol.*, **11**, 353–64.

Jacobs, A. (1984). Serum ferritin and malignant tumours, *Med. Oncol. Tumor Pharmacother.*, **1**, 149–56.

Morstyn, G., and Burgess, A. W. (1988). Hemopoietic growth factors: a review, *Cancer Res.*, **48**, 5624–37.

Potaznik, D., Groshen, S., Miller, D., Bagin, R., Bhalla, R., Schwartz, M., and de Sousa, M. (1987). Association of serum iron, serum transferrin saturation and serum ferritin with survival in acute lymphocytic leukaemia, *Am. J. Pediatr. Hematol./Oncol.*, **9**, 350–5.

Sachs, L. (1987). The molecular control of blood cell development, *Science*, **238**, 1374–9.

Santambrogio, P., and Massover, W. H. (1989). Rabbit serum alpha-2-macroglobulin binds to liver ferritin: association causes a heterogeneity of ferritin molecules, *Br. J. Haematol.*, **71**, 281–90.

Torok-Storb, B. (1988). Cellular interactions, *Blood*, **72**, 373–85.

Worwood, M. (1974). Iron and the trace metals. In A. Jacobs and M. Worwood *Iron in Biochemistry and Medicine*, pp. 335–67, Academic Press, London.

Wrigglesworth, J. M., and Baum, H. (1980). The biochemical functions of iron. In A. Jacobs and M. Worwood (eds) *Iron in Biochemistry and Medicine*, pp. 29–86, Academic Press, London.

Iron in Immunity, Cancer and Inflammation
Edited by M. de Sousa and J. H. Brock
© 1989 John Wiley & Sons Ltd

Appendix

Problems with Iron and Iron-binding Proteins in Tissue Culture

Jeremy H. Brock

University Department of Bacteriology and Immunology, Western Infirmary, Glasgow G11 6NT, Scotland

INTRODUCTION

Until the late 1970s research on the interaction of iron and iron-binding proteins with cells was largely confined to short-term incubations with erythroid precursors, principally reticulocytes, which were carried out in relatively simple buffered salt solutions. The subsequent explosion of interest in the interaction of iron and its carrier proteins with non-erythroid cells has required the use of much more sophisticated culture systems, and has inevitably increased the possibilities of introducing methodological artifacts. Many new workers have entered the field during this period who, while extremely experienced in other areas, may not have appreciated some of the peculiar technical problems presented by working with iron and iron-binding proteins in biological systems. Such information is often not easy to find in the literature, as critical minor details are often omitted from papers which are essentially non-methodological. This appendix is intended to point out some of the problems that may arise when working with iron and iron-binding proteins in cell culture systems, and suggest ways in which they may be avoided, drawing largely on the author's own experience. It should be emphasized that this is not intended to provide detailed methodology, but rather to draw attention to potential problems and indicate how they may be solved with reference to appropriate published methods. I do not claim that what follows is the last word on the subejct, and readers may have found other problems (and hopefully some new solutions). If so, I would be pleased to hear about them.

CONTROL OF IRON LEVELS IN CELL CULTURES

Iron in Tissue Culture Media

Most tissue culture media contain iron, even when the presence of this metal is not indicated in the formulation. In our experience RPMI 1640 medium contains between 6 and 12 ng ml^{-1} of iron, there being some variation between batches (this refers to the 1× concentration from Flow Laboratories; we have not examined iron levels in 10× concentrates or powdered media, for which the iron levels in water used for dilution must also be taken into account). It is therefore important to check iron levels in the media by atomic absorption spectroscopy if one wishes to carry out experiments in which low iron levels are required. The form of iron present in culture media is not known, but it may well bind to proteins such as lactoferrin or transferrin if these are added to the medium. The iron levels mentioned above would fully saturate iron-free (apo) transferrin or lactoferrin added to the medium at concentrations up to about 8 μg ml^{-1}. Failure to recognize this problem has led to erroneous values for the binding constant of apotransferrin to transferrin receptors being reported (e.g. Ward, Kushner and Kaplan, 1982; Ward et al., 1983).

One technique often used to render this iron biologically inactive is to add the iron chelator desferrioxamine to the culture medium. Desferrioxamine (marketed by Ciba-Geigy under the trade name Desferal®) is a microbial siderophore used to treat iron overload (see Chapter 17) which binds iron very strongly, and which does not significantly exchange iron with either iron-binding proteins or cells. There are two disadvantages to the use of desferrioxamine. Firstly, although the iron complex does not enter cells to any appreciable extent, the iron-free form can readily do so and may strip cells of iron, thus potentially affecting their function. Addition of a large excess of desferrioxamine may therefore produce artifacts. Secondly, desferrioxamine (though not its iron complex) is unstable in aqueous solution and must be made up immediately before use, and if necessary replenished at regular intervals. An attractive alternative procedure has been reported by Gutteridge (1987) which involves placing a dialysis tube containing chicken apo-ovotransferrin in the medium to scavenge reactive iron prior to use. This method has the advantages of being simple, inexpensive and of actually removing unwanted iron from the medium, rather than leaving it present in a complexed form.

Iron contamination of glass- and plastic-ware

Further contamination can arise from iron present in or on the surface of bottles, flasks, vials, pipette tips, etc. As a general rule contact with glass should be avoided, as the negatively charged surface tends to bind ferric ions. We have not experienced any problems with tissue-culture-grade plastics, but items such as microvials and micropipette tips can sometimes be contaminated. Levels can vary markedly between individual items within a single batch from a single manufacturer; we suspect that the problem may be due to the occasional entry of microscopic iron filings from the moulding press. Manufacturers are usually prepared to supply a small number of items free of charge to allow testing for iron contamination. Determination of iron contamination can be carried out by firstly adding a suitable volume of a solution of 2.5% trichloroacetic acid/0.75% thioglycolic acid/0.5 M HCl to the tube or vial to be tested, and after 30 min adding 0.25-volume of 0.1% ferrozine in saturated sodium acetate (dissolve the ferrozine in a few drops of water before adding the sodium acetate). For large items swirl the liquid around to permit contact with the whole surface; micropipette tips can be tested by sealing the tips in a bed of plasticine. The absorbance is read at 562 nm against a suitable standard curve. This method (Mainou-Fowler, 1985) is modified from a method for determining serum iron (Brittenham, 1979).

If it is not possible to find reliably iron-free plastics then it is necessary to soak the items overnight in 0.1 M HCl (in a plastic beaker) followed by extensive washing with distilled-deionized water.

CONTROL OF LEVELS OF IRON-BINDING PROTEINS

Problems may arise from the possibility that iron-binding proteins, particularly transferrin, are present in cultures even if not deliberately added. Very small amounts of transferrin can significantly affect cell function, as little as 0.5 μg ml^{-1} of transferrin being able to considerably enhance the proliferative response of mouse lymphocytes to concanavalin A in serum-free medium (Brock, 1981). Small amounts of endocytosed transferrin may be carried over following subculture or isolation of cells. This can be minimized by preincubating the cells in transferrin-free medium for 15–30 min to allow exocytosis of any endogenous transferrin to occur. Some cells such as macrophages, activated lymphocytes and various cell lines may synthesize transferrin or transferrin-like proteins (see Chapter 5). Little can be done about this problem when using primary cultures, but for studies involving cell lines it may be worth initially checking whether transferrin transcription or synthesis occurs by immunoprecipitation of culture supernatants or by Northern blotting (see, for example, Lum *et al.*, 1986), if this is not already known.

Tissue culture has traditionally been carried out in media supplemented with serum. This inevitably introduces large amounts of transferrin (and probably small amounts of lactoferrin and ferritin) into the culture system. If human serum is used in human cell cultures, then the amount of transferrin added is likely to be in excess of 150 μg ml^{-1}, which is way beyond the limiting quantity required either for optimal growth or for saturation of transferrin receptors. If fetal calf serum is used, bovine transferrin will be present. Although this binds to human transferrin receptors with much lower affinity than human transferrin (Tsavaler, Stein and Sussman, 1986), the high concentration present normally allows sufficient interaction to occur to permit cell growth, though some contrary results have been reported (Gaston, Bacon and Strober, 1987). For murine cells, human and murine transferrins seem to be virtually interchangeable, with bovine transferrin being significantly less well bound (Brock, Mainou-Fowler and Webster, 1986). However, bovine transferrin may bind non-specifically to cells of other species: for example, only 50% of radiolabelled bovine transferrin bound to rabbit reticulocytes could be displaced by excess unlabelled transferrin (Esparza, 1979). The fate of this non-specifically bound transferrin is unknown, but it might interfere with iron uptake studies from the homologous protein if fetal calf serum is present.

It is therefore evident that use of serum-free culture conditions is generally to be preferred when studying interactions between transferrin and cells. It should, however, be remembered that non-specific interactions between cells and iron-binding proteins may increase if other proteins are not present, and consequently the addition of an excess (e.g. 1 mg ml^{-1}) of albumin is recommended. This introduces a further complication insofar as many commercially available offerings of albumin from various species are contaminated with small amounts of transferrin. Highly purified albumin should therefore be used, and preferably checked for transferrin contamination. This can be done by testing a high concentration (e.g. 20 mg ml^{-1}) against a sensitive radial immunodiffusion plate for transferrin, such as the Behringwerke Partigen-LC Human Transferrin. For other species it may be necessary to develop an ELISA assay. There is now an extensive literature on the use of serum-free media in cell culture, and the subject has been reviewed by Barnes and Sato (1980) and Maurer (1986).

BINDING OF IRON TO TRANSFERRIN

If studies of the interaction of iron-containing transferrin (or lactoferrin) with cells are to be carried out, it is critically important to ensure that all iron is specifically bound to the protein. The two major points of consideration are (1) the possible effect of endogenous iron in the culture medium (see above), and (2) the method used for adding iron to transferrin. Ferric iron readily polymerizes in aqueous solution at neutral or mildly acidic pH. Polymeric ferric iron reacts only slowly with the specific iron-binding sites of transferrin, and may bind non-specifically to the protein. The importance of using a source of iron which readily transfers the metal to transferrin has been discussed in detail elsewhere (Bates and Schlabach, 1973; Workman, Graham and Bates, 1975; Graham and Bates, 1976; Brock, 1985), and some results, e.g. regarding the involvement of lactoferrin in hydroxyl radical production (Ambruso and Johnston, 1981), have been reported in the literature which probably result from the presence of non-specifically bound iron (Halliwell, Gutteridge and Blake, 1985). Bates and Schlabach (1973) recommended the use of the nitrilotriacetate (NTA) complex of Fe^{3+} to specifically donate iron to transferrin, and this has been used in many studies without apparent problems. However, the complex must be carefully prepared from freshly prepared ferric chloride or nitrate and sodium NTA (Graham and Bates, 1976), using at least a 4-fold molar exces of the chelate and ensuring that no precipitation occurs during the preparation. If the Fe:NTA ratio is reduced to 1:2, polynuclear iron complexes may form (Smit, Leijnse and van der Kraan, 1981). The final solution should be pale yellow-green; if it has an orange tint then polymers are present, and these may only react very slowly with transferrin. The FeNTA complex is light-sensitive and should therefore be kept in the dark. Other chelates, notably citrate, have been used, but this requires at least a 20-fold molar excess of citrate to ensure rapid binding (Bates, Billups and Saltman, 1967), and even then some non-specifically-bound iron may result (Berry and Hatton, 1986). Ferric citrate as commercially available normally contains only a 1:1 molar ratio of iron to citrate and rapidly forms unreactive polymers in solution at neutral pH unless additional citrate ions are added. Ferric chloride or other simple ferric salts should be avoided.

A possible problem with the use of FeNTA is that the chelate may itself affect subsequent events. For example, in a study of iron release by macrophages labelled with ^{59}Fe, the addition of 20 μM FeNTA to culture medium in order to saturate all transferrin present resulted in a low-molecular-weight ^{59}Fe complex appearing in the medium, due to the released iron complexing with the added NTA (Brock, Esparza and Logie, 1984). This complex was not found if ferrous ammonium sulphate was used to add iron to the culture medium, as described by Workman, Graham and Bates (1975). This method therefore provides an alternative to the use of ferric chelates, although the ferrous ammonium sulphate must be prepared freshly and at pH 2 if polymer formation and non-specific binding are to be avoided.

REMOVAL OF IRON FROM TRANSFERRINS

Human transferrin is available commercially essentially iron-free, so for most purposes removal of iron should not be necessary if the apo form is required. However, such purified transferrin may contain up to 0.78 mol of aluminium per mol of transferrin (Trapp, 1983; J. H. Brock and S. J. McGregor, unpublished data). To remove iron (or aluminium) from transferrin the standard procedure is to dialyse against citrate buffer at pH 5. However, citrate may remain bound to the protein, and dialysis against 0.1 M $NaClO_4$ before equilibration with the desired buffer is recommended, since the citrate may subsequently bind iron and cause artifacts (Price and Gibson, 1972). Lactoferrin, because of its higher affinity for iron, requires more drastic treatment for removal of iron, and dialysis against 40 mM EDTA pH 4 as described by Mazurier and Spik (1980) is generally satisfactory. In particular, it should be noted that dialysis against citric acid, as originally described by Masson and Heremans (1968), is not recommended as this causes some loss of cell-binding (Van Snick and Masson, 1976) and iron-binding properties (Ainscough *et al.*, 1980).

RADIOLABELLING OF TRANSFERRINS

Many studies require labelling of transferrin with ^{125}I, usually for investigating receptor–ligand interactions. As discussed by Regoeczi (1983), problems may arise due to modification of the structure and properties of the protein. In the first place, it must be emphasized that transferrin (and probably also lactoferrin) should always be iron-saturated before labelling, as the apoproteins are intrinsically more susceptible to denaturation. Furthermore, iodination of residues involved in iron binding may occur if the apoproteins are used. This applies even to mild methods such as the Bolton–Hunter reagent (Bolton and Hunter, 1973), which was found to prevent bovine apotransferrin from subsequently binding iron (unpublished observations), even though it satisfactorily iodinated the iron-saturated protein. Regoeczi (1983) reported that the lactoperoxidase (David and Resifeld, 1974) and iodogen (Fraker and Speck, 1978) methods could both be used satisfactorily for iodinating small amounts of transferrin, though conditions had to be carefully defined when using iodogen. Although Regoeczi (1983) found the iodine monochloride method was less satisfactory, and Workman, Graham and Bates (1975) reported increased non-specific binding to reticulocytes when the chloramine-T method was used, the author has found that transferrin iodinated by chloramine-T can be satisfactorily used for ligand-binding studies provided the protein is labelled at high concentration (≥ 5 mg ml^{-1}) and for a short time (10–15 sec).

Labelling with tritium using sodium borohydride (Jentoft and Dearborn, 1979) has been used as an alternative to iodination and has the advantage of not modifying the iron-binding site (Hatton and Berry, 1987), although this method is more complex to carry out and requires scintillation counting.

Labelling of transferrins with radioisotopes of iron (^{55}Fe or, more usually, ^{59}Fe) is also often required, sometimes in conjunction with iodination. For this the same precautions as mentioned above for iron loading should be observed. It is best not to saturate the protein completely, but to work with transferrin 30–75% saturated, thus avoiding the possibility that endogenous iron in media or reagents already occupying some of the binding sites results in some radioiron remaining unbound. Non-transferrin-bound iron may become cell-associated (though not necessarily internalized) more rapidly than transferrin-bound iron (White and Jacobs, 1978; Brock and Rankin, 1981). As a further safeguard against the presence of non-transferrin-bound iron, the labelled protein should be treated with Chelex 100 resin to remove such iron before use.

LACTOFERRIN

Working with lactoferrin, particularly at low concentrations, can cause additional problems because of the readiness with which it binds to other molecules. The possible effects of this property on the function of lactoferrin are discussed in Chapters 5 and 10. At the technical level, problems may occur because lactoferrin binds to Sephadex G25 (and quite possibly other gel-filtration media) which is often used for separating free and bound ^{125}I after iodination. The binding is relatively weak, however, and the protein is merely retarded rather than retained completely. Lactoferrin also binds to Chelex 100, and brief exposure to the minimum quantity necessary is recommended if the resin has to be used following labelling with radioiron (Oria *et al.*, 1988). Binding to ultrafiltration membranes has also been observed (unpublished observations). In general, the actual concentration of lactoferrin in a standard solution should always be checked before use to allow for possible losses.

Removal of iron from lactoferrin is discussed above.

FERRITIN

Ferritin generally presents fewer potential problems than transferrin for tissue culture work. Commercially available ferritins usually contain about 2000 Fe atoms per molecule, i.e. about half their total iron-binding capacity. Ferritin is a fairly robust protein and can withstand moderate heating;

however, it should be stored refrigerated as a solution, since freezing or freeze-drying tends to cause structural alterations.

Removal of iron from ferritin is usually achieved by dialysis against thioglycollic acid (Chasteen and Theil, 1982; Yang et al., 1987). The latter may tend to remain associated with the protein, and should be removed by dialysis against 0.9% NaCl. Uptake of iron by ferritin is complex (see review by Theil, 1987) and occurs most rapidly if iron is supplied as Fe^{2+}. However, Fe^{3+} (as a 1:20 complex with citrate) can be used for trace-labelling with radioiron where only small amounts of the metal are actually required to be taken up (Treffry and Harrison, 1979).

A number of methods have been used for radioiodination of ferritin (Bolton et al., 1979; Covell and Cook, 1987). Of these the Bolton–Hunter method has been found to be satisfactory in ligand-binding studies (Mack et al., 1985), for which lack of structural modification is more critical than in radioimmunoassays. Ferritin labelled by the chloramine-T or iodogen methods showed structural alterations (Bolton et al., 1979), and chloramine-T-labelled ferritin degraded rapidly on storage (Covell and Cook, 1987).

REFERENCES

Ainscough, E. W., Brodie, A. M., Plowman, J. E., Bloor, S. J., Loehr, J. S., and Loehr, T. M. (1980). Studies on human lactoferrin by electron paramagnetic resonance, fluorescence, and resonance Raman spectroscopy, *Biochemistry*, **19**, 4072–9.

Ambruso, D. R., and Johnston, R. B. (1981). Lactoferrin enhances hydroxyl radical production by human neutrophils, neutrophil particulate fractions, and an enzymatic generating system, *J. Clin. Invest.*, **67**, 352–60.

Barnes, D., and Sato, G. H. (1980). Methods for growth of cultured cells in serum-free medium, *Anal. Biochem.*, **102**, 255–70.

Bates, G. W., Billups, C., and Saltman, P. (1967). The kinetics and mechanism of iron (III) exchange between chelates and transferrin. I. The complexes of citrate and nitrilotriacetate, *J. Biol. Chem.*, **242**, 2810–5.

Bates, G. W., and Schlabach, M. R. (1973). The reaction of ferric salts with transferrin, *J. Biol. Chem.*, **248**, 3228–32.

Berry, L. R., and Hatton, M. W. C. (1986). A comparison of two procedures used for complexing Fe(III) with human apotransferrin: I. Physicochemical properties of the Fe(III)-transferrin products, *Biochem. Cell Biol.*, **64**, 936–45.

Bolton, A. E., and Hunter, W. M. (1973). The labelling of proteins to high specific radioactivities by conjugation to a ^{125}I-containing acylating agent. Application to the radioimmunoassay, *Biochem. J.*, **133**, 529–39.

Bolton, A. E., Lee-Own, V., McLean, R. K., and Challand, G. S. (1979). Three different radioiodination methods for human spleen ferritin compared. *Clin. Chem.*, **25**, 1826–30.

Brittenham, G. (1979). Spectrophotometric plasma iron determination from finger-puncture specimens, *Clin. Chim. Acta*, **91**, 203–11.

Brock, J. H. (1981). The effect of iron and transferrin on the response of serum-free cultures of mouse lymphocytes to concanavalin A and lipopolysaccharide, *Immunology*, **43**, 387–91.

Brock, J. H. (1985). The transferrins. In P. M. Harrison (ed.) *Metalloproteins, Part 2*, pp. 183–262, Macmillan, London.

Brock, J. H., Esparza, I., and Logie, A. C. (1984). The nature of iron released by resident and stimulated mouse peritoneal macrophages, *Biochim. Biophys. Acta*, **797**, 105–111.

Brock, J. H., Mainou-Fowler, T., and Webster, L. M. (1986). Evidence that transferrin may function exclusively as an iron donor in promoting lymphocyte proliferation, *Immunology*, **57**, 105–10.

Brock, J. H., and Rankin, M. C. (1981). Transferrin binding and iron uptake by mouse lymph-node cells during transformation in response to concanavalin A. *Immunology*, **43**, 393–8.

Chasteen, N. D., and Theil, E. C. (1982). Iron binding by horse spleen ferritin. A vanadyl(IV) epr spin probe study, *J. Biol. Chem.*, **257**, 7672–7.

Covell, A. M., and Cook, J. D. (1987). Stability of radioiodinated ferritin, *Clin. Chim. Acta*, **168**, 261–72.

David, G. S., and Resifeld, R. A. (1974). Protein iodination with solid state lactoperoxidase, *Biochemistry*, **13**, 1014–21.

Esparza, I. (1979). Estudio de algunas propiedades estructurales y biológicas de la transferrina. Doctoral Thesis, University of Zaragoza.

Fraker, P. J., and Speck, J. C. (1978). Protein and cell membrane iodination with a sparingly soluble chloramide, 1,3,4,6-tetrachloro-3a,6a-diphenylglycoluril, *Biochem. Biophys. Res. Commun.*, **80**, 849–57.

Gaston, J. S. H., Bacon, P. A., and Strober, S. (1987). Enhancement of human T-lymphocyte growth by human transferrin in the presence of fetal bovine serum, *Cell. Immunol.*, **106**, 366–75.

Graham, G., and Bates, G. W. (1976). Approaches to the standardization of serum unsaturated iron binding capacity, *J. Lab. Clin. Med.*, **88**, 477–86.

Gutteridge, J. M. C. (1987). A method for removal of trace iron contamination from biological buffers, *FEBS Lett.*, **214**, 362–4.

Halliwell, B., Gutteridge, J. M. C., and Blake, D. (1985). Metal ions and oxygen radical reactions in human inflammatory joint disease, *Phil. Trans. R. Soc. Lond. B*, **311**, 659–71.

Hatton, M. W. C., and Berry, L. R. (1987). A comparison of two procedures used for complexing Fe(III) with human apotransferrin. II. Uptake of Fe(III) by K-562 cells from [55]Fe-transferrins and Fe-[^{3}H]transferrins, *Biochem. Cell Biol.*, **65**, 271–9.

Jentoft, N., and Dearborn, D. G. (1979). Labeling of proteins by reductive methylation using sodium borohydride, *J. Biol. Chem.*, **254**, 4359–65.

Lum, J. B., Infante, A. J., Makker, D. M., Yang, F., and Bowman, B. H. (1986). Transferrin synthesis by inducer T lymphocytes, *J. Clin. Invest.*, **77**, 841–9.

Mack, U., Storey, E. L., Powell, L. W., and Halliday, J. W. (1985). Characterization of the binding of ferritin to the rat liver ferritin receptor, *Biochim. Biophys. Acta*, **843**, 164–70.

Mainou-Fowler, T. (1985). The importance of transferrin-bound iron for the proliferation of mouse T-lymphocytes *in vitro*, Doctoral Thesis, University of Glasgow.

Masson, P. L., and Heremans, J. F. (1968). Metal combining properties of human lactoferrin (red milk protein). I. The involvement of bicarbonate in the reaction, *Eur. J. Biochem.*, **6**. 579–84.

Maurer, H. R. (1986). Towards chemically-defined, serum-free media for mammalian cell culture. In R. I. Freshney (ed.) *Animal Cell Culture*, pp. 13–39, IRL Press, Oxford.

Mazurier, J., and Spik, G. (1980). Comparative study of the iron-binding properties of human transferrins. I. Complete and sequential iron saturation and desaturation of the lactotransferrin, *Biochim. Biophys. Acta*, **629**, 399–408.

Oria, R., Alvarez-Hernández, X., Licéaga, J., and Brock, J. H. (1988). Uptake and handling of iron from transferrin, lactoferrin and immune complexes by a macrophage cell line, *Biochem. J.*, **251**, 221–5.

Price, E. M., and Gibson, J. F. (1972). A re-interpretation of bicarbonate-free transferrin e.p.r. spectra, *Biochem. Biophys. Res. Commun.*, **46**, 646–51.

Regoeczi, E. (1983). Iodogen-catalyzed iodination of transferrin, *Int. J. Peptide Protein Res.*, **22**, 422–33.

Smit, S., Leijnse, B., and van der Kraan, A. M. (1981). Polynuclear iron complexes in human transferrin preparations, *J. Inorg. Biochem.*, **15**, 329–38.

Theil, E. C. (1987). Ferritin structure, gene regulation, and cellular function in animals, plants and microorganisms, *Annu. Rev. Biochem.*, **56**, 289–315.

Trapp, G. A. (1983). Plasma aluminium is bound to transferrin, *Life Sci.*, **33**, 311–6.

Treffry, A., and Harrison, P. M. (1979). The binding of ferric iron by ferritin, *Biochem. J.*, **181**, 709–16.

Tsavaler, L., Stein, B. S., and Sussman, H. H. (1986). Demonstration of the specific binding of bovine transferrin to the human transferrin receptor in K562 cells: evidence for interspecies transferrin internalization, *J. Cell. Physiol.*, **128**, 1–8.

Van Snick, J. L., and Masson, P. L. (1976). The binding of human lactoferrin to mouse peritoneal cells, *J. Exp. Med.*, **144**, 1568–80.

Ward, J. H., Kushner, J. P., and Kaplan, J. (1982). Regulation of HeLa cell transferrin receptors, *J. Biol. Chem.*, **257**, 10317–23.

Ward, J. H., Kushner, J. P., Ray, F. A., and Kaplan, J. (1983). Transferrin receptor function in hereditary hemochromatosis, *J. Lab. Clin. Med.*, **103**, 246–54.

White, G. P., and Jacobs, A. (1978). Iron uptake by Chang cells from transferrin, nitrilotriacetate and citrate complexes, *Biochim. Biophys. Acta*, **543**, 217–25.

Workman, E. F., Graham, G., and Bates, G. W. (1975). The effect of serum and experimental variables on the transferrin and reticulocyte interaction. *Biochim. Biophys. Acta*, **399**, 254–64.

Yang, C.-Y., Meaghan, A., Huynh, B. H., Sayers, D. E., and Theil, E. C. (1987). Iron(III) clusters bound to horse spleen apoferritin: an X-ray absorption and Mössbauer spectroscopy study that shows that iron nuclei can form on the protein, *Biochemistry*, **26**, 497–503.

Index

Acidic isoferritins, see Ferritin
Aconitase 46
Adjuvant arthritis
   desferrioxamine 151
   ^{111}In in diagnosis of 331
   iron deficiency in 151
   iron dextran in 148
Adriamycin 358, 379, 396
Air pouch 150
Allergic encephalomyelitis 374
Allopurinol 370, 371
Alpha-fetoprotein (AFP)
   in chronic liver disease 309
   in primary heptocarcinoma (PHC) 310
Alpha-2 macroglobulin 131, 395
Aluminium 377
Alveolar macrophages, see Macrophage(s)
Amidophosphoribosyl transferase 48
Anaemia
   mechanism of hypoferraemia of inflammation 111
   of malignant disease 111
   role of T cells in BCG-induced 117
Antibiotics
   daunorubicin 396
   tetracycline 381
Arthritis
   role of iron overload 146
   (see also Rheumatoid arthritis)

B lymphocytes, see Lymphocyte(s)
Beta-thalassaemia intermedia
   mitogen responses 251
   T cell sets 249
Beta-thalassaemia major
   clinical features of iron overload 366
   compliance with therapy 366

   IgG on red blood cells 24
   iron overload 361
   mitogen responses 251
   mixed lymphocyte reaction (MLR) 251
   natural killer (NK) activity 248
   T cells 249
Blood transfusion
   immunosuppressive effect of 5
Blym-1 40, 62, 63
Breast cancer
   ferritin-bearing lymphocytes 291
Butylated hydroxyanisole (BHA)
   action in oxidant stress 184
   protection against cerebral malaria 188

Cachectin, see Tumour necrosis factor
Caeruloplasmin, in synovial fluid 159
Catalase 45, 156
Cell cycle 268
   role of iron in 270
Cell differentiation, iron and 271
Chemotaxis 98, 121
Chronic myeloid leukaemia
   chromosome translocations in 232
   lactoferrin in 232
   (see also Leukaemia)
Clathrin-coated pits
   endocytosis of transferrin 43
Collagenase
   action of IL-1 on 189
   action of TNF on 189
   in rheumatoid disease 156
Complement, C5a in inflammation 121
Conalbumin, see Ovotransferrin

Daunorubicin 396
Desferrioxamine (DFO)
   absorption 265

Desferrioxamine (DFO) (cont.)
  effect on
    adjuvant arthritis 151
    allergic encephalomyelitis 374
    bleomycin-induced fibrosis 376
    cell proliferation 270
    faecal iron excretion 367
    graft-versus-host disease 375
    infections 380
    ischaemia 370
    leukaemia 205
    mammary epithelial cancer cells 270
    pancreatic transplants 375
    paraquat toxicity 375, 376
    Plasmodium growth 380
    pulmonary vasculitis 373
    rheumatoid arthritis 373
    thalassaemia 366
    TNF production 185
  half-life 367
  ocular toxicity 373, 382
  origin 362
  removal of iron from tissue culture media 400
  toxicity of 382
Diferric transferrin reductase 85
Down's syndrome
  hepatitis B antigen in 303
  red blood cells and 24

Elastase
  binding of lactoferrin to macrophages 90
  rheumatoid arthritis 155
  inhibitor, inactivation of 156
Endocytosis, *see* Receptor-mediated endocytosis
Endogenous pyrogen 182
  (*see also* Interleukin 1)
Endotoxin 112, 119
Enterochelin 36
Erythropoietin
  anaemia of inflammation 113
  regulation by haemoglobin 114
  serum levels in iron-deficiency anaemia 113

^{52}Fe, clinical use of 320
Fenton reaction 368
  (*see also* Haber–Weiss reaction and free radicals)

Ferritin
  acidic (H-subunit)
    action *in vivo* 204, 205
    amino acid composition 57
    binding to K562 cells 276
    cDNA 57, 58
    ferroxidase activity 57
    glycosylation 202
    inhibition of colony formation 201
    inhibition of T cell proliferation 290
    receptor for 205
    recombinant 204
    release by monocytes 203
    role in iron storage 58
    suppression of colony formation 201, 237
    T cells, effect on release of 202
  antibodies to in hepatoma therapy 327
  basic (L-subunit)
    amino acid composition 57
    cDNA 58
    chromosomal localization of gene 59
    role in iron storage 58
  carcinofetal 287
  inhibition of E-rosette formation 290
  in chronic liver disease 309, 311
  in cirrhosis 309
  in free radical production 154
  in liver cancer 307, 311
  in milk 42
  in pregnancy 290
  iron detoxification by 42, 58
  iron uptake by 40
  iron removal from 41, 406
  placental 283, 294
  radiolabelling of 406
  receptors for 264, 276
  secretion of 251
  serum, *see* Serum ferritin
  subunits 40, 56
    homology between 58
  synthesis
    inflammation 124, 148
    lymphocytes 87
    macrophages 91, 126
    regulation of 61
    tumours 307
  three-dimensional structure 56

Index

uptake of labelled antibodies to by tumours 327, 328
Fever, red blood cell survival and 113
Free radicals 179, 368
  damage to proteins by 157
  effect on lymphocytes 163
  iron chelators and 369
  joint disease 153
  lactoferrin and production of 228
  senescent red cells and 26, 29

^{67}Ga citrate
  binding to transferrin 321
  half-life 320
  in inflammation 329
  tumours
    imaging 319, 325
    mechanism of accumulation in 324
^{68}Ga, half-life of 320
GM-CSF production, effect of
  IL-1 225
  lactoferrin 232
  TNF 225
Granuloma formation 188

H ferritin, see Ferritin
Haber–Weiss reaction 228, 368
Haem
  proteins 45
  synthesis 272
Haemarthrosis 145, 146
Haemochromatosis (idiopathic, hereditary)
  HLA and 252
  iron in macrophages 253
  life span in neonatal 10
  NK activity in 248
  thermostable E-rosette formation 249
Haemoglobin 45
Haemopexin 146
Haemosiderin
  in inflammation 119
  oxidative damage and 369
  staining by Perl's reagent 41
  structure of 41
Hepatitis B virus infection
  chronic carriers 301, 302
  liver cancer 301, 305
  serum iron levels 304

Hepatocytes 38, 131, 252, 265, 369
Historical references 3, 4, 145, 187
HLA, relationship to
  ferritin secretion by macrophages 251
  inhibition of mixed lympocyte reaction by iron 251
Hodgkin's disease 287, 289, 294, 295, 329
Hyaluronic acid, breakdown of 158
Hydroxyurea 379

IgA
  faecal and iron-fortified formula 11
  iron-deficiency and mucosal 96
IgE, see Mast cells
IgG
  damage by free radicals 157
  removal of red blood cells 17, 19, 22
IgM
  iron-deficiency and mucosal 96
  removal of red blood cells 17, 19
IL-1
  lactoferrin action on 206
  inhibition of erythropoiesis 116
  production in iron deficiency 97
  role in hypoferraemia of inflammation 122, 131
IL-2
  effect on TNF release 186
  regulation of transferrin receptor expression 83
IL-3 200, 203, 210
IL-4 200
Immunotoxins 353
^{111}In
  binding to transferrin 321
  half-life 320
  in inflammation 330
  tumour imaging 325
Interferon-α 277
Interferon-β 276
Interferon-γ
  effect on TNF and IL-1 production 186, 188
  in malaria 188
  regulation of macrophage transferrin receptors 276
  response to acidic ferritin 204
Iron
  absorption 6, 47

Iron (cont.)
  chelators (see also Desferrioxamine)
    clinical use of 365
    definition 36, 362
    orally active 364
    types of 363
  chemistry of 35
  deficiency, effect on
    antibody response 95, 152
    cell-mediated immunity 95, 152
    joint disease 150
    lymphocyte mitochondria 96
    lymphocyte proliferation 95
    macrophage function 97
    neutrophil function 97, 152
    NK activity 96
  excretion 48
  losses in menstruation and
      pregnancy 5
  overload (see also Beta-thalassaemia,
      Haemochromatosis)
    arthritis 146, 147
    chelation therapy 365
    endemic 92, 253
    Kaschin Beck's disease 147
    liver cancer 301
    phagocytosis, impairment of 254
    superoxide production in 254
  recycling of 5, 6, 48
  suppression of mixed lymphocyte
      reaction 6
  tissue distribution 6
  uptake of non-transferrin bound 266
Iron–sulphur proteins 45
Ischaemia
  cerebral 371
  inflamed joint 160
  intestinal 371
  myocardial 370

Kaschin Beck's disease, see Iron
    overload

L ferritin, see Ferritin
Lactoferrin
  antibody response, inhibition of 225
  antimicrobial activity 49, 93, 124,
      207
  binding to
    cells 89, 230
    DNA 231

    gel filtration media 405
  chromosomal localisation of gene
      71
  enhancement of phagocytosis 90
  glycan chains 39
  hypoferraemia of inflammation, role
      in 122, 123
  IL-1, suppression of 206
  iron absorption, effect on 47
  iron-binding properties 39, 63, 228
  isoelectric point 39
  myelopoiesis, regulation of 205, 224
    in humans 234
    in mice 233
  plasma concentration 230
  superoxide production, effect on
      124
  synthesis by myeloid cells 93
Leukaemia
  acidic isoferritins in 201
  iron and treatment of 395
  lactoferrin in 207, 231
  low-affinity iron uptake system 83
  monoclonal antibodies to transferrin
      receptor, effect of 348
  placental ferritin in 295
Lipid peroxidation (see also Free
    radicals)
  in red blood cells 27
  in rheumatoid disease 155
Lymphocyte(s)
  B, transferrin and immunoglobulin
      synthesis by 84
  E-rosette formation in iron overload
      248
  ferritin-bearing
    in breast cancer 291
    in other malignancies 294
  migration 11
  mitochondrial abnormalities in iron
      deficiency 96
  proliferation of
    ferritin, suppression by 275, 290
    in thalassaemia 250
    iron and iron chelates, effect on
        83, 162, 378
    iron uptake in 266
    transferrin, role of 83
T
  anaemia of inflammation, role in
      116

CD4/CD8 ratios and transferrin
  saturation 64
 ferritin synthesis by 87
 in iron overload 248
 transferrin synthesis by 84, 87,
  236, 274

Macrophage(s)
 alveolar
  ferritin content 91
  transferrin receptor expression 88
 ferritin secretion 91, 203
 ferritin synthesis 90
 haem oxygenase in 92
 haemochromatosis, absence of iron
  loading in 252
 inflammation 119, 121
 iron absorption, role of mucosal 47
 iron overload, effect on 254
 iron release by 92
 lactoferrin binding by 89, 230
 red blood cells, removal by 6, 12, 19
 transferrin receptors, expression of
  88, 276
 transferrin synthesis by 91
Malaria 166, 187, 380
 (*see also Plasmodium*)
Mannitol 372
Mast cells, effect of transferrin on IgE
  release 94
Melanotransferrin 37, 40, 62, 266
 amino acid sequence 63
 chromosomal localization of gene 71
 regulation of gene expression 66
Metallothionein 130
Mixed lymphocyte reaction 5, 251
 (*see also* Lymphocyte)
Monoamine oxidase 46
Monocyte(s), *see* Macrophage(s)
Myobacterium tuberculosis 189
Myeloperoxidase 97, 232
Myoglobin 45

NADH dehydrogenase 46
Neuroblastoma 307
Neutrophil(s)
 adherence of pollen grains to, role of
  transferrin 93
 iron deficiency, function in 97, 152
 iron overload, function in 254
 lactoferrin in 49, 93, 229

 lactoferrin-deficient 207
NK cells
 CFU-C, action on 117
 iron overload, effect on activity 248
 transferrin, role of 275
 transferrin receptor as target
  structure 85

Ovotransferrin 37, 63, 65, 400
Oxidant stress, TNF release in 184
Oxygen radicals, *see* Free radicals

p97, *see* Melanotransferrin
Parabactin 379
Paraquat 375
Parenchymal cells, *see* Hepatocytes
Phagocytosis of senescent red blood
  cells 17
Peroxidase 45
 (*see also* Myeloperoxidase)
Peptides, iron-containing 46
Pigmented villonodular synovitis 146
Plasmodium 187, 380
 inhibition of growth by
  desferrioxamine 380
Platelet activating factor 182, 185
P_{O_2}, in rheumatoid synovium 161
Porphyria cutanea tarda 377
Post-ischaemic reperfusion injury 370
Prostanoids 180
Proteases, *see* Cathepsin, Collagenase,
  Elastase
Proteoglycans 274

Receptors, *see under individual ligands*
Receptor-mediated endocytosis of
  transferrin 43
Red blood cells
 band 3 25, 29
 bromelain-treated 9
 IgG in removal of 19
 life span
  human 6
  inflammation 112
  mouse 19, 23
  senescent 17
  young 17, 18
 phagocytosis of 17
 vitamin E deficiency and 27
Renal dialysis
 anaemia in 377

Renal dialysis (*cont.*)
  hepatitis in 303
  phagocytosis in 254
Ribonucleotide reductase 38, 46, 82
  in lymphocyte proliferation 42
  mode of action of hydroxyurea 379
Rheumatoid arthritis
  BFU-E and CFU-E in 115
  desferrioxamine, use of in 373
  imaging with ^{67}Ga and ^{111}In 330
  iron deposits in joints 148
  transferrin receptor-bearing lymphocytes 163
  (*see also* Arthritis)

Sarcoidosis 189
Schistosomiasis 189
Serum ferritin, levels in
  breast cancer 291
  haemochromatosis 252
  inflammation 128
  liver cancer 304, 306
Siderophores 49, 362
Succinate dehydrogenase 46
Superoxide, *see* Free radicals
Superoxide dismutase 158
Synovial fluid, iron in 148

T lymphocytes, *see* Lymphocyte(s)
Tetracycline 381
Thalassaemia, *see* Beta-thalassaemia
Thromboxane A$_2$ 180
Transferrin
  binding of pollen grains to neutrophils 94
  chronic alcoholism, changes in 37
  endocytosis of 43, 265
  gene
    chromosomal localization 65, 71
    regulation of expression 65, 66
  iron-binding 37, 38, 402
  isoelectric point 39
  mast cells, effect on 94
  microbial growth, effect on 48
  molecular weight 37
  phylogeny 62
  radiolabelling 404
  rat-into-mouse chimaeras 8
  receptor, *see* Transferrin-receptor
  removal of iron from 404
  suppression of myelopoiesis by 211, 235
  synthesis by
    lymphocytes 84, 87
    macrophages 91
  three-dimensional structure of 62
  tissue culture media, presence of 401
Transferrin-receptor
  affinity constants 43, 67
  amino acid sequence of domains 67, 68
  ^{67}Ga uptake, role in 324
  gene
    chromosomal localization 68, 71
    regulation of expression 70, 82, 273
  IL-2 and expression of 83
  interferons, effect on expression 277
  lymphocytes, expression by 82, 83
  molecular characteristics 66
  monoclonal antibodies to 323, 342
    cell growth, effect of 348
    immunoglobulin class and activity of 347
    immunotherapy with 342, 348
    iron uptake, inhibition of 343, 346
  NK activity, role in 85
  phosphorylation of 43, 67
  placenta, expression by 66, 263
  proliferation, role in 82, 267
  reticulocytes, expression by 67
Transplantation reperfusion 372
Trypanosoma cruzi 381
Tumour necrosis factor (TNF)
  antibodies to 187
  GM-CSF, effect on 225
  iron release from macrophages, effect on 92
  MHC antigens, effect on expression of 186
  oxidant stress and production of 184
  pathological effects 187
  production in
    malaria 187
    meningococcal septicaemia 181
    mycobacteria-infected macrophages 189

Uteroferrin 37, 40

Vitamin E deficiency
  haemolytic anaemia in 27

red blood cells in 28, 29
schistosomiasis and 189

Xanthine oxidase 46, 160, 370

^{90}Y, labelling of antiferritin antibodies 329

Zinc, in inflammation 130